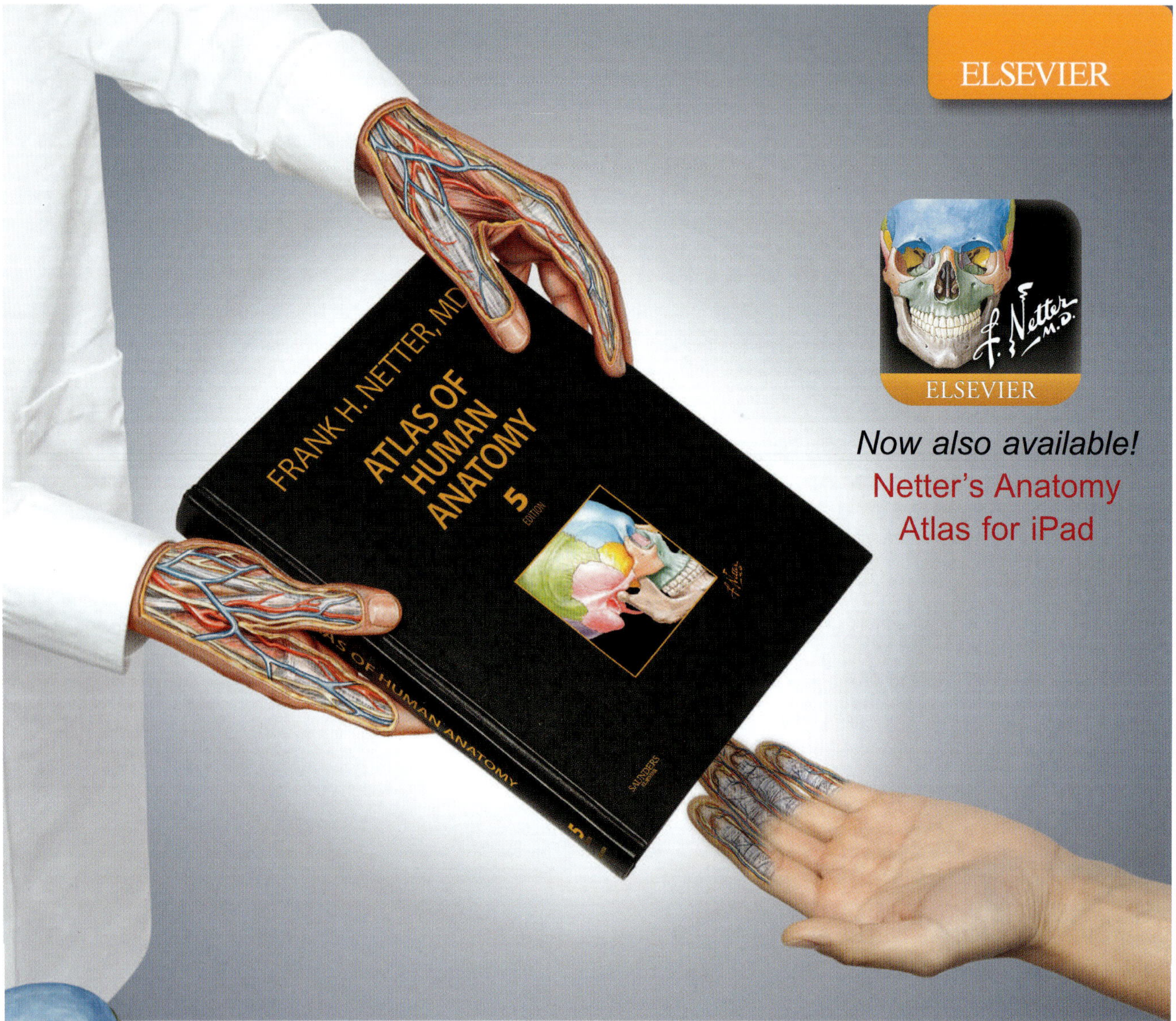
ELSEVIER
FRANK H. NETTER, MD
ATLAS OF HUMAN ANATOMY
5 EDITION
Now also available!
Netter's Anatomy
Atlas for iPad

NETTER'S

Correlative Imaging: Cardiothoracic Anatomy

Volume Editor

MICHAEL B. GOTWAY, MD

Department of Radiology
Mayo Clinic
Scottsdale, Arizona;
Clinical Associate Professor, Diagnostic Radiology/Biomedical Imaging and Pulmonary/Critical Care Medicine
Department of Radiology
University of California, San Francisco
San Francisco, California;
Clinical Professor, University of Arizona College of Medicine
Adjunct Professor, Department of Biomedical Informatics
Arizona State University
Phoenix, Arizona

Series Editor

NANCY M. MAJOR, MD

Director of Diagnostic Imaging
Orthopaedic Associates of Allentown
Allentown, Pennsylvania

Illustrations by
Frank H. Netter, MD

Contributing Illustrators
Kristen Wienandt Marzejon, MS, MFA
Carlos A.G. Machado, MD

SAUNDERS
ELSEVIER

ELSEVIER
SAUNDERS

1600 John F. Kennedy Blvd.
Ste 1800
Philadelphia, PA 19103-2899

NETTER'S CORRELATIVE IMAGING: CARDIOTHORACIC ANATOMY ISBN: 978-1-4377-0440-2

Library of Congress Cataloging-in-Publication Data

Gotway, Michael B.
Netter's correlative imaging: cardiothoracic anatomy / Michael B. Gotway; illustrations by Frank H. Netter; contributing illustrators, Kristen Wienandt Marzejon, Carlos A.G. Machado.
p. ; cm.
Correlative imaging: cardiothoracic anatomy
Includes bibliographical references and index.
ISBN 978-1-4377-0440-2 (hardcover: alk. paper)
I. Netter, Frank H. (Frank Henry), 1906-1991. II. Title. III. Title:
Correlative imaging: cardiothoracic anatomy.
[DNLM: 1. Lung--anatomy & histology--Atlases. 2. Thorax--anatomy & histology--Atlases.
3. Diagnostic Imaging--Atlases. 4. Heart--anatomy & histology--Atlases. WF 17]
612.2'4--dc23 2011047534

Senior Content Strategist: Elyse O'Grady
Content Development Manager: Marybeth Thiel
Publishing Services Manager: Anne Altepeter
Project Managers: Cheryl Abbott and Jessica Becher
Design Direction: Louis Forgione

Printed in China
Last digit is the print number: 9 8 7 6 5 4 3 2 1

About the Artists

FRANK H. NETTER, MD

Frank H. Netter was born in 1906 in New York City. He studied art at the Art Student's League and the National Academy of Design before entering medical school at New York University, where he received his MD degree in 1931. During his student years, Dr. Netter's notebook sketches attracted the attention of the medical faculty and other physicians, allowing him to augment his income by illustrating articles and textbooks. He continued illustrating as a sideline after establishing a surgical practice in 1933, but he ultimately opted to give up his practice in favor of a full-time commitment to art. After service in the U.S. Army during World War II, Dr. Netter began his long collaboration with the CIBA Pharmaceutical Company (now Novartis Pharmaceuticals). This 45-year partnership resulted in the production of the extraordinary collection of medical art so familiar to physicians and other medical professionals worldwide.

In 2005 Elsevier, Inc., purchased the Netter Collection and all publications from Icon Learning Systems. There are now more than 50 publications featuring the art of Dr. Netter available through Elsevier, Inc. (in the United States: www.us.elsevierhealth.com/Netter and outside the United States: www.elsevierhealth.com)

Dr. Netter's works are among the finest examples of the use of illustration in the teaching of medical concepts. The 13-book *Netter Collection of Medical Illustrations*, which includes the greater part of the more than 20,000 paintings created by Dr. Netter, became and remains one of the most famous medical works ever published. *The Netter Atlas of Human Anatomy*, first published in 1989, presents the anatomical paintings from the Netter Collection. Now translated into 16 languages, it is the anatomy atlas of choice among medical and health professions students the world over.

The Netter illustrations are appreciated not only for their aesthetic qualities but, more important, for their intellectual content. As Dr. Netter wrote in 1949, "... clarification of a subject is the aim and goal of illustration. No matter how beautifully painted or how delicately and subtly rendered a subject may be, it is of little value as a *medical illustration* if it does not serve to make clear some medical point." Dr. Netter's planning, conception, point of view, and approach are what inform his paintings and what makes them so intellectually valuable.

Frank H. Netter, MD, physician and artist, died in 1991.

Learn more about the physician-artist whose work has inspired the Netter Reference collection:

http://www.netterimages.com/artist/netter.htm

CARLOS MACHADO, MD

Carlos Machado was chosen by Novartis to be Dr. Netter's successor. He continues to be the main artist who contributes to the Netter collection of medical illustrations.

Self-taught in medical illustration, cardiologist Carlos Machado has contributed meticulous updates to some of Dr. Netter's original plates and has created many paintings of his own in the style of Netter as an extension of the Netter collection. Dr. Machado's photorealistic expertise and his keen insight into the physician/patient relationship inform his vivid and unforgettable visual style. His dedication to researching each topic and subject he paints places him among the premier medical illustrators at work today.

Learn more about his background and see more of his art at:

http://www.netterimages.com/artist/machado.htm

KRISTEN WIENANDT MARZEJON, MS, MFA

Kristen Wienandt Marzejon is a certified medical illustrator with an MS degree from the University of Illinois at Chicago's Biomedical Visualization graduate program. Her passion for both art and science from an early age makes her perfectly suited to this gratifying profession. She started her career as a staff illustrator at Rush University Medical Center in Chicago and then committed to self-employed status in 2001. She offers medical illustration and graphic design services to a variety of clients in the medical arena.

The work of Frank Netter has been a valuable part of Kristen's medical library throughout her 20-year career. That said, she is honored to continue the Netter tradition by producing work authentic to his distinctive style.

About the Author

Michael B. Gotway, MD, is a cardiopulmonary radiologist at the Mayo Clinic in Scottsdale, Arizona. Dr. Gotway completed his medical school training at the University of Illinois at Chicago, after which he performed his diagnostic radiology residency training at the University of California, San Francisco (UCSF), where he was presented with the Elmer Ng, MD award as outstanding diagnostic radiology resident. Dr. Gotway subsequently performed his cardiopulmonary imaging fellowship at UCSF, after which he joined the faculty at UCSF in cardiopulmonary imaging, based at San Francisco General Hospital (SFGH). Dr. Gotway was presented with the Outstanding Teacher Award by the Department of Medicine, section of Pulmonary and Critical Care Medicine, in 1999 and the Hideyo Minagi Outstanding Teacher Award by the UCSF Diagnostic Radiology Residency Program in 2002. Dr. Gotway held the position of Radiology Residency Program Director at UCSF from 2001 to 2005, as well as the Body Imaging Fellowship Director at SFGH from 2002 to 2004. From 2004 to 2005, Dr. Gotway was acting Vice-Chair for the Department of Radiology at UCSF, as well as the acting Chief of Radiology at SFGH. Before joining the Mayo Clinic, Dr. Gotway was a radiologist partner at Scottsdale Medical Imaging, Ltd, an affiliate of Southwest Diagnostic Imaging, from 2005 to 2012.

Preface

Thoracic computed tomography (CT) is a commonly performed procedure and an integral part of modern medical practice. Like most CT imaging, thoracic CT is performed and interpreted in the *transverse* plane. The transverse plane, or as more commonly referred to in daily practice, the *axial* plane, is perpendicular to the long axis of the body, dividing the body into cranial and caudal portions. When viewing axial supine CT sections, by convention, the patient's right side is on the viewer's left, with anterior structures at the "top" of the image. With multislice CT, serial, contiguous axial sections are acquired as a volume and can be displayed at various slice thicknesses, depending on the desired spatial resolution. The image data are commonly presented as a cephalocaudad "stack" of images that the user can actively scroll through. This display convention has been adopted in this volume. In clinical practice, anatomy is often tracked from image to image when scrolling in a cephalocaudad direction, allowing the reader to develop a three-dimensional impression of the structure of interest. The user is encouraged to adopt this approach when reviewing the thoracic and cardiac images to foster a three-dimensional understanding of cardiothoracic anatomy.

The thoracic CT images in this volume are displayed in both "soft tissue" and "lung" windows. The term "windowing" refers to manipulation of the display parameters (window width and window level) whereby the user changes the grayscale of an image to facilitate visualization of various anatomical structures. In the thoracic CT section of this volume, at each level, two images are shown: one displayed using a lung window, the other displayed using a soft-tissue window. These displays are created from the same source image; the display is merely changed to a lung window to optimize visualization of lung anatomy and to a soft tissue window to highlight mediastinal anatomy. In practice, several different window width and level settings are employed during review of CT images, each tailored to show the anatomy of interest to advantage.

Cardiac computed tomographic angiography (CTA) is a relatively recent development in the continual improvement of CT technology. Cardiac CTA is performed during the bolus administration of intravenous contrast material and during a breath hold, and the scan is performed in conjunction with electrocardiographic (ECG) gating to control for cardiac motion. CTA examinations performed using retrospective ECG gating allow for the reconstruction of CT data at various time points during the cardiac cycle. Because CT is sensitive to motion, and even minimal motion may compromise the quality of a cardiac CTA examination, ECG gating is an integral part of the performance of cardiac CTA. Images obtained when heart motion is relatively minimized, typically during diastole when the heart is undergoing isovolumic relaxation, provide relatively motion-free images for interpretation.

A typical cardiac CTA examination is performed in the axial plane and contains hundreds of images. The interpreter reviews these images and actively interacts with the data, creating various images that highlight particular aspects of cardiac anatomy or pathology. For cardiac imaging, the axial plane is not the only imaging plane, or even the primary imaging plane, used for interpretation. Rather, other imaging planes are created with reference to the axis of the heart: *2-chamber views (vertical long axis), 4-chamber views (horizontal long axis), and short axis* views of the heart are commonly employed. These planes are easily constructed from the axial data, and several examples of these imaging planes are presented at the end of the cardiac CTA section and in the cardiac MRI section. The axial plane is used for anatomical illustration in the cardiac CTA plates because it is the plane in which the data are acquired and an appreciation of non-axial cardiac anatomy is facilitated by first gaining an understanding of cardiovascular anatomy in the axial plane. After axial anatomy is understood, using a dedicated workstation to actively manipulate the data and visualize cardiac anatomy in various projections is the best method to gain a firm understanding of cardiovascular anatomy.

Note that right ventricular anatomy is not particularly well illustrated in the cardiac CTA study shown in these plates. This is because cardiac CTA examinations are often performed with injection of saline following the injection of iodinated intravenous contrast media, effectively "washing contrast" from the right cardiac chambers. This is done because dense intravenous contrast within the right heart chambers may create artifacts that impair visualization of important cardiovascular structures, particularly the right coronary artery. The reader is referred to the magnetic resonance imaging plates for details regarding right atrial and ventricular anatomy.

The number of images acquired in a typical cardiac CTA examination can be large. Because of space limitations, all the images acquired in the examination used for these plates cannot be shown, but relevant sections (roughly every sixth image from the actual examination) are presented to illustrate normal cardiovascular anatomy.

The information displayed in the cardiac anatomy plates is primarily geared toward cardiovascular anatomy. Some non–cardiovascular structures are illustrated because they are well seen during cardiac CTA examinations and those interpreting these studies must possess a detailed knowledge of non–cardiovascular thoracic anatomy because pathological conditions affecting non–cardiovascular structures are commonly encountered at cardiac CTA examinations. The reader is referred to the thoracic anatomy plates for a more detailed review of non–cardiovascular anatomy, particularly pulmonary anatomy.

Magnetic resonance imaging (MRI, or MR) is a technology that also produces cross-sectional images of thoracic and cardiovascular structures but operates using a completely different physical basis than CT imaging—MRI does not employ ionizing radiation to generate image data. MR can provide exquisite visualization of mediastinal anatomy, but the MR images in this volume are restricted to cardiac anatomy because of space limitations. MR imaging can be performed using a wide variety of techniques, each of which has specific benefits and limitations. In this volume, basic "black-blood" and "white-blood" imaging sequences are shown side by side. Although the anatomy shown in image sequence pairs coincides very closely, unlike the process of windowing with CT images, creation of these images does require separate scans, so very slight differences in the anatomical details of these image pairs may be evident to the astute observer. Although white-blood imaging depicts flowing blood as bright, this imaging sequence does not require the use of intravenous contrast.

MR imaging can be acquired in any plane. As with cardiac CTA, axial data are often obtained, but the cardiac imaging planes constitute the primary imaging planes used for clinical interpretation. The MRI plates in this volume are obtained in the axial plane and supplemented with cardiac imaging planes similar to the cardiac CTA plates.

Finally, several plates illustrating minor anatomical variations are shown. These variations include often incidentally detected tracheobronchial, fissure, and venous anomalies. In addition, the axial data chosen for the MRI plates show a minor vascular aberrancy—the aberrant right subclavian artery. The anatomical variations displayed in this volume generally carry little clinical significance. However, it is anticipated that the display of such variations will enhance the appreciation of the "normal" anatomy shown in the other plates while highlighting the power of imaging to demonstrate human anatomy.

Michael B. Gotway, MD

Contents

PART 1 THORACIC ANATOMY

Chapter 1 OVERVIEW OF THORACIC ANATOMY

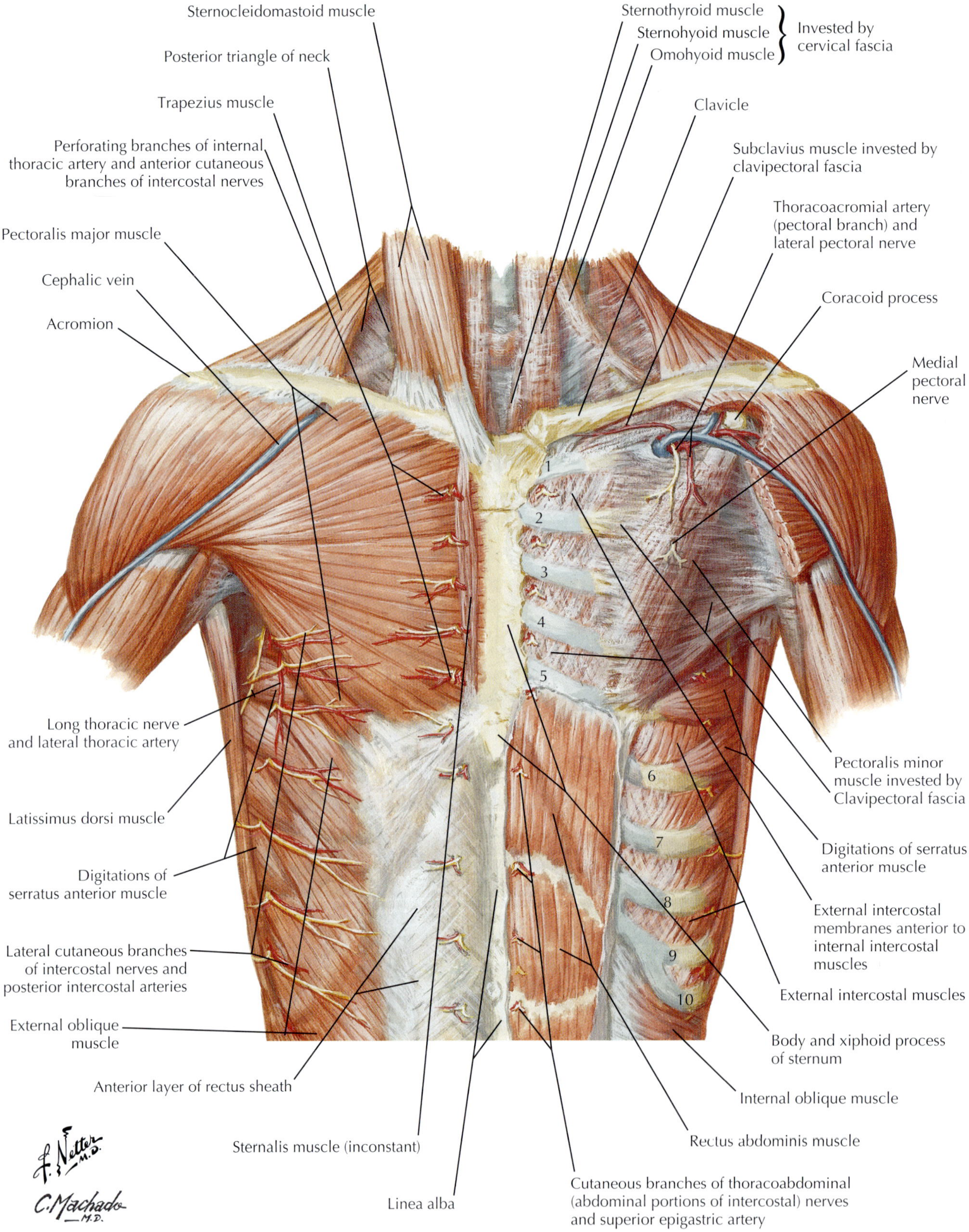

Sternocleidomastoid muscle
Posterior triangle of neck
Trapezius muscle
Perforating branches of internal thoracic artery and anterior cutaneous branches of intercostal nerves
Pectoralis major muscle
Cephalic vein
Acromion
Long thoracic nerve and lateral thoracic artery
Latissimus dorsi muscle
Digitations of serratus anterior muscle
Lateral cutaneous branches of intercostal nerves and posterior intercostal arteries
External oblique muscle
Anterior layer of rectus sheath
Sternalis muscle (inconstant)
Linea alba
Sternothyroid muscle
Sternohyoid muscle
Omohyoid muscle
Invested by cervical fascia
Clavicle
Subclavius muscle invested by clavipectoral fascia
Thoracoacromial artery (pectoral branch) and lateral pectoral nerve
Coracoid process
Medial pectoral nerve
Pectoralis minor muscle invested by Clavipectoral fascia
Digitations of serratus anterior muscle
External intercostal membranes anterior to internal intercostal muscles
External intercostal muscles
Body and xiphoid process of sternum
Internal oblique muscle
Rectus abdominis muscle
Cutaneous branches of thoracoabdominal (abdominal portions of intercostal) nerves and superior epigastric artery
1
2
3
4
5
6
7
8
9
10
F. Netter M.D.
C. Machado M.D.

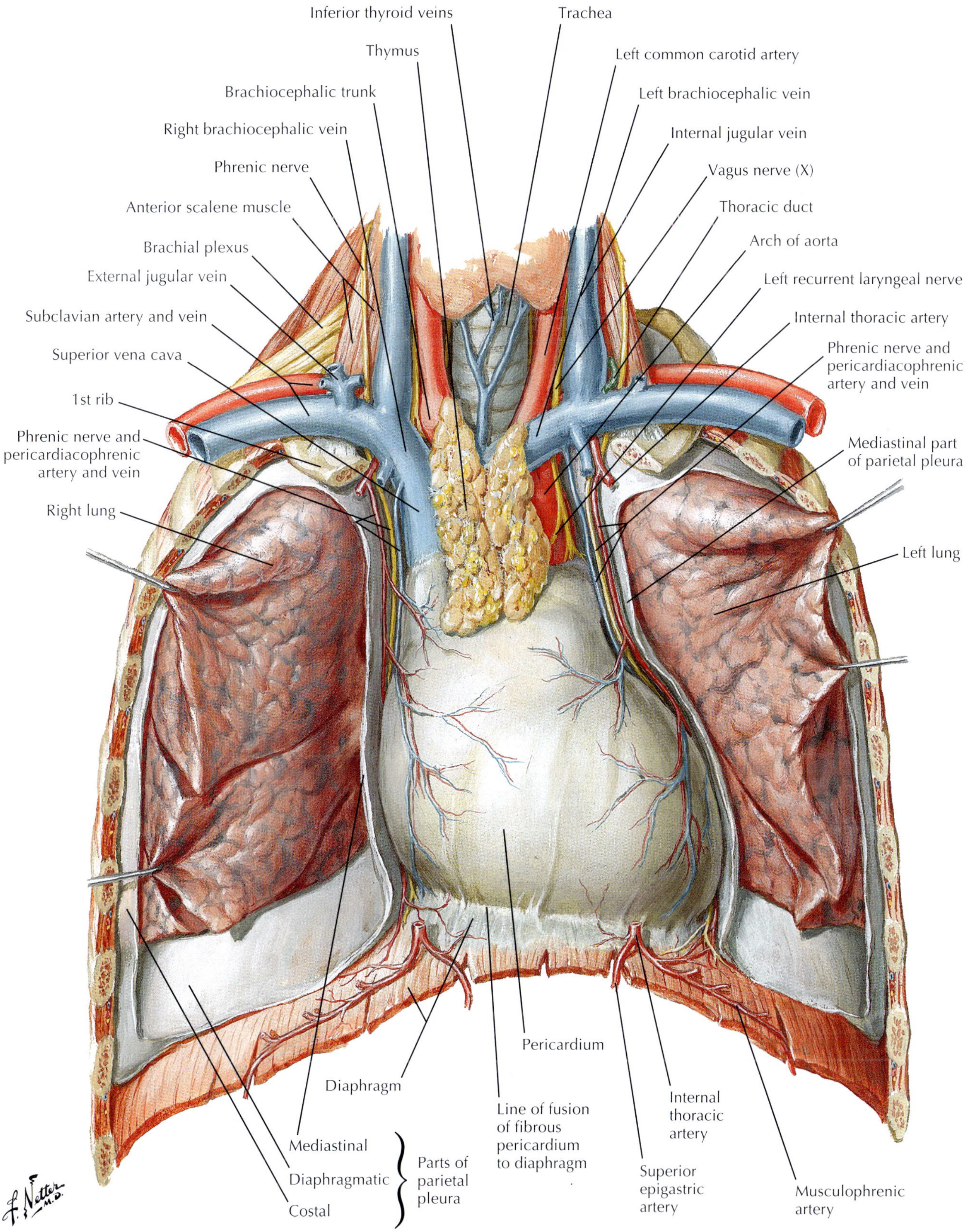
Inferior thyroid veins
Trachea
Thymus
Left common carotid artery
Brachiocephalic trunk
Left brachiocephalic vein
Right brachiocephalic vein
Internal jugular vein
Phrenic nerve
Vagus nerve (X)
Anterior scalene muscle
Thoracic duct
Brachial plexus
Arch of aorta
External jugular vein
Left recurrent laryngeal nerve
Subclavian artery and vein
Internal thoracic artery
Superior vena cava
Phrenic nerve and pericardiacophrenic artery and vein
1st rib
Mediastinal part of parietal pleura
Phrenic nerve and pericardiacophrenic artery and vein
Right lung
Left lung
Pericardium
Diaphragm
Line of fusion of fibrous pericardium to diaphragm
Internal thoracic artery
Mediastinal
Diaphragmatic
Costal
Parts of parietal pleura
Superior epigastric artery
Musculophrenic artery
F. Netter M.D.

GREAT VESSELS OF SUPERIOR MEDIASTINUM

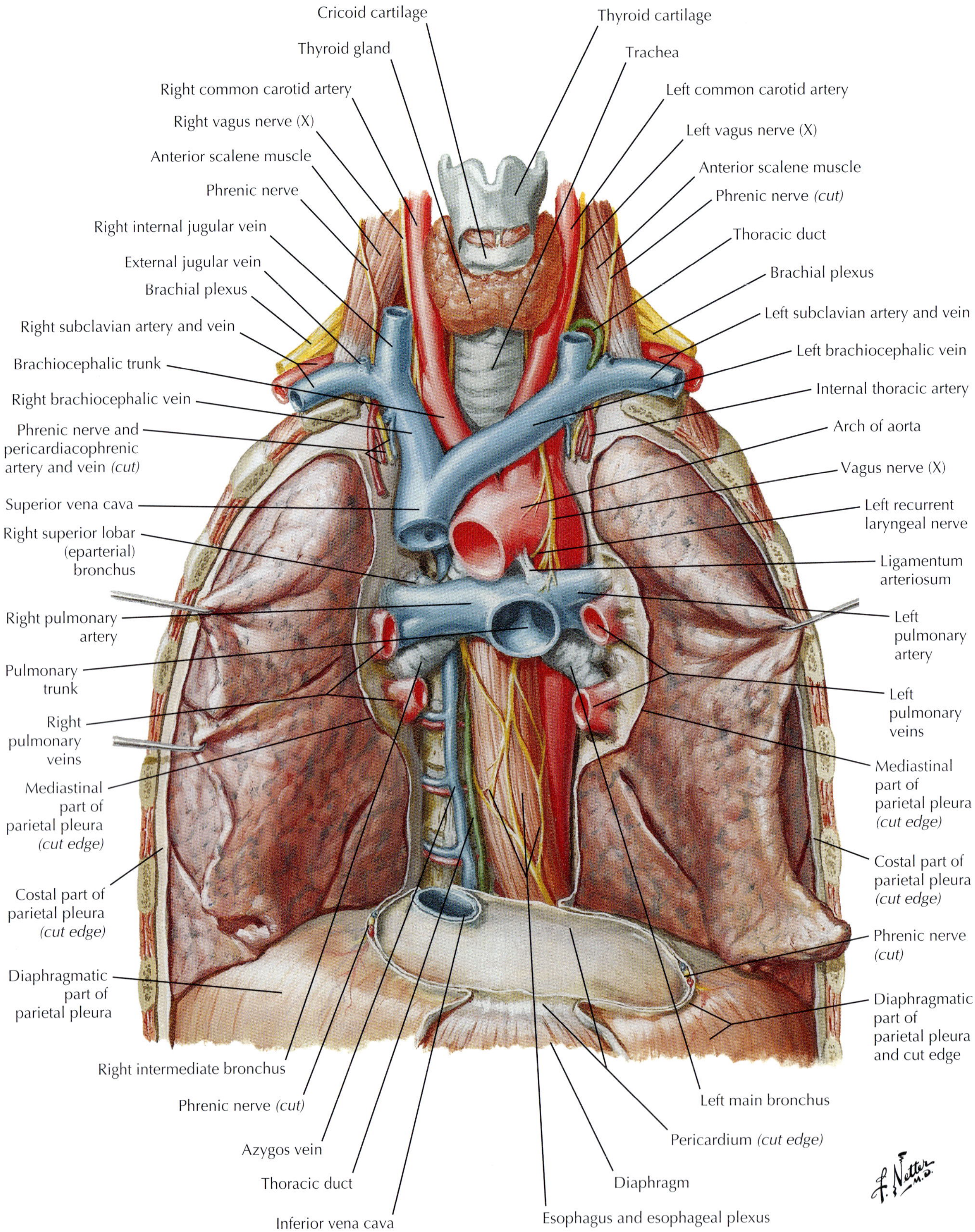

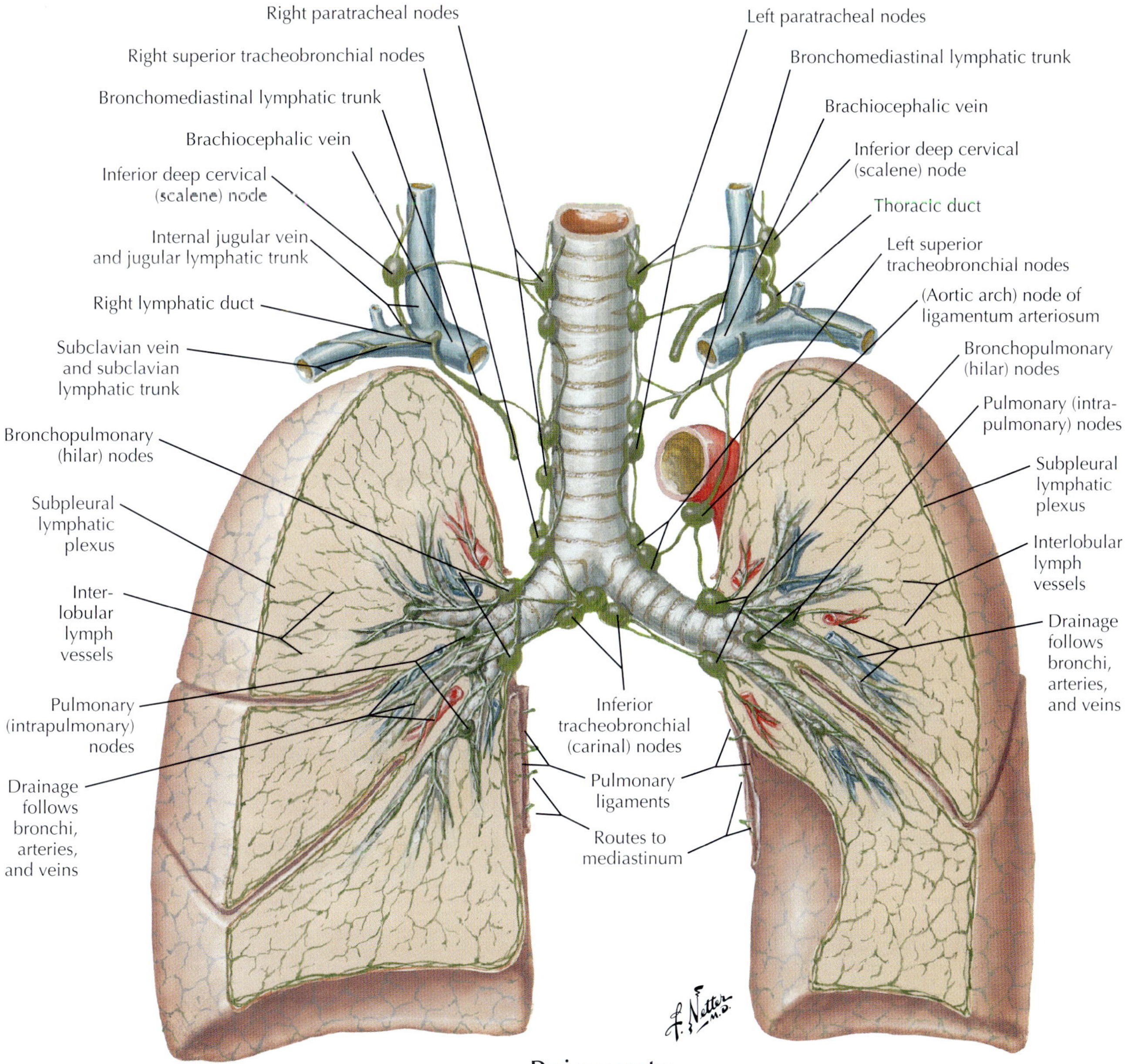

Drainage routes

Right lung: All lobes drain to pulmonary and bronchopulmonary (hilar) nodes, then to inferior tracheobronchial (carinal) nodes, right superior tracheobronchial nodes, and right paratracheal nodes on the way to the brachiocephalic vein via the bronchomediastinal lymphatic trunk and/or inferior deep cervical (scalene) node.

Left lung: The superior lobe drains to pulmonary and bronchopulmonary (hilar) nodes, inferior tracheobronchial (carinal) nodes, left superior tracheobronchial nodes, left paratracheal nodes and/or (aortic arch) node of ligamentum arteriosum, then to the brachiocephalic vein via the left bronchomediastinal trunk and thoracic duct. The left inferior lobe also drains to the pulmonary and bronchopulmonary (hilar) nodes and to inferior tracheobronchial (carinal) nodes, but then mostly to right superior tracheobronchial nodes, where it follows the same route as lymph from the right lung.

Lymph Vessels and Nodes of Esophagus

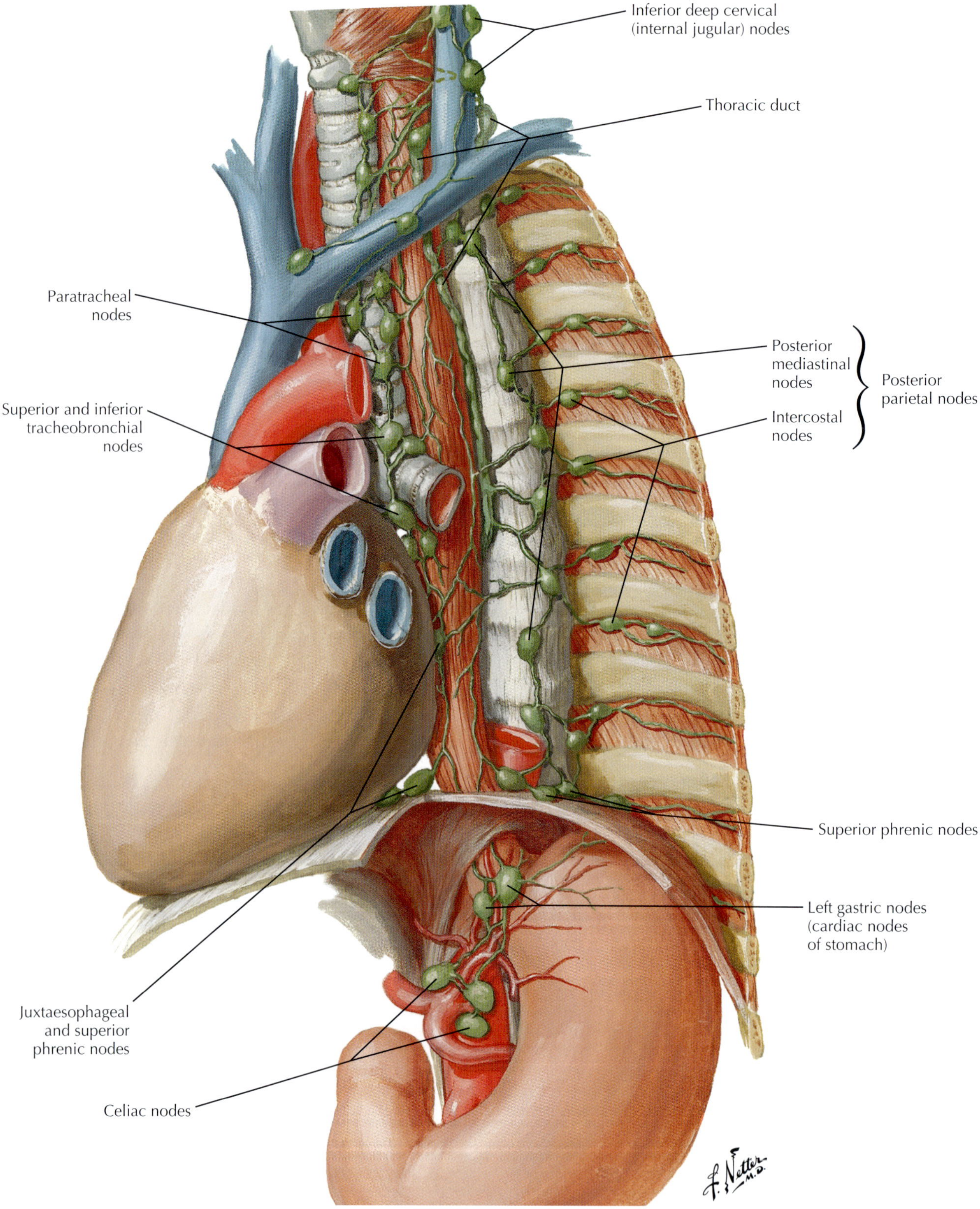

Veins of Esophagus

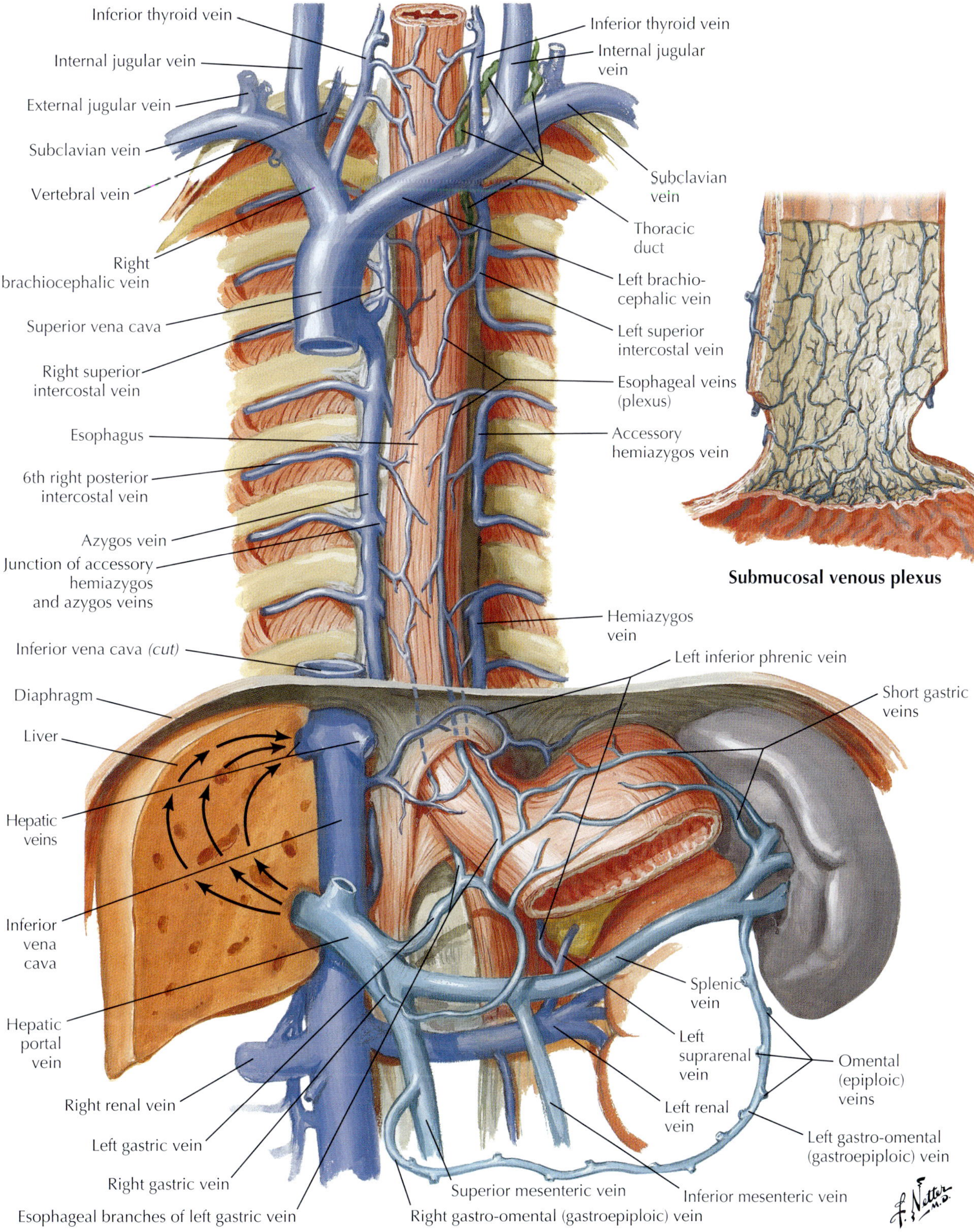

Submucosal venous plexus

Thorax: Four Chambers of Heart

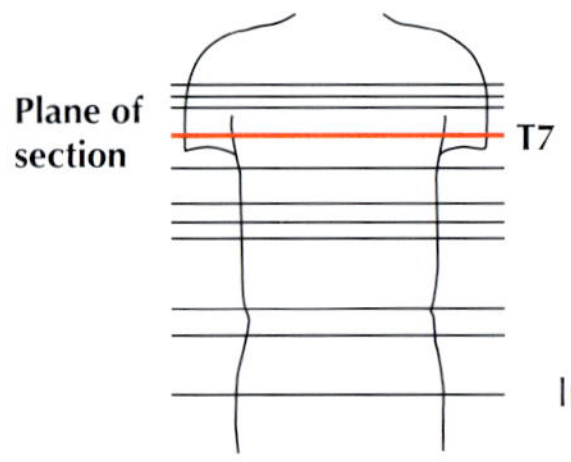

Transverse Section: Level of T7, 3rd Interchondral Space

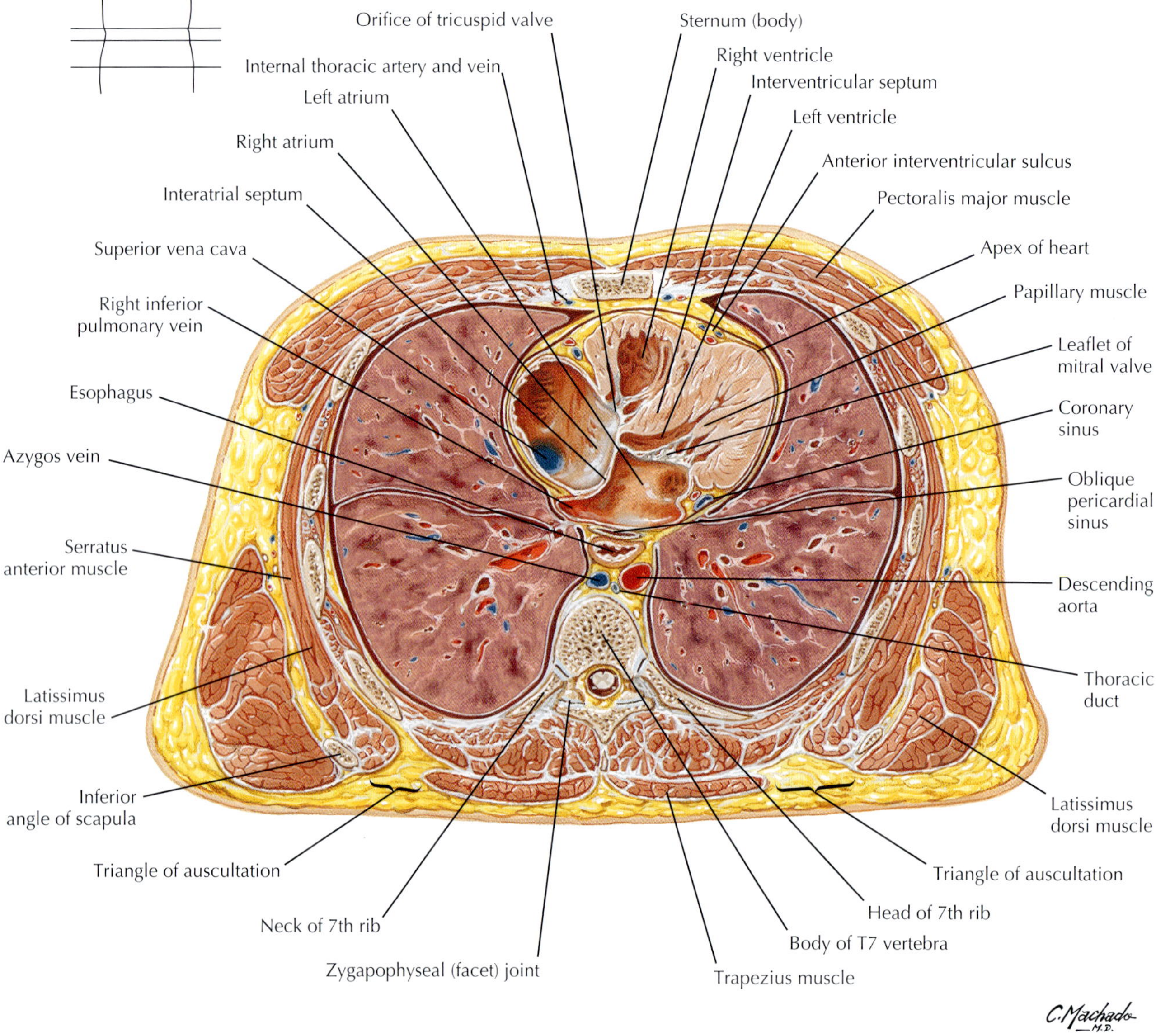

Chapter 2 THORACIC SOFT TISSUE AND LUNG

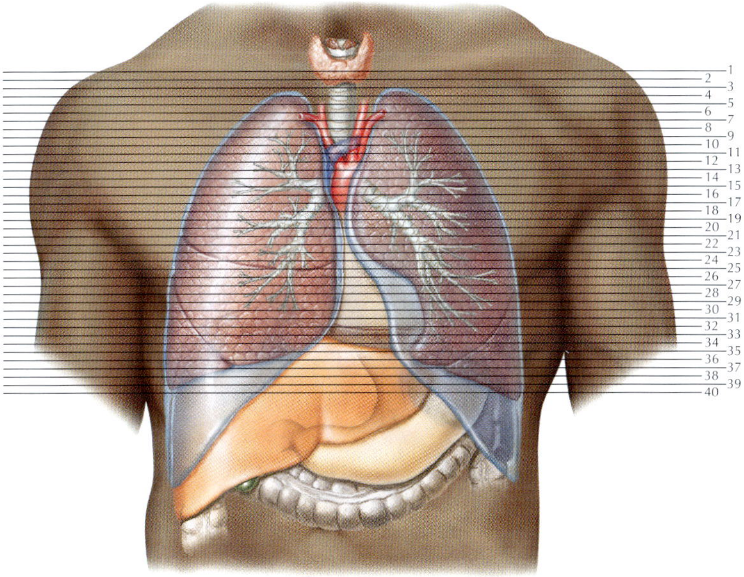

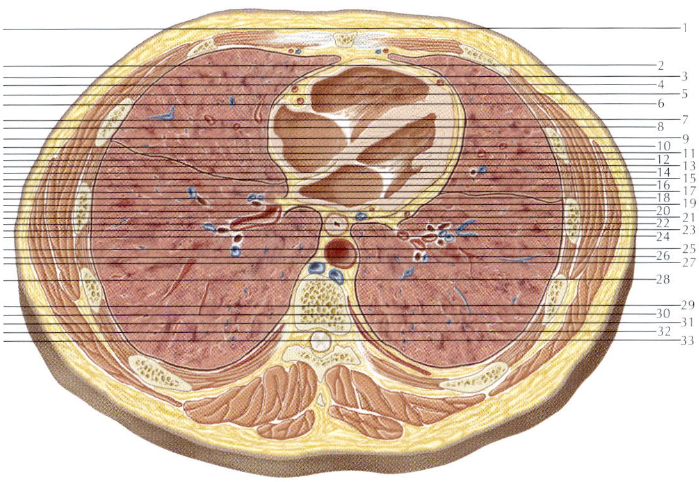

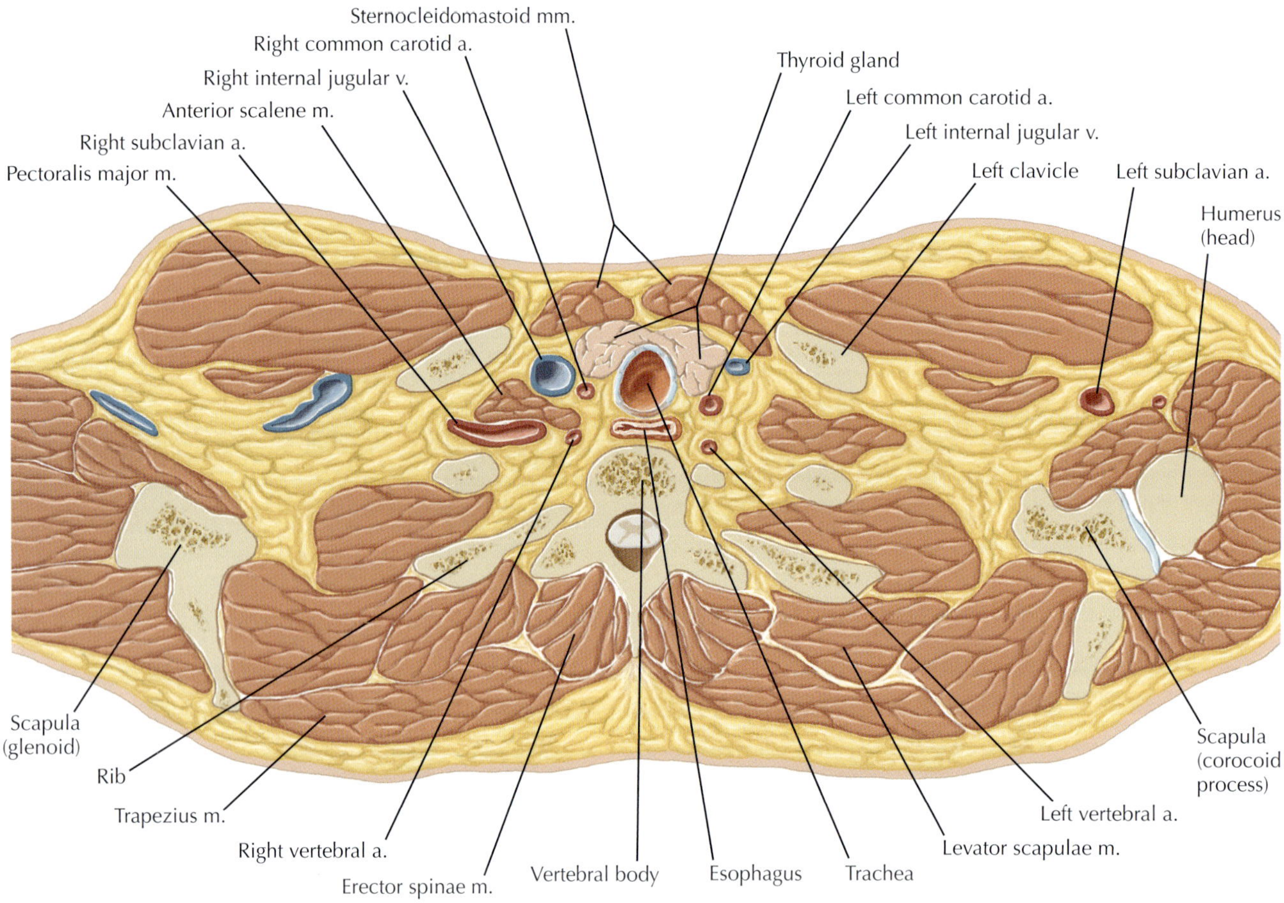
Sternocleidomastoid mm.
Right common carotid a.
Right internal jugular v.
Anterior scalene m.
Right subclavian a.
Pectoralis major m.
Thyroid gland
Left common carotid a.
Left internal jugular v.
Left clavicle
Left subclavian a.
Humerus (head)
Scapula (glenoid)
Rib
Trapezius m.
Right vertebral a.
Erector spinae m.
Vertebral body
Esophagus
Trachea
Levator scapulae m.
Left vertebral a.
Scapula (corocoid process)

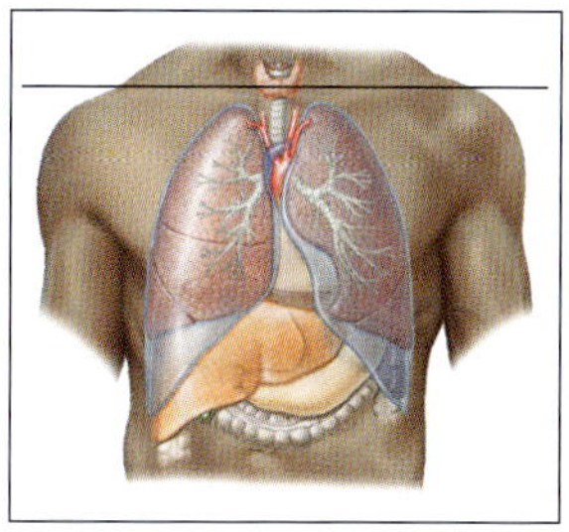

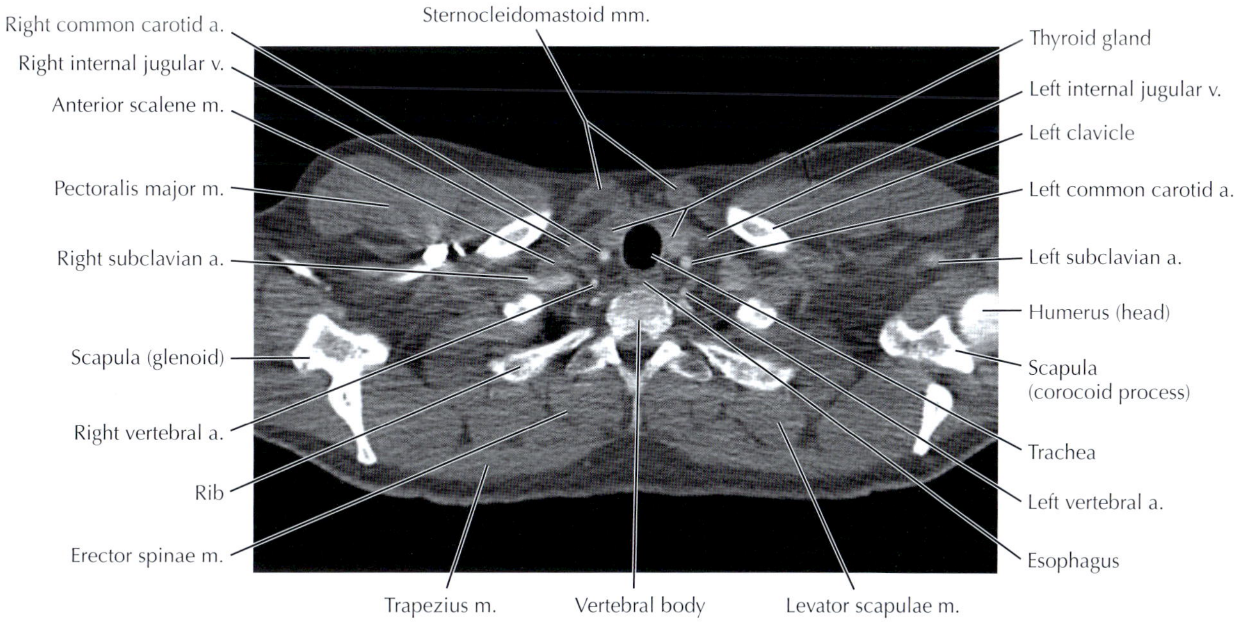
Right common carotid a.
Right internal jugular v.
Anterior scalene m.
Pectoralis major m.
Right subclavian a.
Scapula (glenoid)
Right vertebral a.
Rib
Erector spinae m.
Sternocleidomastoid mm.
Thyroid gland
Left internal jugular v.
Left clavicle
Left common carotid a.
Left subclavian a.
Humerus (head)
Scapula (corocoid process)
Trachea
Left vertebral a.
Esophagus
Trapezius m.
Vertebral body
Levator scapulae m.

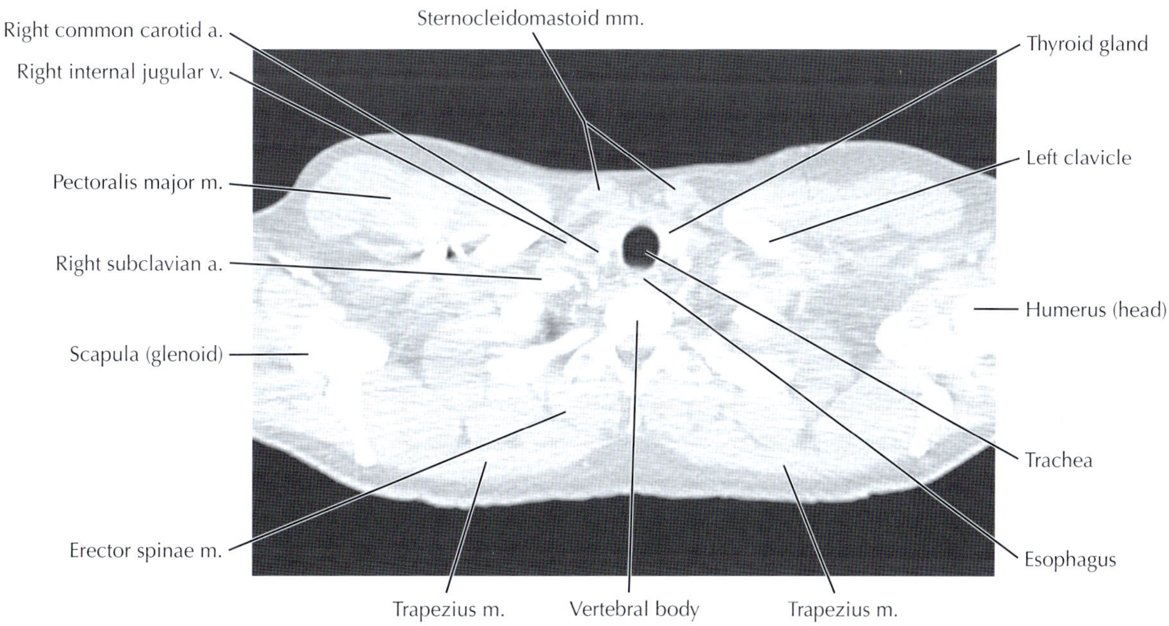
Right common carotid a.
Right internal jugular v.
Pectoralis major m.
Right subclavian a.
Scapula (glenoid)
Erector spinae m.
Sternocleidomastoid mm.
Thyroid gland
Left clavicle
Humerus (head)
Trachea
Esophagus
Trapezius m.
Vertebral body
Trapezius m.

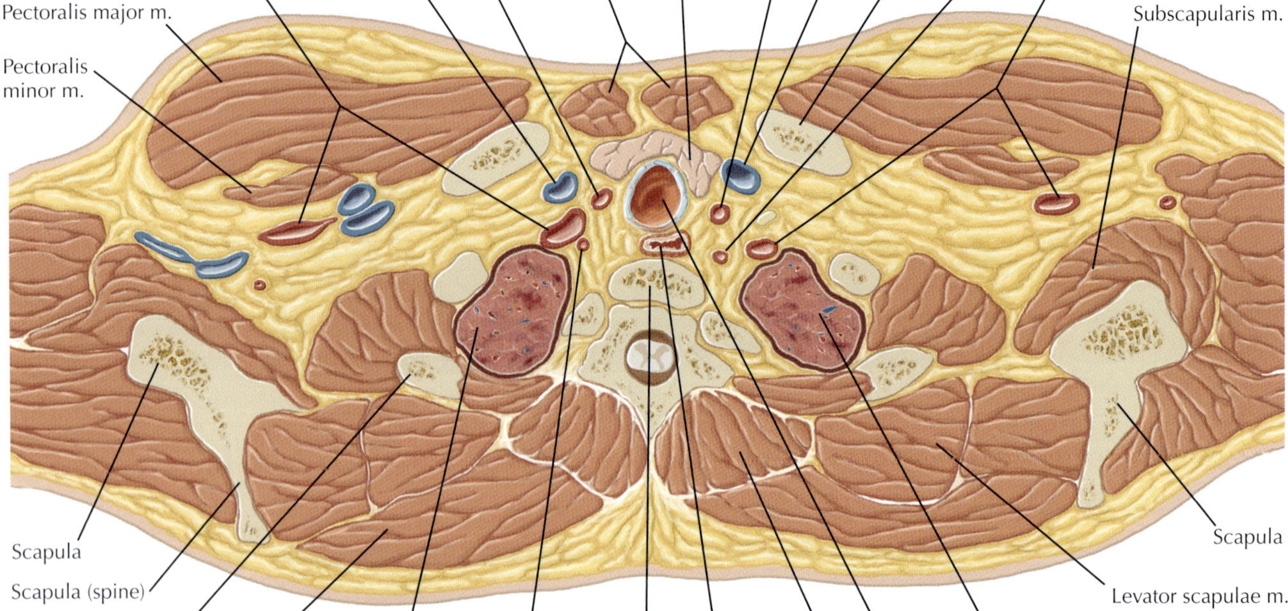
Sternocleidomastoid mm.
Thyroid gland
Left common carotid a.
Right common carotid a.
Left internal jugular v.
Right internal jugular v.
Left clavicle
Left vertebral a.
Right subclavian a.
Left subclavian a.
Pectoralis major m.
Subscapularis m.
Pectoralis minor m.
Scapula
Scapula
Scapula (spine)
Levator scapulae m.
Rib
Left lung apex (left upper lobe, apical-posterior segment)
Trapezius m.
Trachea
Right lung apex (right upper lobe, apical segment)
Right vertebral a.
Vertebral body
Esophagus
Erector spinae m.

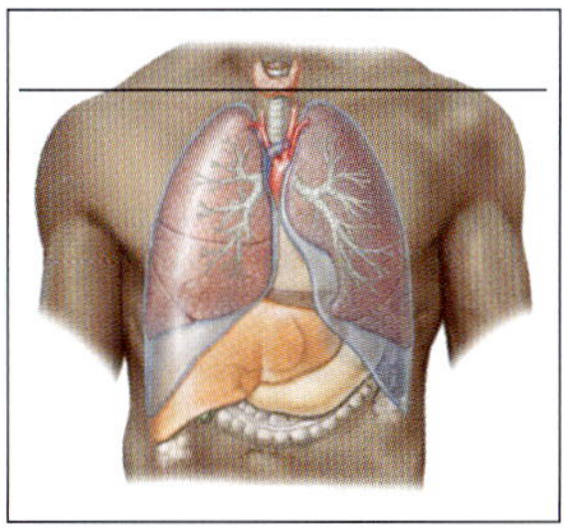

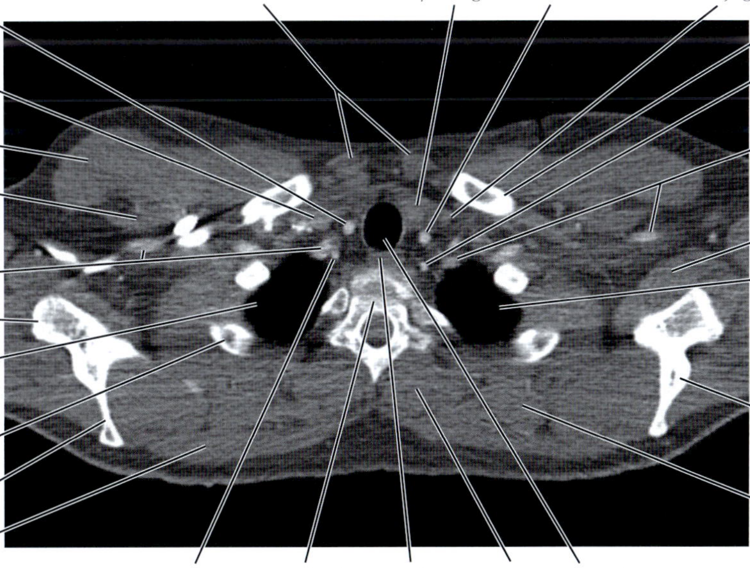
Right common carotid a.
Right internal jugular v.
Pectoralis major m.
Pectoralis minor m.
Right subclavian a.
Scapula
Right lung apex (right upper lobe, apical segment)
Rib
Scapula (spine)
Trapezius m.
Sternocleidomastoid mm.
Thyroid gland
Left common carotid a.
Left internal jugular v.
Left clavicle
Left vertebral a.
Left subclavian a.
Subscapularis m.
Left lung apex (left upper lobe, apical-posterior segment)
Scapula
Levator scapulae m.
Right vertebral a.
Vertebral body
Esophagus
Erector spinae m.
Trachea

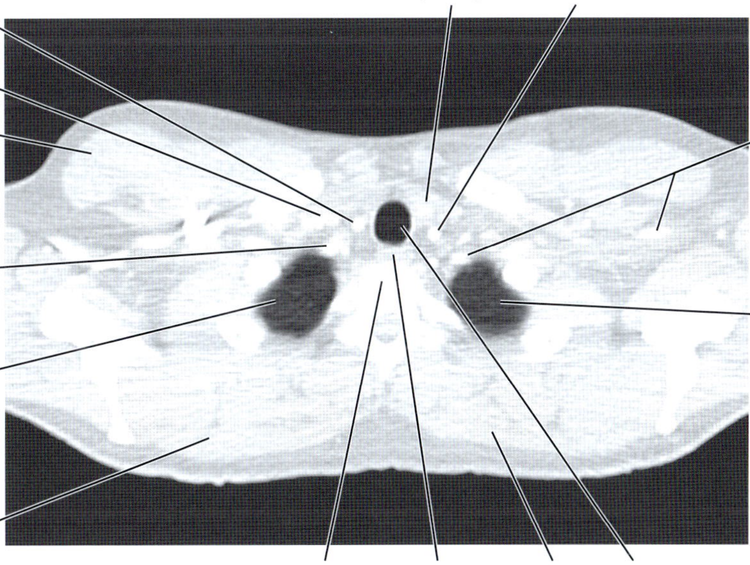
Right common carotid a.
Right internal jugular v.
Pectoralis major m.
Right subclavian a.
Right lung apex (right upper lobe, apical segment)
Trapezius m.
Thyroid gland
Left common carotid a.
Left subclavian a.
Left lung apex (left upper lobe, apical-posterior segment)
Vertebral body
Esophagus
Trapezius m.
Trachea

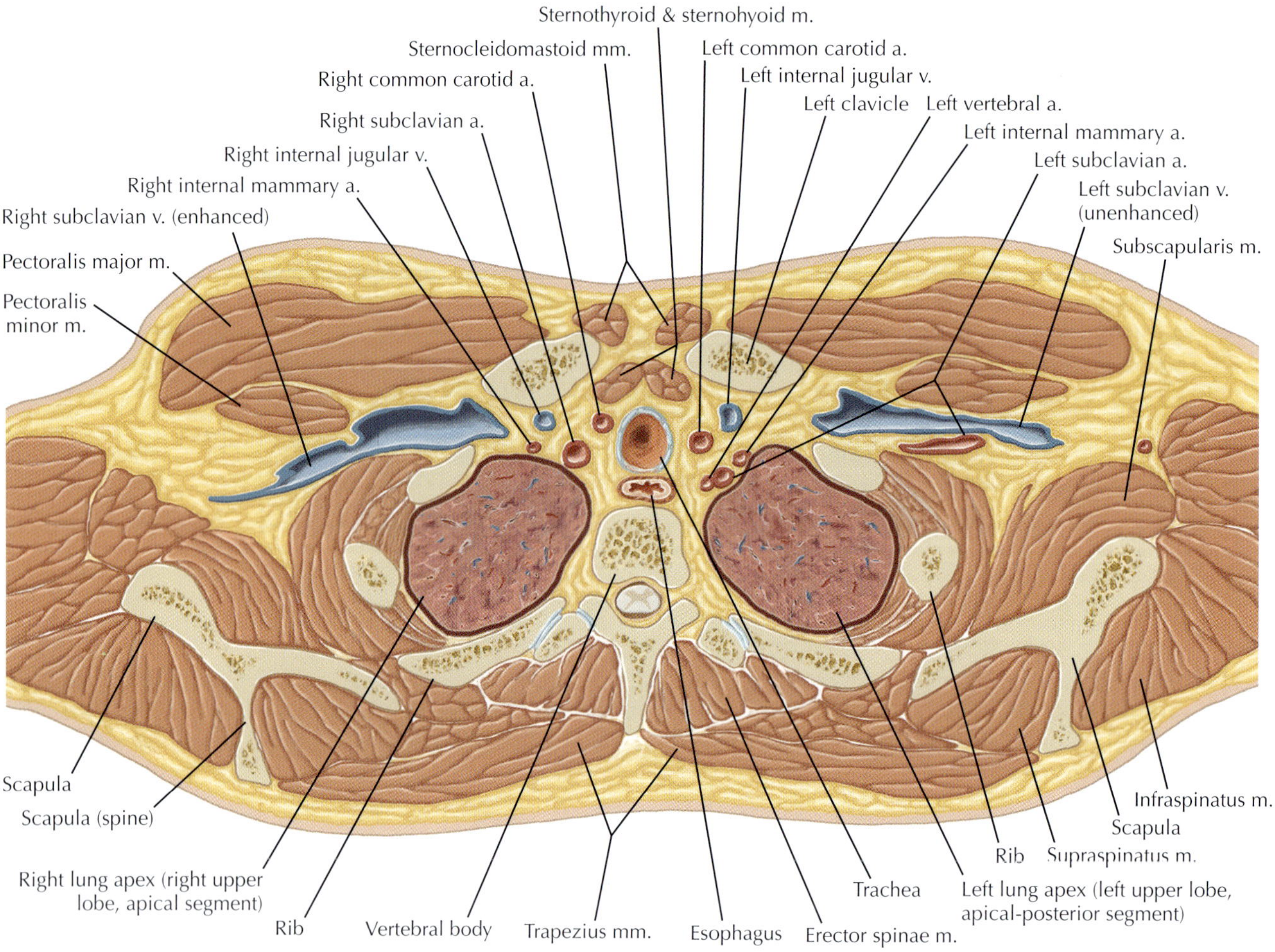

DIAGNOSTIC CONSIDERATION

Thoracic CT scans may be performed with or without the intravenous injection of iodinated contrast. Contrast-enhanced thoracic CT scanning is usually performed following injection into an upper extremity vein, with imaging started at 30 to 40 seconds after the injection is begun, depending on the specific application. In this patient, contrast was injected via the right upper extremity, resulting in dense enhancement of the *right subclavian vein* (and the *right brachiocephalic vein* on Axial 5 and subsequent images); the *left subclavian vein* (and *left brachiocephalic vein* on Axial 5 and subsequent images) remains unenhanced in this patient because imaging was begun before injected contrast had sufficient time to circulate throughout the body and reach the left subclavian vein.

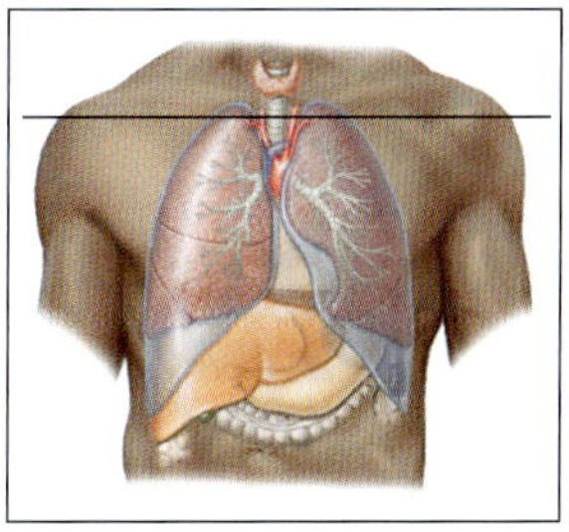

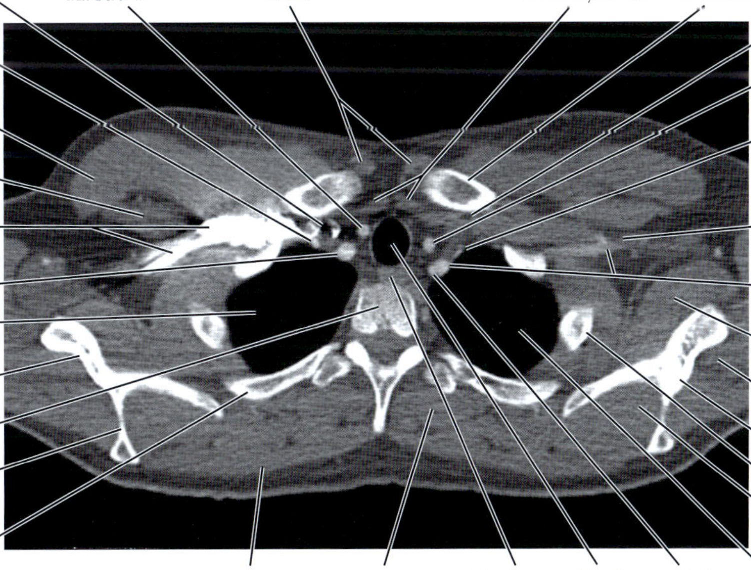
Right internal jugular v.
Right common carotid a.
Sternocleidomastoid mm.
Sternothyroid & sternohyoid m.
Left clavicle
Right internal mammary a.
Pectoralis major m.
Pectoralis minor m.
Right subclavian v. (enhanced)
Right subclavian a.
Right lung apex (right upper lobe, apical segment)
Scapula
Vertebral body
Scapula (spine)
Rib
Left internal jugular v.
Left common carotid a.
Left internal mammary a.
Left subclavian v. (unenhanced)
Left subclavian a.
Subscapularis m.
Infraspinatus m.
Scapula
Rib
Supraspinatus m.
Left lung apex (left upper lobe, apical-posterior segment)
Trapezius m.
Erector spinae m.
Esophagus
Trachea
Left vertebral a.

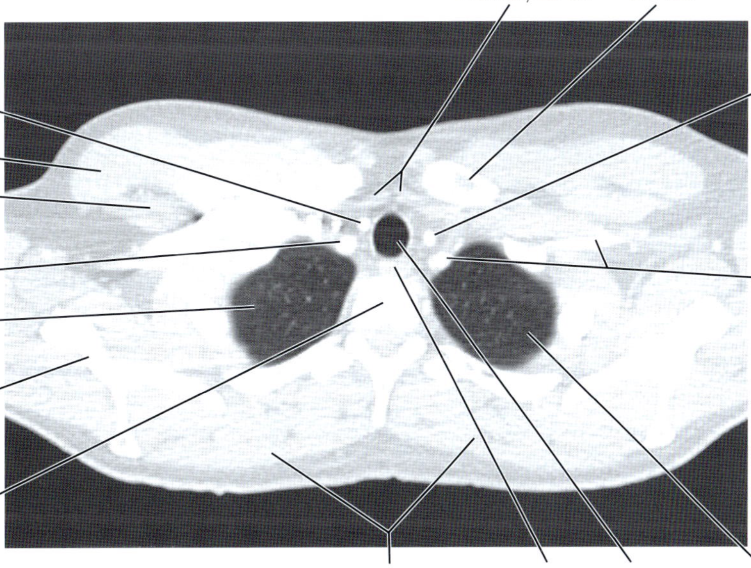
Sternothyroid & sternohyoid m.
Left clavicle
Right common carotid a.
Pectoralis major m.
Pectoralis minor m.
Right subclavian a.
Right lung apex (right upper lobe, apical segment)
Scapula
Vertebral body
Left common carotid a.
Left subclavian a.
Left lung apex (left upper lobe, apical-posterior segment)
Trapezius mm.
Esophagus
Trachea

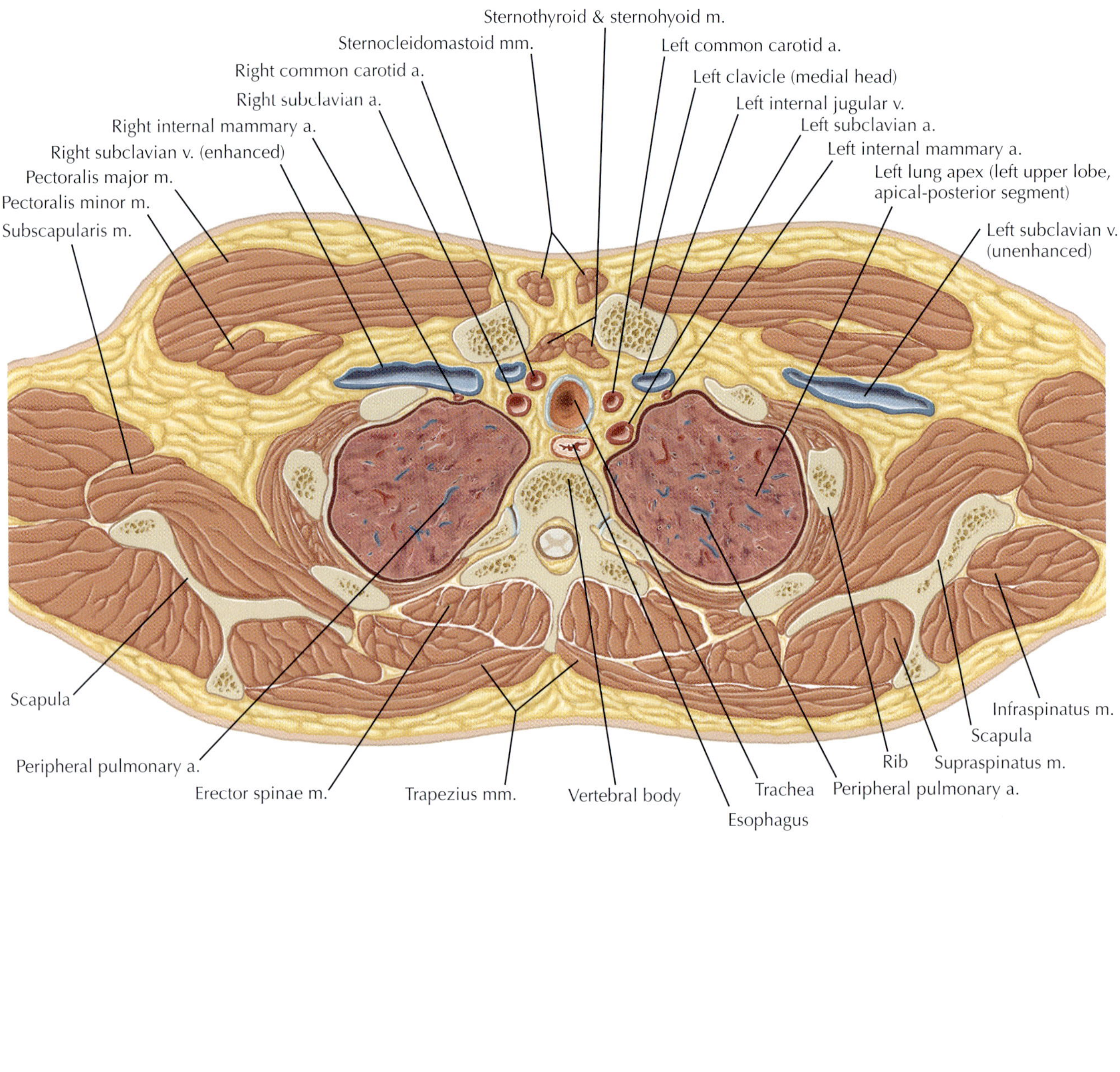
Sternothyroid & sternohyoid m.
Sternocleidomastoid mm.
Left common carotid a.
Right common carotid a.
Left clavicle (medial head)
Right subclavian a.
Left internal jugular v.
Right internal mammary a.
Left subclavian a.
Right subclavian v. (enhanced)
Left internal mammary a.
Pectoralis major m.
Left lung apex (left upper lobe, apical-posterior segment)
Pectoralis minor m.
Subscapularis m.
Left subclavian v. (unenhanced)
Scapula
Infraspinatus m.
Scapula
Peripheral pulmonary a.
Rib
Supraspinatus m.
Erector spinae m.
Trapezius mm.
Vertebral body
Trachea
Peripheral pulmonary a.
Esophagus

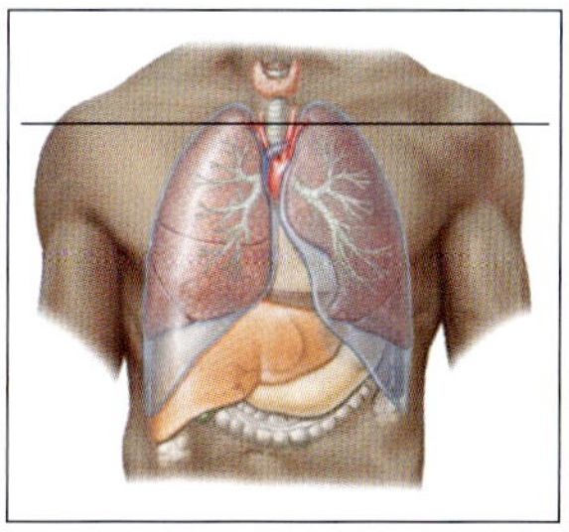

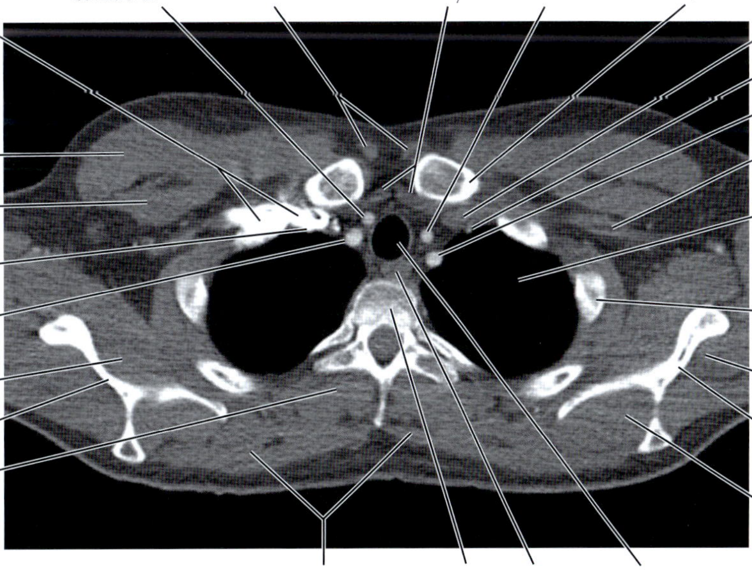
Right common carotid a.
Sternocleidomastoid mm.
Sternothyroid & sternohyoid m.
Left common carotid a.
Left clavicle (medial head)
Right subclavian v. (enhanced)
Left internal jugular v.
Left internal mammary a.
Left subclavian a.
Pectoralis major m.
Left subclavian v. (unenhanced)
Pectoralis minor m.
Left lung apex (left upper lobe, apical-posterior segment)
Right internal mammary a.
Right subclavian a.
Rib
Subscapularis m.
Infraspinatus m.
Scapula
Scapula
Erector spinae m.
Supraspinatus m.
Trapezius mm.
Vertebral body
Esophagus
Trachea

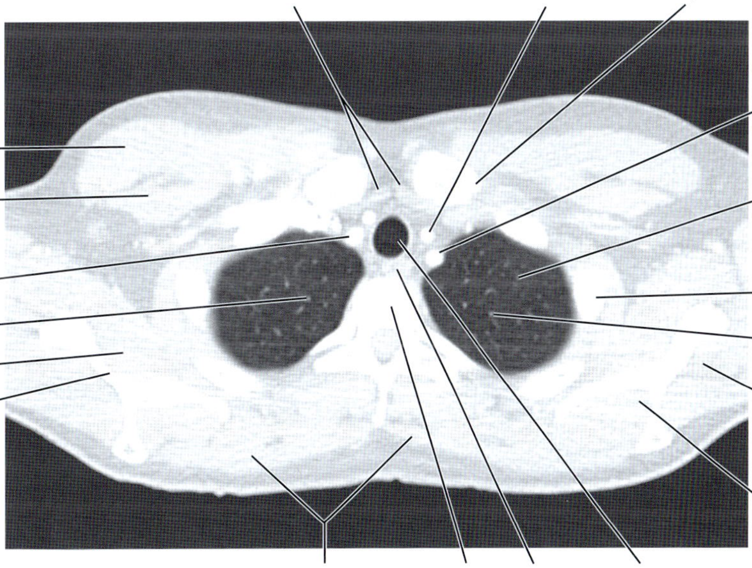
Sternocleidomastoid mm.
Left common carotid a.
Left clavicle (medial head)
Left subclavian a.
Pectoralis major m.
Pectoralis minor m.
Left lung apex (left upper lobe, apical-posterior segment)
Right subclavian a.
Rib
Peripheral pulmonary a.
Peripheral pulmonary a.
Subscapularis m.
Infraspinatus m.
Scapula
Supraspinatus m.
Trapezius mm.
Vertebral body
Esophagus
Trachea

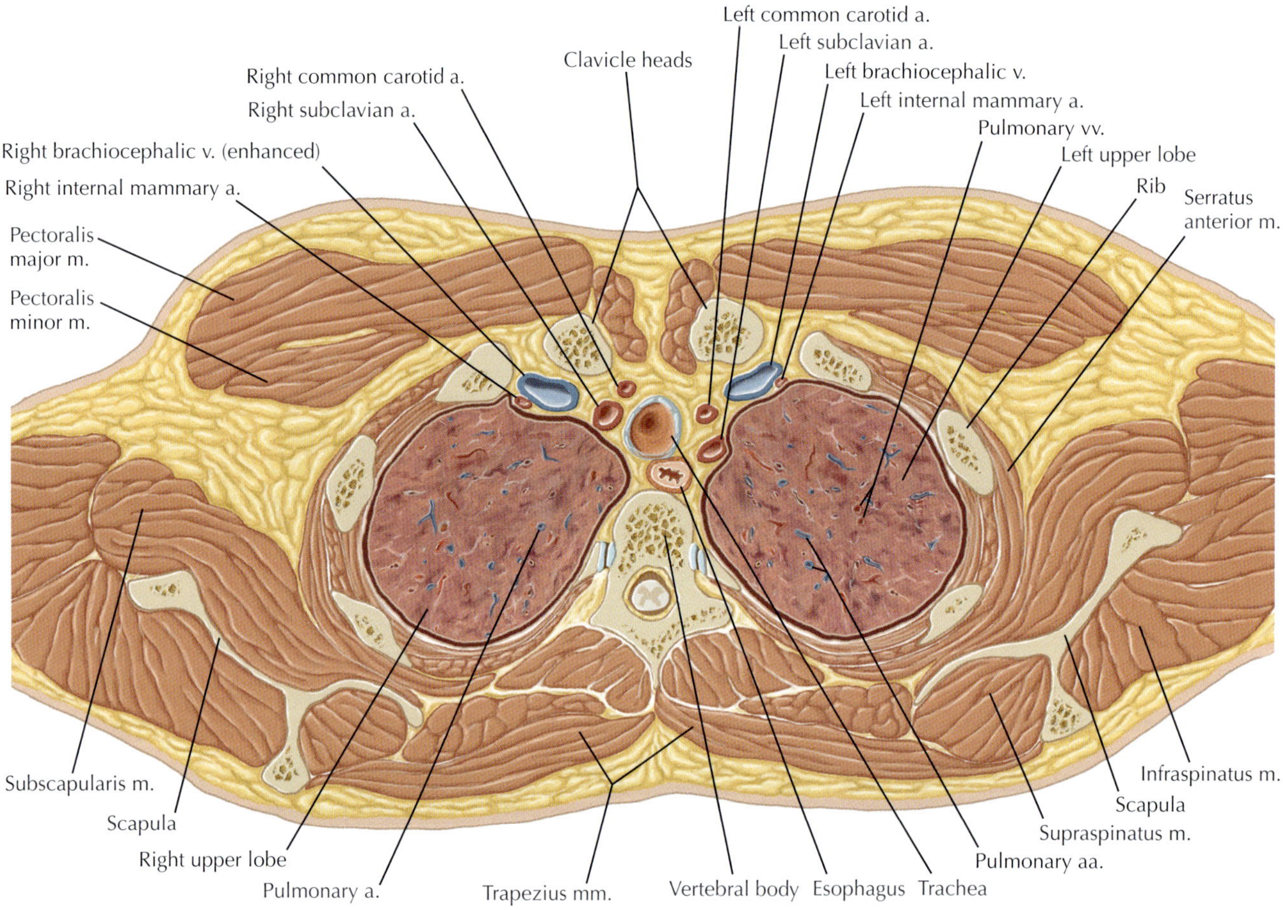
Left common carotid a.
Left subclavian a.
Clavicle heads
Left brachiocephalic v.
Right common carotid a.
Left internal mammary a.
Right subclavian a.
Pulmonary vv.
Right brachiocephalic v. (enhanced)
Left upper lobe
Right internal mammary a.
Rib
Serratus anterior m.
Pectoralis major m.
Pectoralis minor m.
Subscapularis m.
Scapula
Right upper lobe
Pulmonary a.
Trapezius mm.
Vertebral body
Esophagus
Trachea
Pulmonary aa.
Supraspinatus m.
Scapula
Infraspinatus m.

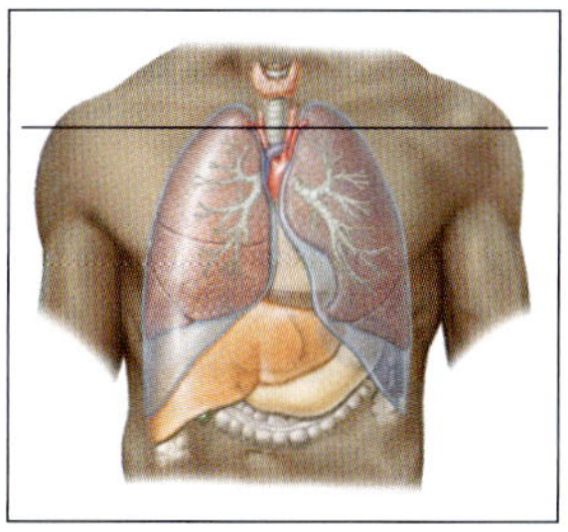

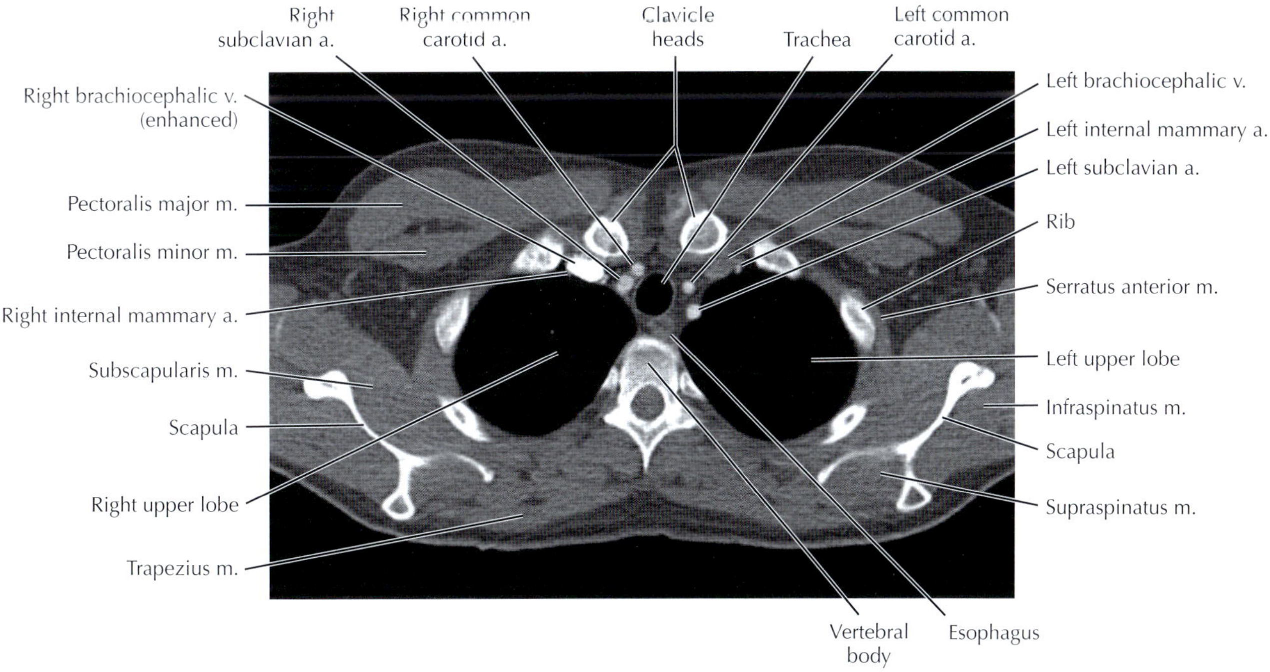
Right subclavian a.
Right common carotid a.
Clavicle heads
Trachea
Left common carotid a.
Right brachiocephalic v. (enhanced)
Left brachiocephalic v.
Left internal mammary a.
Left subclavian a.
Pectoralis major m.
Rib
Pectoralis minor m.
Serratus anterior m.
Right internal mammary a.
Left upper lobe
Subscapularis m.
Infraspinatus m.
Scapula
Scapula
Right upper lobe
Supraspinatus m.
Trapezius m.
Vertebral body
Esophagus

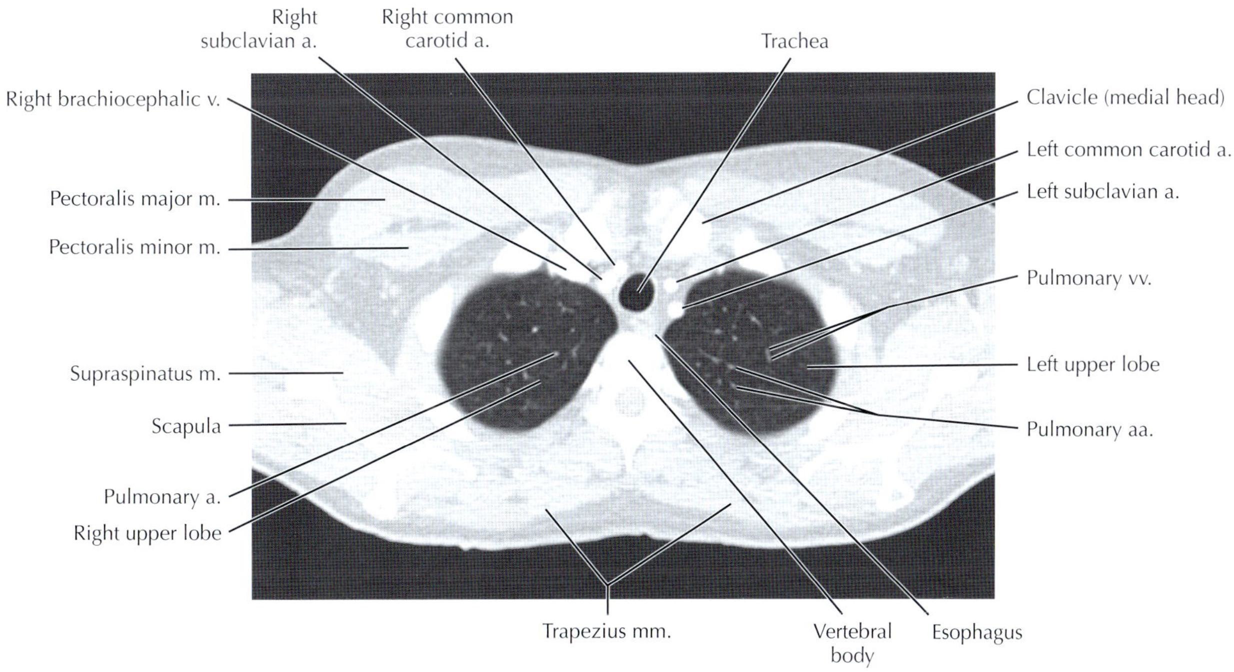
Right subclavian a.
Right common carotid a.
Trachea
Right brachiocephalic v.
Clavicle (medial head)
Left common carotid a.
Pectoralis major m.
Left subclavian a.
Pectoralis minor m.
Pulmonary vv.
Left upper lobe
Supraspinatus m.
Pulmonary aa.
Scapula
Pulmonary a.
Right upper lobe
Trapezius mm.
Vertebral body
Esophagus

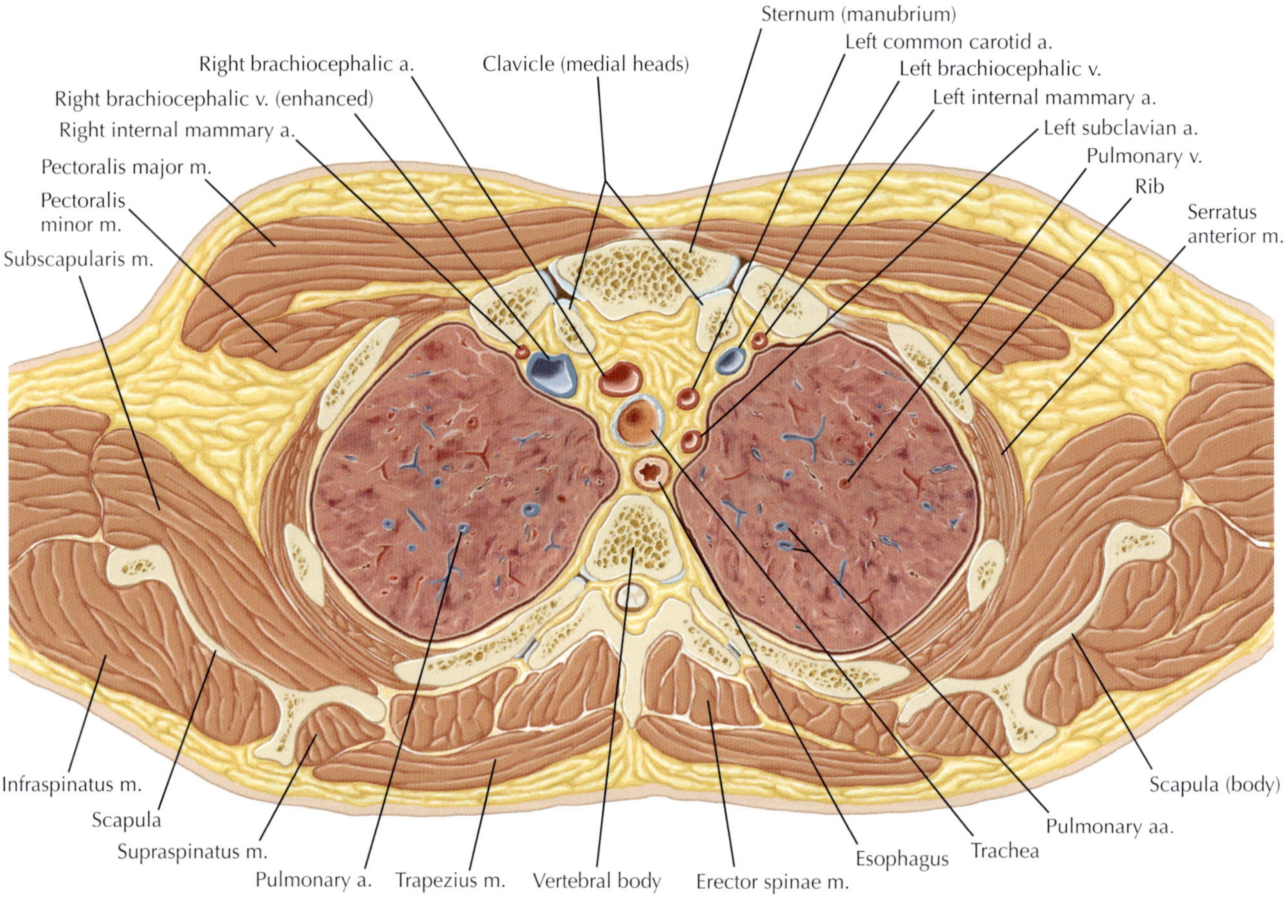

Sternum (manubrium)
Left common carotid a.
Right brachiocephalic a.
Clavicle (medial heads)
Left brachiocephalic v.
Right brachiocephalic v. (enhanced)
Left internal mammary a.
Right internal mammary a.
Left subclavian a.
Pulmonary v.
Pectoralis major m.
Rib
Pectoralis minor m.
Serratus anterior m.
Subscapularis m.
Infraspinatus m.
Scapula (body)
Scapula
Pulmonary aa.
Supraspinatus m.
Esophagus
Trachea
Pulmonary a.
Trapezius m.
Vertebral body
Erector spinae m.

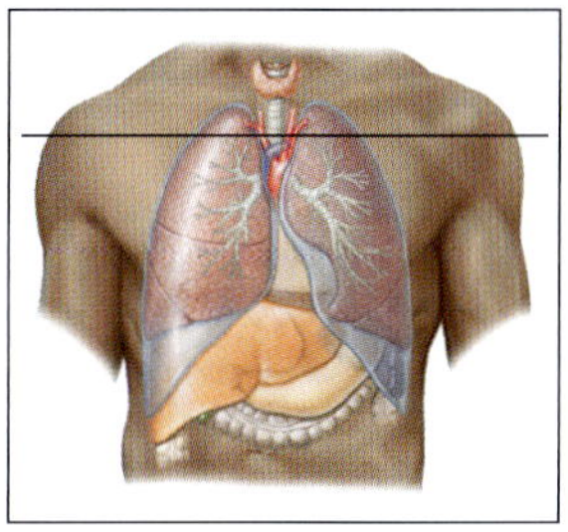

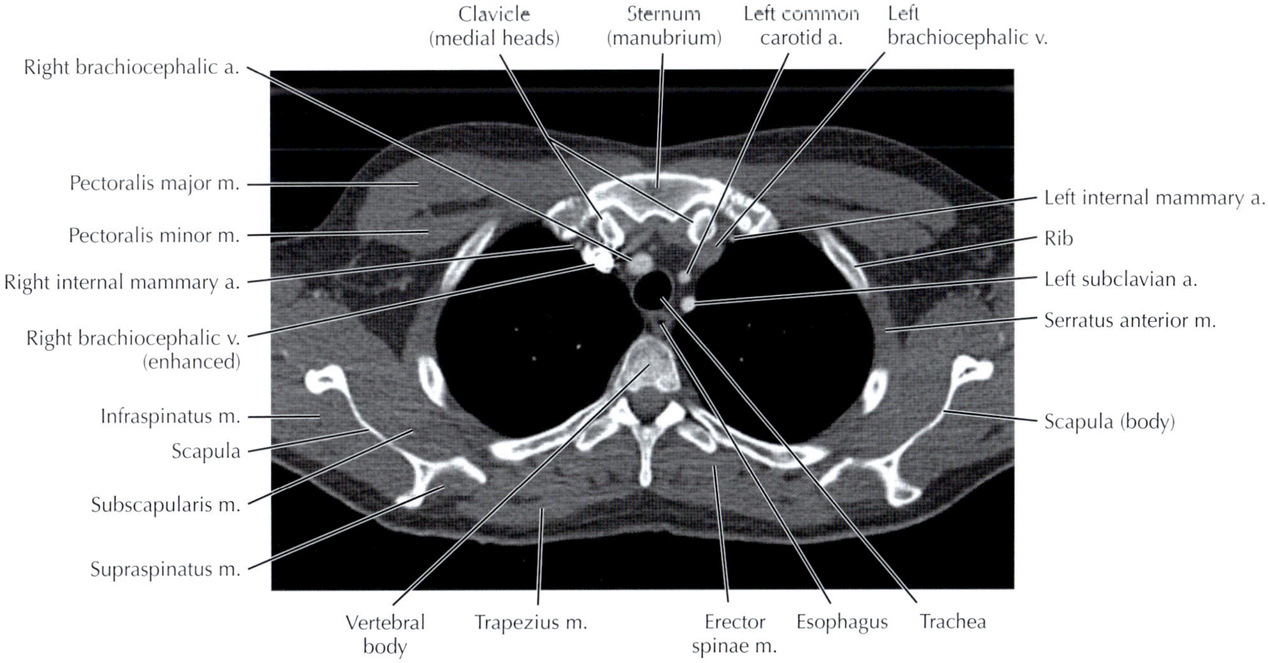
Clavicle (medial heads)
Sternum (manubrium)
Left common carotid a.
Left brachiocephalic v.
Right brachiocephalic a.
Pectoralis major m.
Pectoralis minor m.
Right internal mammary a.
Right brachiocephalic v. (enhanced)
Infraspinatus m.
Scapula
Subscapularis m.
Supraspinatus m.
Left internal mammary a.
Rib
Left subclavian a.
Serratus anterior m.
Scapula (body)
Vertebral body
Trapezius m.
Erector spinae m.
Esophagus
Trachea

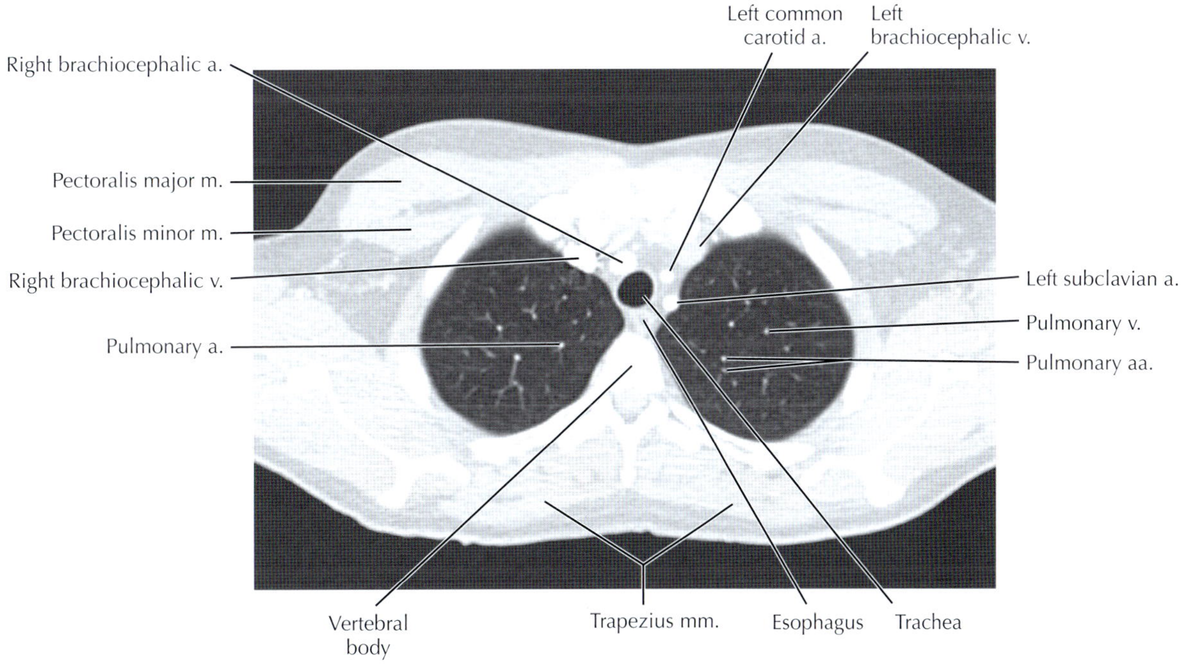
Left common carotid a.
Left brachiocephalic v.
Right brachiocephalic a.
Pectoralis major m.
Pectoralis minor m.
Right brachiocephalic v.
Pulmonary a.
Left subclavian a.
Pulmonary v.
Pulmonary aa.
Vertebral body
Trapezius mm.
Esophagus
Trachea

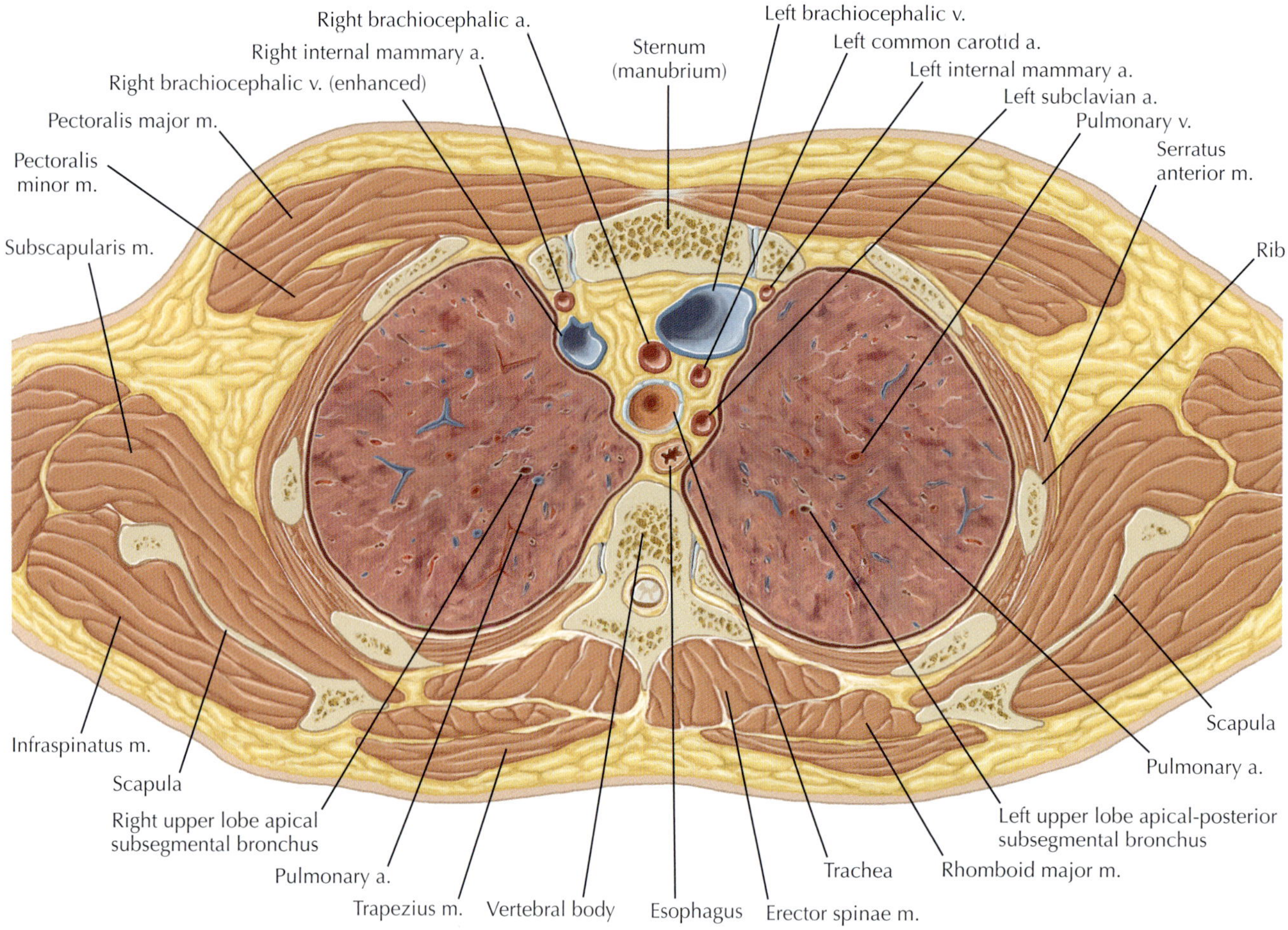
Right brachiocephalic a.
Right internal mammary a.
Right brachiocephalic v. (enhanced)
Pectoralis major m.
Pectoralis minor m.
Subscapularis m.
Sternum (manubrium)
Left brachiocephalic v.
Left common carotid a.
Left internal mammary a.
Left subclavian a.
Pulmonary v.
Serratus anterior m.
Rib
Infraspinatus m.
Scapula
Right upper lobe apical subsegmental bronchus
Pulmonary a.
Trapezius m.
Vertebral body
Esophagus
Erector spinae m.
Trachea
Rhomboid major m.
Left upper lobe apical-posterior subsegmental bronchus
Pulmonary a.
Scapula

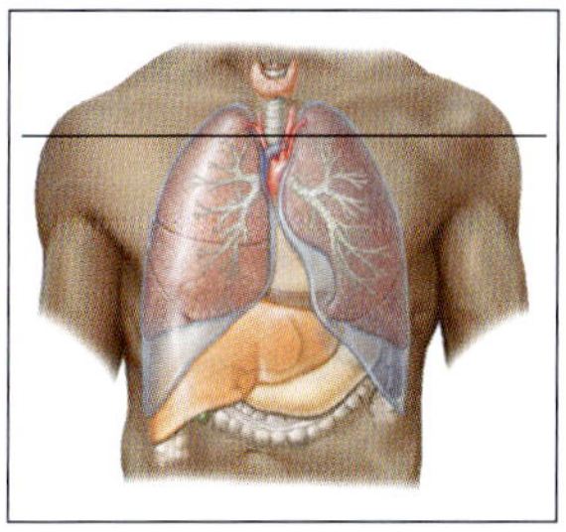

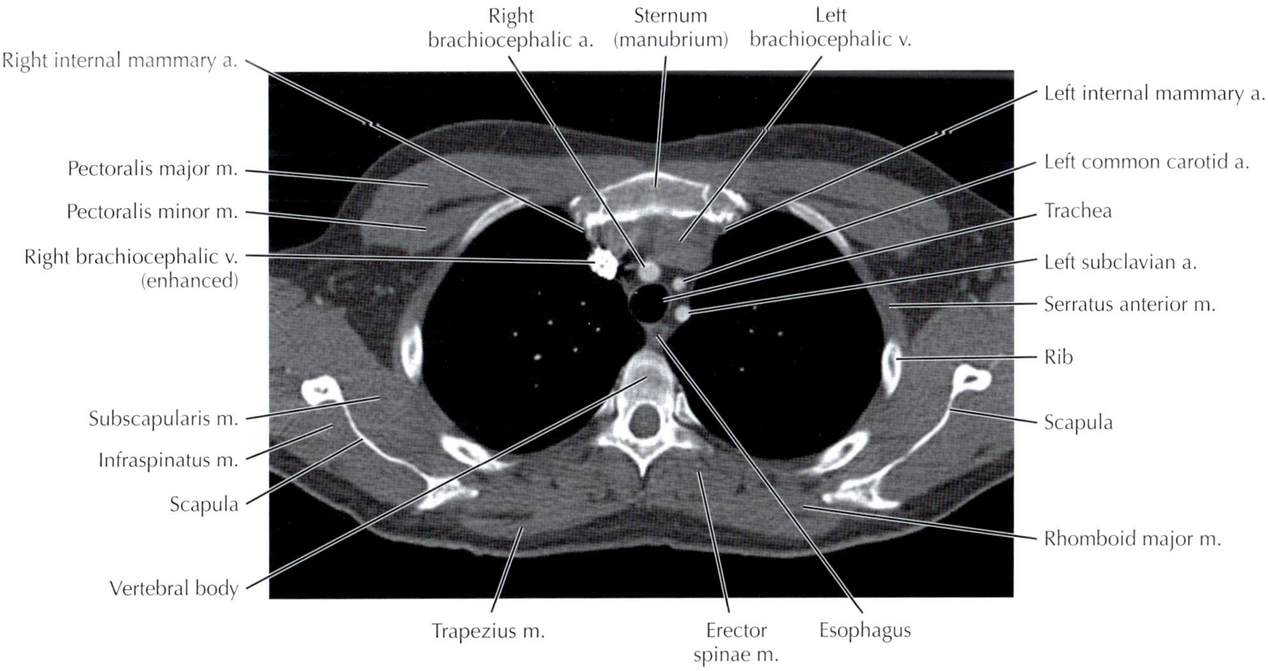
Right brachiocephalic a.
Sternum (manubrium)
Left brachiocephalic v.
Right internal mammary a.
Pectoralis major m.
Pectoralis minor m.
Right brachiocephalic v. (enhanced)
Subscapularis m.
Infraspinatus m.
Scapula
Vertebral body
Trapezius m.
Erector spinae m.
Esophagus
Left internal mammary a.
Left common carotid a.
Trachea
Left subclavian a.
Serratus anterior m.
Rib
Scapula
Rhomboid major m.

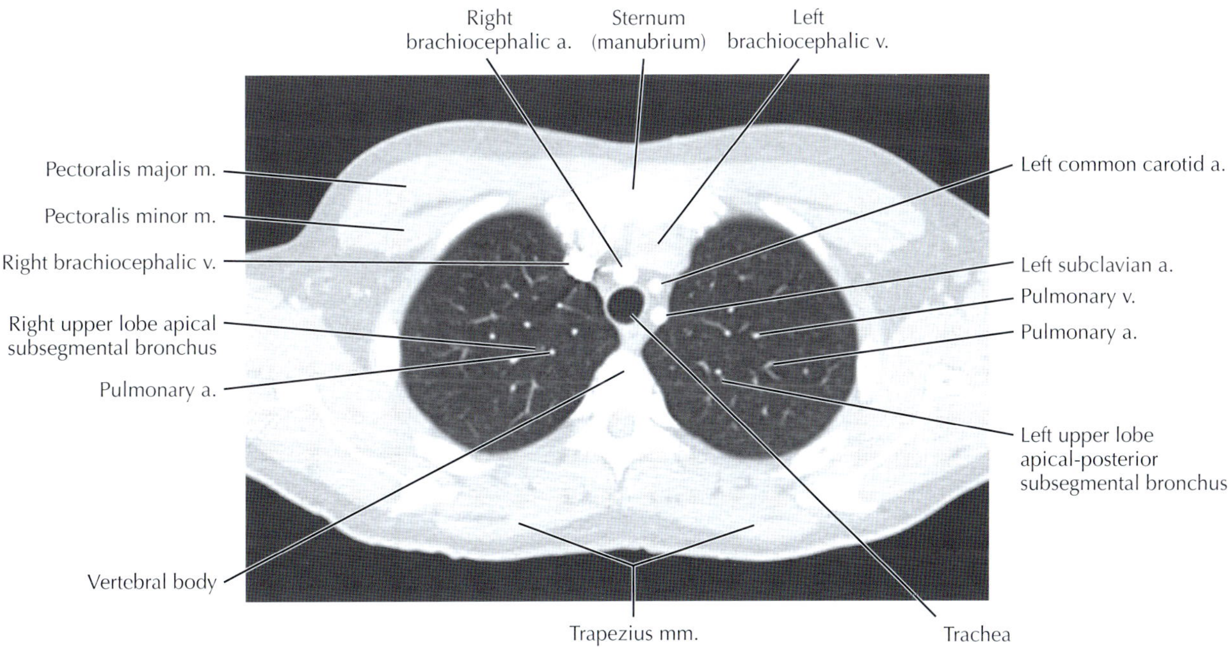
Right brachiocephalic a.
Sternum (manubrium)
Left brachiocephalic v.
Pectoralis major m.
Pectoralis minor m.
Right brachiocephalic v.
Right upper lobe apical subsegmental bronchus
Pulmonary a.
Vertebral body
Trapezius mm.
Trachea
Left common carotid a.
Left subclavian a.
Pulmonary v.
Pulmonary a.
Left upper lobe apical-posterior subsegmental bronchus

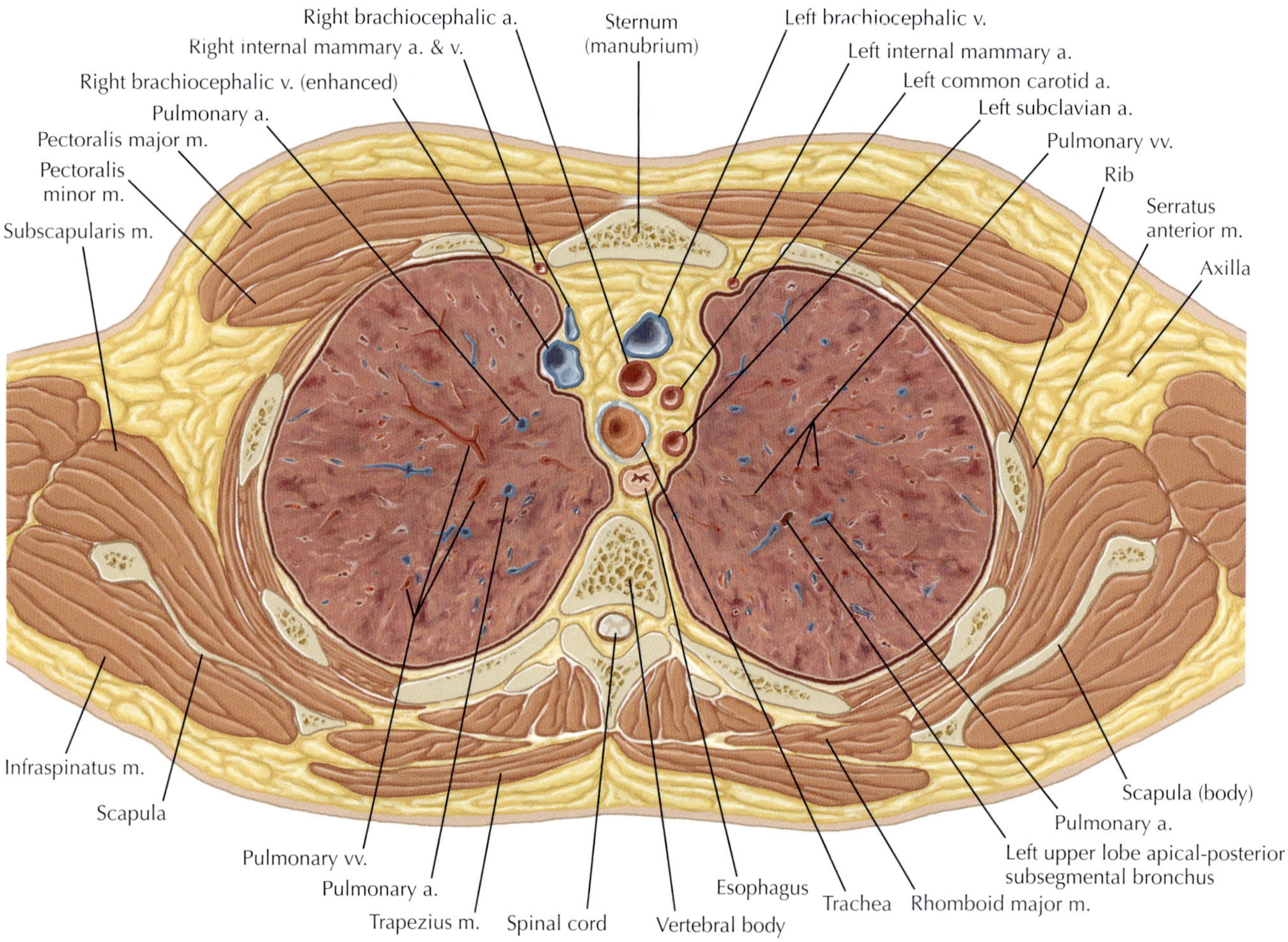
Right brachiocephalic a.
Right internal mammary a. & v.
Right brachiocephalic v. (enhanced)
Pulmonary a.
Pectoralis major m.
Pectoralis minor m.
Subscapularis m.
Sternum (manubrium)
Left brachiocephalic v.
Left internal mammary a.
Left common carotid a.
Left subclavian a.
Pulmonary vv.
Rib
Serratus anterior m.
Axilla
Infraspinatus m.
Scapula
Pulmonary vv.
Pulmonary a.
Trapezius m.
Spinal cord
Vertebral body
Esophagus
Trachea
Rhomboid major m.
Scapula (body)
Pulmonary a.
Left upper lobe apical-posterior subsegmental bronchus

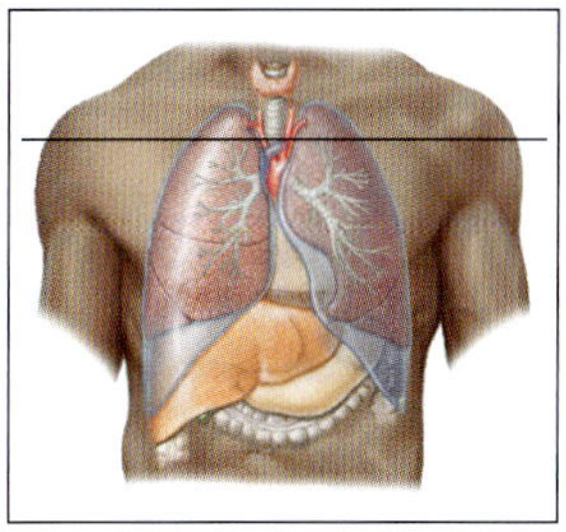

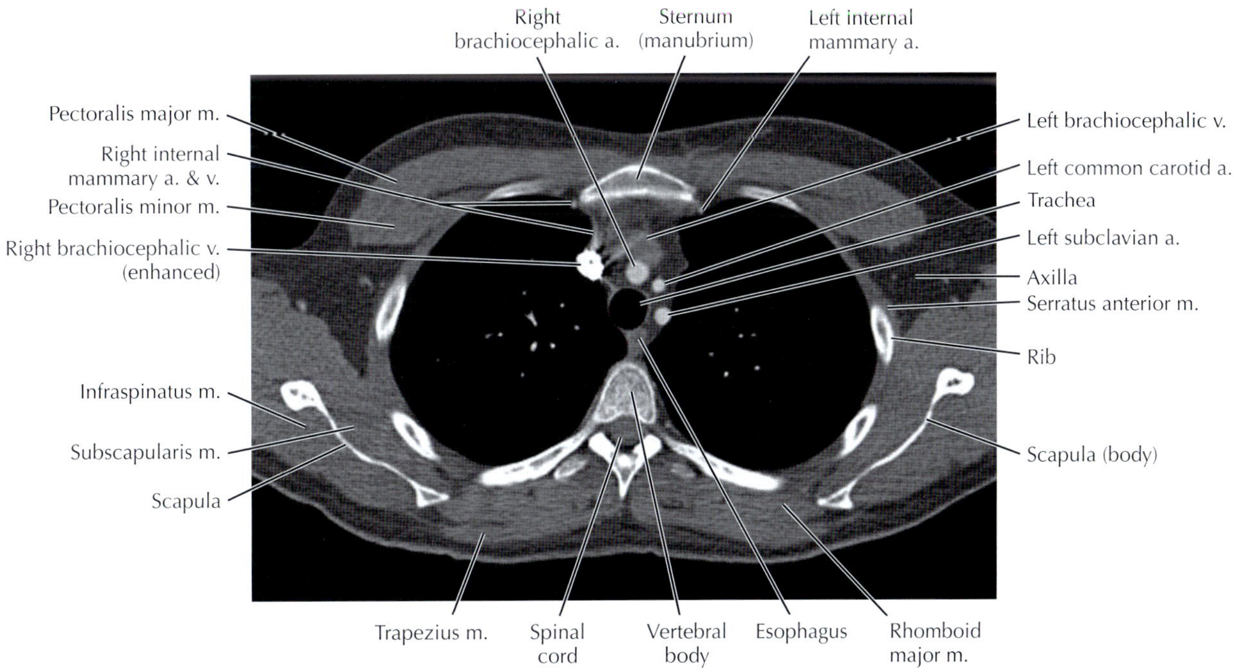
Right brachiocephalic a.
Sternum (manubrium)
Left internal mammary a.
Pectoralis major m.
Right internal mammary a. & v.
Pectoralis minor m.
Right brachiocephalic v. (enhanced)
Infraspinatus m.
Subscapularis m.
Scapula
Left brachiocephalic v.
Left common carotid a.
Trachea
Left subclavian a.
Axilla
Serratus anterior m.
Rib
Scapula (body)
Trapezius m.
Spinal cord
Vertebral body
Esophagus
Rhomboid major m.

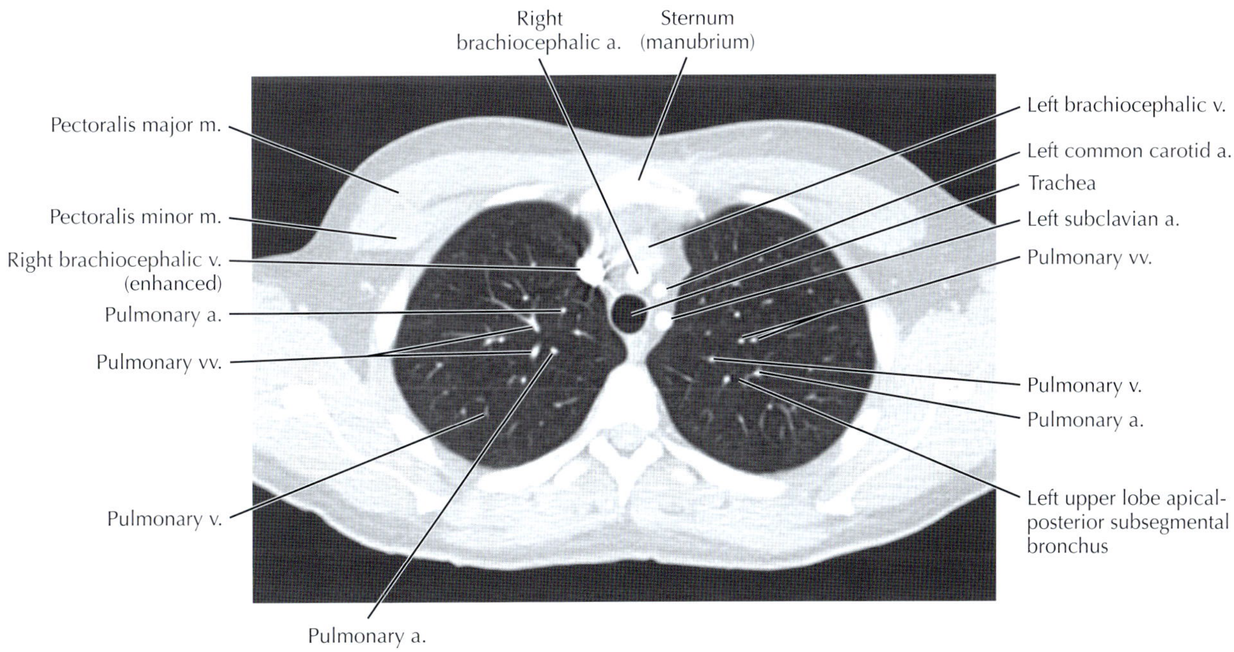
Right brachiocephalic a.
Sternum (manubrium)
Pectoralis major m.
Pectoralis minor m.
Right brachiocephalic v. (enhanced)
Pulmonary a.
Pulmonary vv.
Pulmonary v.
Pulmonary a.
Left brachiocephalic v.
Left common carotid a.
Trachea
Left subclavian a.
Pulmonary vv.
Pulmonary v.
Pulmonary a.
Left upper lobe apical-posterior subsegmental bronchus

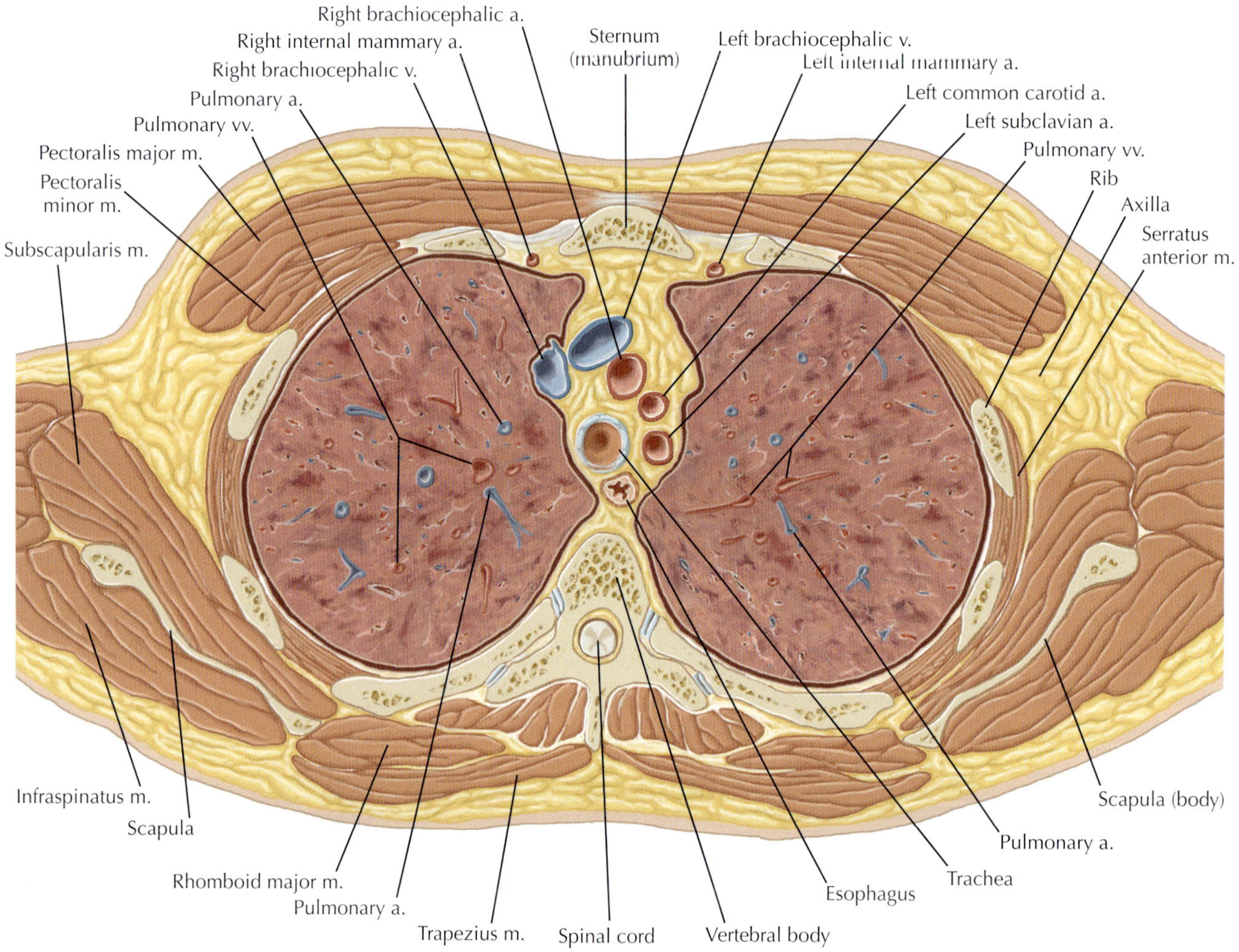
Right brachiocephalic a.
Right internal mammary a.
Right brachiocephalic v.
Pulmonary a.
Pulmonary vv.
Pectoralis major m.
Pectoralis minor m.
Subscapularis m.
Sternum (manubrium)
Left brachiocephalic v.
Left internal mammary a.
Left common carotid a.
Left subclavian a.
Pulmonary vv.
Rib
Axilla
Serratus anterior m.
Infraspinatus m.
Scapula
Rhomboid major m.
Pulmonary a.
Trapezius m.
Spinal cord
Vertebral body
Esophagus
Trachea
Pulmonary a.
Scapula (body)

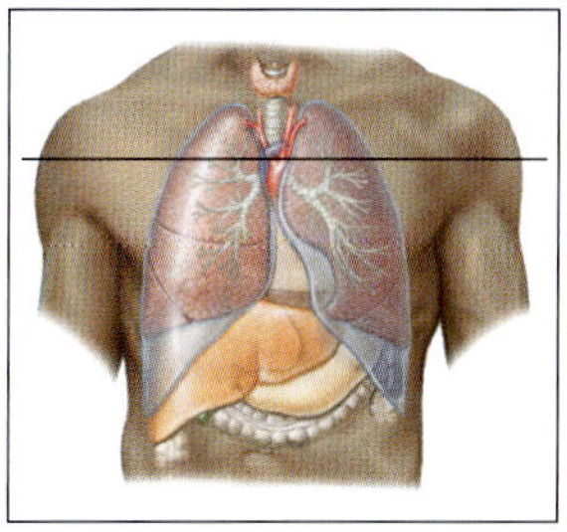

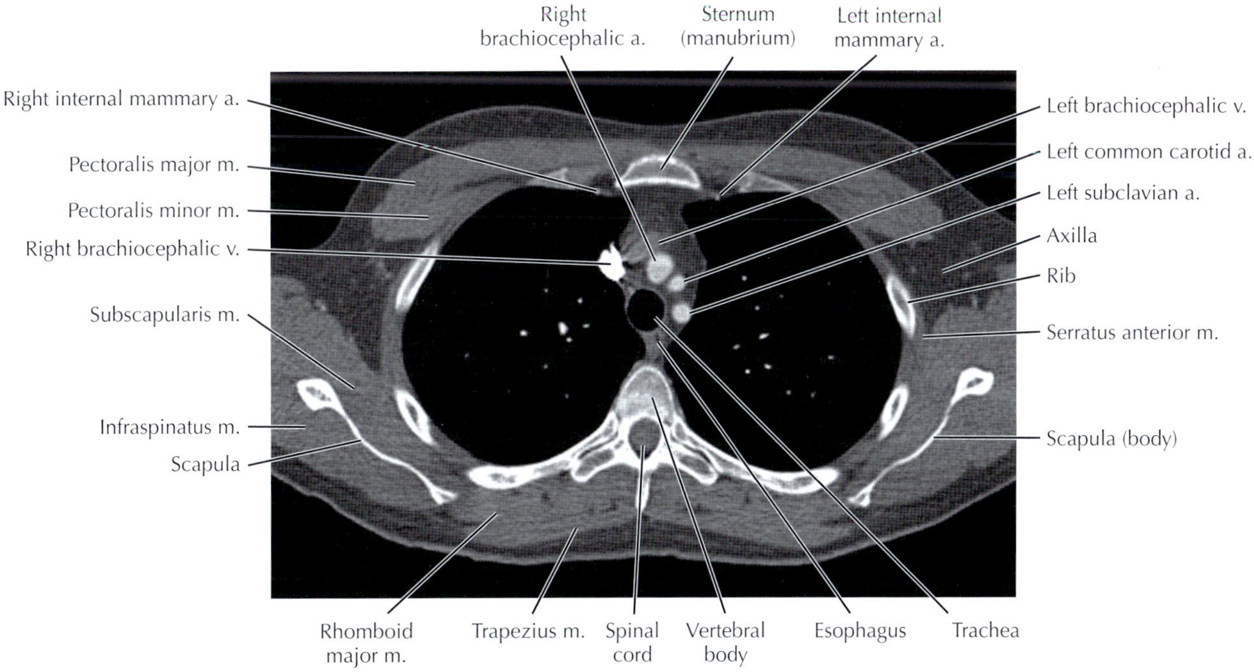
Right brachiocephalic a.
Sternum (manubrium)
Left internal mammary a.
Right internal mammary a.
Pectoralis major m.
Pectoralis minor m.
Right brachiocephalic v.
Subscapularis m.
Infraspinatus m.
Scapula
Left brachiocephalic v.
Left common carotid a.
Left subclavian a.
Axilla
Rib
Serratus anterior m.
Scapula (body)
Rhomboid major m.
Trapezius m.
Spinal cord
Vertebral body
Esophagus
Trachea

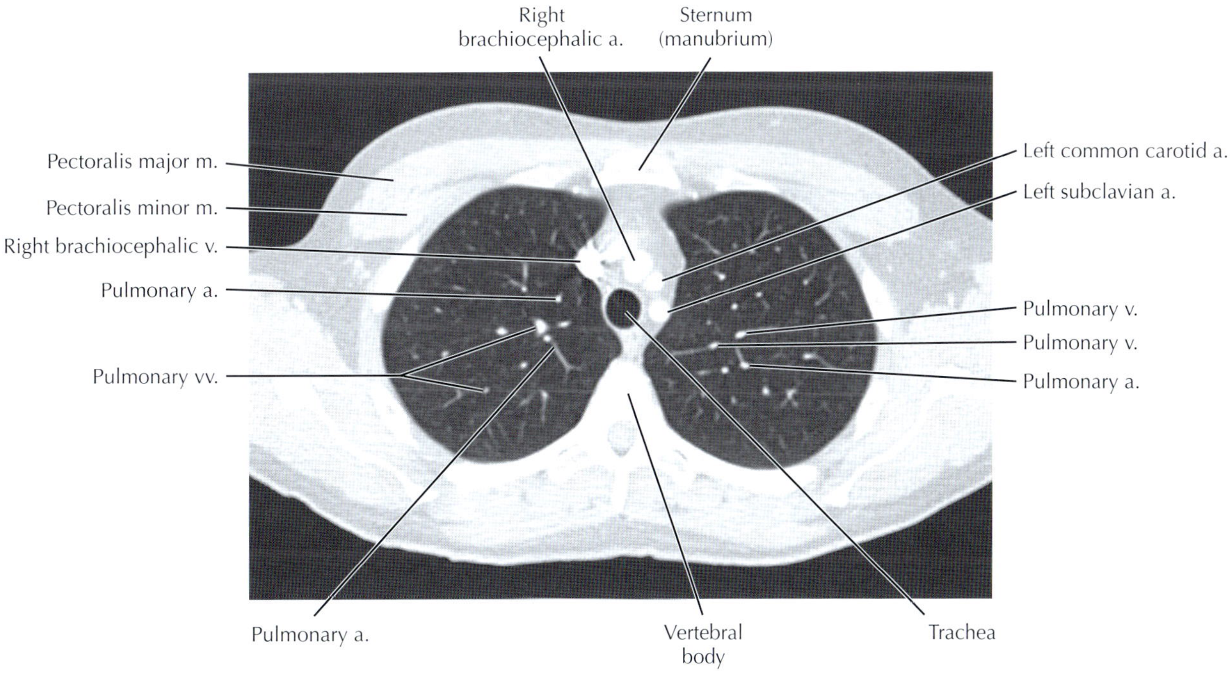
Right brachiocephalic a.
Sternum (manubrium)
Pectoralis major m.
Pectoralis minor m.
Right brachiocephalic v.
Pulmonary a.
Pulmonary vv.
Left common carotid a.
Left subclavian a.
Pulmonary v.
Pulmonary v.
Pulmonary a.
Pulmonary a.
Vertebral body
Trachea

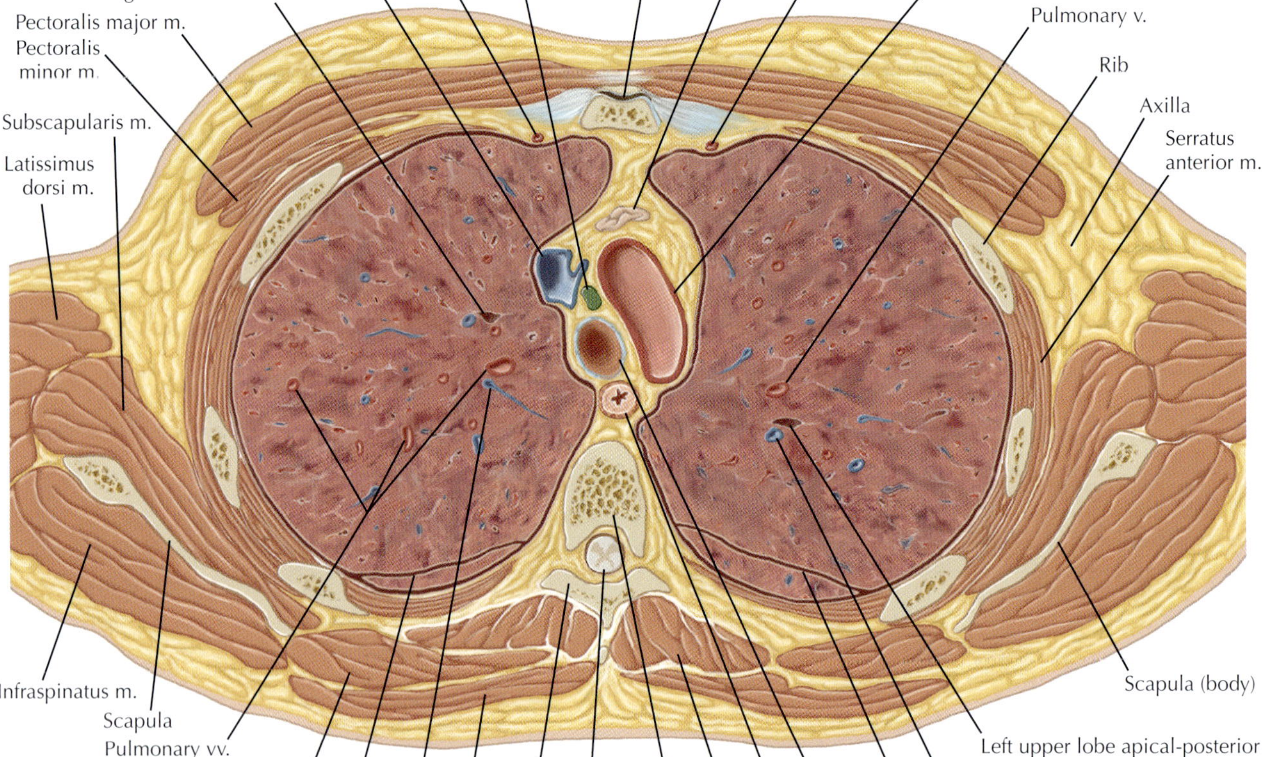

DIAGNOSTIC CONSIDERATION

At this level, in lung windows, a small *apical-posterior segment left upper lobe bronchus* and *artery* are visible adjacent to one another. This relationship aids in the identification of small, peripheral pulmonary vessels—arteries course adjacent to bronchi, whereas pulmonary veins course separately. Note this relationship on subsequent images and in the peripheral aspects of the lower lobes.

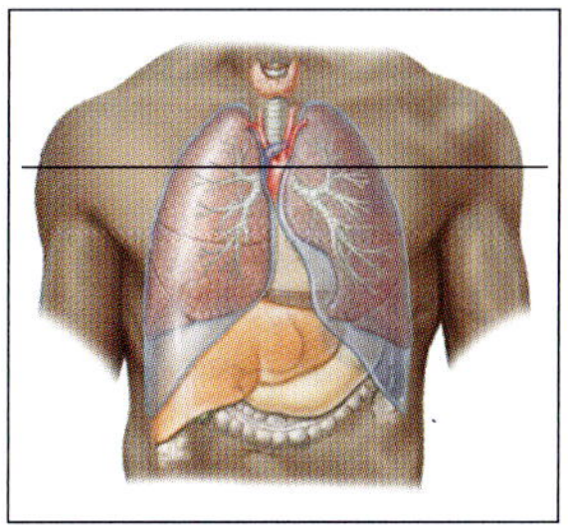

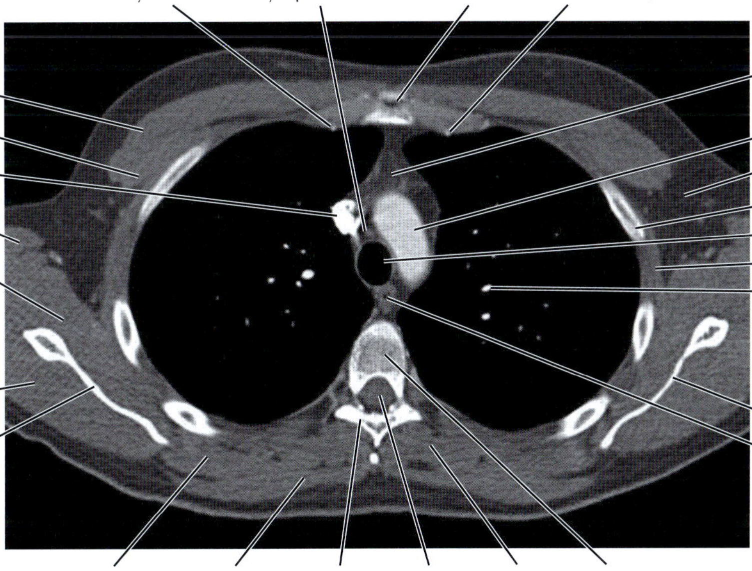
Sternum (joint between manubrium & body)
Right internal mammary a.
Right paratracheal lymph node
Left internal mammary a.
Pectoralis major m.
Pectoralis minor m.
Superior vena cava
Latissimus dorsi m.
Subscapularis m.
Infraspinatus m.
Scapula
Anterior mediastinum (residual thymus)
Aortic arch
Axilla
Rib
Trachea
Serratus anterior m.
Pulmonary v.
Scapula (body)
Esophagus
Rhomboid major m.
Trapezius m.
Vertebral lamina
Spinal cord
Erector spinae m.
Vertebral body

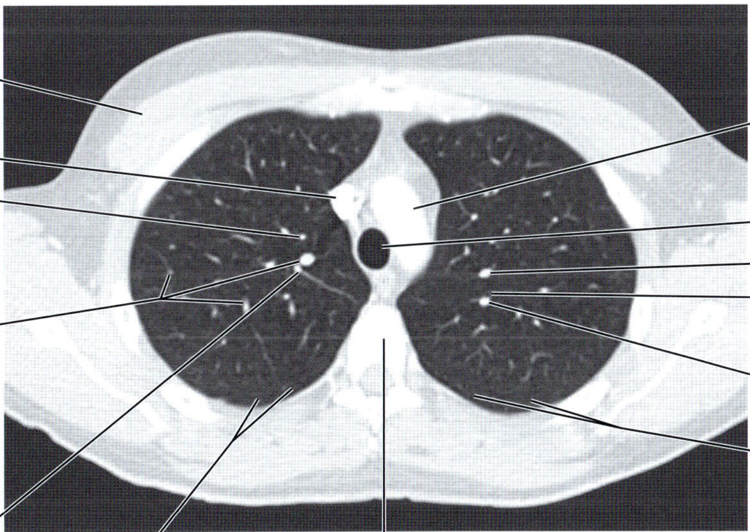
Pectoralis major m.
Superior vena cava
Right upper lobe apical subsegmental bronchus
Pulmonary v.
Pulmonary a.
Right oblique (major) fissure
Vertebral body
Aortic arch
Trachea
Pulmonary v.
Left upper lobe apical-posterior subsegmental bronchus
Pulmonary a.
Left oblique (major) fissure

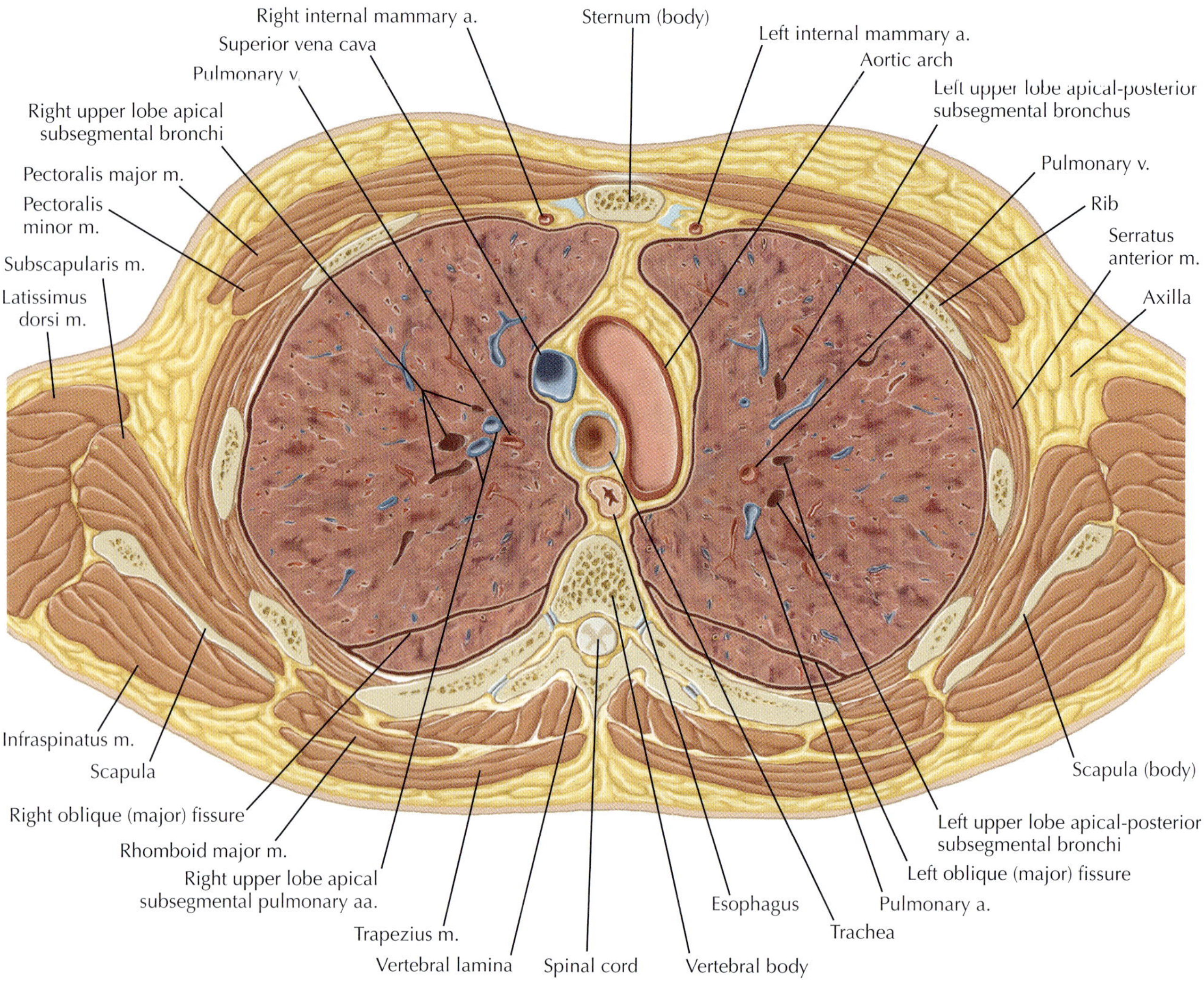
Right internal mammary a.
Superior vena cava
Pulmonary v.
Right upper lobe apical subsegmental bronchi
Pectoralis major m.
Pectoralis minor m.
Subscapularis m.
Latissimus dorsi m.
Sternum (body)
Left internal mammary a.
Aortic arch
Left upper lobe apical-posterior subsegmental bronchus
Pulmonary v.
Rib
Serratus anterior m.
Axilla
Infraspinatus m.
Scapula
Right oblique (major) fissure
Rhomboid major m.
Right upper lobe apical subsegmental pulmonary aa.
Trapezius m.
Vertebral lamina
Spinal cord
Vertebral body
Esophagus
Trachea
Pulmonary a.
Left oblique (major) fissure
Left upper lobe apical-posterior subsegmental bronchi
Scapula (body)

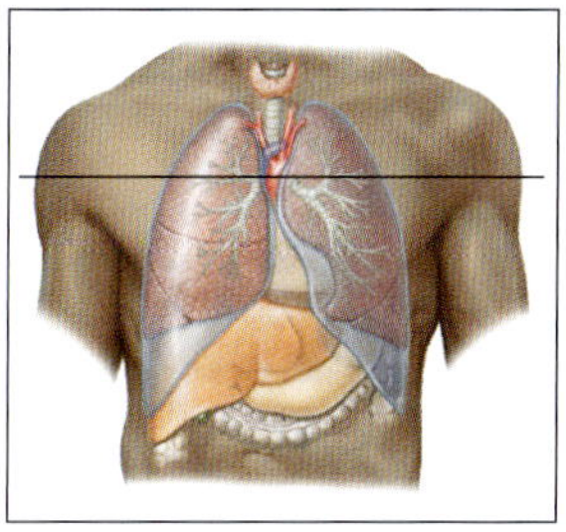

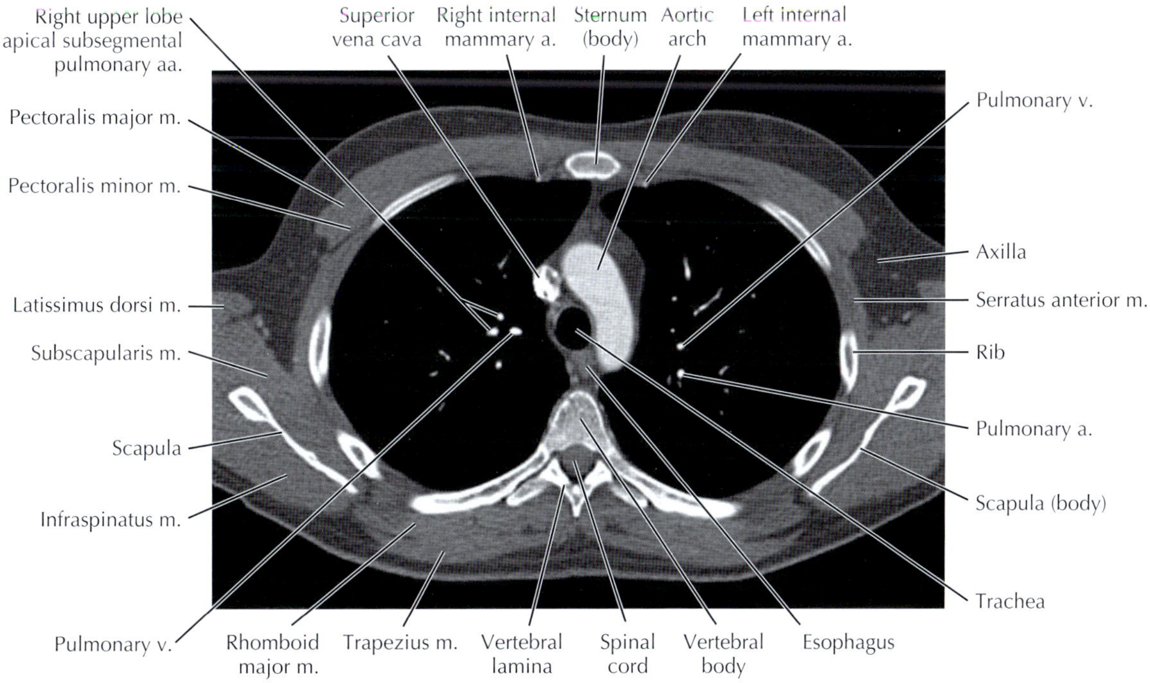
Right upper lobe apical subsegmental pulmonary aa.
Superior vena cava
Right internal mammary a.
Sternum (body)
Aortic arch
Left internal mammary a.
Pulmonary v.
Pectoralis major m.
Pectoralis minor m.
Axilla
Latissimus dorsi m.
Serratus anterior m.
Subscapularis m.
Rib
Scapula
Pulmonary a.
Infraspinatus m.
Scapula (body)
Trachea
Pulmonary v.
Rhomboid major m.
Trapezius m.
Vertebral lamina
Spinal cord
Vertebral body
Esophagus

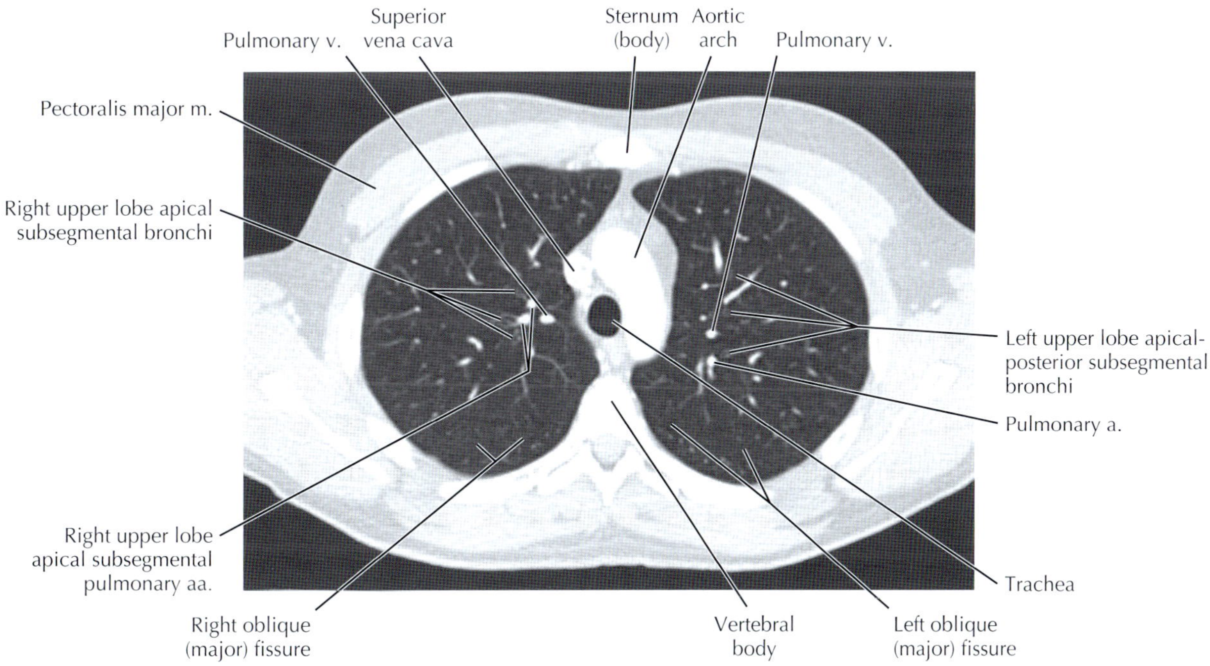
Pulmonary v.
Superior vena cava
Sternum (body)
Aortic arch
Pulmonary v.
Pectoralis major m.
Right upper lobe apical subsegmental bronchi
Left upper lobe apical-posterior subsegmental bronchi
Pulmonary a.
Right upper lobe apical subsegmental pulmonary aa.
Trachea
Right oblique (major) fissure
Vertebral body
Left oblique (major) fissure

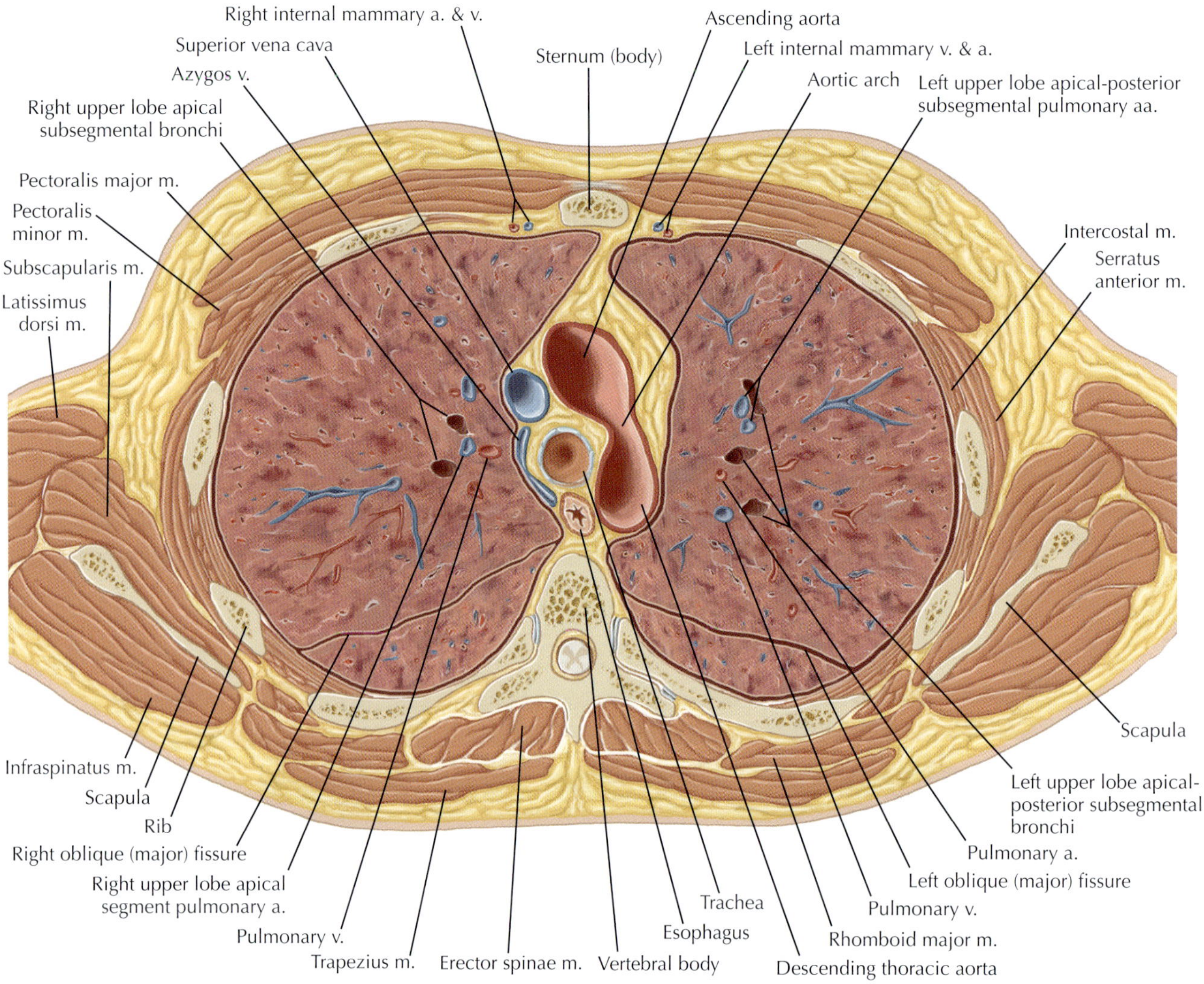
Right internal mammary a. & v.
Superior vena cava
Azygos v.
Right upper lobe apical subsegmental bronchi
Pectoralis major m.
Pectoralis minor m.
Subscapularis m.
Latissimus dorsi m.
Sternum (body)
Ascending aorta
Left internal mammary v. & a.
Aortic arch
Left upper lobe apical-posterior subsegmental pulmonary aa.
Intercostal m.
Serratus anterior m.
Scapula
Left upper lobe apical-posterior subsegmental bronchi
Pulmonary a.
Left oblique (major) fissure
Pulmonary v.
Rhomboid major m.
Descending thoracic aorta
Trachea
Esophagus
Vertebral body
Erector spinae m.
Trapezius m.
Pulmonary v.
Right upper lobe apical segment pulmonary a.
Right oblique (major) fissure
Rib
Scapula
Infraspinatus m.

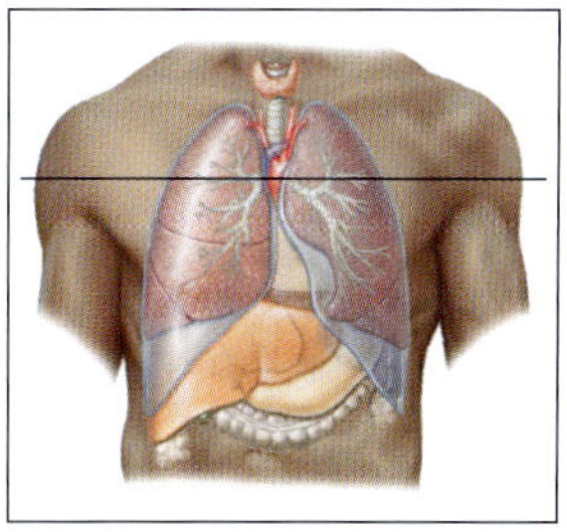

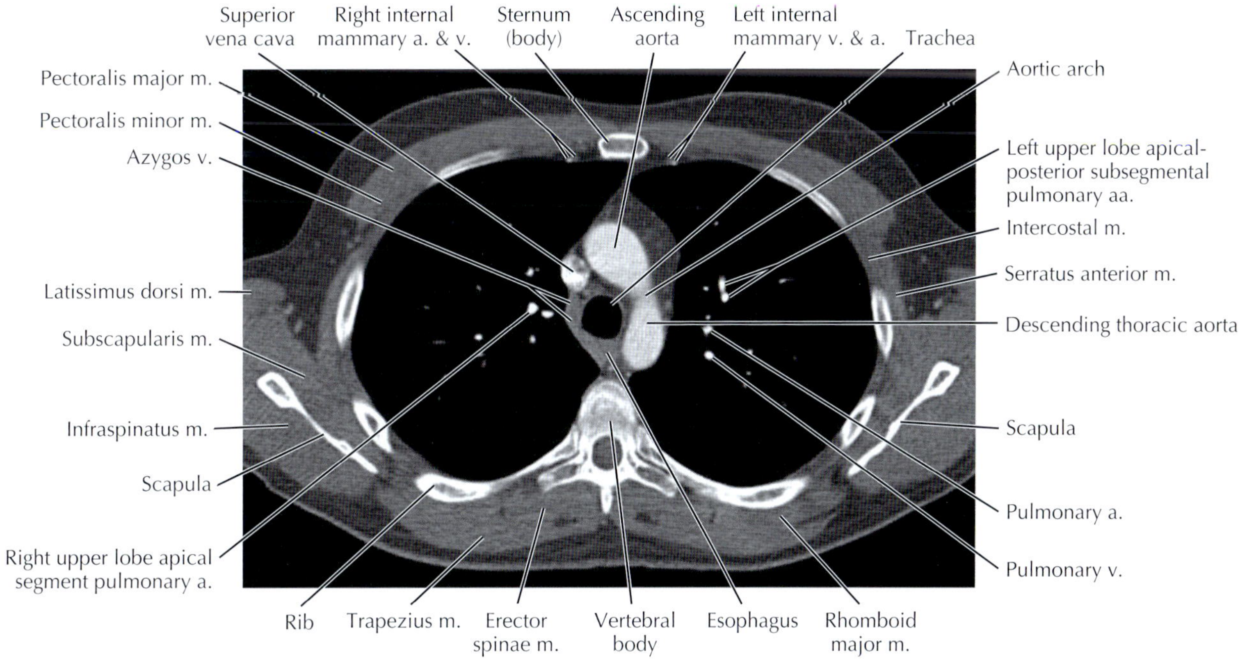
Superior vena cava
Right internal mammary a. & v.
Sternum (body)
Ascending aorta
Left internal mammary v. & a.
Trachea
Pectoralis major m.
Pectoralis minor m.
Azygos v.
Latissimus dorsi m.
Subscapularis m.
Infraspinatus m.
Scapula
Right upper lobe apical segment pulmonary a.
Aortic arch
Left upper lobe apical-posterior subsegmental pulmonary aa.
Intercostal m.
Serratus anterior m.
Descending thoracic aorta
Scapula
Pulmonary a.
Pulmonary v.
Rib
Trapezius m.
Erector spinae m.
Vertebral body
Esophagus
Rhomboid major m.

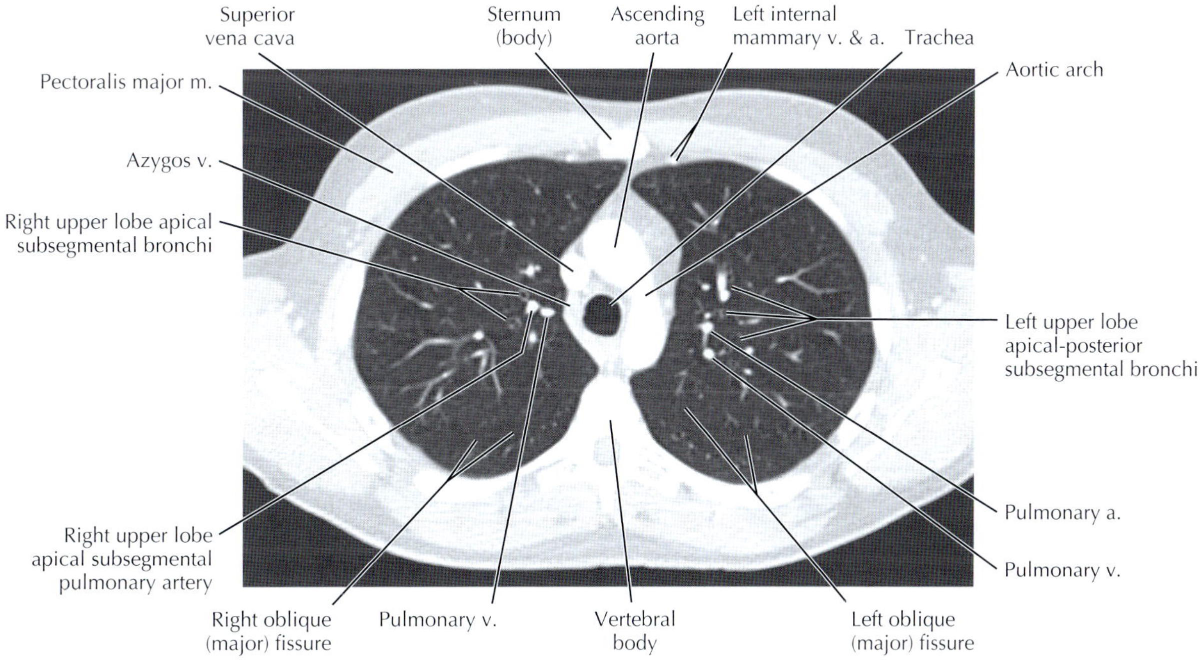
Superior vena cava
Sternum (body)
Ascending aorta
Left internal mammary v. & a.
Trachea
Pectoralis major m.
Azygos v.
Right upper lobe apical subsegmental bronchi
Aortic arch
Left upper lobe apical-posterior subsegmental bronchi
Right upper lobe apical subsegmental pulmonary artery
Pulmonary a.
Pulmonary v.
Right oblique (major) fissure
Pulmonary v.
Vertebral body
Left oblique (major) fissure

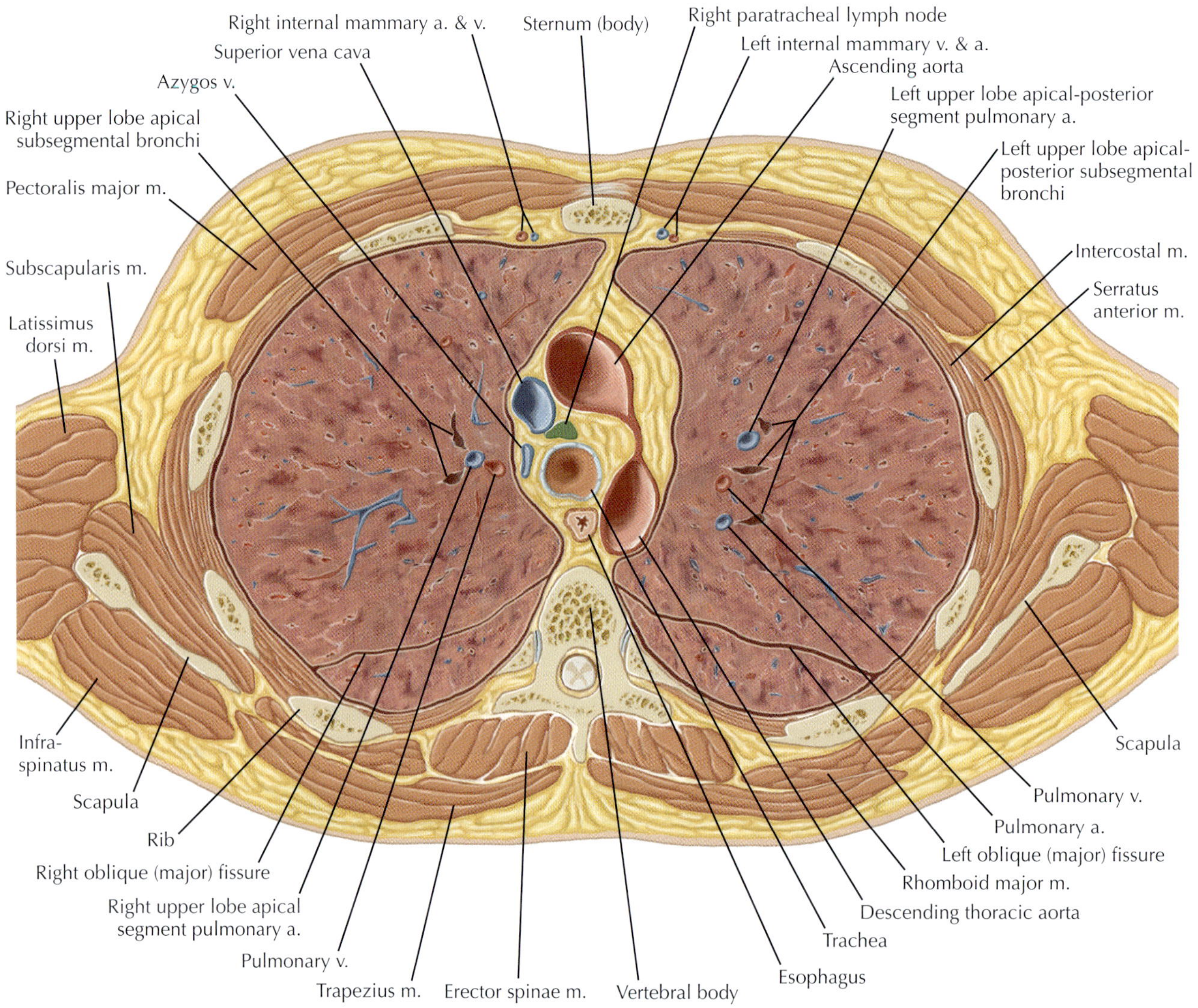
Right internal mammary a. & v.
Sternum (body)
Right paratracheal lymph node
Left internal mammary v. & a.
Superior vena cava
Ascending aorta
Azygos v.
Left upper lobe apical-posterior segment pulmonary a.
Right upper lobe apical subsegmental bronchi
Left upper lobe apical-posterior subsegmental bronchi
Pectoralis major m.
Intercostal m.
Subscapularis m.
Serratus anterior m.
Latissimus dorsi m.
Infra-spinatus m.
Scapula
Scapula
Rib
Right oblique (major) fissure
Right upper lobe apical segment pulmonary a.
Pulmonary v.
Trapezius m.
Erector spinae m.
Vertebral body
Esophagus
Trachea
Descending thoracic aorta
Rhomboid major m.
Left oblique (major) fissure
Pulmonary a.
Pulmonary v.

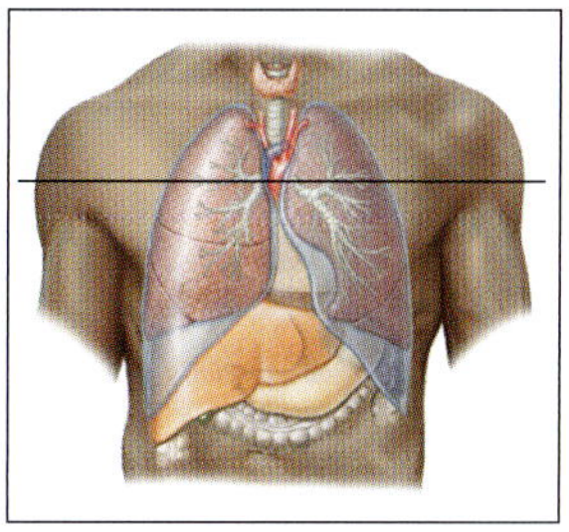

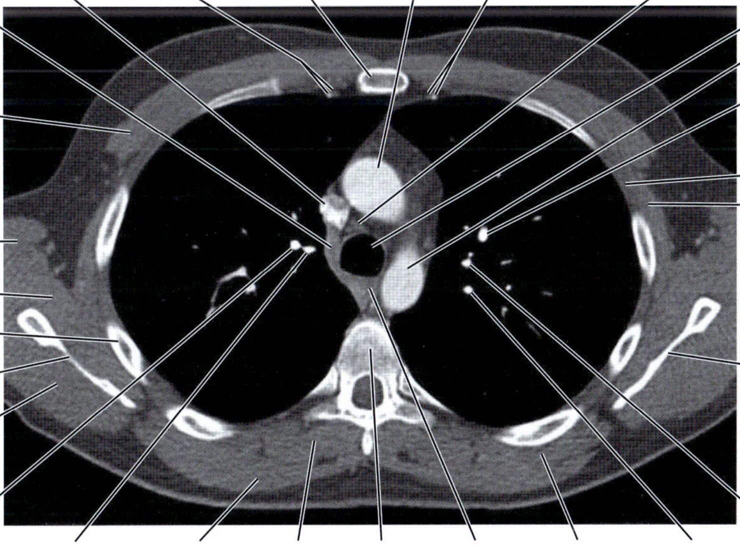

Superior vena cava
Right internal mammary a. & v.
Sternum (body)
Ascending aorta
Left Internal mammary v. & a.
Right paratracheal lymph node
Azygos v.
Trachea
Descending thoracic aorta
Pectoralis major m.
Left upper lobe apical-posterior segment pulmonary a.
Intercostal m.
Serratus anterior m.
Latissimus dorsi m.
Subscapularis m.
Rib
Scapula
Scapula
Infraspinatus m.
Right upper lobe apical segment pulmonary a.
Pulmonary v.
Pulmonary v.
Trapezius m.
Erector spinae m.
Vertebral body
Esophagus
Rhomboid major m.
Pulmonary a.

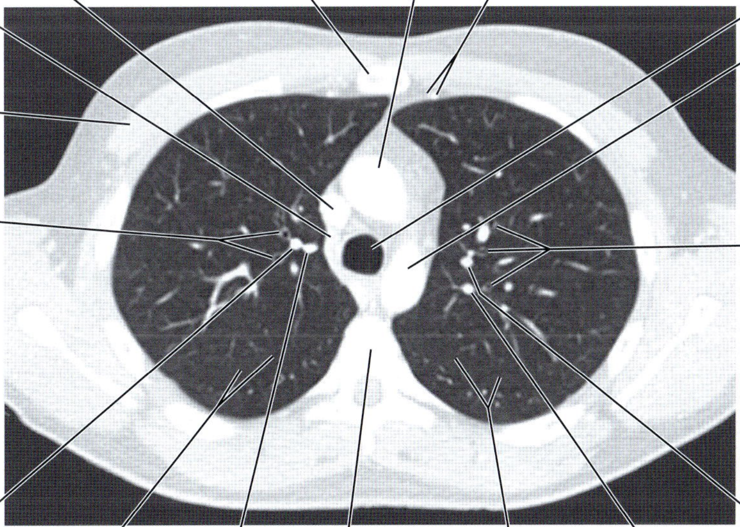

Superior vena cava
Sternum (body)
Ascending aorta
Left internal mammary v. & a.
Azygos v.
Trachea
Descending thoracic aorta
Pectoralis major m.
Right upper lobe apical subsegmental bronchi
Left upper lobe apical-posterior subsegmental bronchi
Right upper lobe apical segment pulmonary a.
Pulmonary v.
Right oblique (major) fissure
Pulmonary v.
Vertebral body
Left oblique (major) fissure
Pulmonary a.

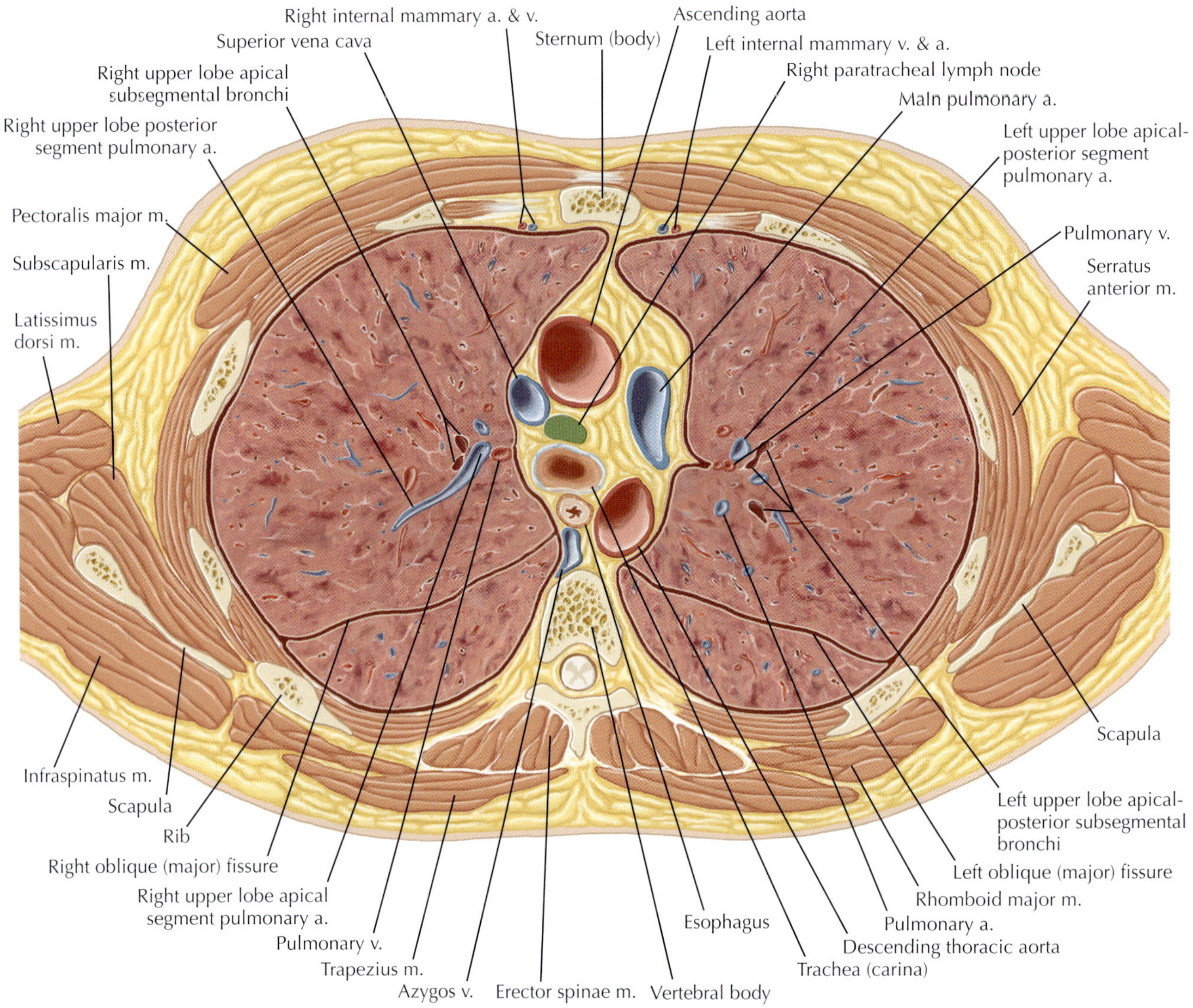
Right internal mammary a. & v.
Superior vena cava
Sternum (body)
Ascending aorta
Left internal mammary v. & a.
Right paratracheal lymph node
Main pulmonary a.
Right upper lobe apical subsegmental bronchi
Right upper lobe posterior segment pulmonary a.
Left upper lobe apical-posterior segment pulmonary a.
Pectoralis major m.
Pulmonary v.
Subscapularis m.
Serratus anterior m.
Latissimus dorsi m.
Scapula
Infraspinatus m.
Scapula
Rib
Right oblique (major) fissure
Right upper lobe apical segment pulmonary a.
Pulmonary v.
Trapezius m.
Azygos v.
Erector spinae m.
Vertebral body
Esophagus
Left upper lobe apical-posterior subsegmental bronchi
Left oblique (major) fissure
Rhomboid major m.
Pulmonary a.
Descending thoracic aorta
Trachea (carina)

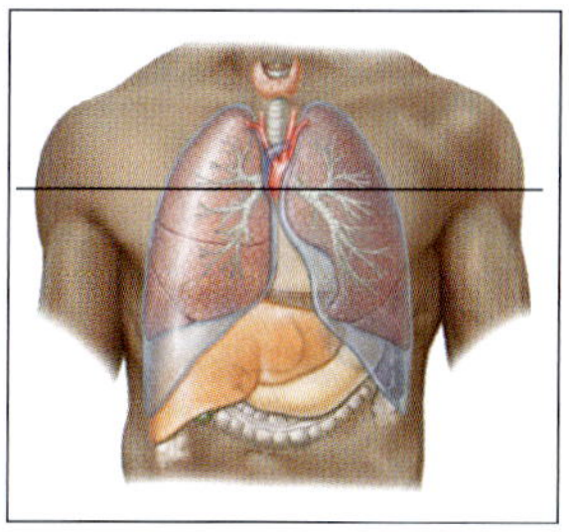

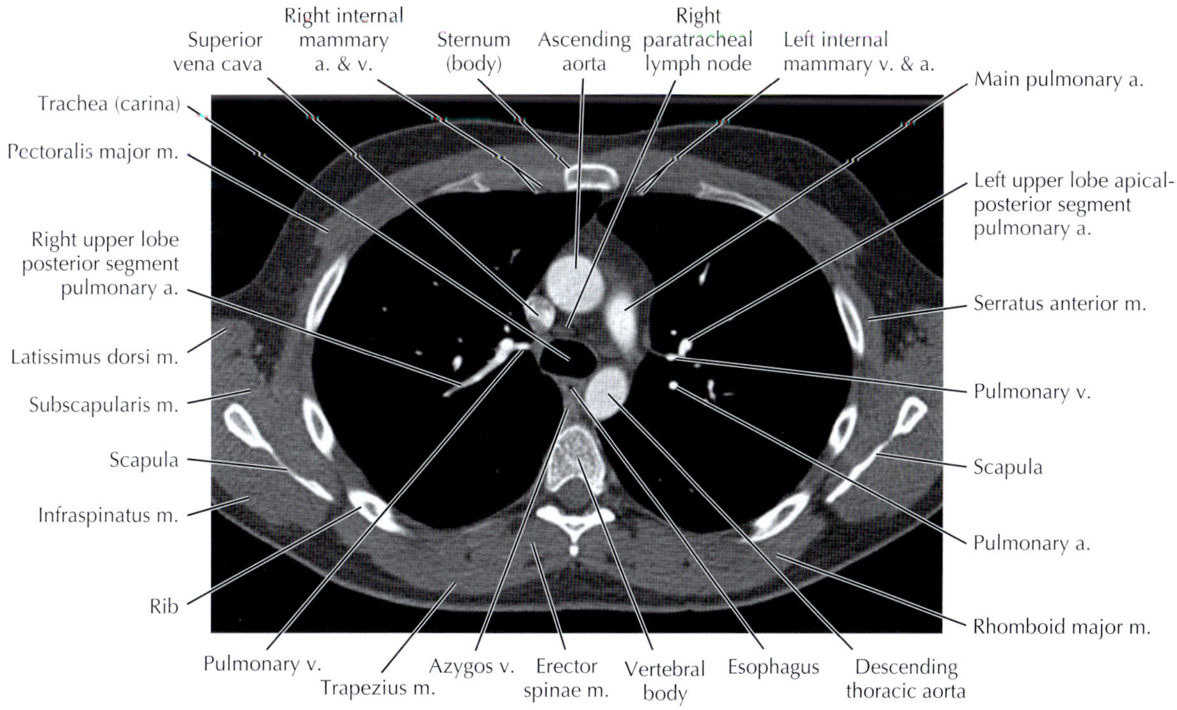
Superior vena cava
Right internal mammary a. & v.
Sternum (body)
Ascending aorta
Right paratracheal lymph node
Left internal mammary v. & a.
Main pulmonary a.
Trachea (carina)
Pectoralis major m.
Right upper lobe posterior segment pulmonary a.
Latissimus dorsi m.
Subscapularis m.
Scapula
Infraspinatus m.
Rib
Left upper lobe apical-posterior segment pulmonary a.
Serratus anterior m.
Pulmonary v.
Scapula
Pulmonary a.
Rhomboid major m.
Pulmonary v.
Trapezius m.
Azygos v.
Erector spinae m.
Vertebral body
Esophagus
Descending thoracic aorta

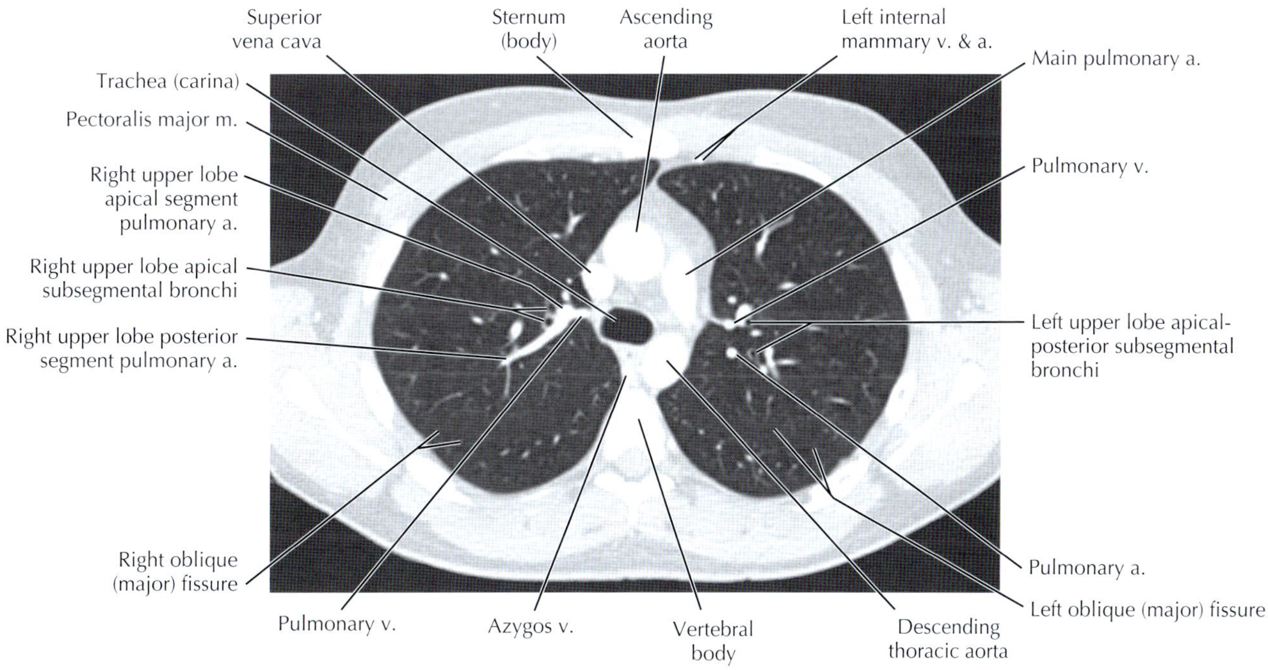
Superior vena cava
Sternum (body)
Ascending aorta
Left internal mammary v. & a.
Main pulmonary a.
Trachea (carina)
Pectoralis major m.
Right upper lobe apical segment pulmonary a.
Right upper lobe apical subsegmental bronchi
Right upper lobe posterior segment pulmonary a.
Right oblique (major) fissure
Pulmonary v.
Left upper lobe apical-posterior subsegmental bronchi
Pulmonary a.
Left oblique (major) fissure
Pulmonary v.
Azygos v.
Vertebral body
Descending thoracic aorta

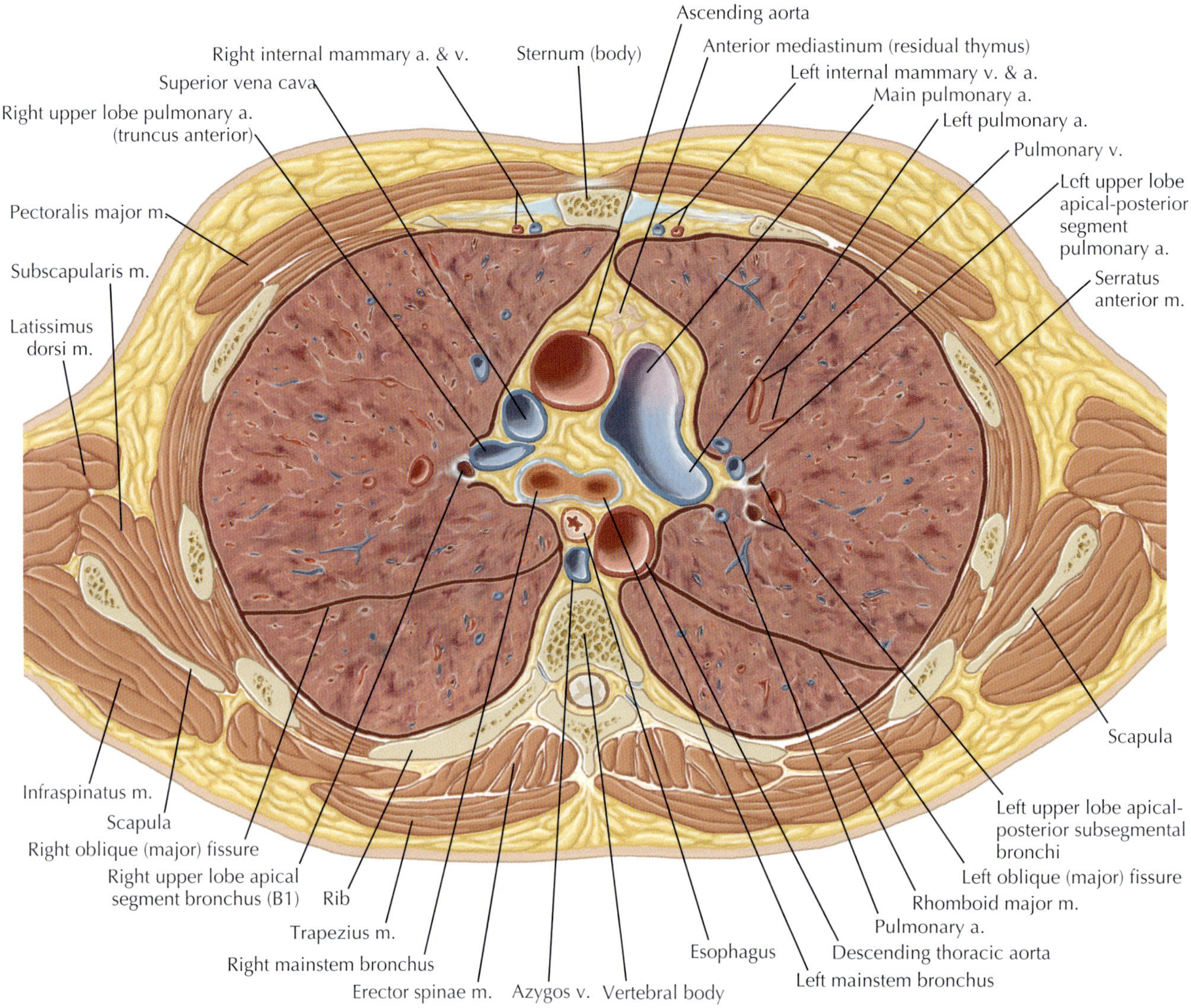

DIAGNOSTIC CONSIDERATION

The composition of the anterior mediastinum varies substantially with age. In younger patients (particularly infants and children), abundant soft tissue, representing *thymus* residing within anterior mediastinal fat, is often readily visible on thoracic CT. As individuals age, the thymus normally involutes and becomes more fatty replaced, and progressively less soft tissue is visible within the anterior mediastinal fat. The pace at which thymic involution occurs is variable, and a fairly wide variation in the appearance of "normal thymus" at various ages is recognized.

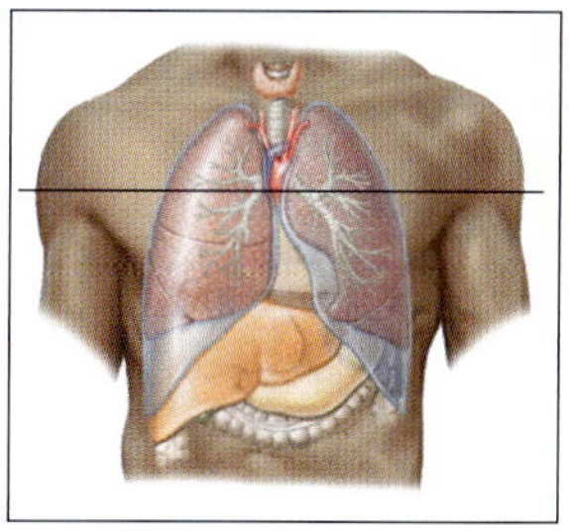

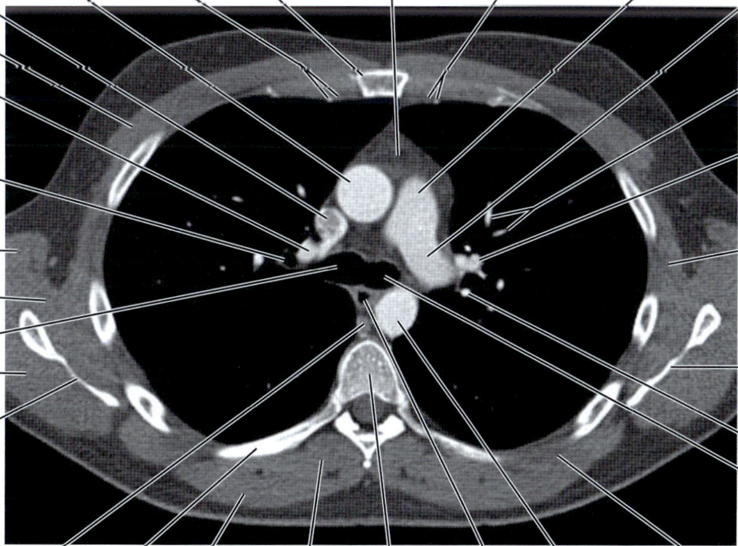
Ascending aorta
Right internal mammary a. & v.
Sternum (body)
Anterior mediastinum (residual thymus)
Left internal mammary v. & a.
Main pulmonary a.
Left pulmonary a.
Superior vena cava
Pectoralis major m.
Right upper lobe pulmonary a. (truncus anterior)
Right upper lobe apical segment bronchus (B1)
Latissimus dorsi m.
Subscapularis m.
Right mainstem bronchi
Infraspinatus m.
Scapula
Pulmonary vv.
Left upper lobe apical-posterior segment pulmonary a.
Serratus anterior m.
Scapula
Pulmonary a.
Left mainstem bronchi
Azygos v.
Rib
Trapezius m.
Erector spinae m.
Vertebral body
Esophagus
Descending thoracic aorta
Rhomboid major m.

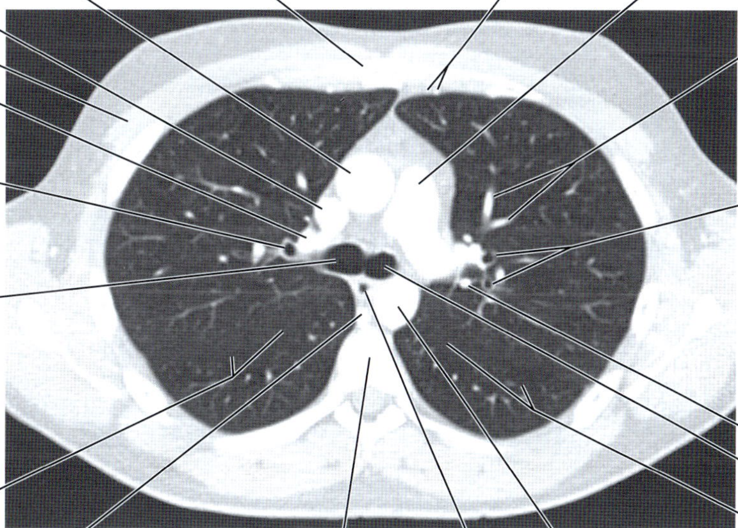
Ascending aorta
Sternum (body)
Left internal mammary v. & a.
Main pulmonary a.
Superior vena cava
Pectoralis major m.
Right upper lobe pulmonary a. (truncus anterior)
Right upper lobe apical segment bronchus (B1)
Right mainstem bronchus
Right oblique (major) fissure
Pulmonary vv.
Left upper lobe apical-posterior subsegmental bronchi
Pulmonary a.
Left mainstem bronchus
Left oblique (major) fissure
Azygos v.
Vertebral body
Esophagus
Descending thoracic aorta

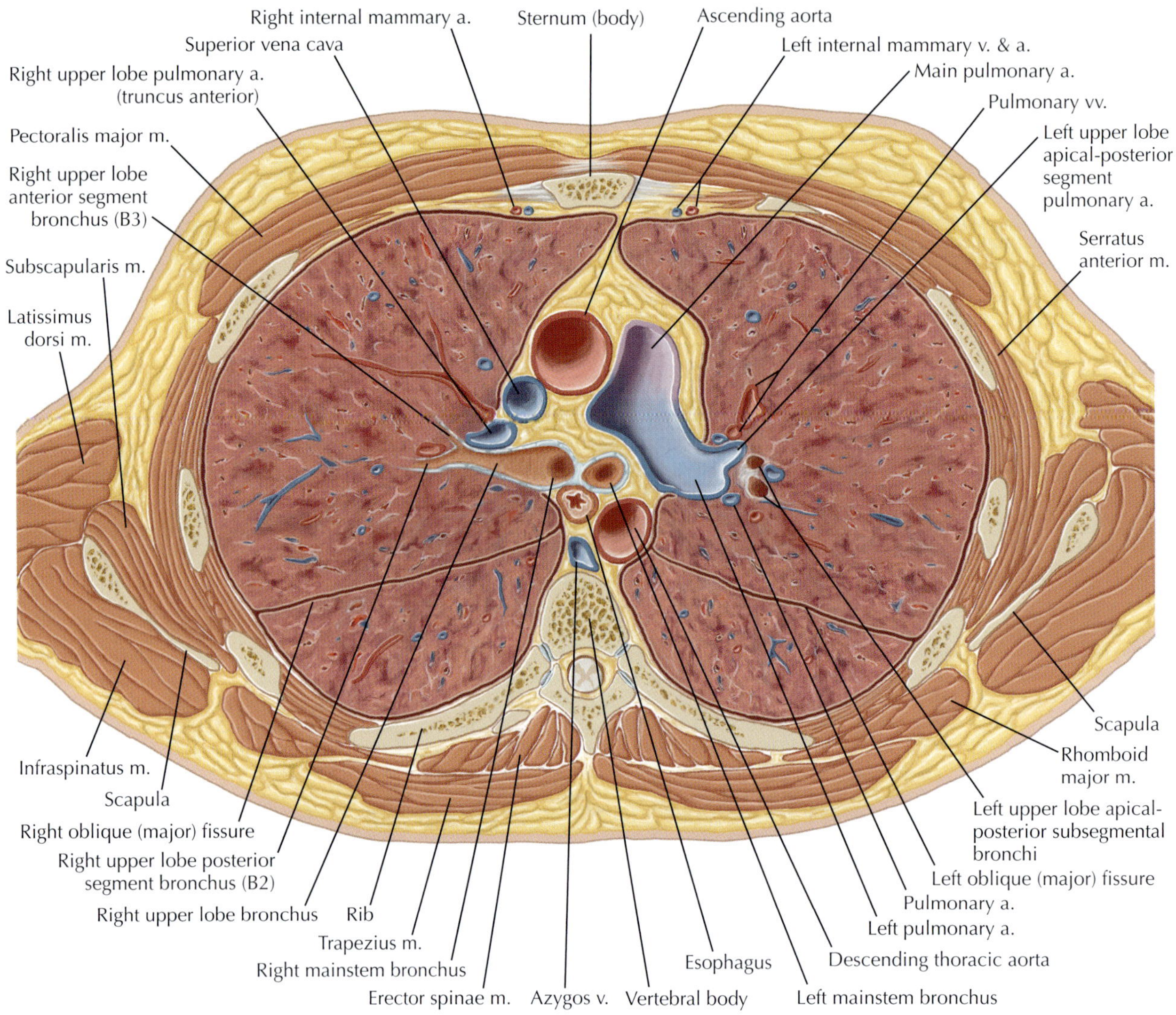

NORMAL ANATOMY

At this level, the *segmental bronchi* within the right upper lobe are now visible. Segmental bronchi are commonly named for the anatomic segment they supply (e.g., apical segment right upper lobe bronchus). Another nomenclature system for segmental bronchi may occasionally be encountered, as described by the Federative Committee on Anatomical Terminology in *Terminologia Anatomica*. This terminology identifies the segmental bronchi according to numbers (e.g., B1 = apical segment right upper lobe bronchus, B1+2 = apical-posterior segment left upper lobe bronchus; see Axial 19). Both nomenclature systems are illustrated in this text.

NORMAL VARIANT

A number of variations in the branching pattern of the pulmonary arteries are recognized. In particular, variations in the branching pattern of the left upper lobe pulmonary artery are commonly encountered in clinical practice. In the most common pattern, the left upper lobe pulmonary artery gives rise to apical-posterior and anterior segmental branches in a manner analogous to the bronchial branching pattern. Less commonly, as in this patient, a posterior left upper lobe subsegmental artery arises directly from the left pulmonary artery. The left upper lobe pulmonary artery can be seen originating from the left pulmonary artery on Axials 17 and 18.

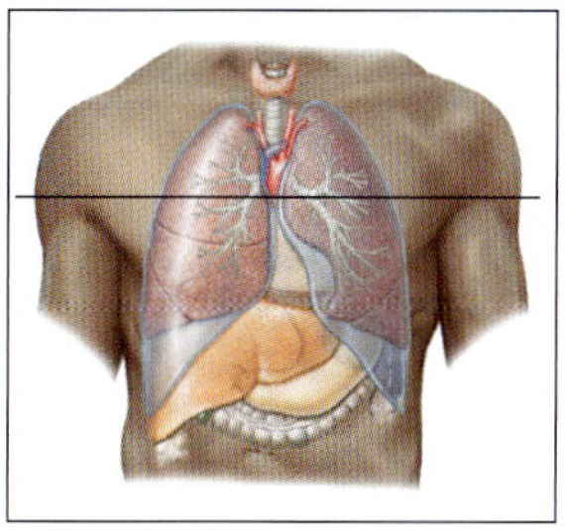

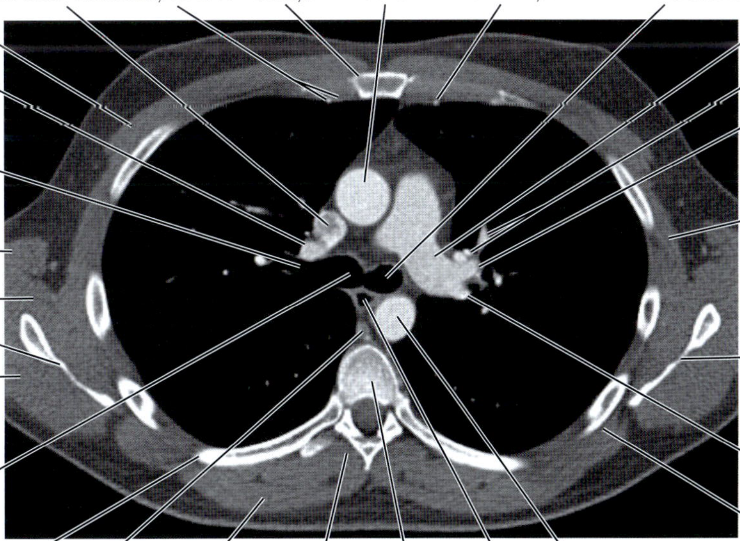
Superior vena cava
Right internal mammary a. & v.
Sternum (body)
Ascending aorta
Left internal mammary a.
Left mainstem bronchus
Pectoralis major m.
Right upper lobe pulmonary a. (truncus anterior)
Right upper lobe bronchus
Latissimus dorsi m.
Subscapularis m.
Scapula
Infraspinatus m.
Right mainstem bronchus
Left pulmonary a.
Pulmonary vv.
Left upper lobe apical-posterior segment pulmonary a.
Serratus anterior m.
Scapula
Pulmonary a.
Rhomboid major m.
Rib
Azygos v.
Trapezius m.
Erector spinae m.
Vertebral body
Esophagus
Descending thoracic aorta

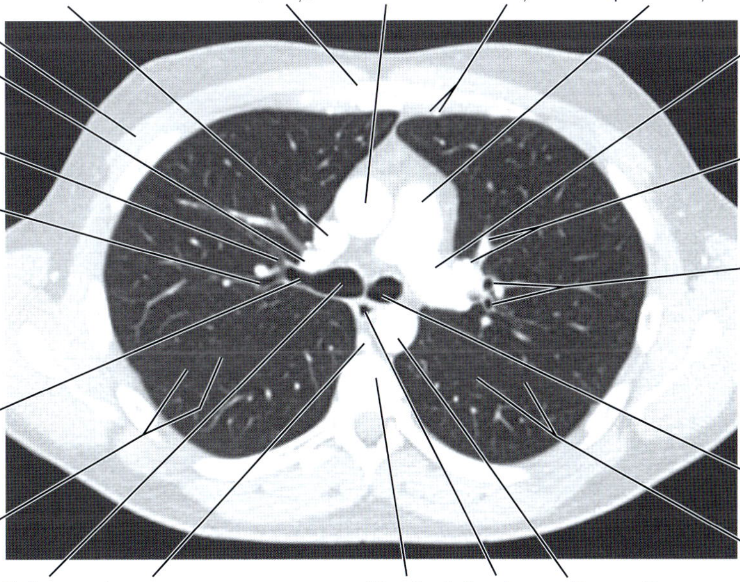
Superior vena cava
Sternum (body)
Ascending aorta
Left internal mammary v. & a.
Main pulmonary a.
Pectoralis major m.
Right upper lobe pulmonary a. (truncus anterior)
Right upper lobe anterior segment bronchus (B3)
Right upper lobe posterior segment bronchus (B2)
Right upper lobe apical segment bronchus (B1)
Right oblique (major) fissure
Left pulmonary a.
Pulmonary vv.
Left upper lobe apical-posterior subsegmental bronchi
Left mainstem bronchus
Left oblique (major) fissure
Right mainstem bronchus
Azygos v.
Vertebral body
Esophagus
Descending thoracic aorta

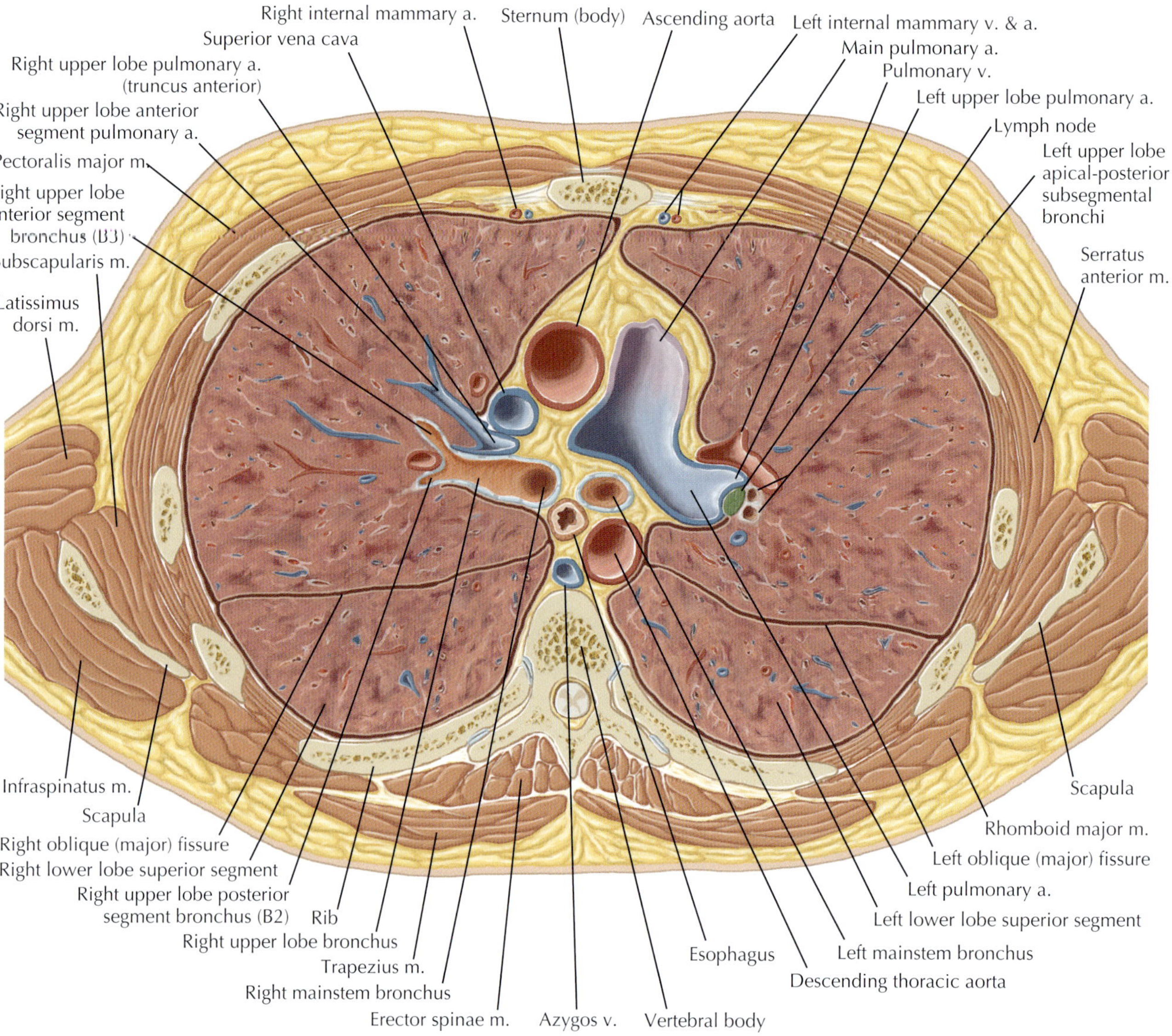

DIAGNOSTIC CONSIDERATION

The artery supplying the right upper lobe is visible. This vessel is usually simply referred to as "the right upper lobe pulmonary artery"; however, the term *truncus anterior* is occasionally used as well and is equivalent in meaning.

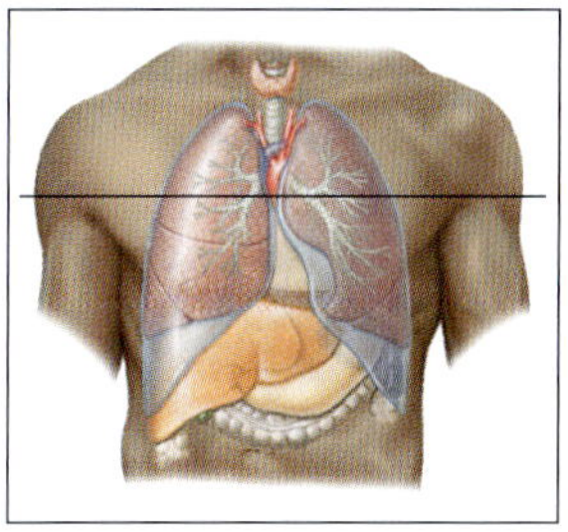

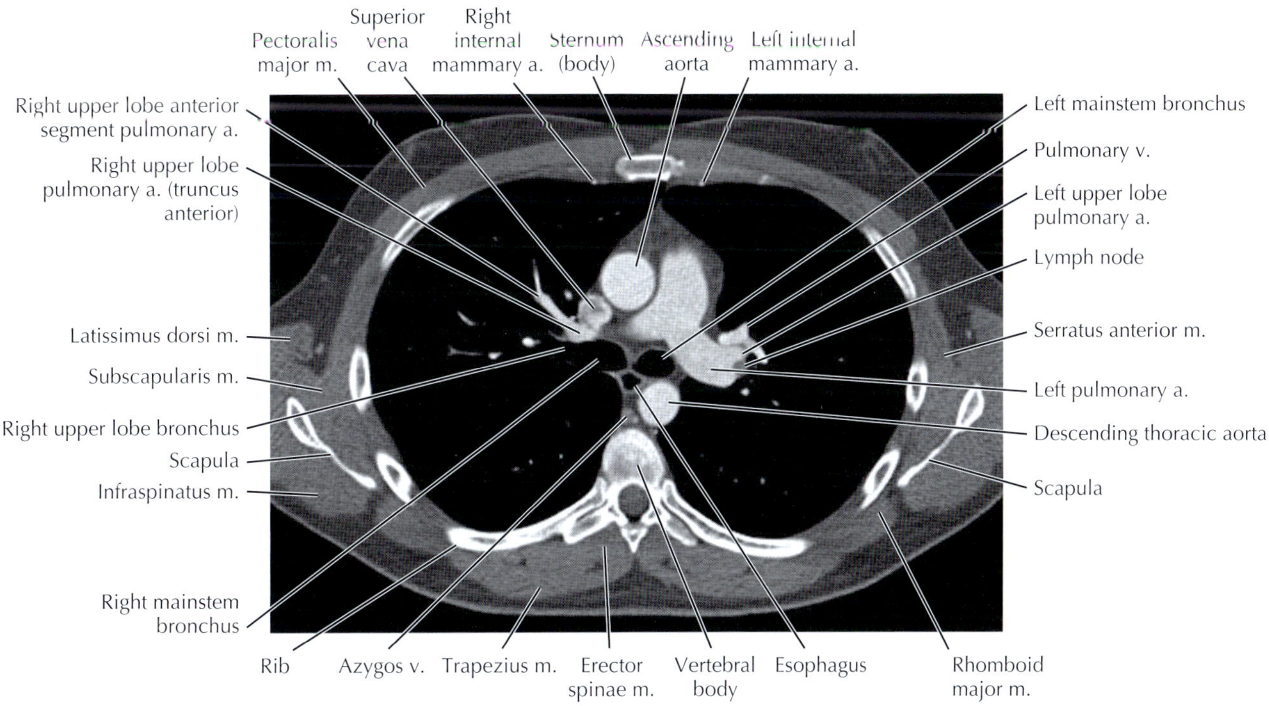
Pectoralis major m.
Superior vena cava
Right internal mammary a.
Sternum (body)
Ascending aorta
Left internal mammary a.
Right upper lobe anterior segment pulmonary a.
Right upper lobe pulmonary a. (truncus anterior)
Latissimus dorsi m.
Subscapularis m.
Right upper lobe bronchus
Scapula
Infraspinatus m.
Right mainstem bronchus
Left mainstem bronchus
Pulmonary v.
Left upper lobe pulmonary a.
Lymph node
Serratus anterior m.
Left pulmonary a.
Descending thoracic aorta
Scapula
Rib
Azygos v.
Trapezius m.
Erector spinae m.
Vertebral body
Esophagus
Rhomboid major m.

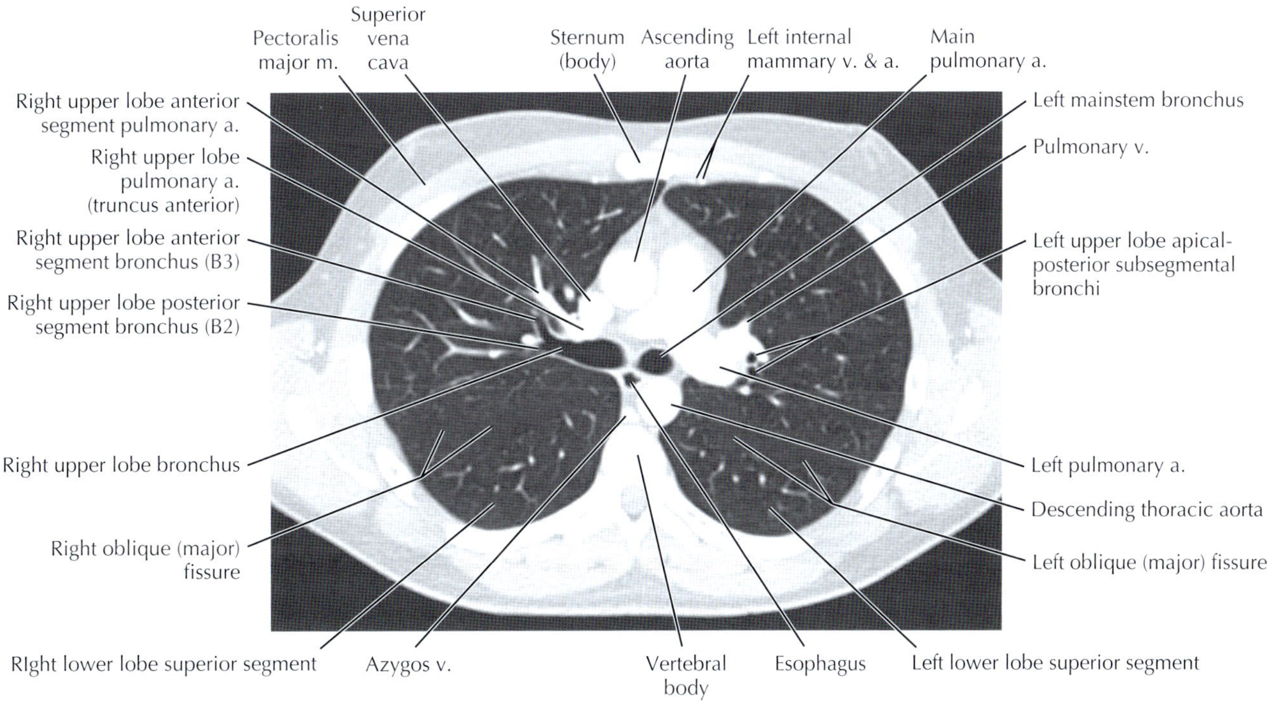
Pectoralis major m.
Superior vena cava
Sternum (body)
Ascending aorta
Left internal mammary v. & a.
Main pulmonary a.
Right upper lobe anterior segment pulmonary a.
Right upper lobe pulmonary a. (truncus anterior)
Right upper lobe anterior segment bronchus (B3)
Right upper lobe posterior segment bronchus (B2)
Right upper lobe bronchus
Right oblique (major) fissure
Left mainstem bronchus
Pulmonary v.
Left upper lobe apical-posterior subsegmental bronchi
Left pulmonary a.
Descending thoracic aorta
Left oblique (major) fissure
RIght lower lobe superior segment
Azygos v.
Vertebral body
Esophagus
Left lower lobe superior segment

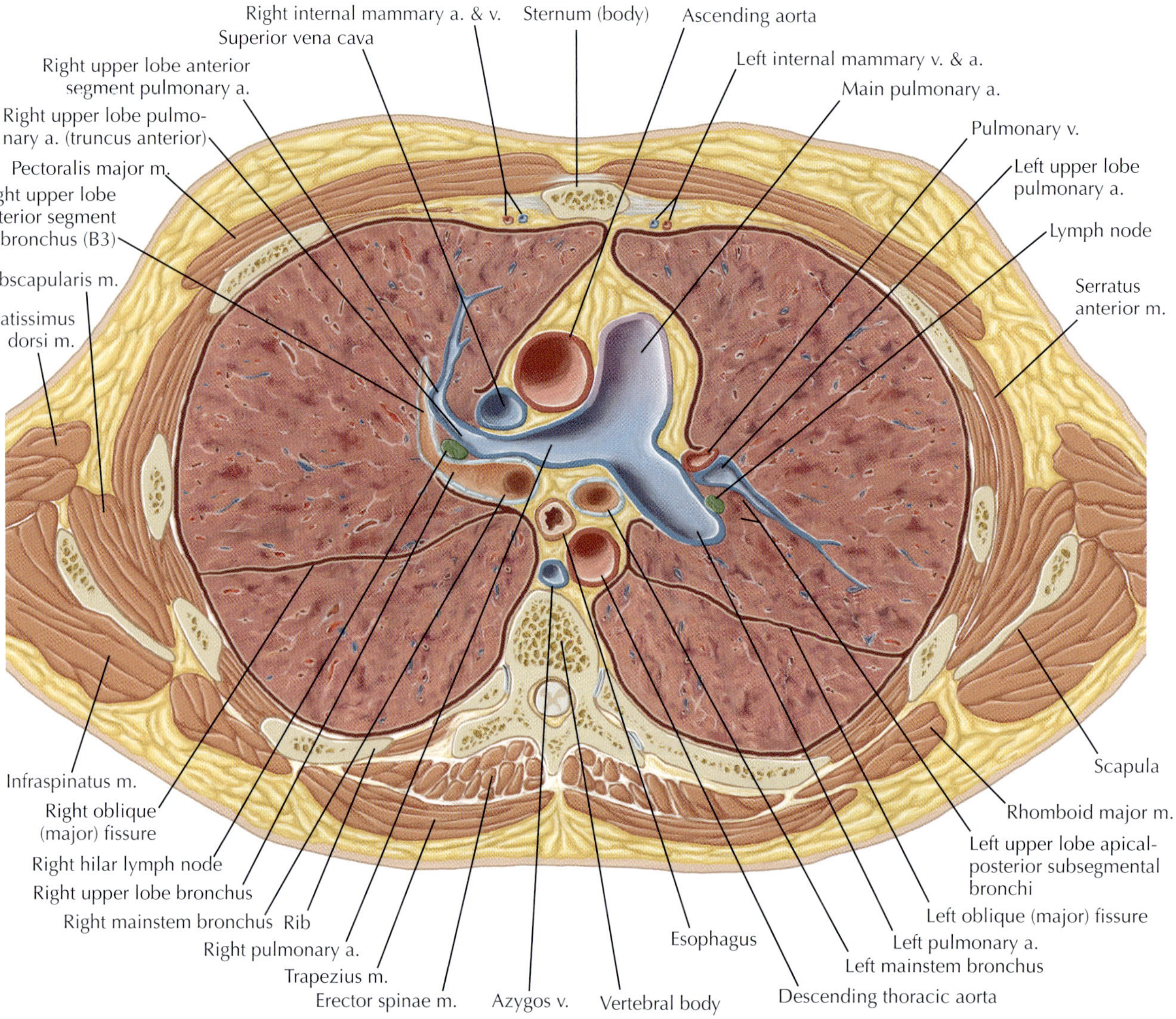
Right internal mammary a. & v.
Sternum (body)
Ascending aorta
Superior vena cava
Left internal mammary v. & a.
Right upper lobe anterior segment pulmonary a.
Main pulmonary a.
Right upper lobe pulmonary a. (truncus anterior)
Pulmonary v.
Pectoralis major m.
Left upper lobe pulmonary a.
Right upper lobe anterior segment bronchus (B3)
Lymph node
Subscapularis m.
Serratus anterior m.
Latissimus dorsi m.
Scapula
Infraspinatus m.
Rhomboid major m.
Right oblique (major) fissure
Left upper lobe apical-posterior subsegmental bronchi
Right hilar lymph node
Right upper lobe bronchus
Left oblique (major) fissure
Right mainstem bronchus
Rib
Left pulmonary a.
Esophagus
Right pulmonary a.
Left mainstem bronchus
Trapezius m.
Descending thoracic aorta
Erector spinae m.
Azygos v.
Vertebral body

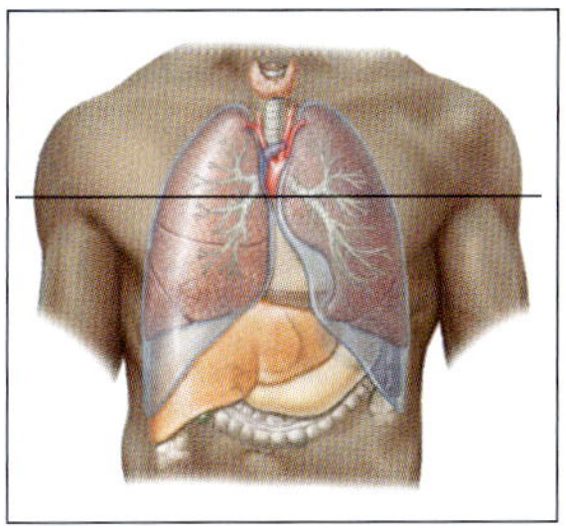

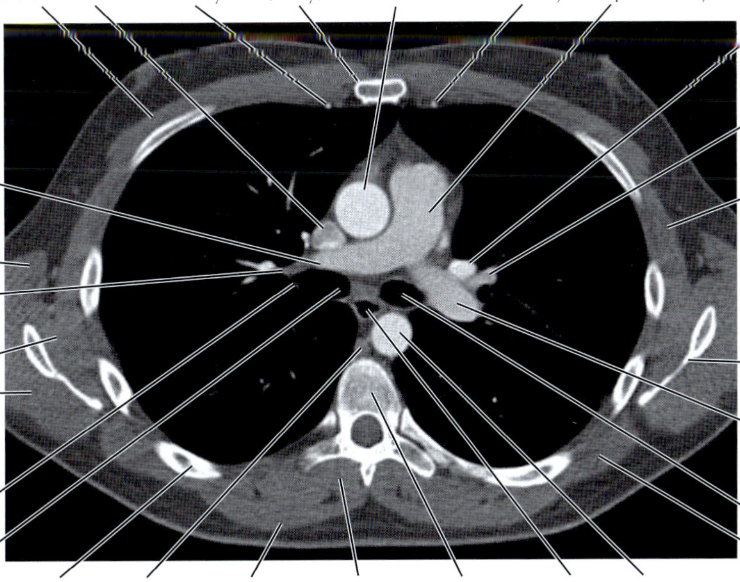

Pectoralis major m.
Superior vena cava
Right internal mammary a.
Sternum (body)
Ascending aorta
Left internal mammary a.
Main pulmonary a.
Pulmonary vein
Left upper lobe pulmonary a.
Serratus anterior m.
Right upper lobe pulmonary a. (truncus anterior)
Latissimus dorsi m.
Right hilar lymph node
Subscapularis m.
Infraspinatus m.
Scapula
Left interlobar pulmonary artery
Right upper lobe bronchus
Right mainstem bronchus
Left mainstem bronchus
Rhomboid major m.
Rib
Azygos v.
Trapezius m.
Erector spinae m.
Vertebral body
Esophagus
Descending thoracic aorta

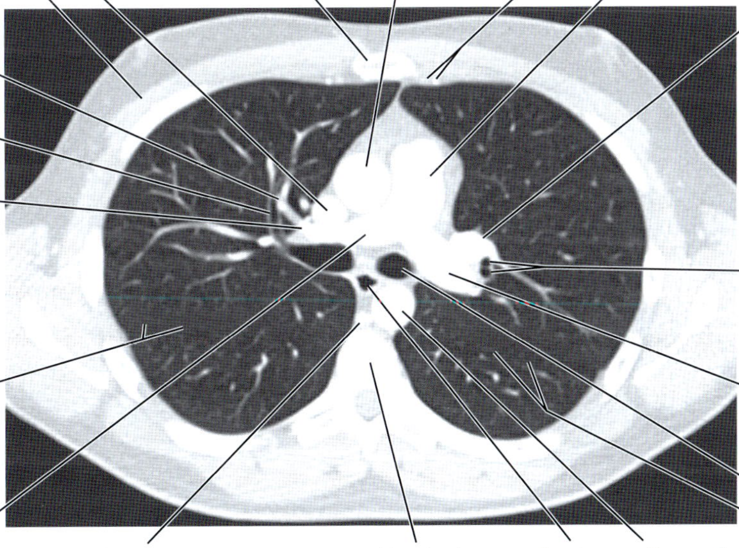

Pectoralis major m.
Superior vena cava
Sternum (body)
Ascending aorta
Left internal mammary v. & a.
Main pulmonary a.
Pulmonary v.
Right upper lobe anterior segmental pulmonary a.
Right upper lobe anterior segment bronchus (B3)
Right upper lobe pulmonary a. (truncus anterior)
Left upper lobe apical-posterior subsegmental bronchi
Right oblique (major) fissure
Left pulmonary a.
Left mainstem bronchus
Left oblique (major) fissure
Right pulmonary a.
Azygos v.
Vertebral body
Esophagus
Descending thoracic aorta

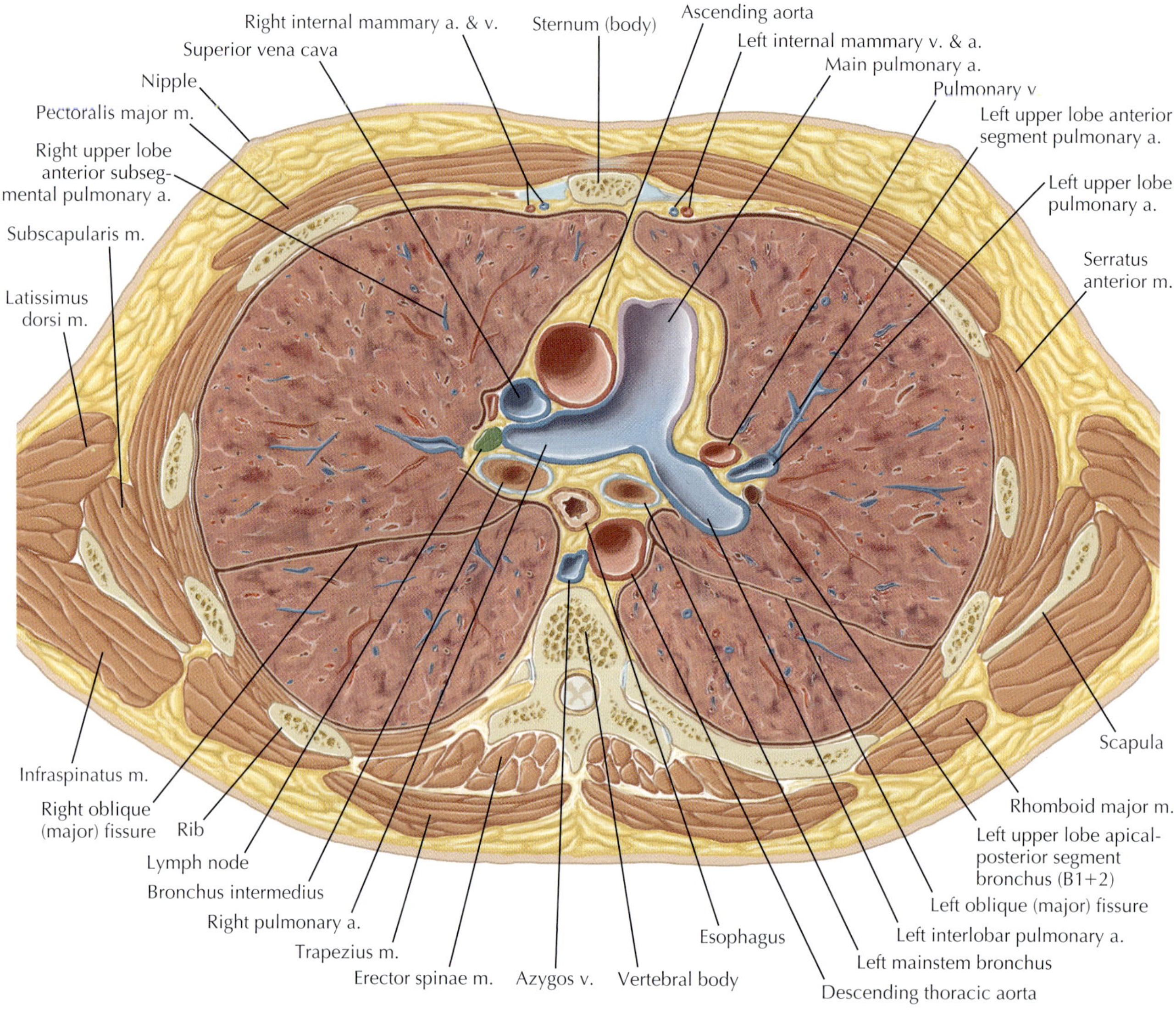
Right internal mammary a. & v.
Sternum (body)
Ascending aorta
Left internal mammary v. & a.
Main pulmonary a.
Superior vena cava
Nipple
Pulmonary v
Pectoralis major m.
Left upper lobe anterior segment pulmonary a.
Right upper lobe anterior subsegmental pulmonary a.
Left upper lobe pulmonary a.
Subscapularis m.
Serratus anterior m.
Latissimus dorsi m.
Scapula
Infraspinatus m.
Right oblique (major) fissure
Rib
Rhomboid major m.
Left upper lobe apical-posterior segment bronchus (B1+2)
Lymph node
Bronchus intermedius
Left oblique (major) fissure
Right pulmonary a.
Left interlobar pulmonary a.
Esophagus
Trapezius m.
Left mainstem bronchus
Erector spinae m.
Azygos v.
Vertebral body
Descending thoracic aorta

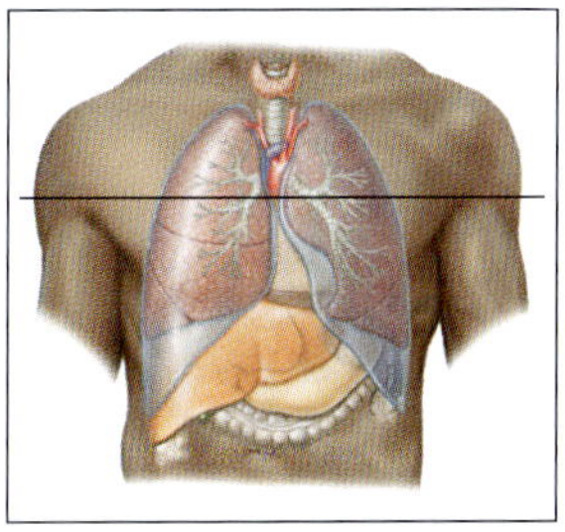

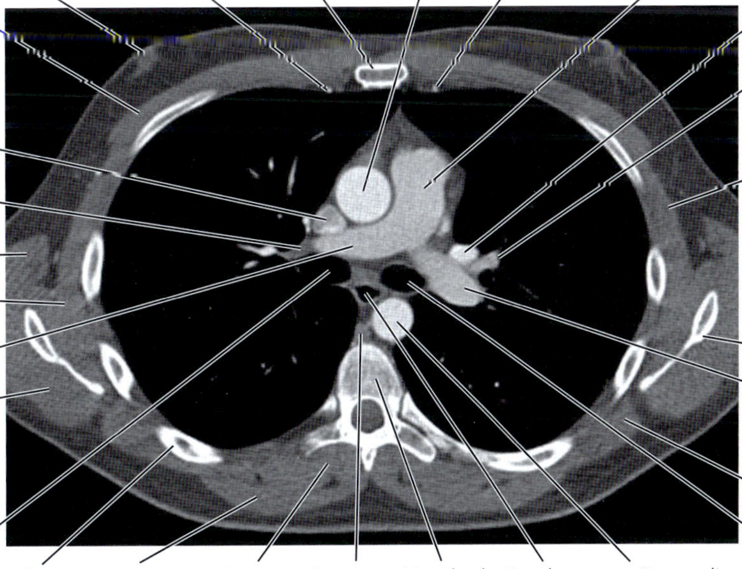
Nipple
Right internal mammary a.
Sternum (body)
Ascending aorta
Left internal mammary a.
Main pulmonary a.
Pectoralis major m.
Pulmonary v.
Left upper lobe pulmonary a.
Superior vena cava
Serratus anterior m.
Lymph node
Latissimus dorsi m.
Subscapularis m.
Right pulmonary a.
Scapula
Infraspinatus m.
Left interlobar pulmonary artery
Rhomboid major m.
Bronchus intermedius
Left mainstem bronchus
Rib
Trapezius m.
Erector spinae m.
Azygos v.
Vertebral body
Esophagus
Descending thoracic aorta

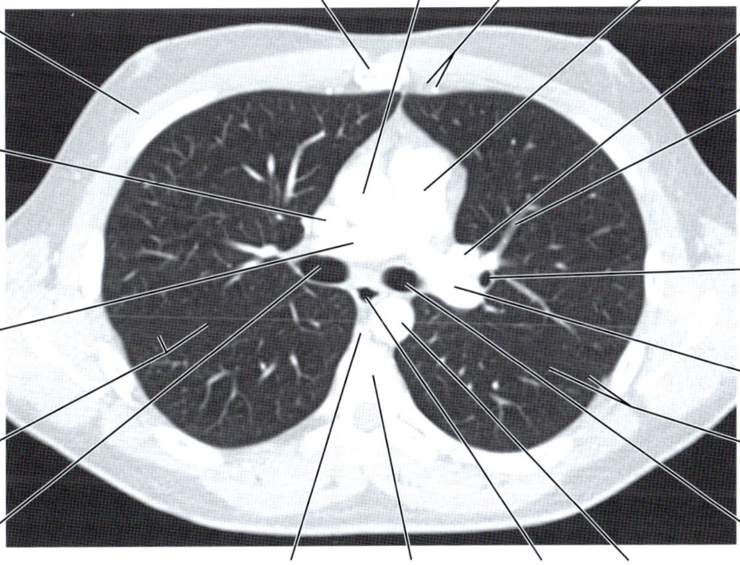
Sternum (body)
Ascending aorta
Left internal mammary v. & a.
Main pulmonary a.
Pectoralis major m.
Pulmonary v.
Left upper lobe anterior segment pulmonary a.
Superior vena cava
Left upper lobe apical-posterior segment bronchus (B1+2)
Right pulmonary artery
Left interlobar pulmonary a.
Right oblique (major) fissure
Left oblique (major) fissure
Bronchus intermedius
Left mainstem bronchus
Azygos v.
Vertebral body
Esophagus
Descending thoracic aorta

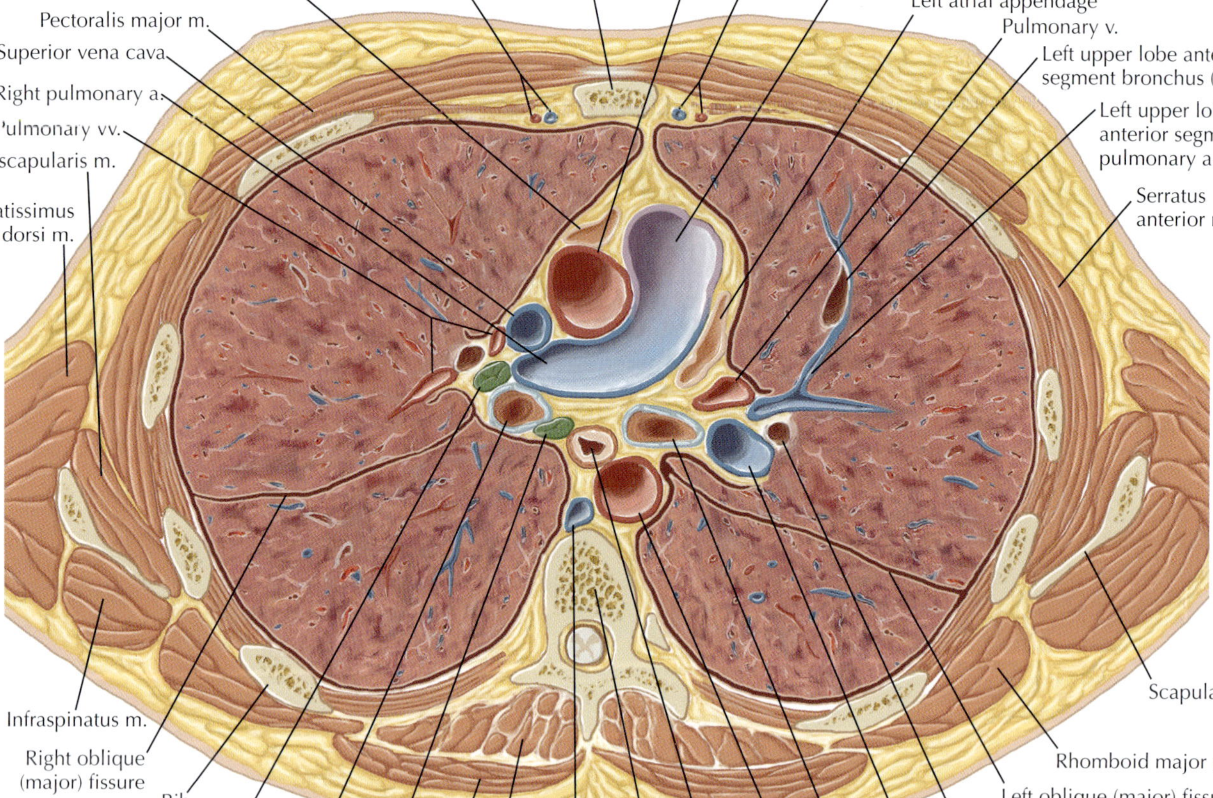

NORMAL ANATOMY

On this and a number of cranially and caudally located images displayed in lung windows, the *oblique fissures* are visible as thin, hypovascular planes extending transversely across the lungs bilaterally. The oblique fissures sweep anteriorly from the posterior toward the anterior chest wall. The oblique fissures are also often commonly referred to as the *major* fissures.

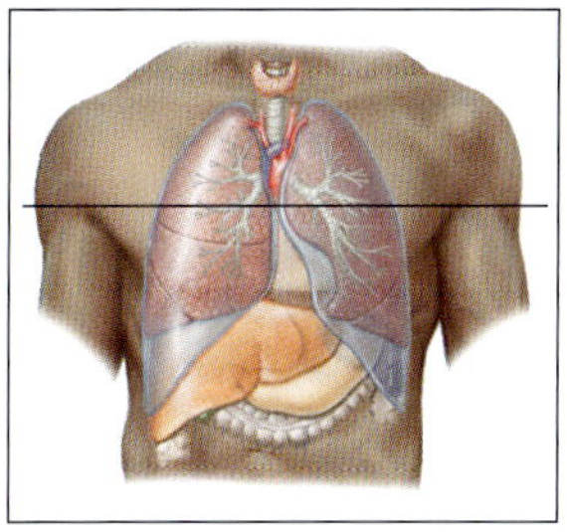

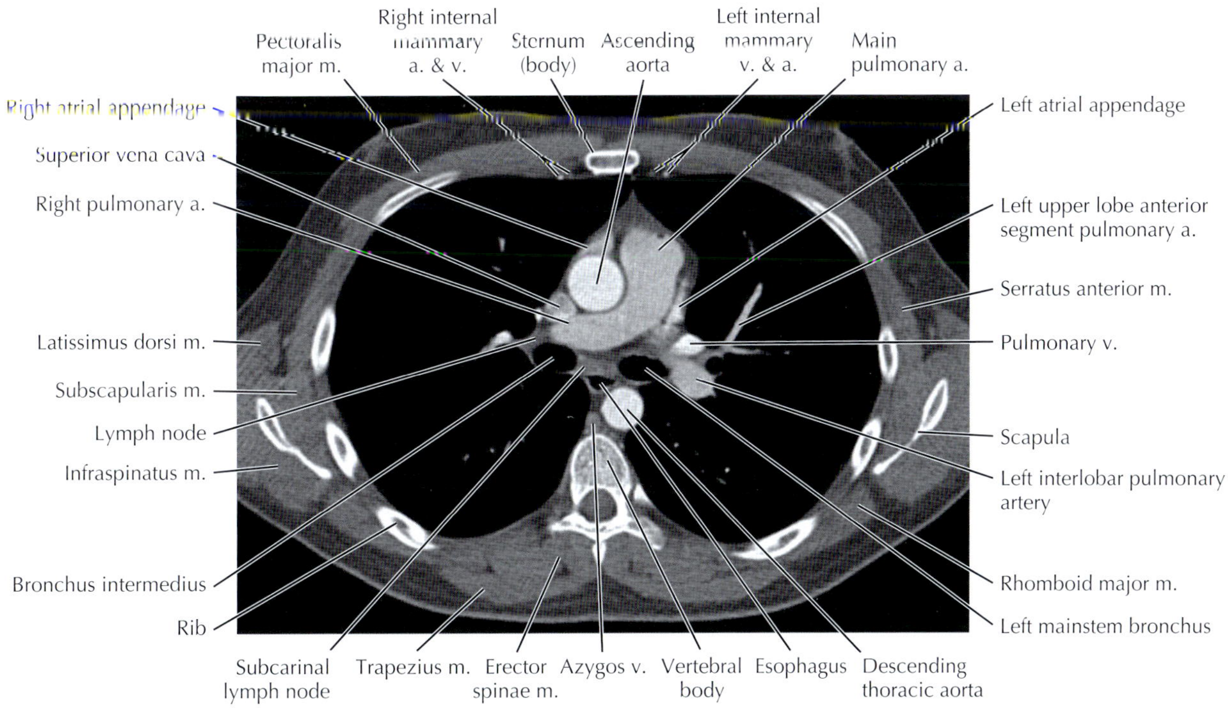
Pectoralis major m.
Right internal mammary a. & v.
Sternum (body)
Ascending aorta
Left internal mammary v. & a.
Main pulmonary a.
Right atrial appendage
Superior vena cava
Right pulmonary a.
Latissimus dorsi m.
Subscapularis m.
Lymph node
Infraspinatus m.
Bronchus intermedius
Rib
Subcarinal lymph node
Trapezius m.
Erector spinae m.
Azygos v.
Vertebral body
Esophagus
Descending thoracic aorta
Left atrial appendage
Left upper lobe anterior segment pulmonary a.
Serratus anterior m.
Pulmonary v.
Scapula
Left interlobar pulmonary artery
Rhomboid major m.
Left mainstem bronchus

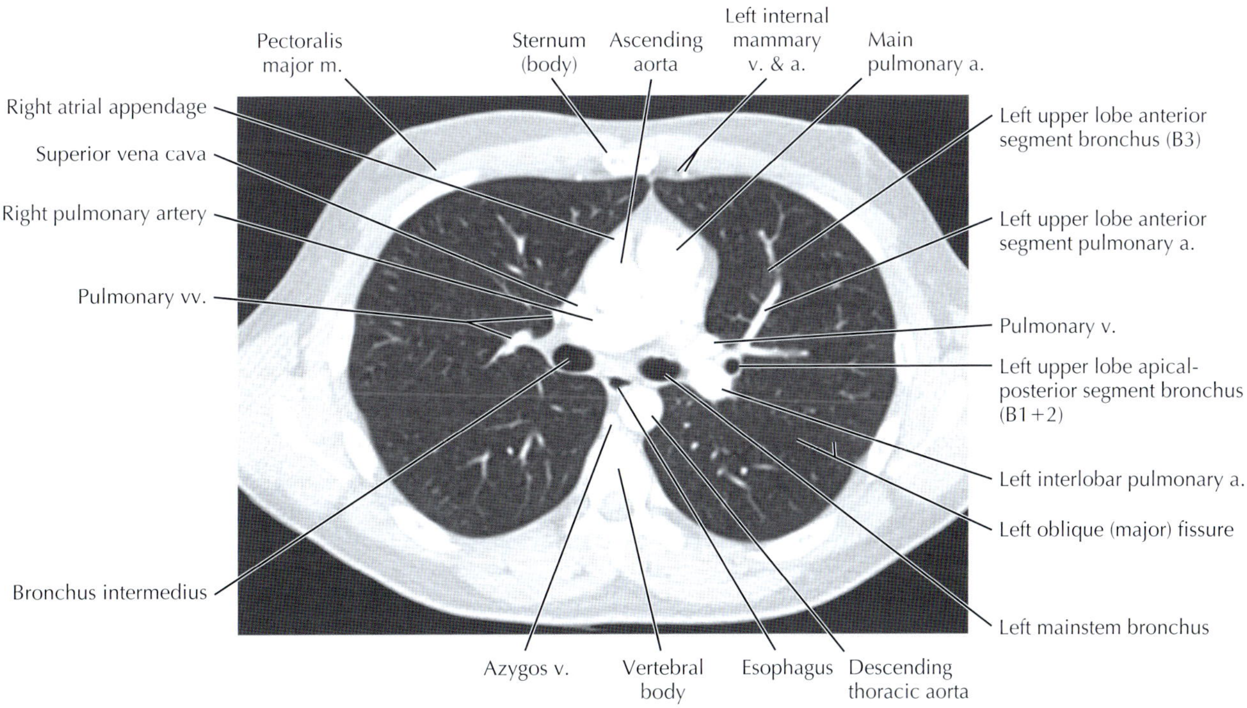
Pectoralis major m.
Sternum (body)
Ascending aorta
Left internal mammary v. & a.
Main pulmonary a.
Right atrial appendage
Superior vena cava
Right pulmonary artery
Pulmonary vv.
Bronchus intermedius
Azygos v.
Vertebral body
Esophagus
Descending thoracic aorta
Left upper lobe anterior segment bronchus (B3)
Left upper lobe anterior segment pulmonary a.
Pulmonary v.
Left upper lobe apical-posterior segment bronchus (B1+2)
Left interlobar pulmonary a.
Left oblique (major) fissure
Left mainstem bronchus

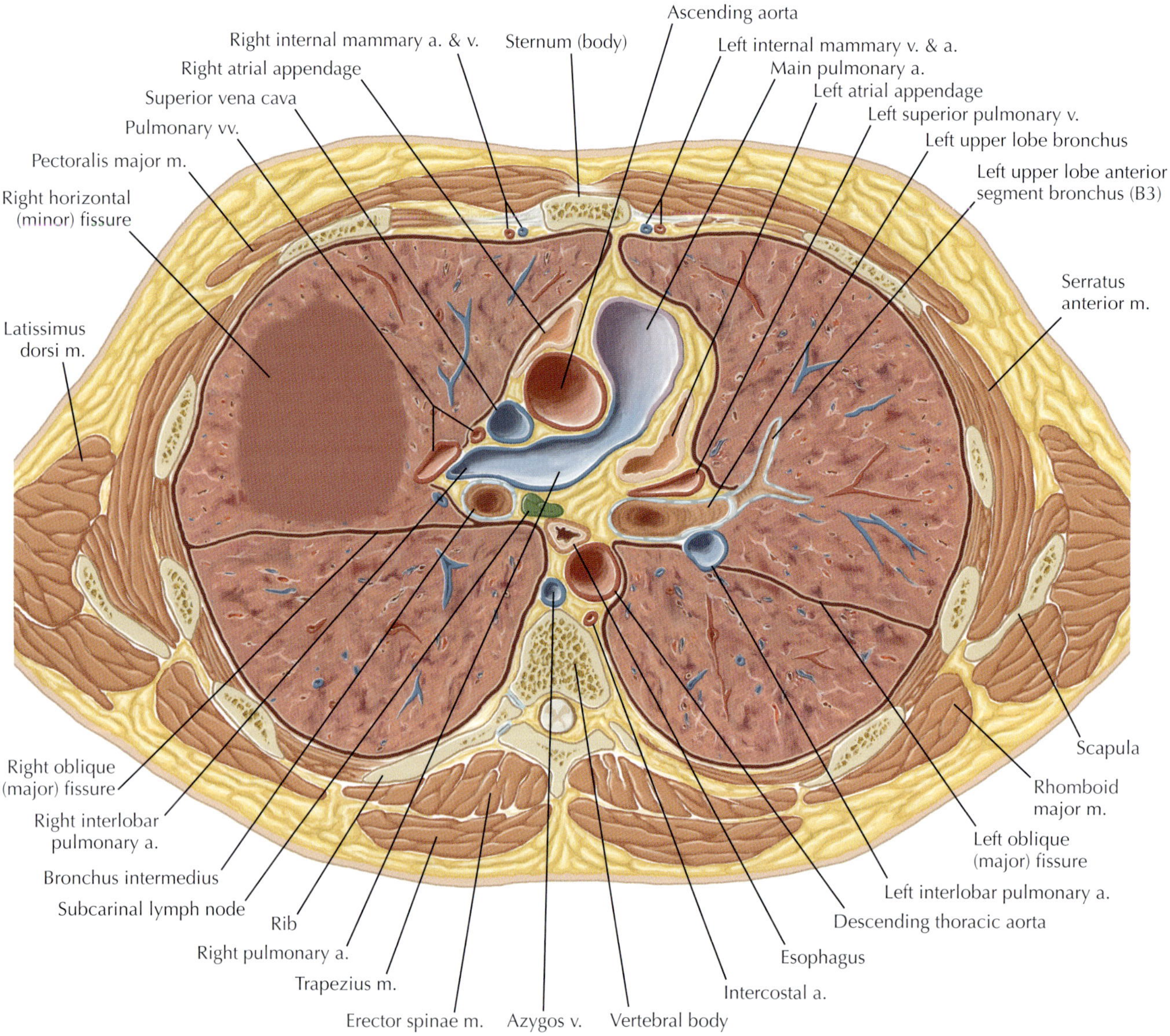

NORMAL ANATOMY

In lung windows, the *horizontal fissure* is visible on the right as a hypovascular area anteriorly. The horizontal fissure separates the right upper and middle lobes, and is also commonly referred to as the *minor* fissure.

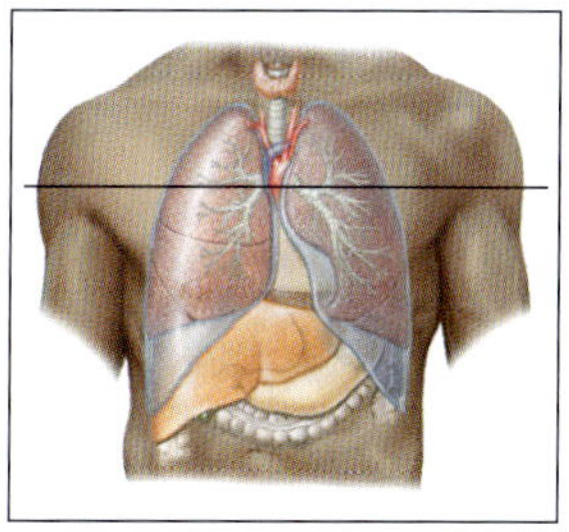

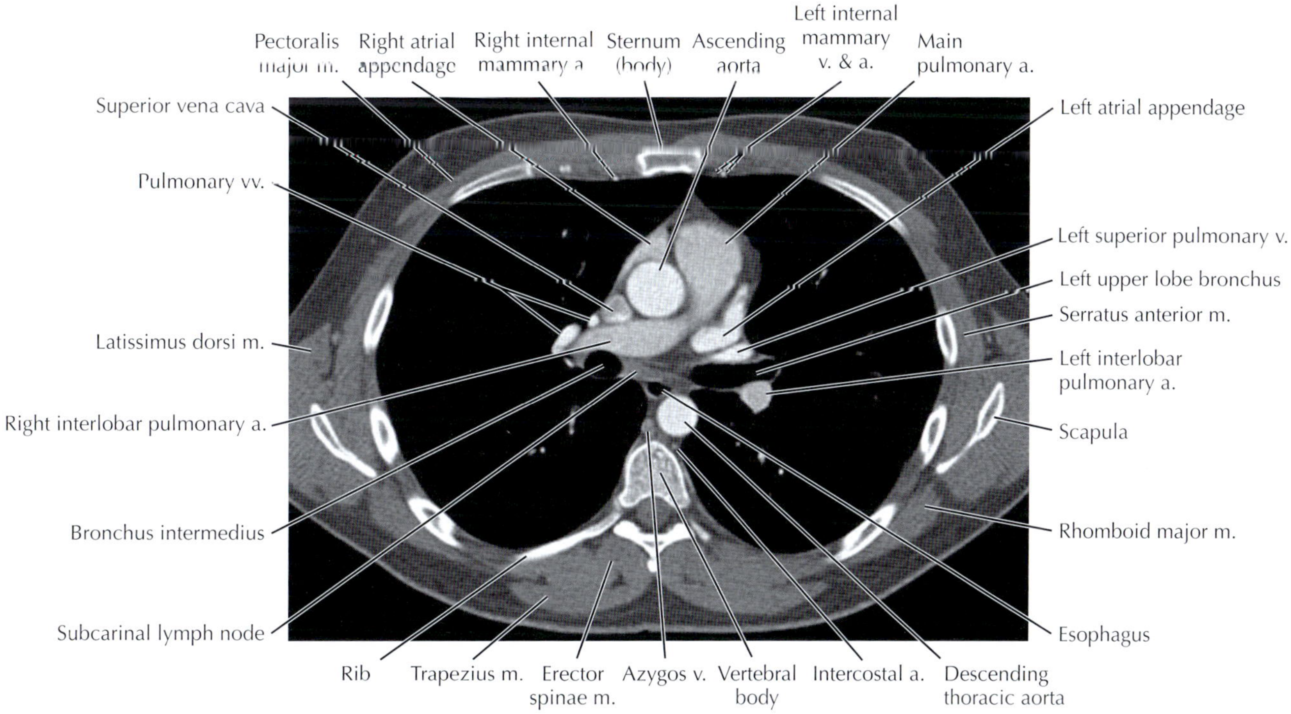
Pectoralis major m.
Right atrial appendage
Right internal mammary a.
Sternum (body)
Ascending aorta
Left internal mammary v. & a.
Main pulmonary a.
Superior vena cava
Pulmonary vv.
Latissimus dorsi m.
Right interlobar pulmonary a.
Bronchus intermedius
Subcarinal lymph node
Left atrial appendage
Left superior pulmonary v.
Left upper lobe bronchus
Serratus anterior m.
Left interlobar pulmonary a.
Scapula
Rhomboid major m.
Esophagus
Rib
Trapezius m.
Erector spinae m.
Azygos v.
Vertebral body
Intercostal a.
Descending thoracic aorta

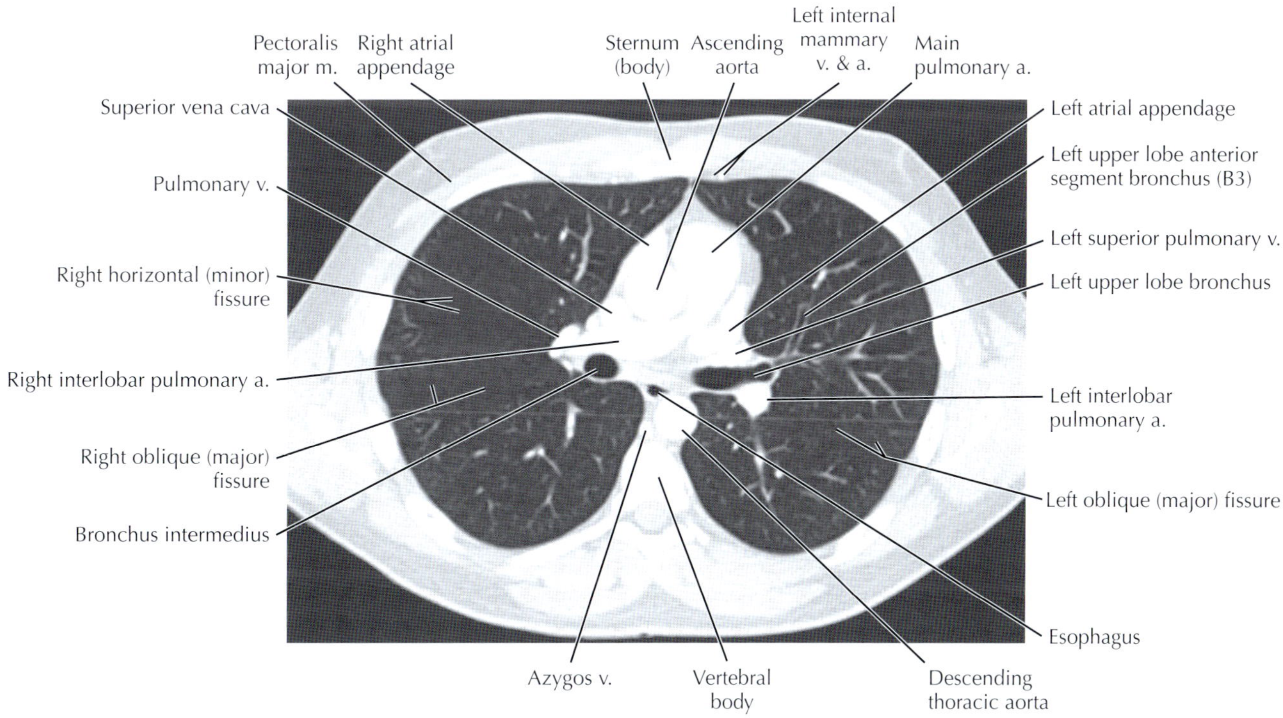
Pectoralis major m.
Right atrial appendage
Sternum (body)
Ascending aorta
Left internal mammary v. & a.
Main pulmonary a.
Superior vena cava
Pulmonary v.
Right horizontal (minor) fissure
Right interlobar pulmonary a.
Right oblique (major) fissure
Bronchus intermedius
Left atrial appendage
Left upper lobe anterior segment bronchus (B3)
Left superior pulmonary v.
Left upper lobe bronchus
Left interlobar pulmonary a.
Left oblique (major) fissure
Esophagus
Azygos v.
Vertebral body
Descending thoracic aorta

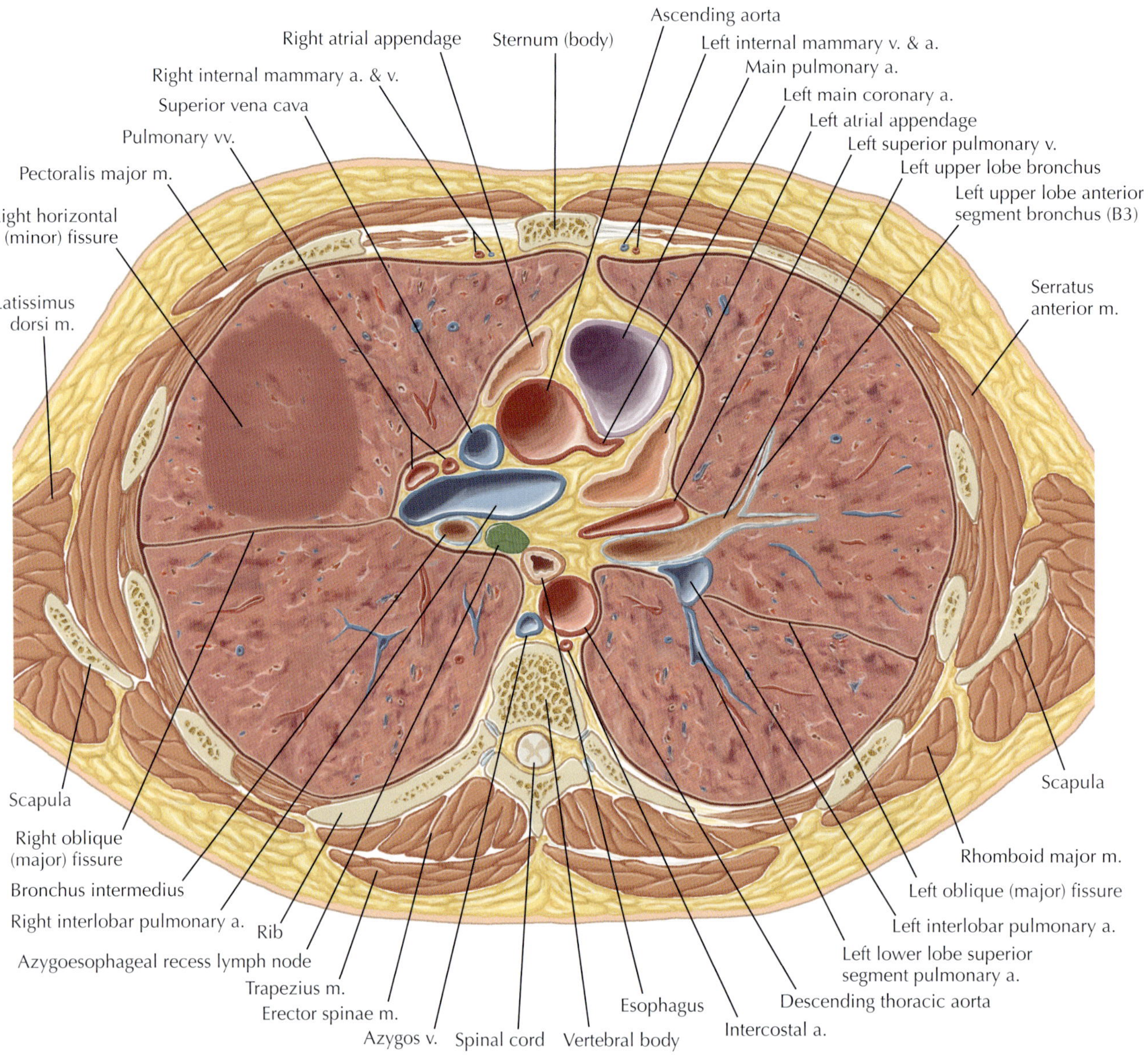
Ascending aorta
Right atrial appendage
Sternum (body)
Left internal mammary v. & a.
Main pulmonary a.
Right internal mammary a. & v.
Left main coronary a.
Superior vena cava
Left atrial appendage
Pulmonary vv.
Left superior pulmonary v.
Left upper lobe bronchus
Pectoralis major m.
Left upper lobe anterior segment bronchus (B3)
Right horizontal (minor) fissure
Serratus anterior m.
Latissimus dorsi m.
Scapula
Scapula
Right oblique (major) fissure
Rhomboid major m.
Bronchus intermedius
Left oblique (major) fissure
Right interlobar pulmonary a.
Rib
Left interlobar pulmonary a.
Azygoesophageal recess lymph node
Left lower lobe superior segment pulmonary a.
Trapezius m.
Descending thoracic aorta
Erector spinae m.
Esophagus
Azygos v.
Spinal cord
Vertebral body
Intercostal a.

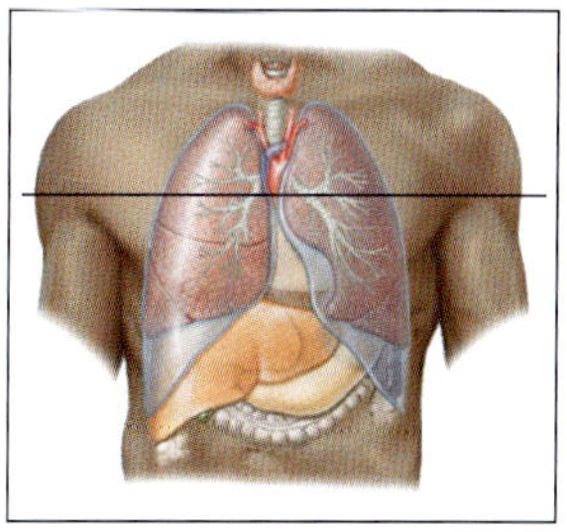

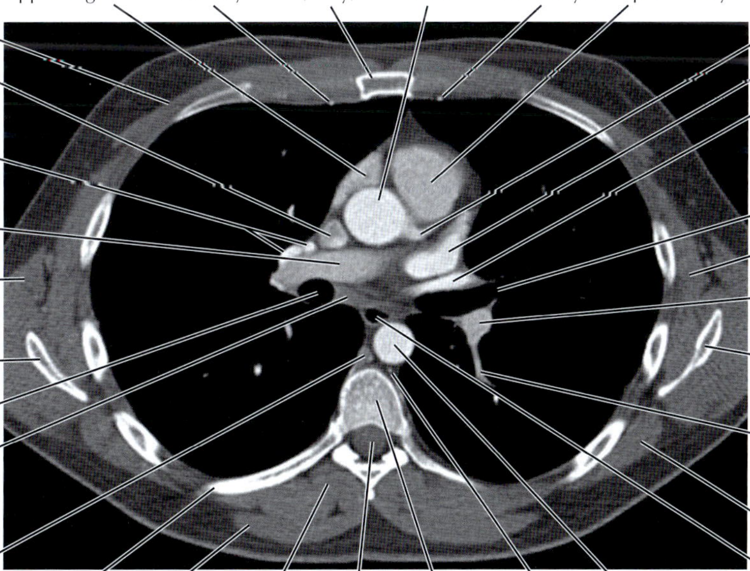
Right atrial appendage
Right internal mammary a.
Sternum (body)
Ascending aorta
Left internal mammary a.
Main pulmonary a.
Pectoralis major m.
Superior vena cava
Pulmonary v.
Right interlobar pulmonary a.
Latissimus dorsi m.
Scapula
Bronchus intermedius
Azygoesophageal recess lymph node
Azygos v.
Left main coronary a.
Left atrial appendage
Left superior pulmonary v.
Left upper lobe bronchus
Serratus anterior m.
Left interlobar pulmonary a.
Scapula
Left lower lobe superior segment pulmonary a.
Rhomboid major m.
Esophagus
Rib
Trapezius m.
Erector spinae m.
Spinal cord
Vertebral body
Intercostal a.
Descending thoracic aorta

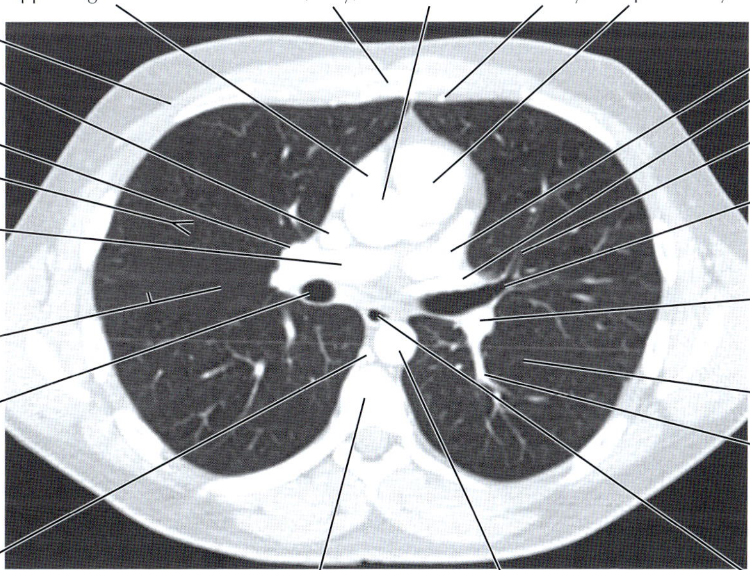
Right atrial appendage
Sternum (body)
Ascending aorta
Left internal mammary a.
Main pulmonary a.
Pectoralis major m.
Superior vena cava
Pulmonary v.
Right horizontal (minor) fissure
Right interlobar pulmonary a.
Right oblique (major) fissure
Bronchus intermedius
Azygos v.
Left atrial appendage
Left superior pulmonary v.
Left upper lobe anterior segment bronchus (B3)
Left upper lobe bronchus
Left interlobar pulmonary a.
Left oblique (major) fissure
Left lower lobe superior segment pulmonary a.
Esophagus
Vertebral body
Descending thoracic aorta

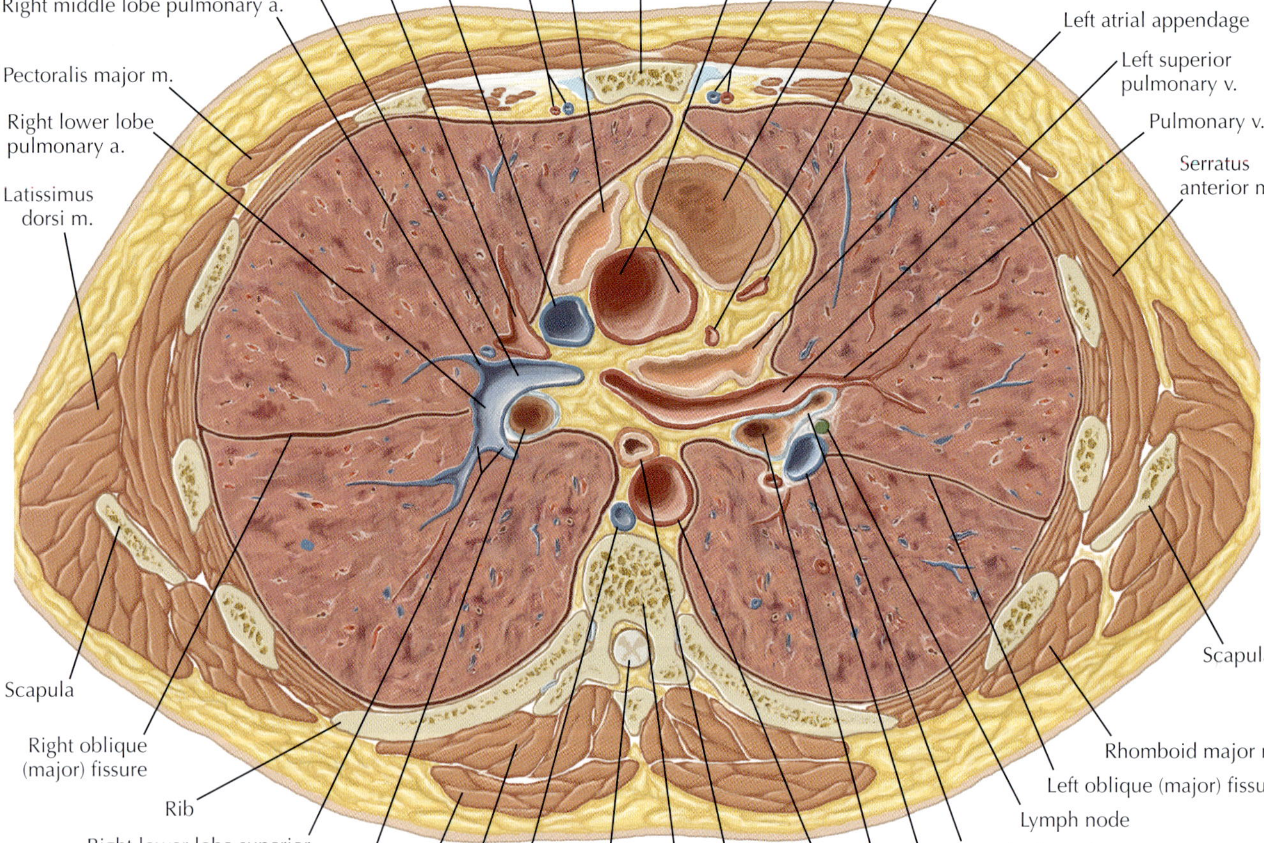

DIAGNOSTIC CONSIDERATION

At this level, the *sinuses of Valsalva* are now visible. The sinuses of Valsalva are three areas of mild dilation of the aortic root located between the aortic valve annulus and sinotubular junction. Each sinus of Valsalva is associated with its corresponding aortic valve cusp. Occasionally abnormal enlargement of one of the sinuses of Valsalva may be encountered, representing a sinus of Valsalva aneurysm. Aneurysms of the sinus of Valsalva require attention because they may result in rupture—a potentially catastrophic event.

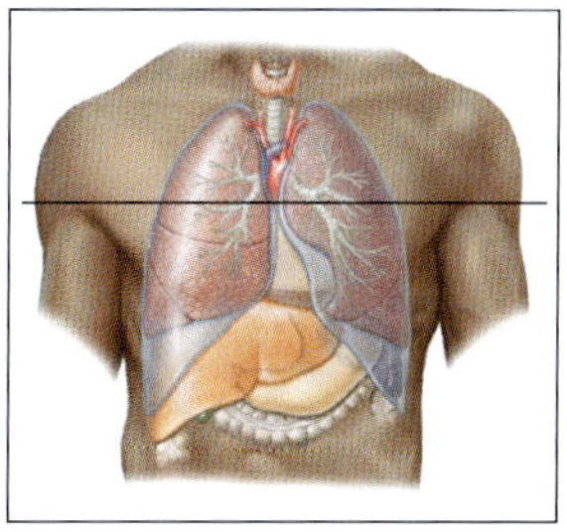

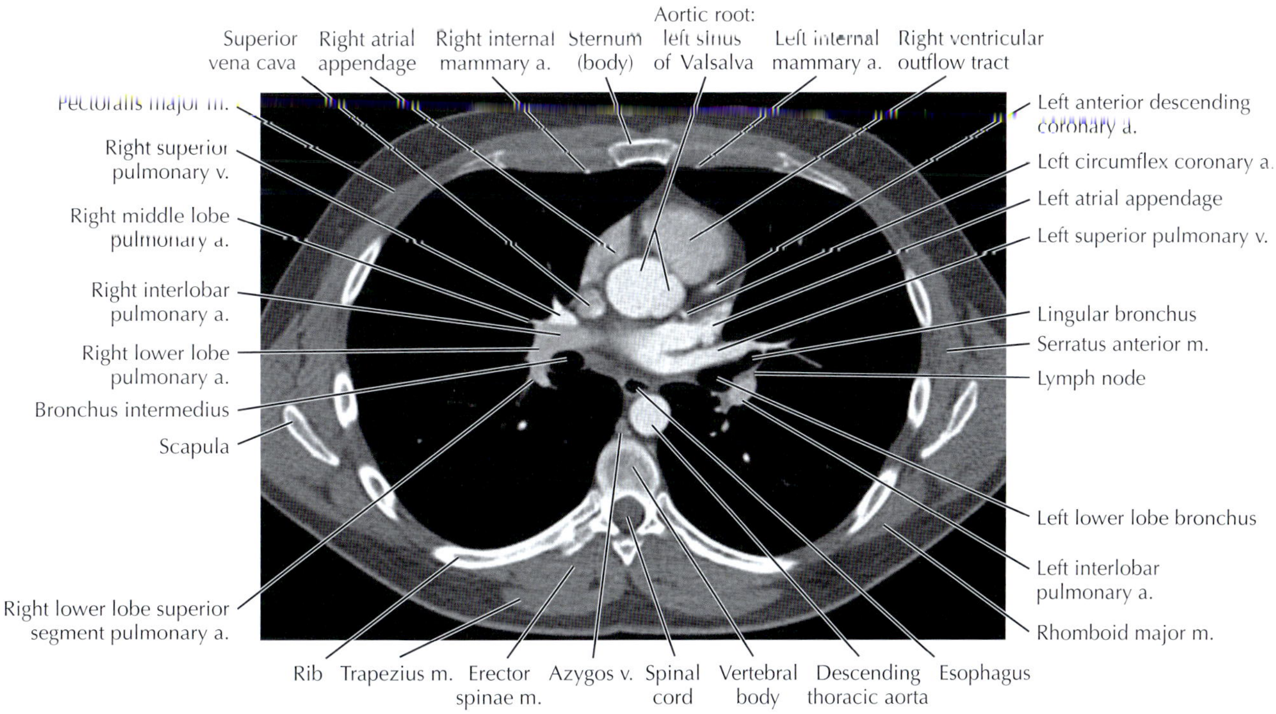
Superior vena cava
Right atrial appendage
Right internal mammary a.
Sternum (body)
Aortic root: left sinus of Valsalva
Left internal mammary a.
Right ventricular outflow tract
Pectoralis major m.
Right superior pulmonary v.
Right middle lobe pulmonary a.
Right interlobar pulmonary a.
Right lower lobe pulmonary a.
Bronchus intermedius
Scapula
Right lower lobe superior segment pulmonary a.
Left anterior descending coronary a.
Left circumflex coronary a.
Left atrial appendage
Left superior pulmonary v.
Lingular bronchus
Serratus anterior m.
Lymph node
Left lower lobe bronchus
Left interlobar pulmonary a.
Rhomboid major m.
Rib
Trapezius m.
Erector spinae m.
Azygos v.
Spinal cord
Vertebral body
Descending thoracic aorta
Esophagus

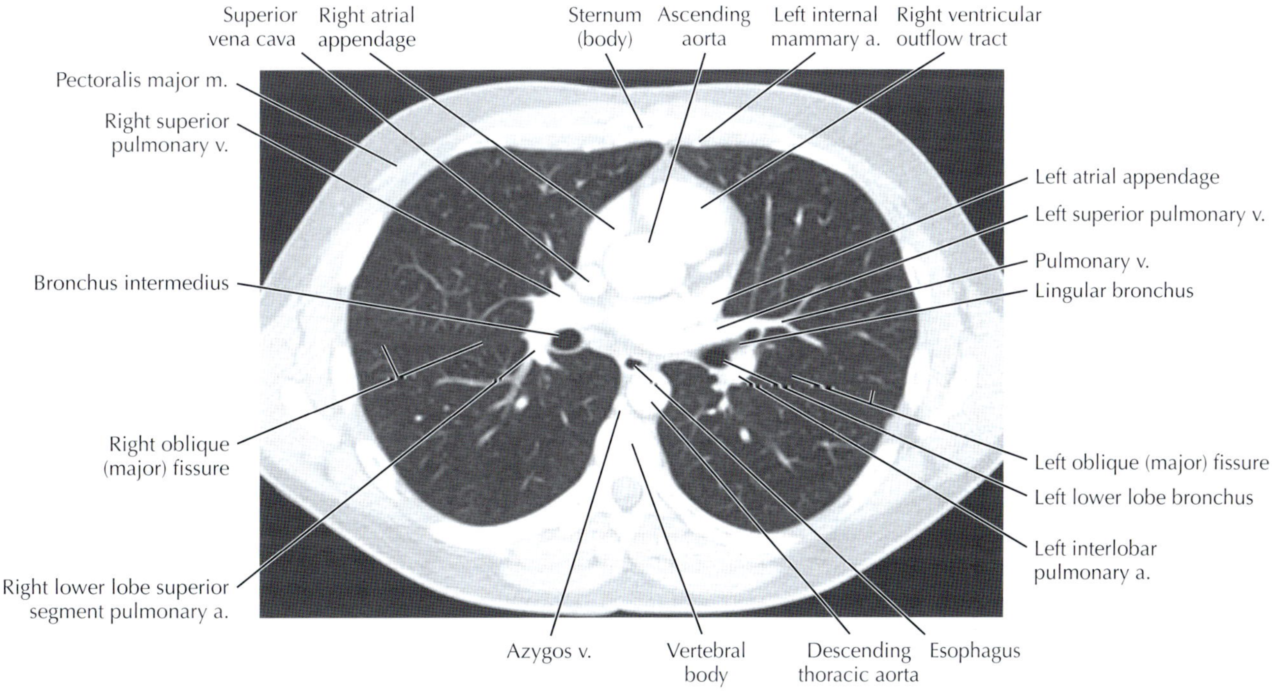
Superior vena cava
Right atrial appendage
Sternum (body)
Ascending aorta
Left internal mammary a.
Right ventricular outflow tract
Pectoralis major m.
Right superior pulmonary v.
Bronchus intermedius
Right oblique (major) fissure
Right lower lobe superior segment pulmonary a.
Left atrial appendage
Left superior pulmonary v.
Pulmonary v.
Lingular bronchus
Left oblique (major) fissure
Left lower lobe bronchus
Left interlobar pulmonary a.
Azygos v.
Vertebral body
Descending thoracic aorta
Esophagus

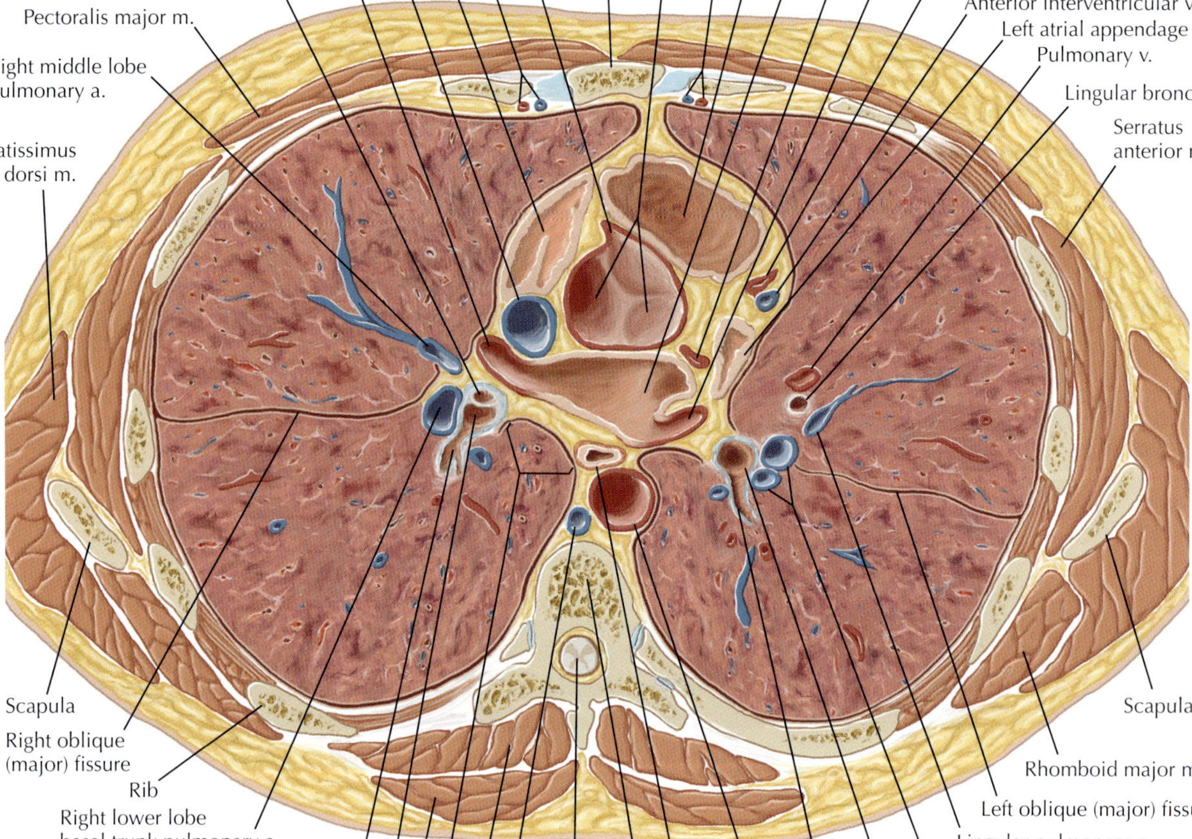

DIAGNOSTIC CONSIDERATION

The *azygoesophageal recess* is the region of the retocardiac mediastinum outlined by the right lower lobe, extending from the arch of the azygos vein to the diaphragm. This space is an important area because various types of pathology, including mediastinal masses and lymphadenopathy, may occur in this area.

NORMAL ANATOMY

The undivided lower lobe bronchi are short structures giving rise to the *superior segment bronchi (B6)* of the lower lobes; these airways are readily visible in lung windows. Inferior to the superior segmental bronchi, the lower lobe airways continue as *lower lobe bronchial trunks* but are also sometimes referred to as *truncus basalis*. Bilaterally, the basal bronchial trunks give rise to the basal segmental bronchi.

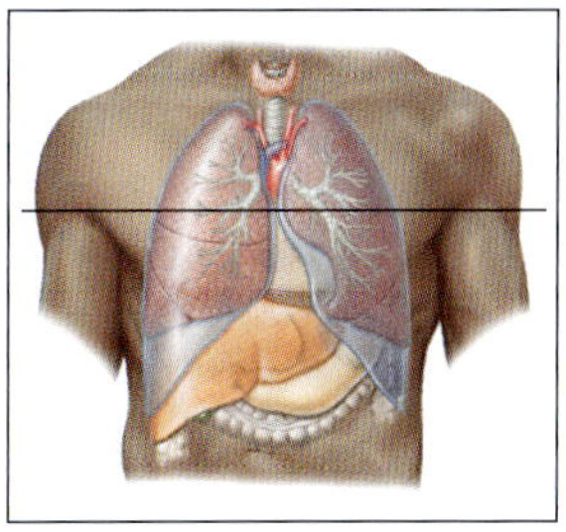

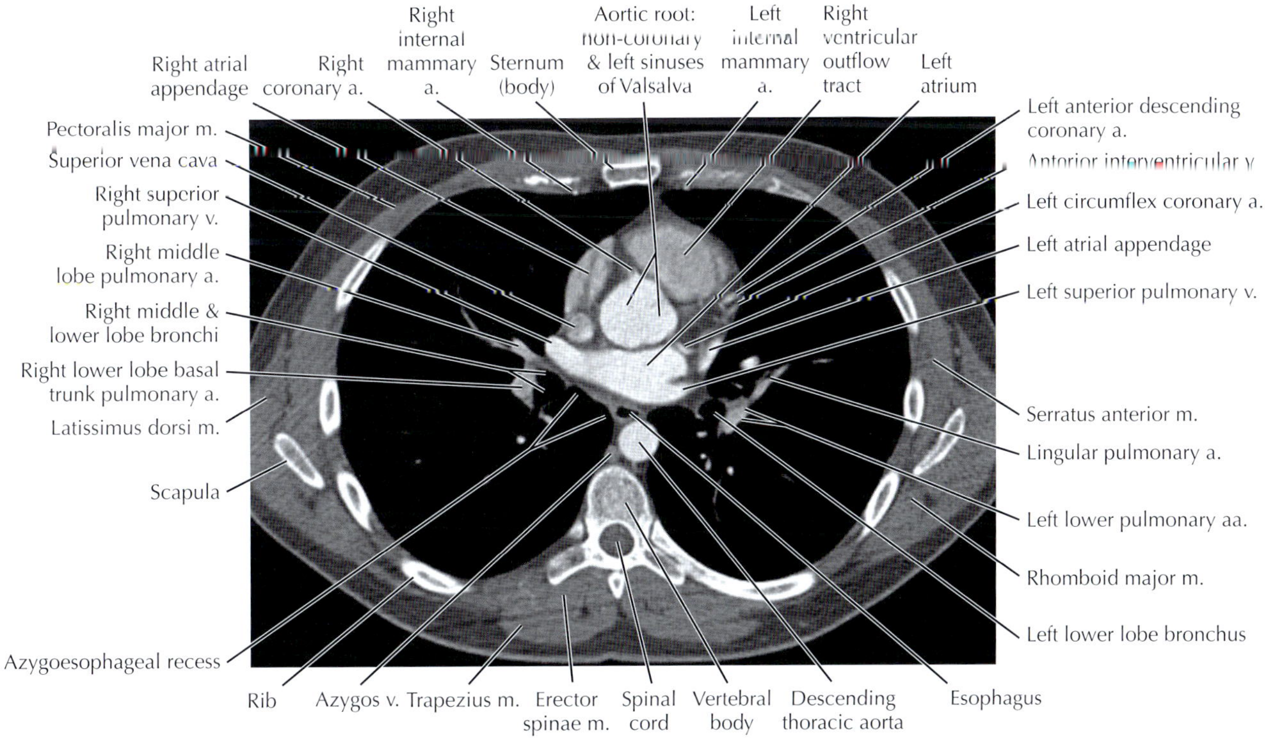
Right atrial appendage
Right coronary a.
Right internal mammary a.
Sternum (body)
Aortic root: non-coronary & left sinuses of Valsalva
Left internal mammary a.
Right ventricular outflow tract
Left atrium
Left anterior descending coronary a.
Anterior interventricular v.
Left circumflex coronary a.
Left atrial appendage
Left superior pulmonary v.
Serratus anterior m.
Lingular pulmonary a.
Left lower pulmonary aa.
Rhomboid major m.
Left lower lobe bronchus
Esophagus
Descending thoracic aorta
Vertebral body
Spinal cord
Erector spinae m.
Trapezius m.
Azygos v.
Rib
Azygoesophageal recess
Scapula
Latissimus dorsi m.
Right lower lobe basal trunk pulmonary a.
Right middle & lower lobe bronchi
Right middle lobe pulmonary a.
Right superior pulmonary v.
Superior vena cava
Pectoralis major m.

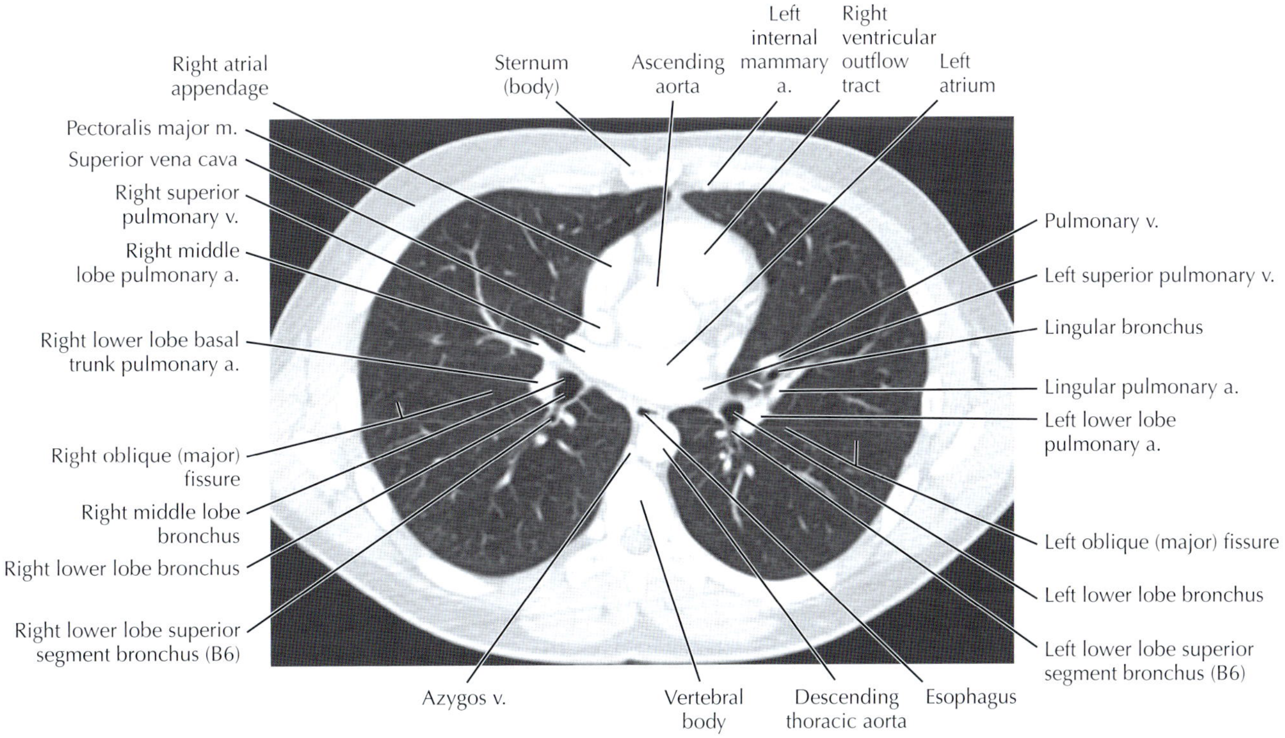
Right atrial appendage
Sternum (body)
Ascending aorta
Left internal mammary a.
Right ventricular outflow tract
Left atrium
Pulmonary v.
Left superior pulmonary v.
Lingular bronchus
Lingular pulmonary a.
Left lower lobe pulmonary a.
Left oblique (major) fissure
Left lower lobe bronchus
Left lower lobe superior segment bronchus (B6)
Esophagus
Descending thoracic aorta
Vertebral body
Azygos v.
Right lower lobe superior segment bronchus (B6)
Right lower lobe bronchus
Right middle lobe bronchus
Right oblique (major) fissure
Right lower lobe basal trunk pulmonary a.
Right middle lobe pulmonary a.
Right superior pulmonary v.
Superior vena cava
Pectoralis major m.

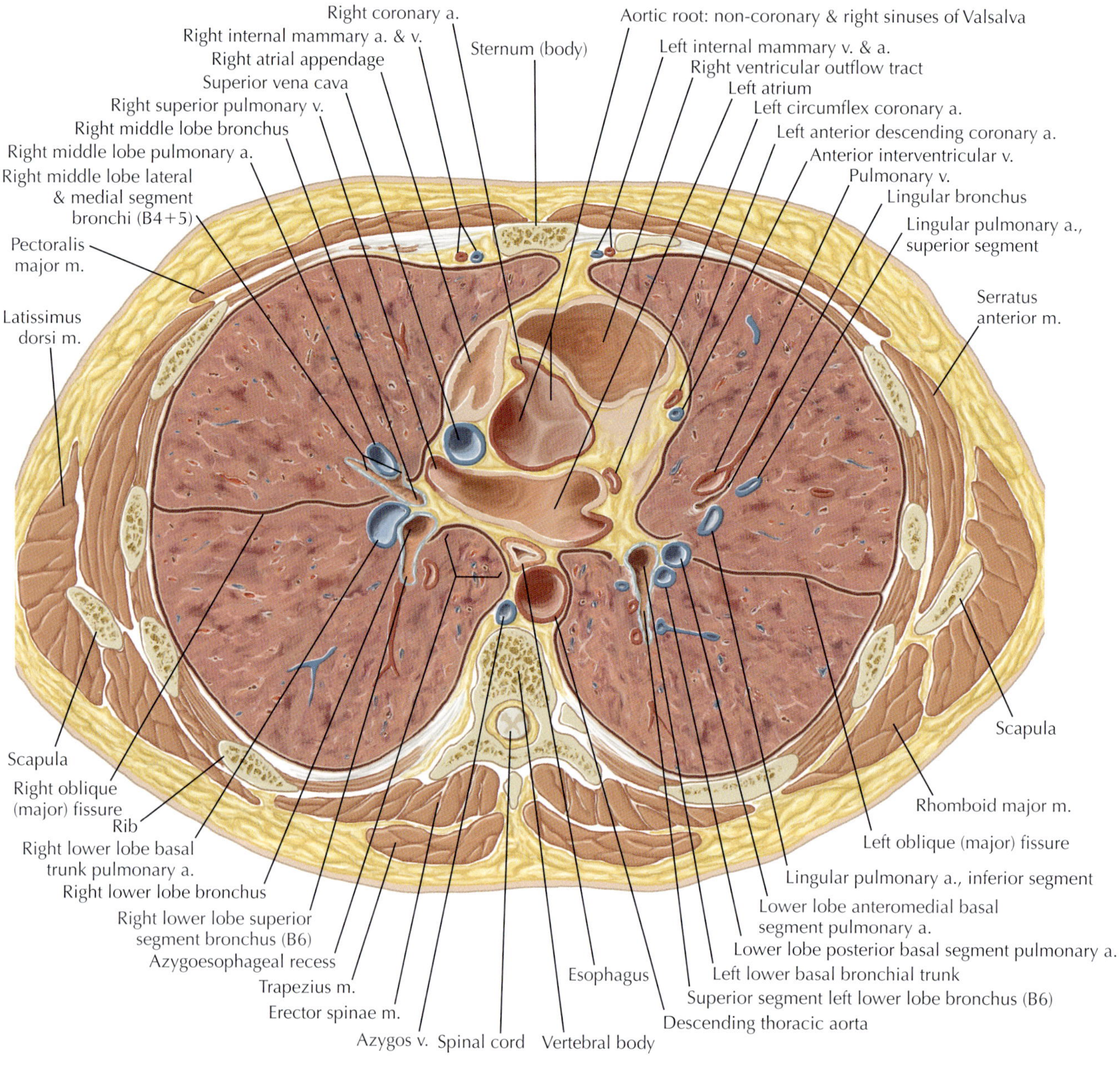

NORMAL VARIANTS

This level marks the origin of the left lower lobe segmental pulmonary arteries. Typically the left basal arterial trunk, inferior to the superior segmental left lower lobe pulmonary artery, branches into the *anteromedial basal*, *lateral basal*, and *posterior basal* segmental pulmonary arteries. In this patient, two, instead of three, basal segmental left lower lobe pulmonary arteries are visible. These vessels can be sequentially followed through Axial 29. On Axial 30, the lateral basal segmental lower lobe pulmonary artery is seen originating from the anteromedial basal segmental vessel. Although this pattern of segmental pulmonary arterial branching is uncommon, variations in the branching patterns of the pulmonary arteries are frequently encountered and usually of no clinical importance.

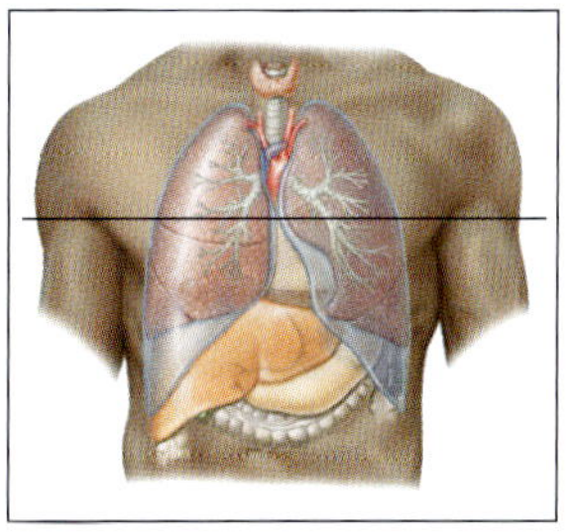

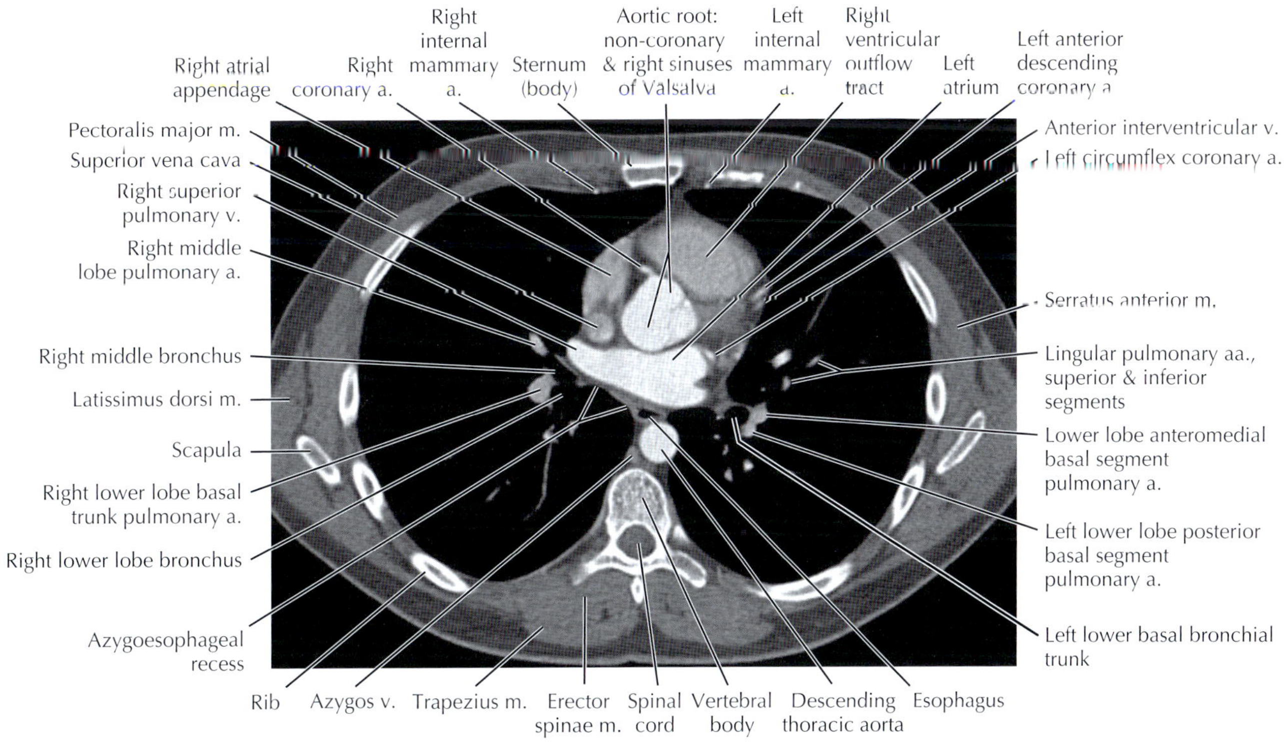
Right atrial appendage
Right coronary a.
Right internal mammary a.
Sternum (body)
Aortic root: non-coronary & right sinuses of Valsalva
Left internal mammary a.
Right ventricular outflow tract
Left atrium
Left anterior descending coronary a.
Pectoralis major m.
Superior vena cava
Right superior pulmonary v.
Right middle lobe pulmonary a.
Right middle bronchus
Latissimus dorsi m.
Scapula
Right lower lobe basal trunk pulmonary a.
Right lower lobe bronchus
Azygoesophageal recess
Anterior interventricular v.
Left circumflex coronary a.
Serratus anterior m.
Lingular pulmonary aa., superior & inferior segments
Lower lobe anteromedial basal segment pulmonary a.
Left lower lobe posterior basal segment pulmonary a.
Left lower basal bronchial trunk
Rib
Azygos v.
Trapezius m.
Erector spinae m.
Spinal cord
Vertebral body
Descending thoracic aorta
Esophagus

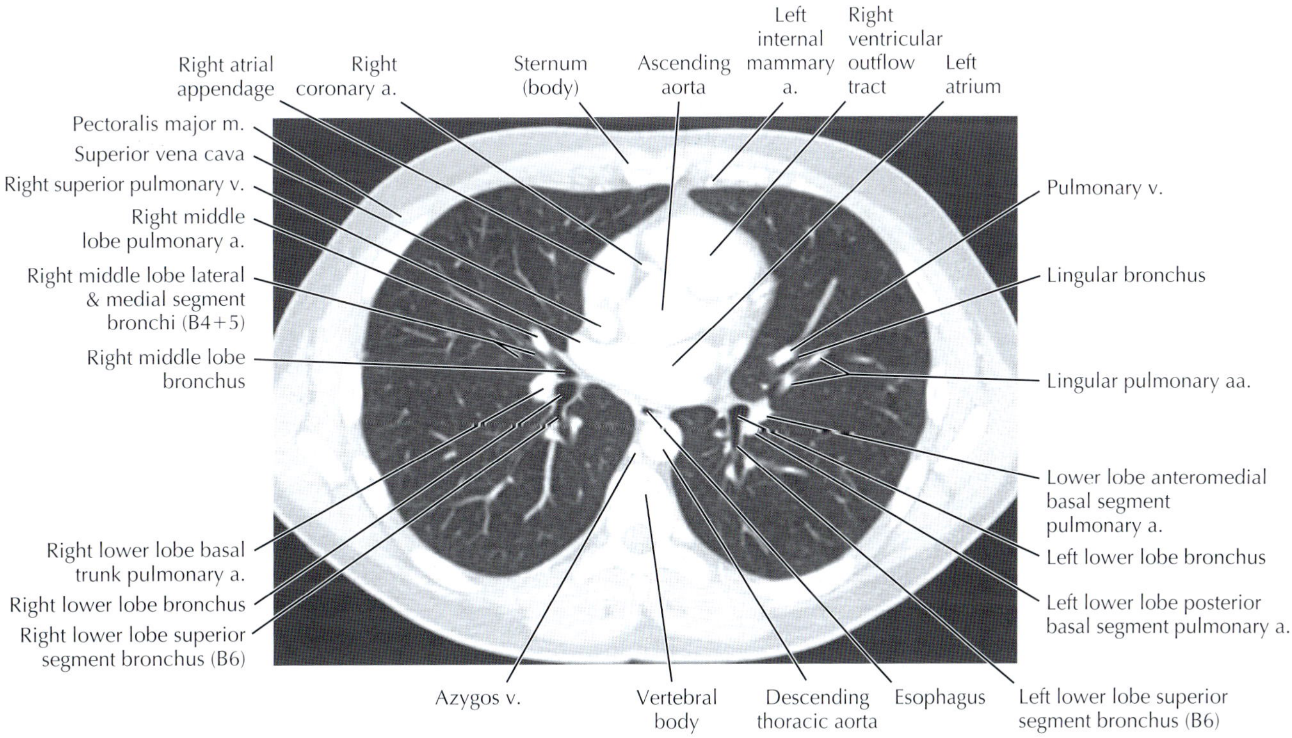
Right atrial appendage
Right coronary a.
Sternum (body)
Ascending aorta
Left internal mammary a.
Right ventricular outflow tract
Left atrium
Pectoralis major m.
Superior vena cava
Right superior pulmonary v.
Right middle lobe pulmonary a.
Right middle lobe lateral & medial segment bronchi (B4+5)
Right middle lobe bronchus
Right lower lobe basal trunk pulmonary a.
Right lower lobe bronchus
Right lower lobe superior segment bronchus (B6)
Pulmonary v.
Lingular bronchus
Lingular pulmonary aa.
Lower lobe anteromedial basal segment pulmonary a.
Left lower lobe bronchus
Left lower lobe posterior basal segment pulmonary a.
Azygos v.
Vertebral body
Descending thoracic aorta
Esophagus
Left lower lobe superior segment bronchus (B6)

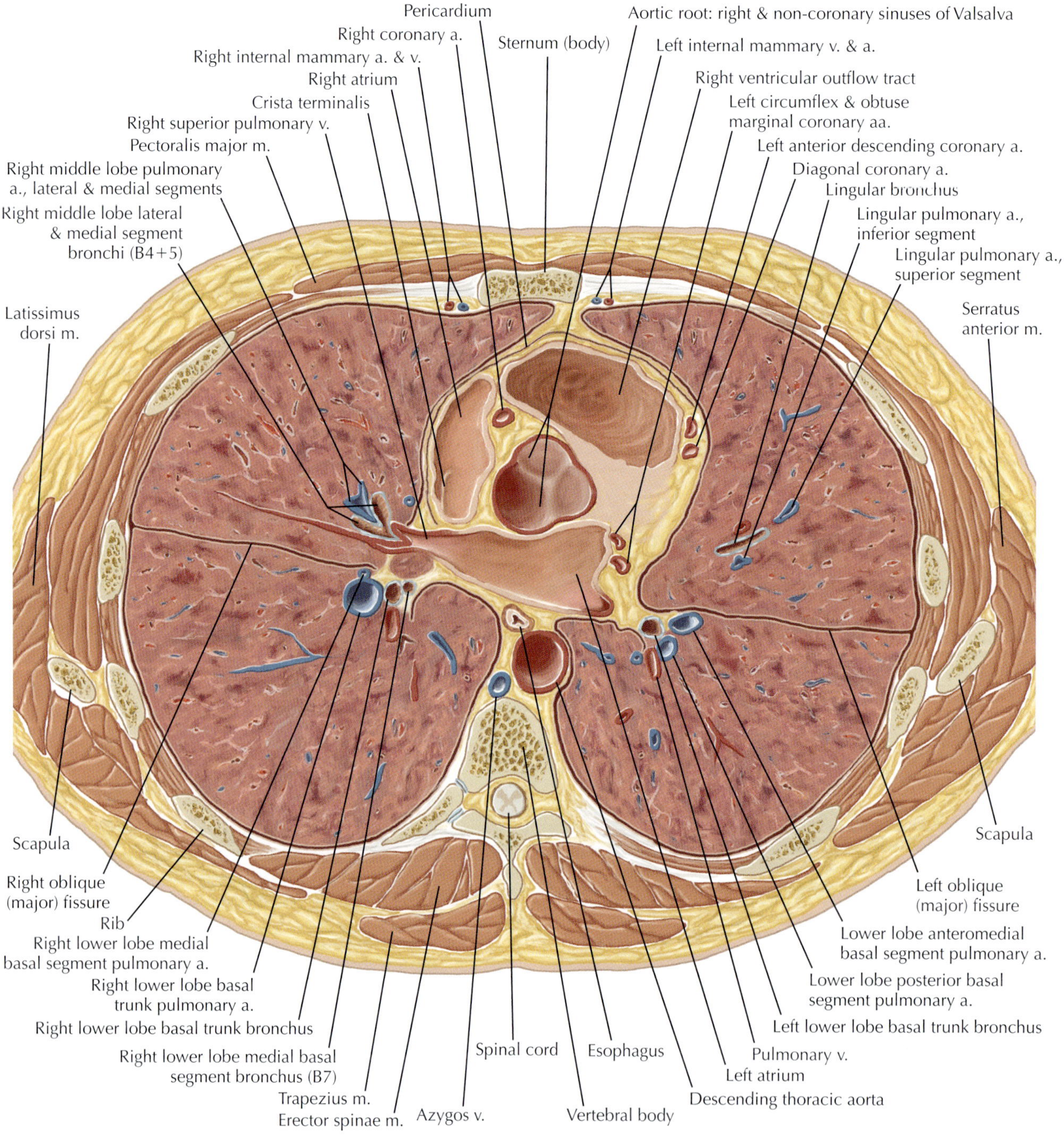

Pericardium
Right coronary a.
Right internal mammary a. & v.
Right atrium
Crista terminalis
Right superior pulmonary v.
Pectoralis major m.
Right middle lobe pulmonary a., lateral & medial segments
Right middle lobe lateral & medial segment bronchi (B4+5)
Latissimus dorsi m.
Sternum (body)
Aortic root: right & non-coronary sinuses of Valsalva
Left internal mammary v. & a.
Right ventricular outflow tract
Left circumflex & obtuse marginal coronary aa.
Left anterior descending coronary a.
Diagonal coronary a.
Lingular bronchus
Lingular pulmonary a., inferior segment
Lingular pulmonary a., superior segment
Serratus anterior m.
Scapula
Right oblique (major) fissure
Rib
Right lower lobe medial basal segment pulmonary a.
Right lower lobe basal trunk pulmonary a.
Right lower lobe basal trunk bronchus
Right lower lobe medial basal segment bronchus (B7)
Trapezius m.
Erector spinae m.
Azygos v.
Spinal cord
Vertebral body
Esophagus
Descending thoracic aorta
Left atrium
Pulmonary v.
Left lower lobe basal trunk bronchus
Lower lobe posterior basal segment pulmonary a.
Lower lobe anteromedial basal segment pulmonary a.
Left oblique (major) fissure
Scapula

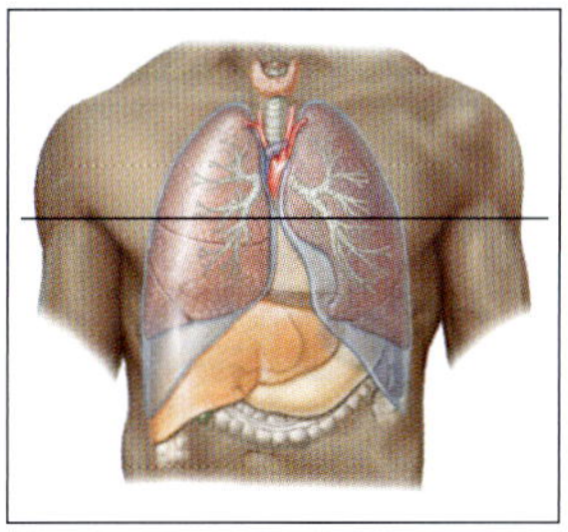

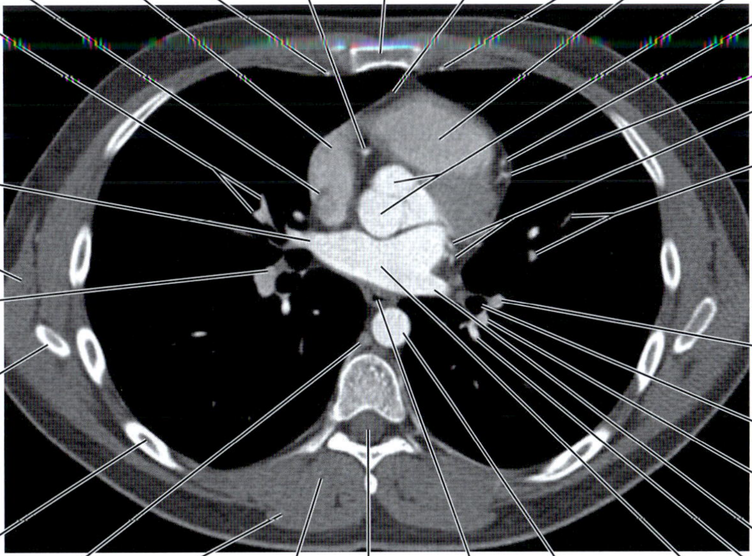
Crista terminalis
Right atrium
Right internal mammary a.
Right coronary a.
Sternum (body)
Pericardium
Left internal mammary a.
Right ventricular outflow tract
Aortic root: non-coronary & right sinuses of Valsalva
Right middle lobe pulmonary a., lateral & medial segments
Right superior pulmonary v.
Latissimus dorsi m.
Right lower lobe medial basal segment pulmonary a.
Scapula
Rib
Left anterior descending coronary a.
Diagonal coronary a.
Left circumflex & obtuse marginal coronary aa.
Lingular pulmonary aa., inferior and superior segments
Left lower lobe antero-medial basal segment pulmonary a.
Left lower basal bronchial trunk
Left lower lobe posterior basal segment pulmonary a.
Left inferior pulmonary v.
Azygos v.
Trapezius m.
Erector spinae m.
Spinal cord
Esophagus
Descending thoracic aorta
Left atrium
Pulmonary v.

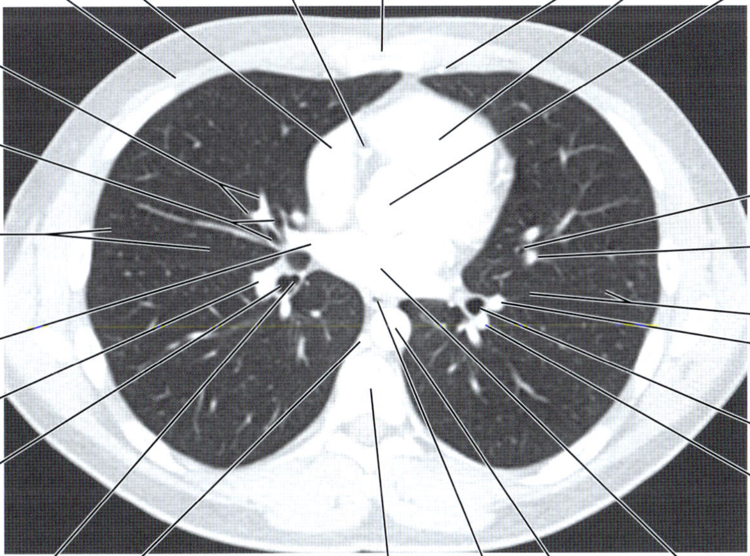
Pectoralis major m.
Right atrium
Right coronary a.
Sternum (body)
Left internal mammary a.
Right ventricular outflow tract
Ascending aorta
Right middle lobe lateral & medial segment pulmonary aa.
Right middle lobe lateral & medial segment bronchi (B4+5)
Right oblique (major) fissure
Right superior pulmonary v.
Right lower lobe basal trunk pulmonary a.
Right lower lobe basal trunk bronchus
Lingular bronchus
Lingular pulmonary a.
Left oblique (major) fissure
Left lower lobe antero-medial basal segment pulmonary a.
Left lower lobe basal trunk bronchus
Left lower lobe posterior basal segment pulmonary a.
Right lower lobe medial basal segment bronchus (B7)
Azygos v.
Vertebral body
Esophagus
Descending thoracic aorta
Left atrium

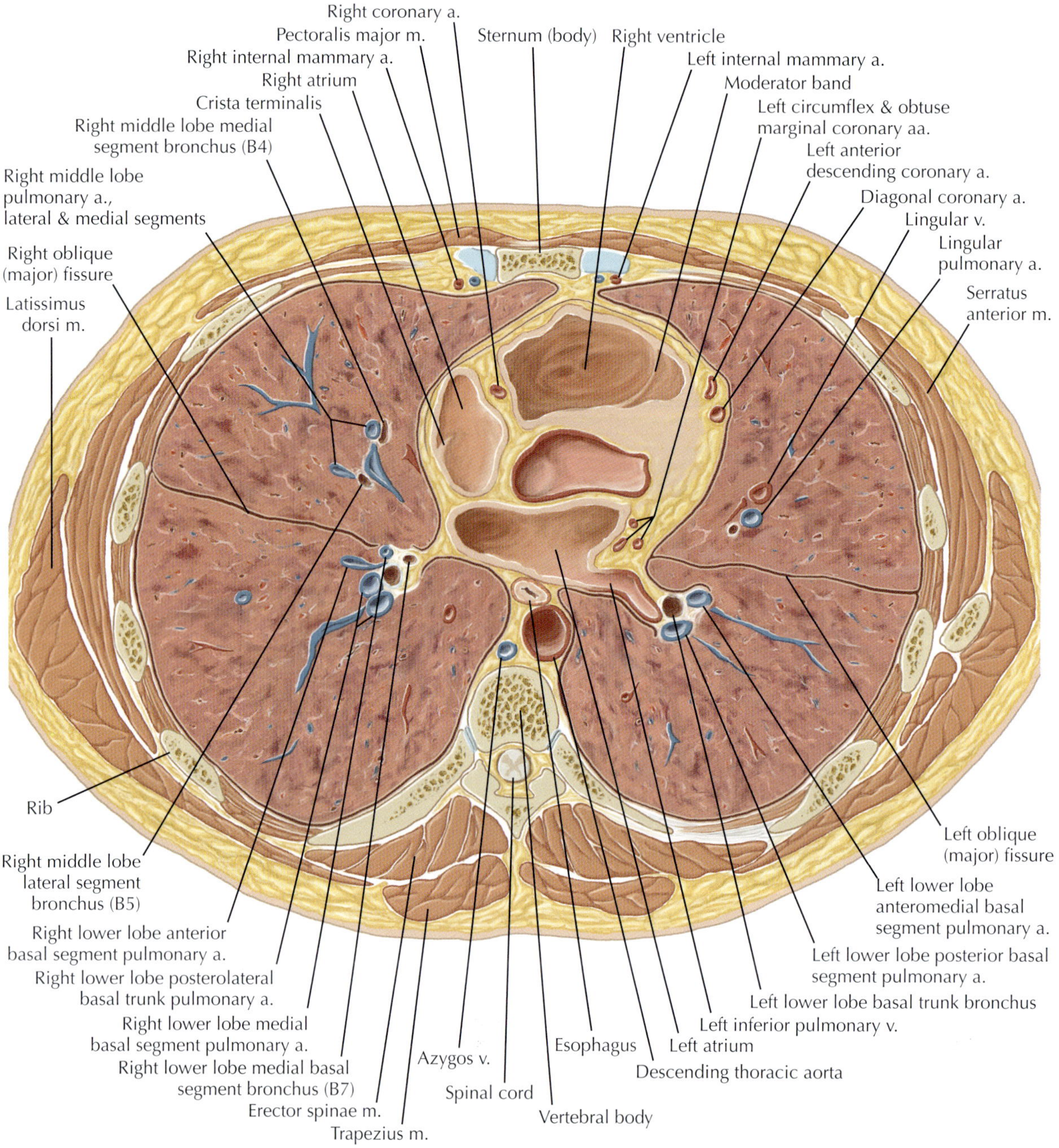

NORMAL VARIANTS

As previously noted, pulmonary artery branching variations are common. In the right lower lobe, the right lower lobe basal arterial trunk usually gives rise first to the medial basal segmental right lower lobe pulmonary artery, followed by a trifurcation into anterior, lateral, and posterior basal segmental arteries. In this patient, however, the medial basal segmental vessel originates first, followed by the anterior basal segmental artery; the lateral and posterior basal segmental vessels remain briefly combined in a posterolateral basal pulmonary arterial trunk. The *right lower lobe posterolateral basal trunk pulmonary artery* subsequently bifurcates into *lateral* and *posterior basal* segmental pulmonary arteries. This variant branching pattern is probably the most commonly encountered variant arterial branching pattern affecting the lower lobe pulmonary arteries, and is of no clinical significance.

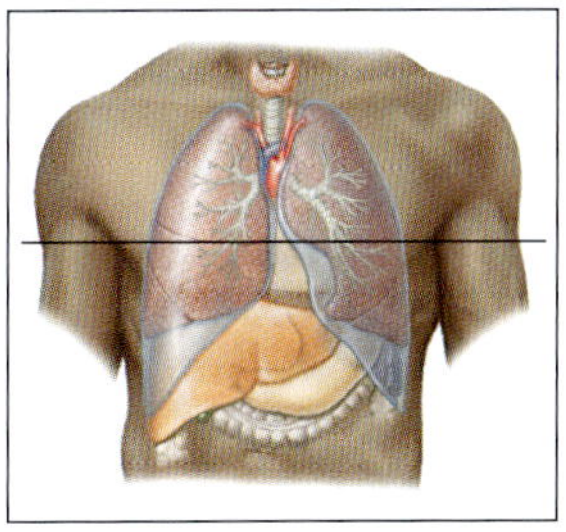

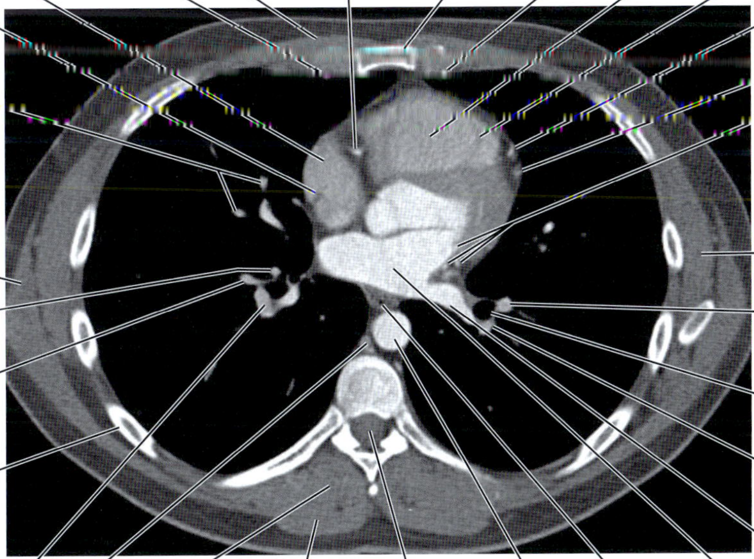
Right atrium
Right internal mammary a.
Pectoralis major m.
Right coronary a.
Sternum (body)
Left internal mammary a.
Right ventricle
Moderator band
Crista terminalis
Right middle lobe lateral & medial segment pulmonary aa.
Latissimus dorsi m.
Right lower lobe medial basal segment pulmonary a.
Right lower lobe anterior basal segment pulmonary a.
Rib
Left anterior descending coronary a.
Diagonal coronary a.
Left circumflex & obtuse marginal coronary aa.
Serratus anterior m.
Left lower lobe antero-medial basal segment pulmonary a.
Left lower lobe basal trunk bronchus
Left lower lobe posterior basal segment pulmonary a.
Left inferior pulmonary v.
Right lower lobe posterolateral basal trunk pulmonary a.
Azygos v.
Erector spinae m.
Trapezius m.
Spinal cord
Descending thoracic aorta
Esophagus
Left atrium

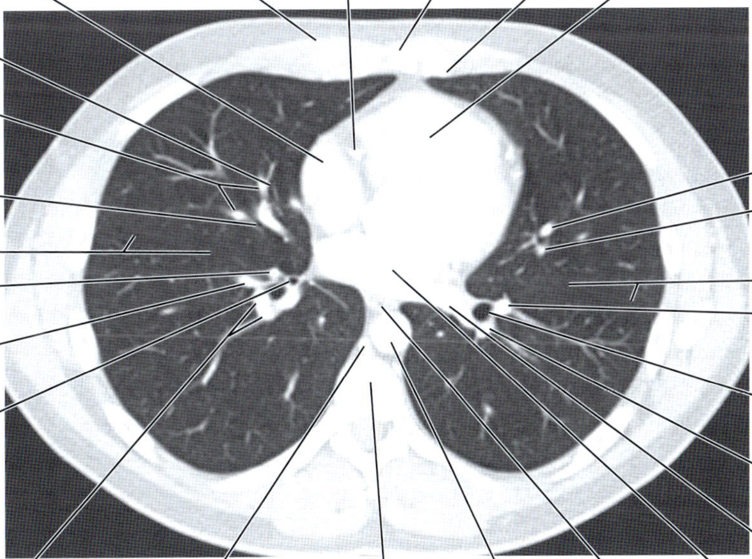
Right atrium
Pectoralis major m.
Right coronary a.
Sternum (body)
Left internal mammary a.
Right ventricle
Right middle lobe medial segment bronchus (B4)
Right middle lobe lateral & medial segment pulmonary aa.
Right middle lobe lateral segment bronchus (B5)
Right oblique (major) fissure
Right lower lobe medial basal segment pulmonary a.
Right lower lobe anterior basal segment pulmonary a.
Right lower lobe medial basal segment bronchus (B7)
Lingular v.
Lingular pulmonary a.
Left oblique (major) fissure
Left lower lobe antero-medial basal segment pulmonary a.
Left lower lobe basal trunk bronchus
Left lower lobe posterior basal segment pulmonary a.
Left inferior pulmonary v.
Right lower lobe lateral & posterior basal segment pulmonary aa.
Azygos v.
Vertebral body
Descending thoracic aorta
Esophagus
Left atrium

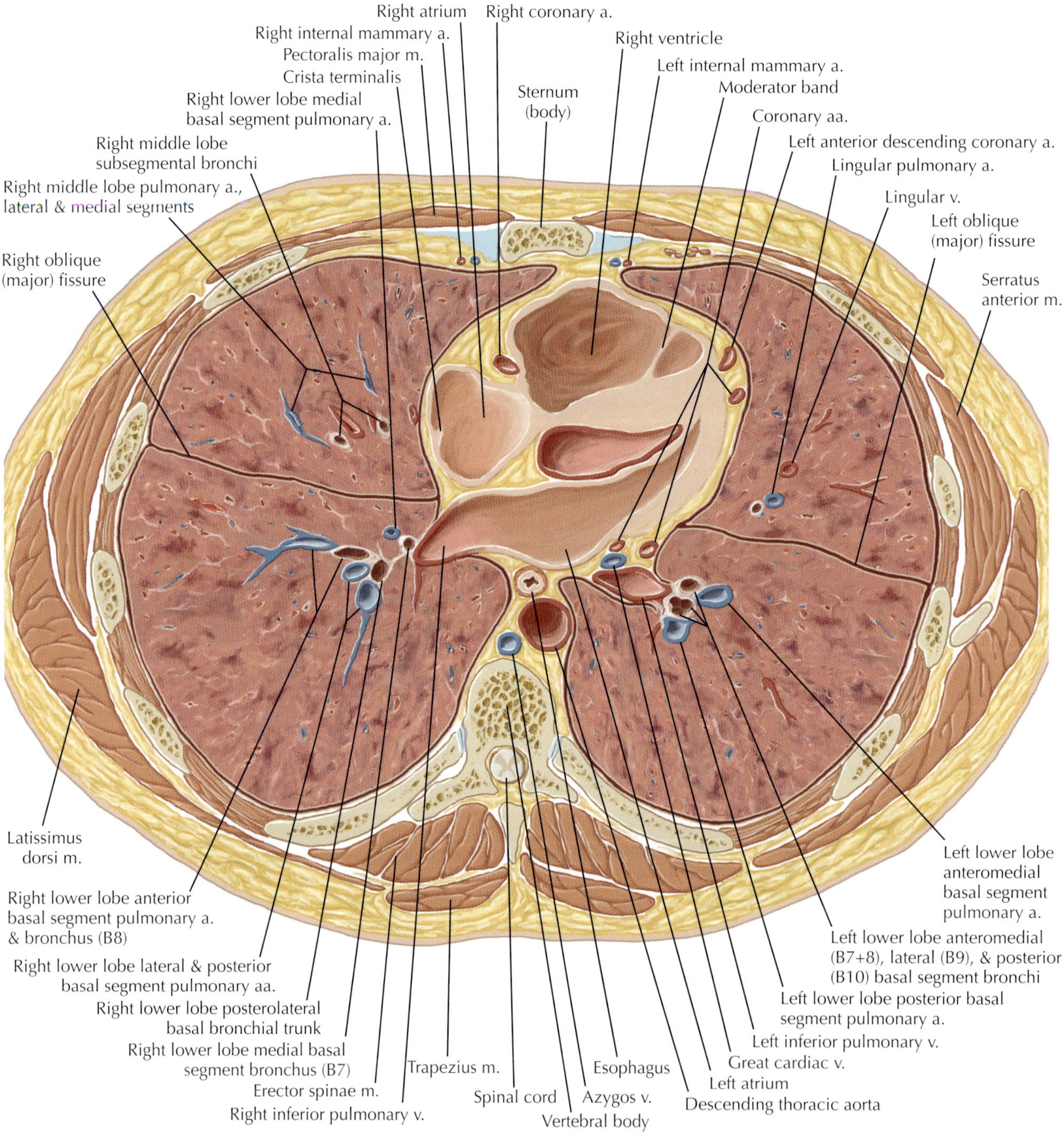
Right atrium
Right coronary a.
Right internal mammary a.
Pectoralis major m.
Crista terminalis
Right lower lobe medial basal segment pulmonary a.
Right middle lobe subsegmental bronchi
Right middle lobe pulmonary a., lateral & medial segments
Right oblique (major) fissure
Sternum (body)
Right ventricle
Left internal mammary a.
Moderator band
Coronary aa.
Left anterior descending coronary a.
Lingular pulmonary a.
Lingular v.
Left oblique (major) fissure
Serratus anterior m.
Latissimus dorsi m.
Right lower lobe anterior basal segment pulmonary a. & bronchus (B8)
Right lower lobe lateral & posterior basal segment pulmonary aa.
Right lower lobe posterolateral basal bronchial trunk
Right lower lobe medial basal segment bronchus (B7)
Erector spinae m.
Right inferior pulmonary v.
Trapezius m.
Spinal cord
Vertebral body
Azygos v.
Esophagus
Descending thoracic aorta
Left atrium
Great cardiac v.
Left inferior pulmonary v.
Left lower lobe posterior basal segment pulmonary a.
Left lower lobe anteromedial (B7+8), lateral (B9), & posterior (B10) basal segment bronchi
Left lower lobe anteromedial basal segment pulmonary a.

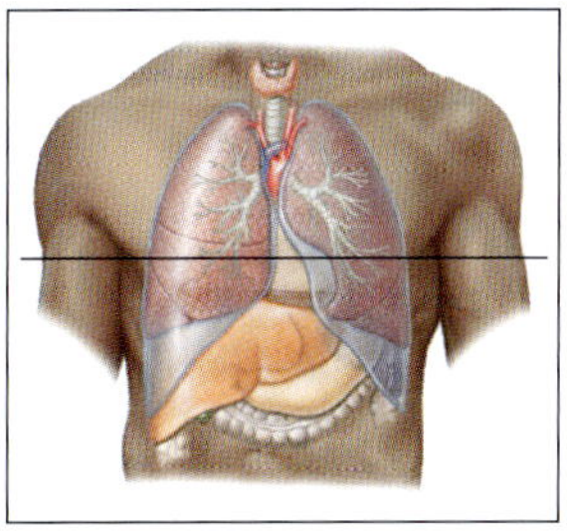

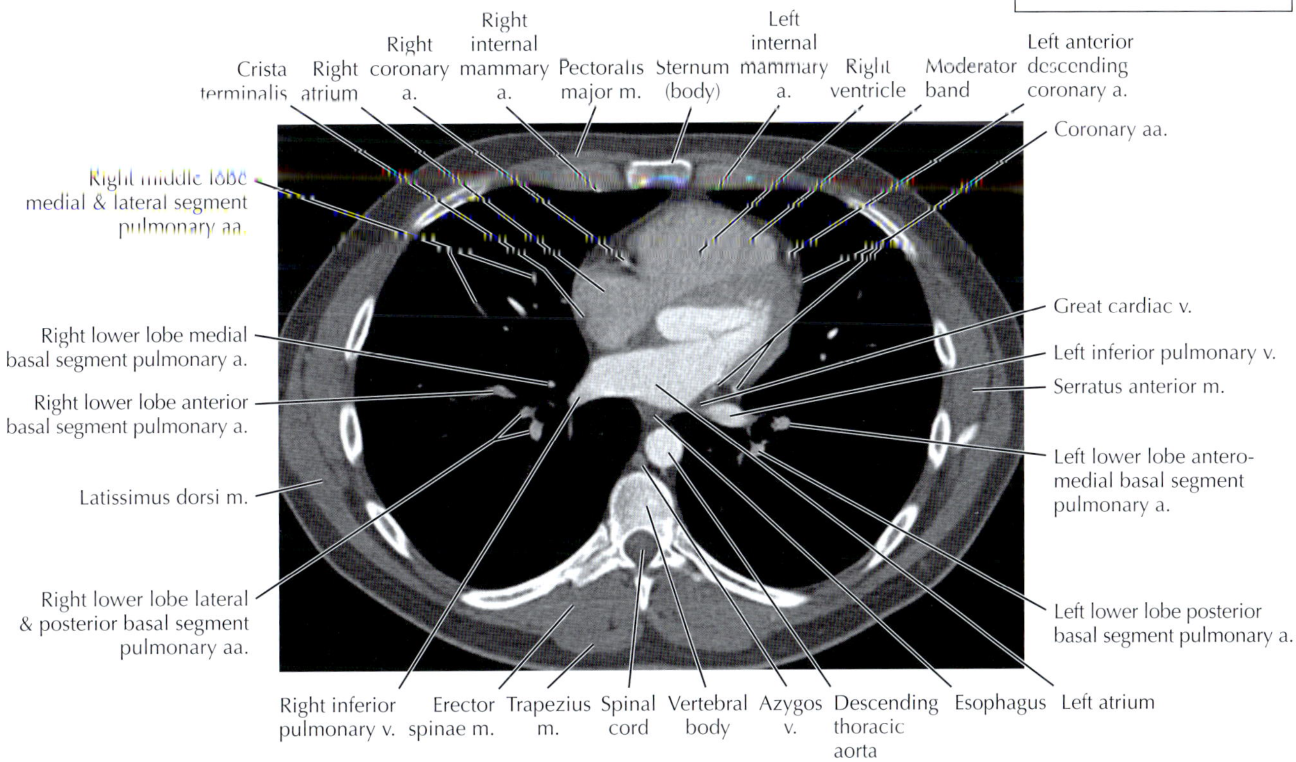
Crista terminalis
Right atrium
Right coronary a.
Right internal mammary a.
Pectoralis major m.
Sternum (body)
Left internal mammary a.
Right ventricle
Moderator band
Left anterior descending coronary a.
Coronary aa.
Right middle lobe medial & lateral segment pulmonary aa.
Right lower lobe medial basal segment pulmonary a.
Right lower lobe anterior basal segment pulmonary a.
Latissimus dorsi m.
Right lower lobe lateral & posterior basal segment pulmonary aa.
Great cardiac v.
Left inferior pulmonary v.
Serratus anterior m.
Left lower lobe antero-medial basal segment pulmonary a.
Left lower lobe posterior basal segment pulmonary a.
Right inferior pulmonary v.
Erector spinae m.
Trapezius m.
Spinal cord
Vertebral body
Azygos v.
Descending thoracic aorta
Esophagus
Left atrium

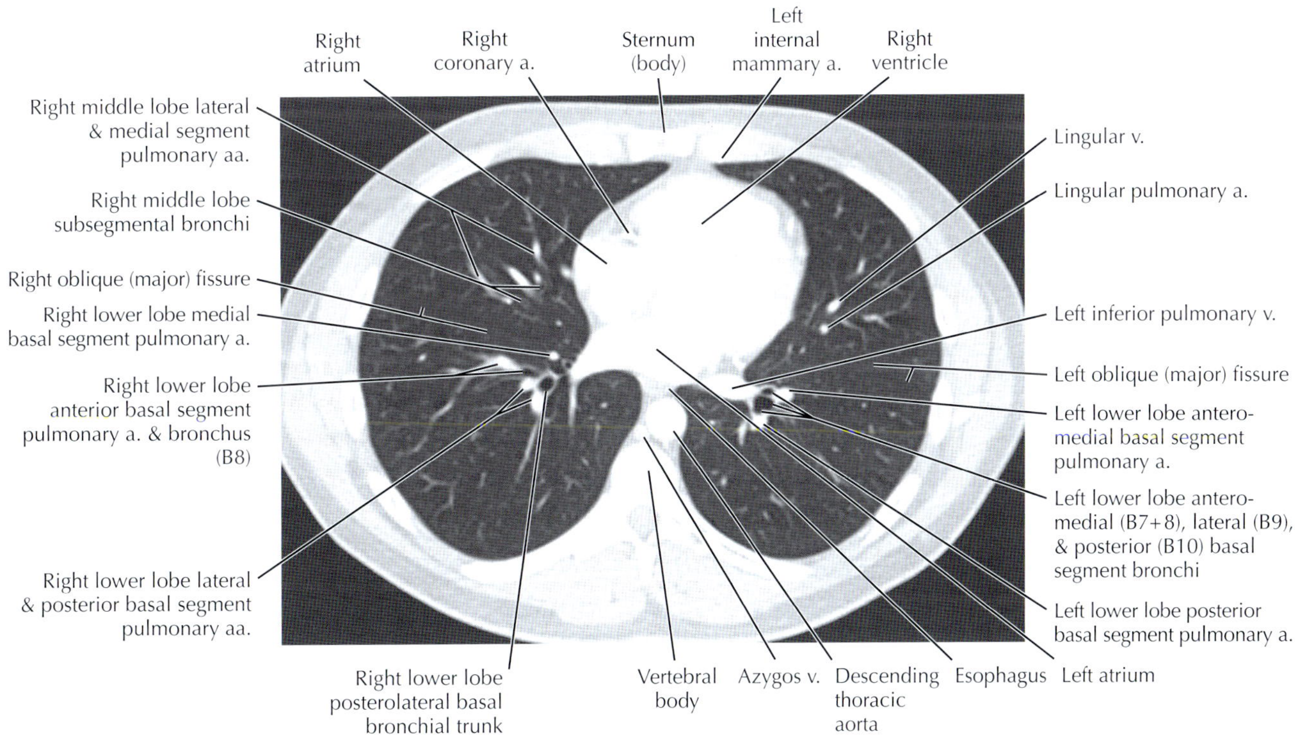
Right atrium
Right coronary a.
Sternum (body)
Left internal mammary a.
Right ventricle
Right middle lobe lateral & medial segment pulmonary aa.
Right middle lobe subsegmental bronchi
Right oblique (major) fissure
Right lower lobe medial basal segment pulmonary a.
Right lower lobe anterior basal segment pulmonary a. & bronchus (B8)
Right lower lobe lateral & posterior basal segment pulmonary aa.
Lingular v.
Lingular pulmonary a.
Left inferior pulmonary v.
Left oblique (major) fissure
Left lower lobe antero-medial basal segment pulmonary a.
Left lower lobe antero-medial (B7+8), lateral (B9), & posterior (B10) basal segment bronchi
Left lower lobe posterior basal segment pulmonary a.
Right lower lobe posterolateral basal bronchial trunk
Vertebral body
Azygos v.
Descending thoracic aorta
Esophagus
Left atrium

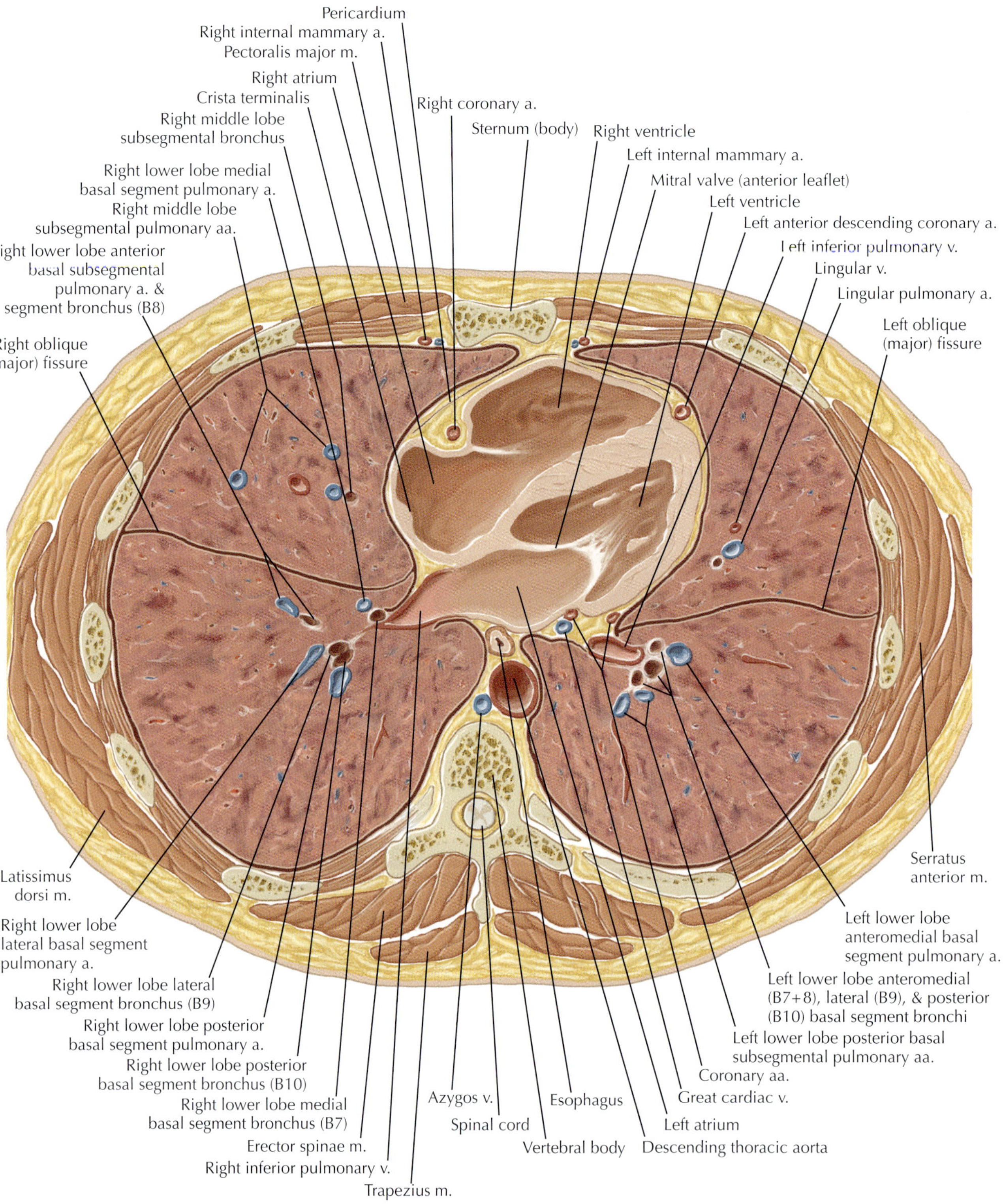
Pericardium
Right internal mammary a.
Pectoralis major m.
Right atrium
Crista terminalis
Right coronary a.
Sternum (body)
Right ventricle
Right middle lobe subsegmental bronchus
Left internal mammary a.
Mitral valve (anterior leaflet)
Right lower lobe medial basal segment pulmonary a.
Left ventricle
Right middle lobe subsegmental pulmonary aa.
Left anterior descending coronary a.
Left inferior pulmonary v.
Right lower lobe anterior basal subsegmental pulmonary a. & segment bronchus (B8)
Lingular v.
Lingular pulmonary a.
Left oblique (major) fissure
Right oblique (major) fissure
Latissimus dorsi m.
Serratus anterior m.
Right lower lobe lateral basal segment pulmonary a.
Left lower lobe anteromedial basal segment pulmonary a.
Right lower lobe lateral basal segment bronchus (B9)
Left lower lobe anteromedial (B7+8), lateral (B9), & posterior (B10) basal segment bronchi
Right lower lobe posterior basal segment pulmonary a.
Left lower lobe posterior basal subsegmental pulmonary aa.
Right lower lobe posterior basal segment bronchus (B10)
Coronary aa.
Azygos v.
Esophagus
Great cardiac v.
Right lower lobe medial basal segment bronchus (B7)
Spinal cord
Left atrium
Erector spinae m.
Vertebral body
Descending thoracic aorta
Right inferior pulmonary v.
Trapezius m.

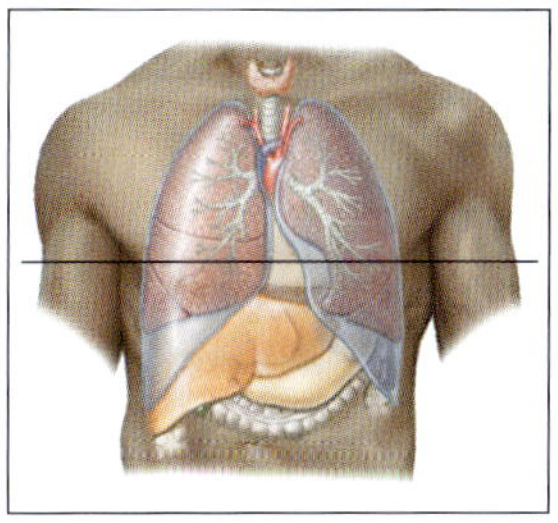

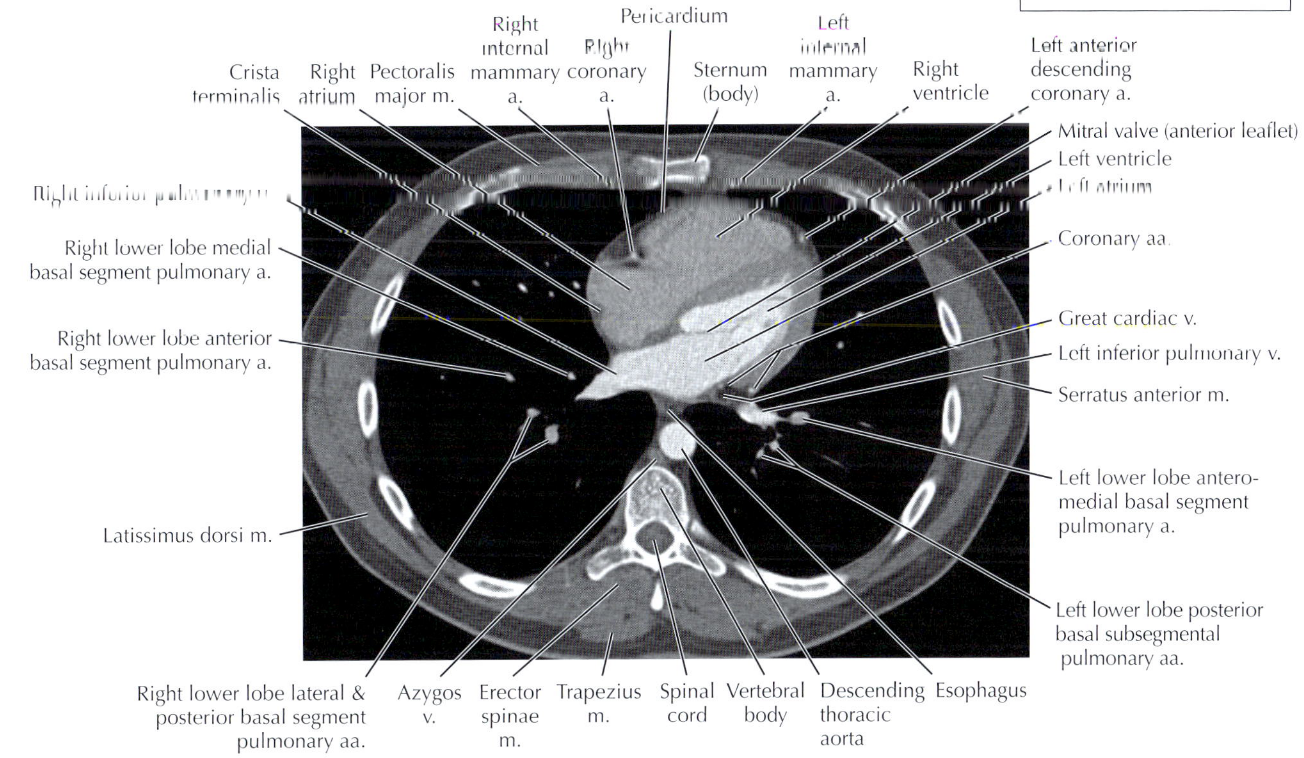
Crista terminalis
Right atrium
Pectoralis major m.
Right internal mammary a.
Right coronary a.
Pericardium
Sternum (body)
Left internal mammary a.
Right ventricle
Left anterior descending coronary a.
Mitral valve (anterior leaflet)
Left ventricle
Coronary aa.
Great cardiac v.
Left inferior pulmonary v.
Serratus anterior m.
Left lower lobe antero-medial basal segment pulmonary a.
Left lower lobe posterior basal subsegmental pulmonary aa.
Right lower lobe medial basal segment pulmonary a.
Right lower lobe anterior basal segment pulmonary a.
Latissimus dorsi m.
Right lower lobe lateral & posterior basal segment pulmonary aa.
Azygos v.
Erector spinae m.
Trapezius m.
Spinal cord
Vertebral body
Descending thoracic aorta
Esophagus

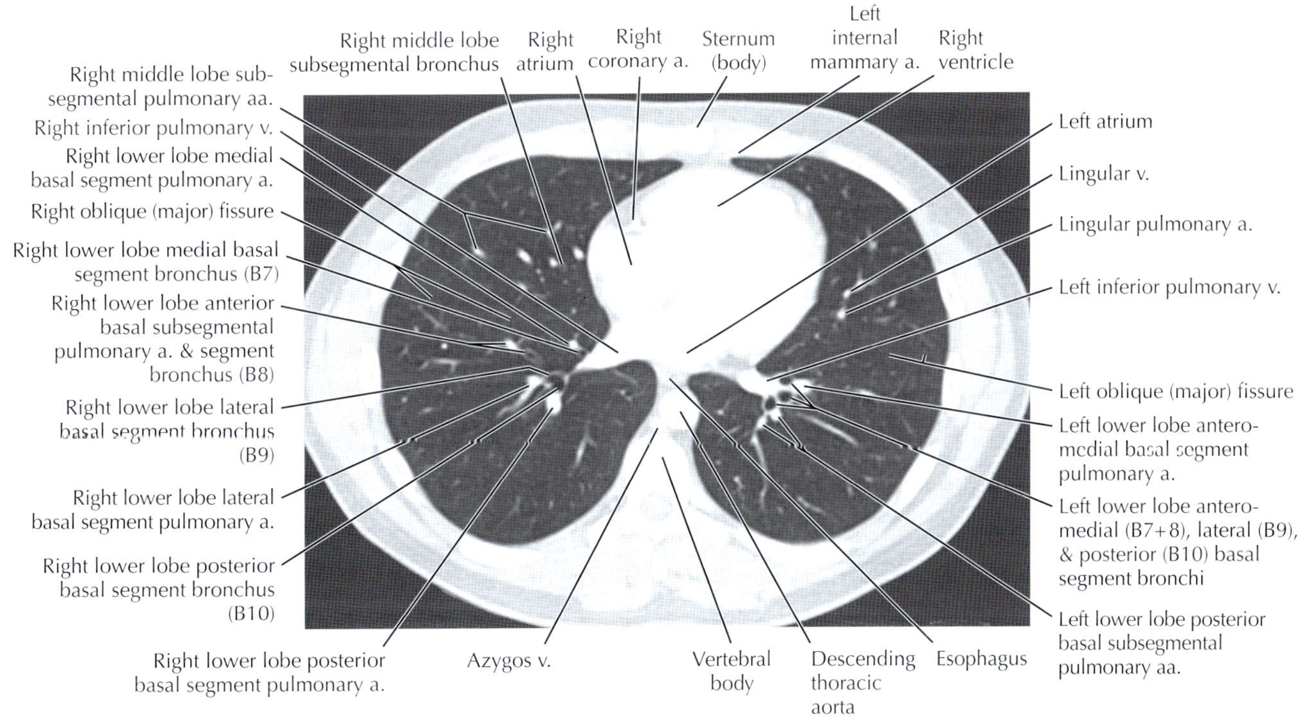
Right middle lobe subsegmental bronchus
Right atrium
Right coronary a.
Sternum (body)
Left internal mammary a.
Right ventricle
Right middle lobe subsegmental pulmonary aa.
Right inferior pulmonary v.
Right lower lobe medial basal segment pulmonary a.
Right oblique (major) fissure
Right lower lobe medial basal segment bronchus (B7)
Right lower lobe anterior basal subsegmental pulmonary a. & segment bronchus (B8)
Right lower lobe lateral basal segment bronchus (B9)
Right lower lobe lateral basal segment pulmonary a.
Right lower lobe posterior basal segment bronchus (B10)
Right lower lobe posterior basal segment pulmonary a.
Azygos v.
Vertebral body
Descending thoracic aorta
Esophagus
Left atrium
Lingular v.
Lingular pulmonary a.
Left inferior pulmonary v.
Left oblique (major) fissure
Left lower lobe antero-medial basal segment pulmonary a.
Left lower lobe antero-medial (B7+8), lateral (B9), & posterior (B10) basal segment bronchi
Left lower lobe posterior basal subsegmental pulmonary aa.

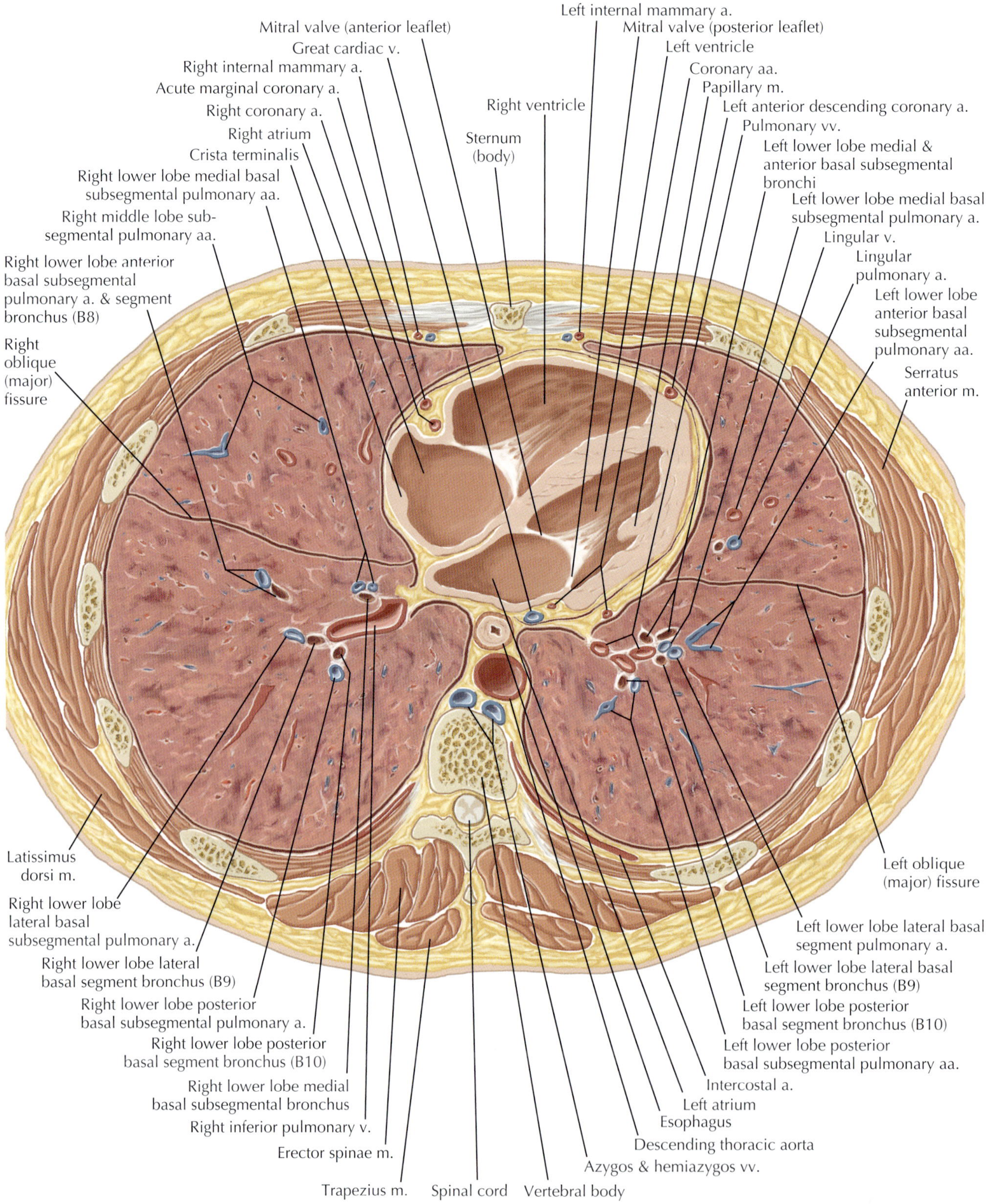
Left internal mammary a.
Mitral valve (anterior leaflet)
Mitral valve (posterior leaflet)
Great cardiac v.
Left ventricle
Right internal mammary a.
Coronary aa.
Acute marginal coronary a.
Papillary m.
Right coronary a.
Right ventricle
Left anterior descending coronary a.
Pulmonary vv.
Right atrium
Sternum (body)
Left lower lobe medial & anterior basal subsegmental bronchi
Crista terminalis
Right lower lobe medial basal subsegmental pulmonary aa.
Left lower lobe medial basal subsegmental pulmonary a.
Right middle lobe sub-segmental pulmonary aa.
Lingular v.
Lingular pulmonary a.
Right lower lobe anterior basal subsegmental pulmonary a. & segment bronchus (B8)
Left lower lobe anterior basal subsegmental pulmonary aa.
Right oblique (major) fissure
Serratus anterior m.
Latissimus dorsi m.
Left oblique (major) fissure
Right lower lobe lateral basal subsegmental pulmonary a.
Left lower lobe lateral basal segment pulmonary a.
Right lower lobe lateral basal segment bronchus (B9)
Left lower lobe lateral basal segment bronchus (B9)
Right lower lobe posterior basal subsegmental pulmonary a.
Left lower lobe posterior basal segment bronchus (B10)
Right lower lobe posterior basal segment bronchus (B10)
Left lower lobe posterior basal subsegmental pulmonary aa.
Right lower lobe medial basal subsegmental bronchus
Intercostal a.
Left atrium
Right inferior pulmonary v.
Esophagus
Erector spinae m.
Descending thoracic aorta
Azygos & hemiazygos vv.
Trapezius m.
Spinal cord
Vertebral body

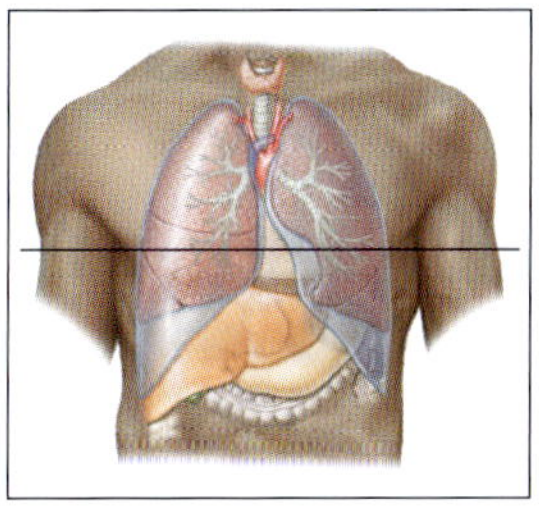

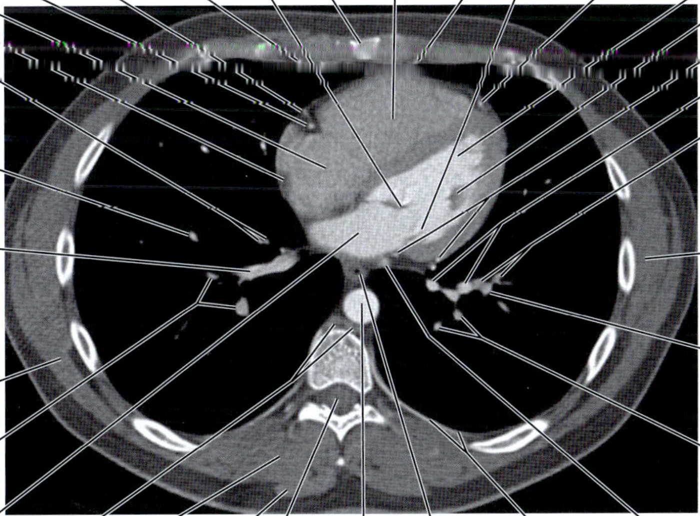
Right atrium
Right coronary a.
Acute marginal coronary a.
Right internal mammary a.
Mitral valve (anterior leaflet)
Sternum (body)
Right ventricle
Left internal mammary a.
Mitral valve (posterior leaflet)
Left anterior descending coronary artery
Left ventricle
Crista terminalis
Right lower lobe medial basal subsegmental pulmonary aa.
Right lower lobe anterior basal segment pulmonary a.
Pulmonary vein
Latissimus dorsi m.
Right lower lobe lateral & posterior basal segment pulmonary aa.
Papillary muscle
Coronary aa.
Pulmonary vv.
Left lower lobe anterior & medial basal subsegmental pulmonary aa.
Serratus anterior m.
Left lower lobe lateral basal segment pulmonary a.
Left lower lobe posterior basal subsegmental pulmonary aa.
Left atrium
Azygos & hemiazygos vv.
Erector spinae m.
Trapezius m.
Spinal cord
Descending thoracic aorta
Esophagus
Intercostal artery
Coronary sinus

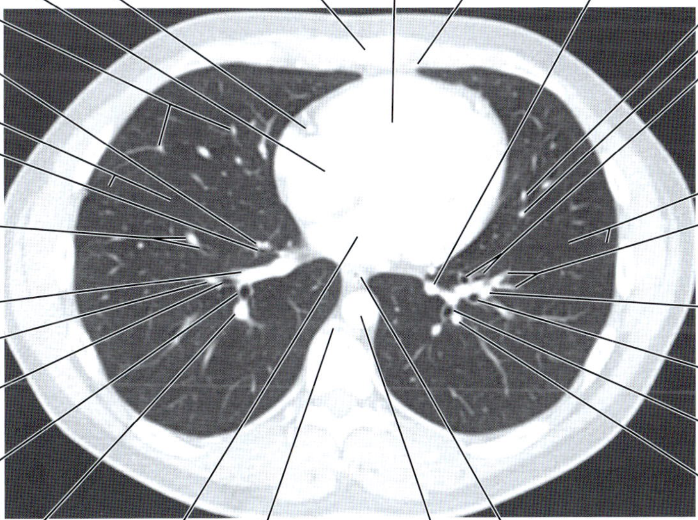
Right atrium
Right coronary a.
Sternum (body)
Right ventricle
Left internal mammary a.
Pulmonary v.
Right middle lobe subsegmental pulmonary aa.
Right lower lobe medial basal subsegmental pulmonary a.
Right oblique (major) fissure
Right lower lobe medial basal subsegmental bronchus
Right lower lobe anterior basal subsegmental pulmonary a. & segment bronchus (B8)
Right inferior pulmonary v.
Right lower lobe lateral basal subsegmental pulmonary a.
Right lower lobe lateral basal segment bronchus (B9)
Right lower lobe posterior basal segment bronchus (B10)
Right lower lobe posterior basal segment pulmonary a.
Lingular v.
Lingular pulmonary a.
Left lower lobe anterior & medial basal subsegmental bronchi
Left oblique (major) fissure
Left lower lobe anteromedial basal subsegmental pulmonary aa.
Left lower lobe lateral basal segment pulmonary a.
Left lower lobe lateral basal segment bronchus (B9)
Left lower lobe posterior basal segment bronchus (B10)
Left lower lobe posterior basal segment pulmonary a.
Left atrium
Azygos v.
Descending thoracic aorta
Esophagus

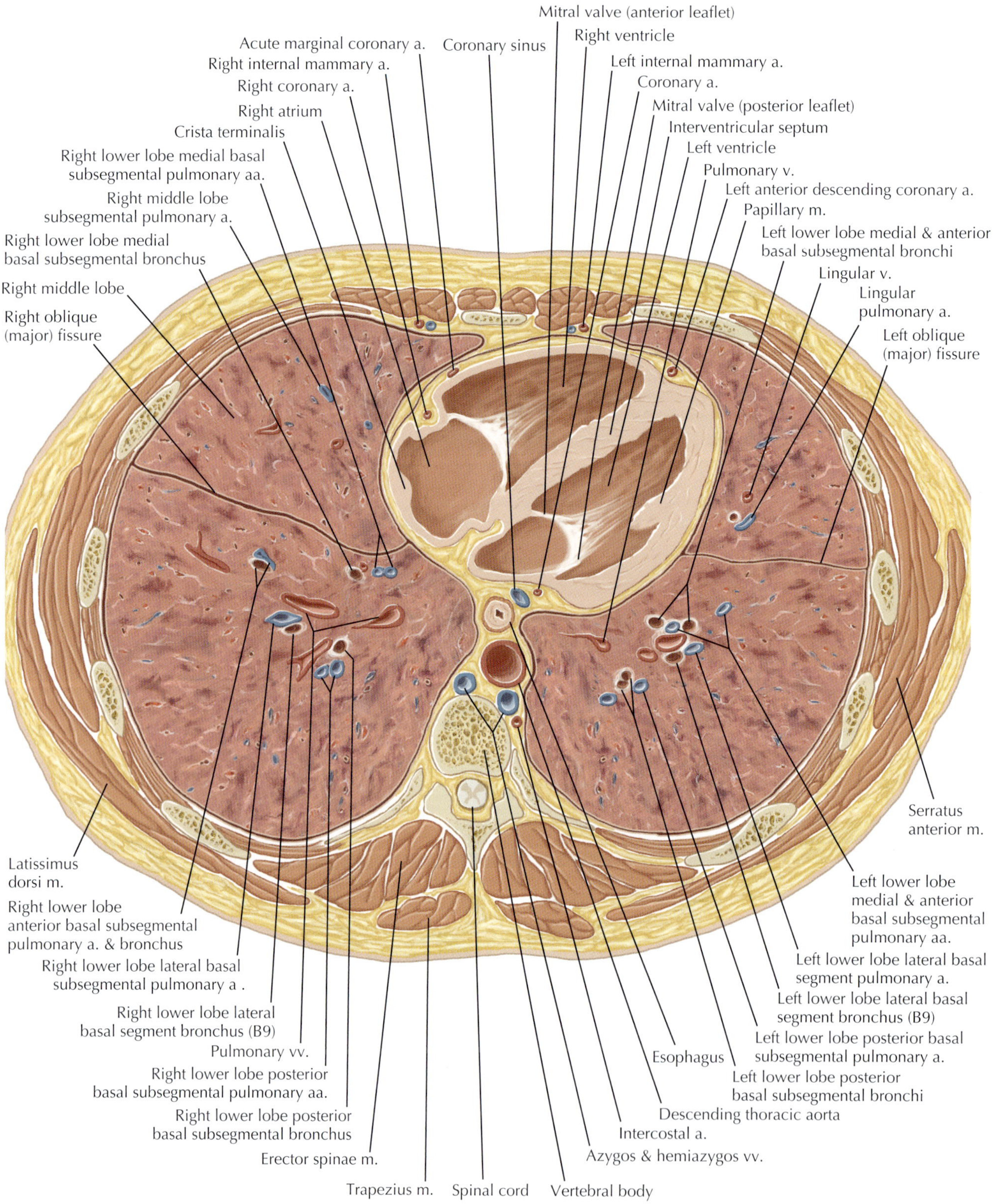
Mitral valve (anterior leaflet)
Right ventricle
Acute marginal coronary a.
Coronary sinus
Right internal mammary a.
Left internal mammary a.
Coronary a.
Right coronary a.
Mitral valve (posterior leaflet)
Right atrium
Interventricular septum
Crista terminalis
Left ventricle
Right lower lobe medial basal subsegmental pulmonary aa.
Pulmonary v.
Left anterior descending coronary a.
Right middle lobe subsegmental pulmonary a.
Papillary m.
Left lower lobe medial & anterior basal subsegmental bronchi
Right lower lobe medial basal subsegmental bronchus
Lingular v.
Right middle lobe
Lingular pulmonary a.
Right oblique (major) fissure
Left oblique (major) fissure
Serratus anterior m.
Latissimus dorsi m.
Left lower lobe medial & anterior basal subsegmental pulmonary aa.
Right lower lobe anterior basal subsegmental pulmonary a. & bronchus
Left lower lobe lateral basal segment pulmonary a.
Right lower lobe lateral basal subsegmental pulmonary a .
Left lower lobe lateral basal segment bronchus (B9)
Right lower lobe lateral basal segment bronchus (B9)
Left lower lobe posterior basal subsegmental pulmonary a.
Pulmonary vv.
Esophagus
Left lower lobe posterior basal subsegmental bronchi
Right lower lobe posterior basal subsegmental pulmonary aa.
Descending thoracic aorta
Right lower lobe posterior basal subsegmental bronchus
Intercostal a.
Erector spinae m.
Azygos & hemiazygos vv.
Trapezius m.
Spinal cord
Vertebral body

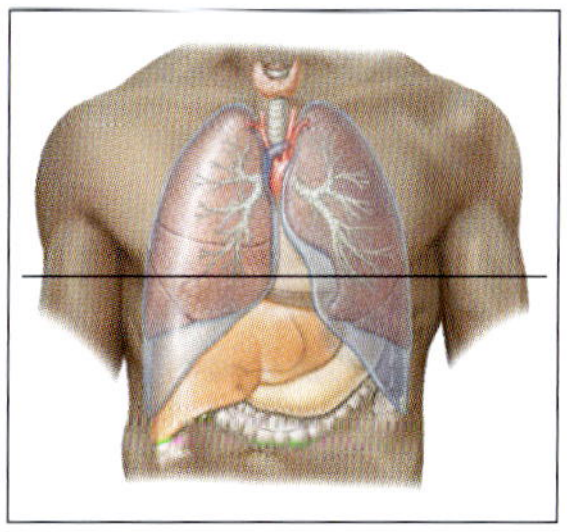

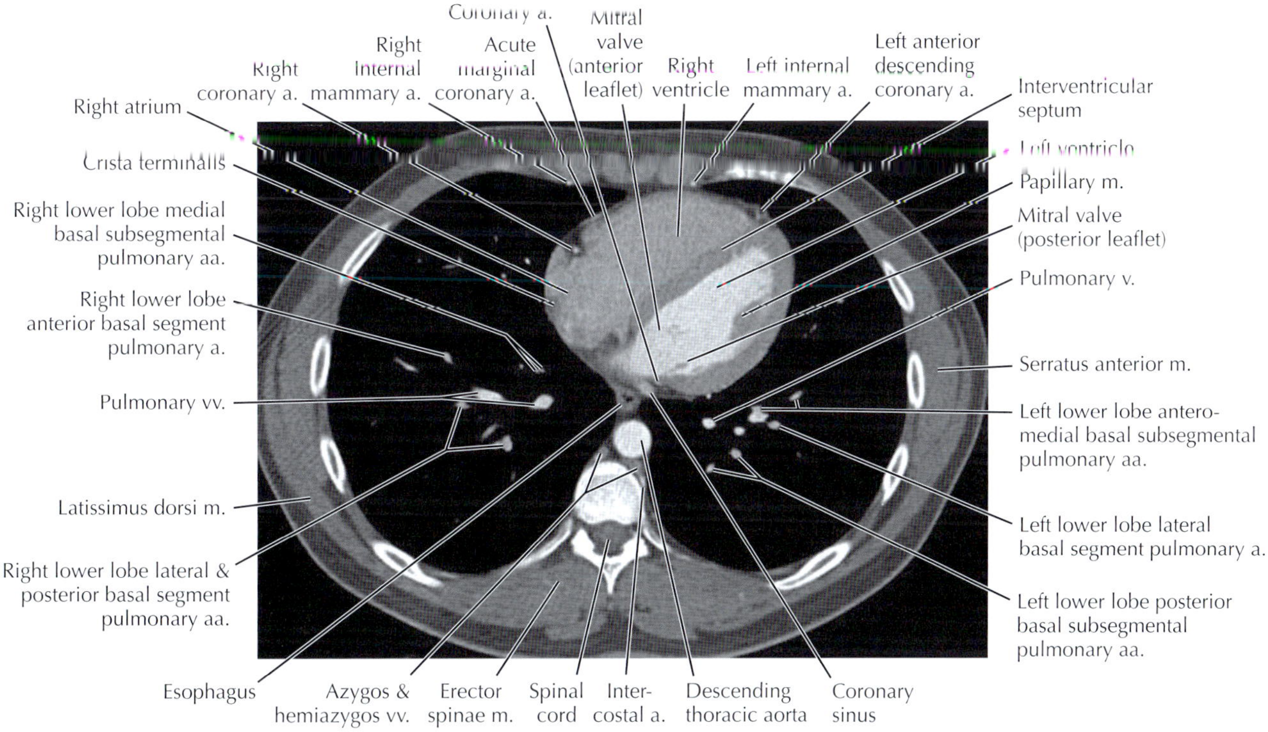
Coronary a.
Right atrium
Right coronary a.
Right internal mammary a.
Acute marginal coronary a.
Mitral valve (anterior leaflet)
Right ventricle
Left internal mammary a.
Left anterior descending coronary a.
Interventricular septum
Left ventricle
Crista terminalis
Papillary m.
Right lower lobe medial basal subsegmental pulmonary aa.
Mitral valve (posterior leaflet)
Pulmonary v.
Right lower lobe anterior basal segment pulmonary a.
Serratus anterior m.
Pulmonary vv.
Left lower lobe antero-medial basal subsegmental pulmonary aa.
Latissimus dorsi m.
Left lower lobe lateral basal segment pulmonary a.
Right lower lobe lateral & posterior basal segment pulmonary aa.
Left lower lobe posterior basal subsegmental pulmonary aa.
Esophagus
Azygos & hemiazygos vv.
Erector spinae m.
Spinal cord
Inter-costal a.
Descending thoracic aorta
Coronary sinus

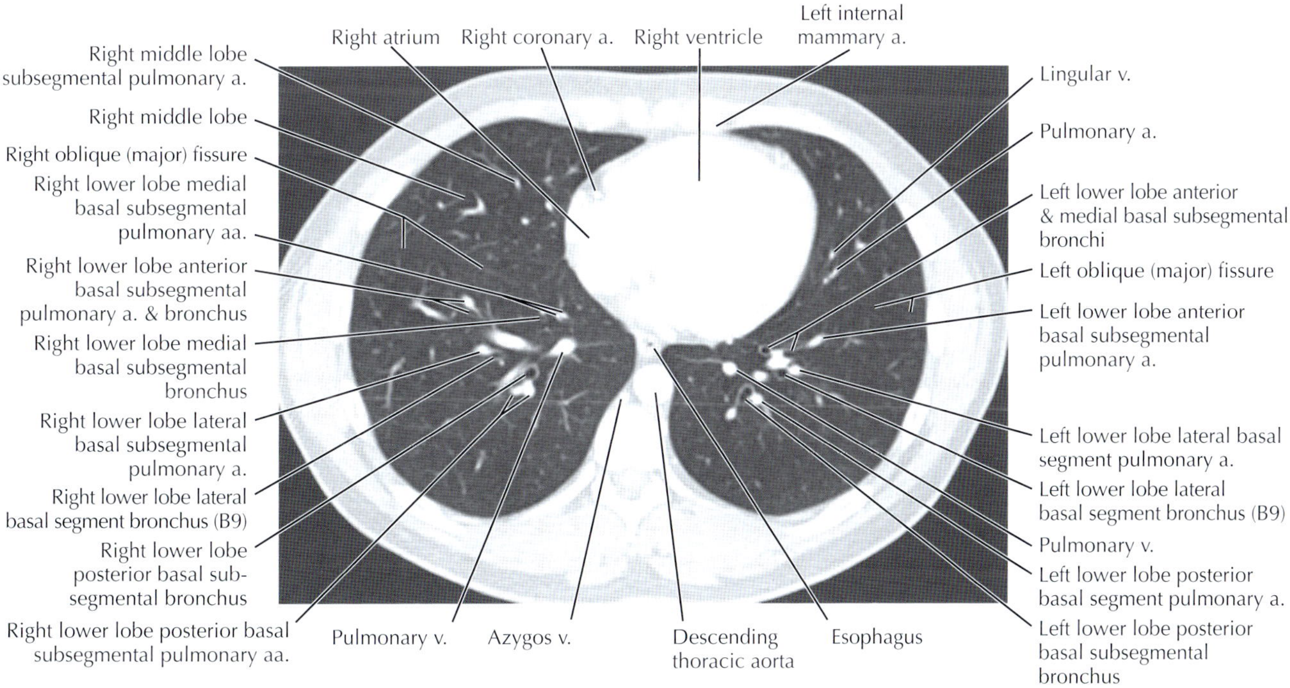
Right atrium
Right coronary a.
Right ventricle
Left internal mammary a.
Right middle lobe subsegmental pulmonary a.
Lingular v.
Right middle lobe
Pulmonary a.
Right oblique (major) fissure
Right lower lobe medial basal subsegmental pulmonary aa.
Left lower lobe anterior & medial basal subsegmental bronchi
Left oblique (major) fissure
Right lower lobe anterior basal subsegmental pulmonary a. & bronchus
Left lower lobe anterior basal subsegmental pulmonary a.
Right lower lobe medial basal subsegmental bronchus
Right lower lobe lateral basal subsegmental pulmonary a.
Left lower lobe lateral basal segment pulmonary a.
Right lower lobe lateral basal segment bronchus (B9)
Left lower lobe lateral basal segment bronchus (B9)
Right lower lobe posterior basal sub-segmental bronchus
Pulmonary v.
Left lower lobe posterior basal segment pulmonary a.
Right lower lobe posterior basal subsegmental pulmonary aa.
Pulmonary v.
Azygos v.
Descending thoracic aorta
Esophagus
Left lower lobe posterior basal subsegmental bronchus

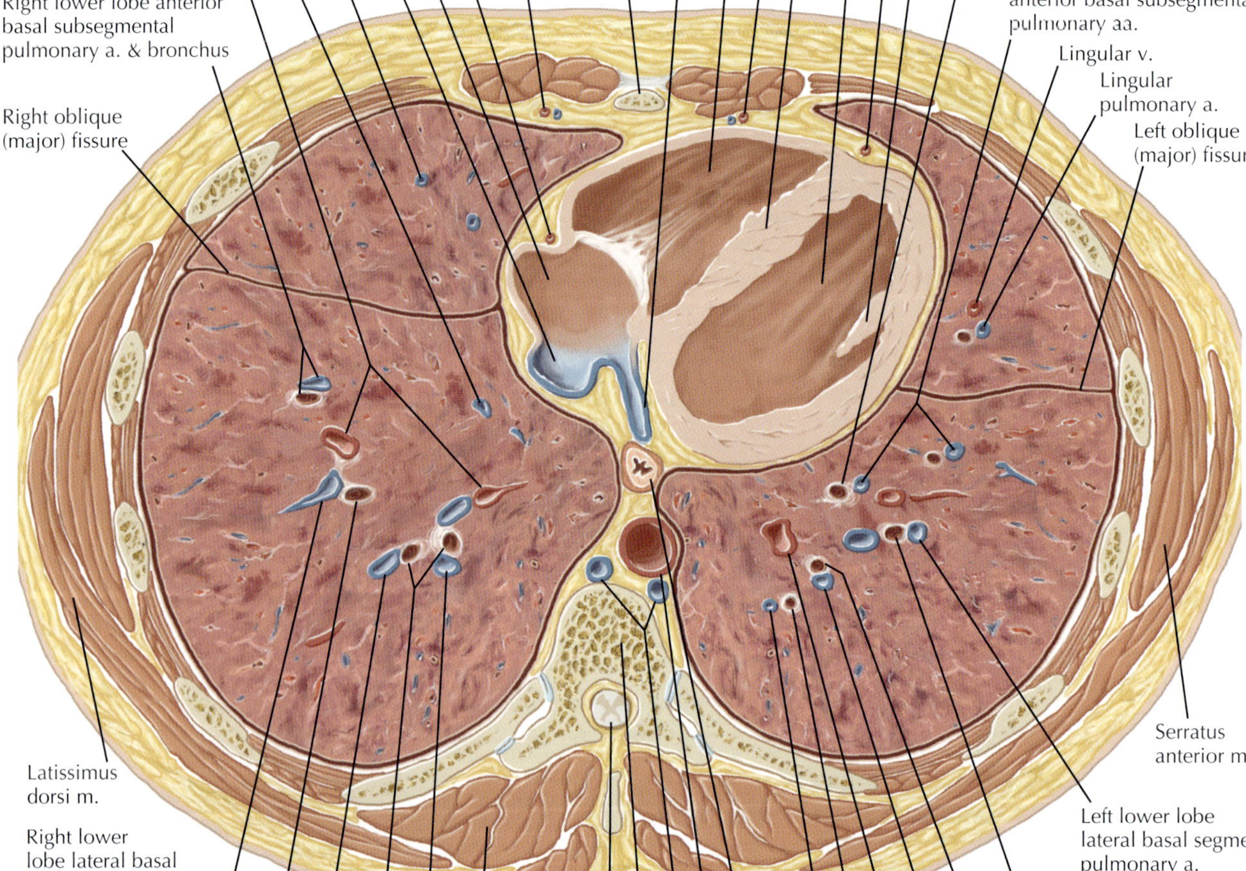
Right internal mammary a.
Right coronary a.
Right atrium
Inferior vena cava
Right middle lobe subsegmental pulmonary a.
Right lower lobe medial basal subsegmental pulmonary a.
Pulmonary vv.
Right lower lobe anterior basal subsegmental pulmonary a. & bronchus
Right oblique (major) fissure
Sternum (Xiphoid)
Coronary sinus
Right ventricle
Left internal mammary a.
Interventricular septum
Left ventricle
Left anterior descending coronary a.
Papillary m.
Left lower lobe medial basal subsegmental bronchus
Left lower lobe medial & anterior basal subsegmental pulmonary aa.
Lingular v.
Lingular pulmonary a.
Left oblique (major) fissure
Serratus anterior m.
Latissimus dorsi m.
Right lower lobe lateral basal subsegmental pulmonary a.
Right lower lobe lateral basal subsegmental bronchus
Right lower lobe posterior basal subsegmental pulmonary a.
Right lower lobe posterior basal subsegmental bronchi
Right lower lobe posterior basal subsegmental pulmonary a.
Erector spinae m.
Trapezius m.
Spinal cord
Vertebral body
Azygos & hemiazygos vv.
Descending thoracic aorta
Esophagus
Left lower lobe lateral basal segment pulmonary a.
Left lower lobe lateral basal segment bronchus (B9)
Left lower lobe posterior basal subsegmental bronchus
Left lower lobe posterior basal subsegmental pulmonary a.
Pulmonary v.
Left lower lobe posterior basal subsegmental bronchus
Left lower lobe posterior basal subsegmental pulmonary a.

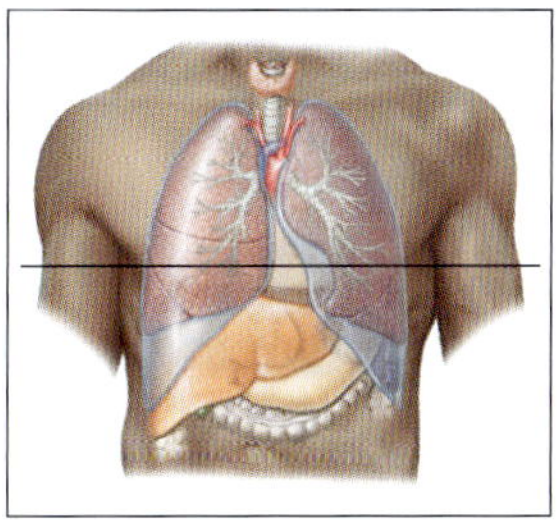

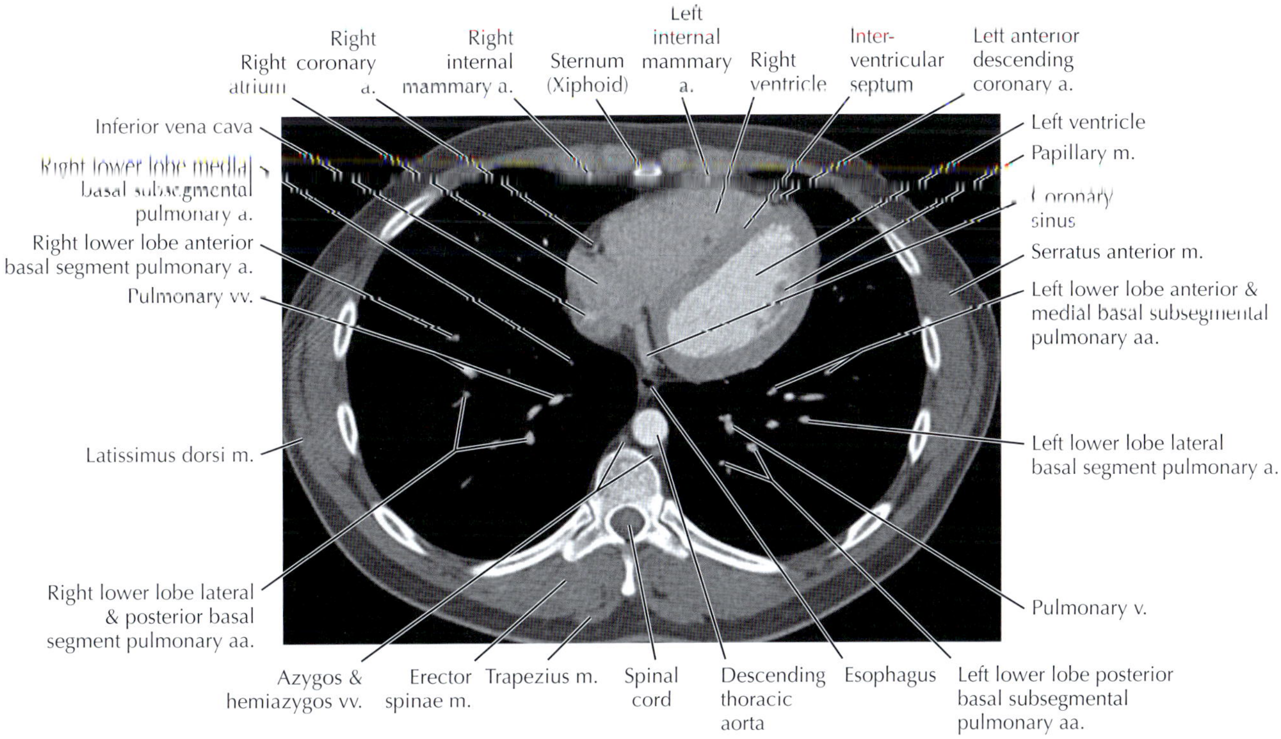
Right atrium
Right coronary a.
Right internal mammary a.
Sternum (Xiphoid)
Left internal mammary a.
Right ventricle
Inter-ventricular septum
Left anterior descending coronary a.
Inferior vena cava
Right lower lobe medial basal subsegmental pulmonary a.
Right lower lobe anterior basal segment pulmonary a.
Pulmonary vv.
Latissimus dorsi m.
Right lower lobe lateral & posterior basal segment pulmonary aa.
Left ventricle
Papillary m.
Coronary sinus
Serratus anterior m.
Left lower lobe anterior & medial basal subsegmental pulmonary aa.
Left lower lobe lateral basal segment pulmonary a.
Pulmonary v.
Azygos & hemiazygos vv.
Erector spinae m.
Trapezius m.
Spinal cord
Descending thoracic aorta
Esophagus
Left lower lobe posterior basal subsegmental pulmonary aa.

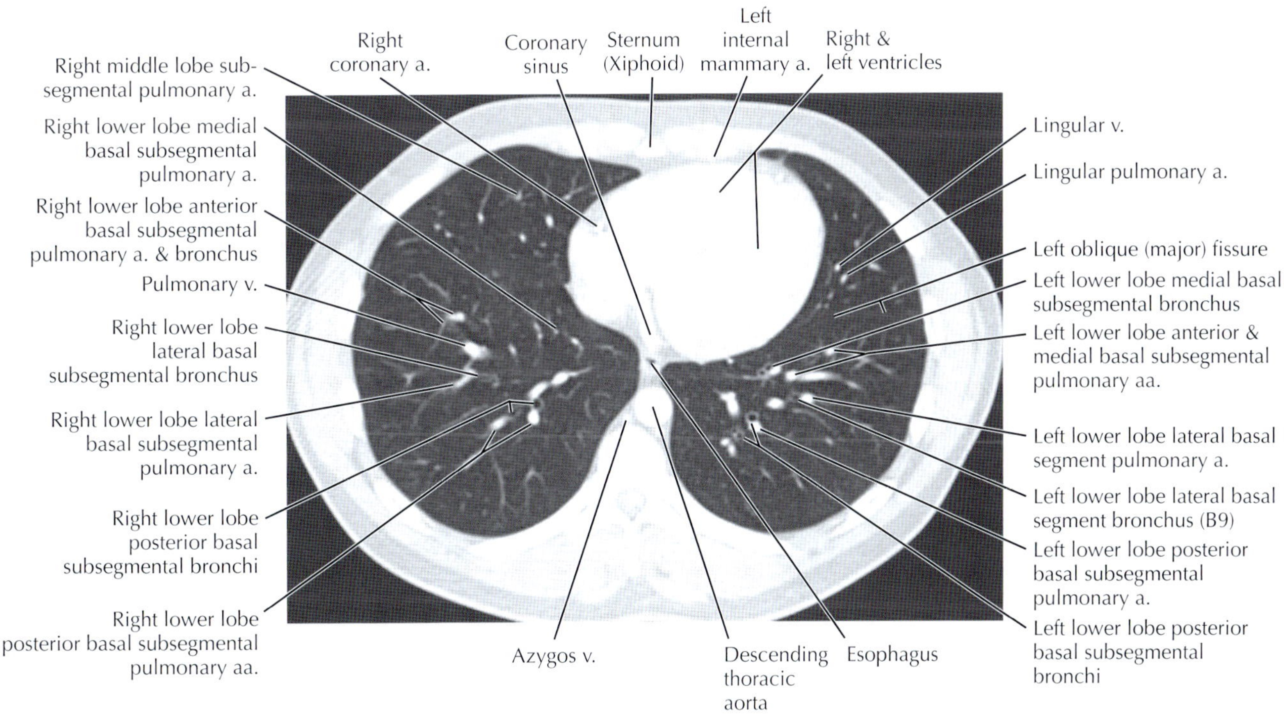
Right middle lobe sub-segmental pulmonary a.
Right coronary a.
Coronary sinus
Sternum (Xiphoid)
Left internal mammary a.
Right & left ventricles
Right lower lobe medial basal subsegmental pulmonary a.
Right lower lobe anterior basal subsegmental pulmonary a. & bronchus
Pulmonary v.
Right lower lobe lateral basal subsegmental bronchus
Right lower lobe lateral basal subsegmental pulmonary a.
Right lower lobe posterior basal subsegmental bronchi
Right lower lobe posterior basal subsegmental pulmonary aa.
Lingular v.
Lingular pulmonary a.
Left oblique (major) fissure
Left lower lobe medial basal subsegmental bronchus
Left lower lobe anterior & medial basal subsegmental pulmonary aa.
Left lower lobe lateral basal segment pulmonary a.
Left lower lobe lateral basal segment bronchus (B9)
Left lower lobe posterior basal subsegmental pulmonary a.
Left lower lobe posterior basal subsegmental bronchi
Azygos v.
Descending thoracic aorta
Esophagus

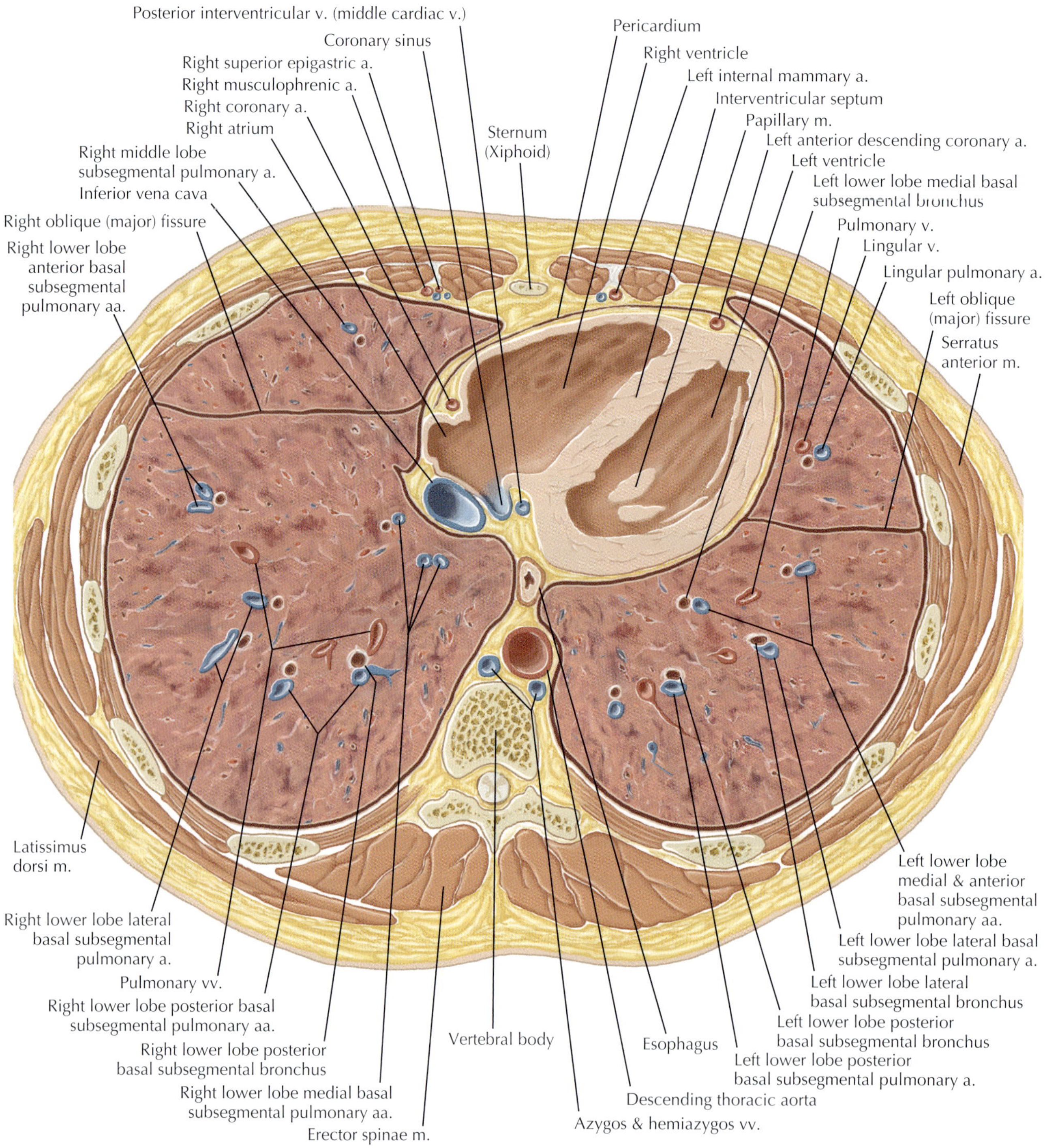
Posterior interventricular v. (middle cardiac v.)
Coronary sinus
Right superior epigastric a.
Right musculophrenic a.
Right coronary a.
Right atrium
Right middle lobe subsegmental pulmonary a.
Inferior vena cava
Right oblique (major) fissure
Right lower lobe anterior basal subsegmental pulmonary aa.
Sternum (Xiphoid)
Pericardium
Right ventricle
Left internal mammary a.
Interventricular septum
Papillary m.
Left anterior descending coronary a.
Left ventricle
Left lower lobe medial basal subsegmental bronchus
Pulmonary v.
Lingular v.
Lingular pulmonary a.
Left oblique (major) fissure
Serratus anterior m.
Latissimus dorsi m.
Right lower lobe lateral basal subsegmental pulmonary a.
Pulmonary vv.
Right lower lobe posterior basal subsegmental pulmonary aa.
Right lower lobe posterior basal subsegmental bronchus
Right lower lobe medial basal subsegmental pulmonary aa.
Erector spinae m.
Vertebral body
Esophagus
Descending thoracic aorta
Azygos & hemiazygos vv.
Left lower lobe medial & anterior basal subsegmental pulmonary aa.
Left lower lobe lateral basal subsegmental pulmonary a.
Left lower lobe lateral basal subsegmental bronchus
Left lower lobe posterior basal subsegmental bronchus
Left lower lobe posterior basal subsegmental pulmonary a.

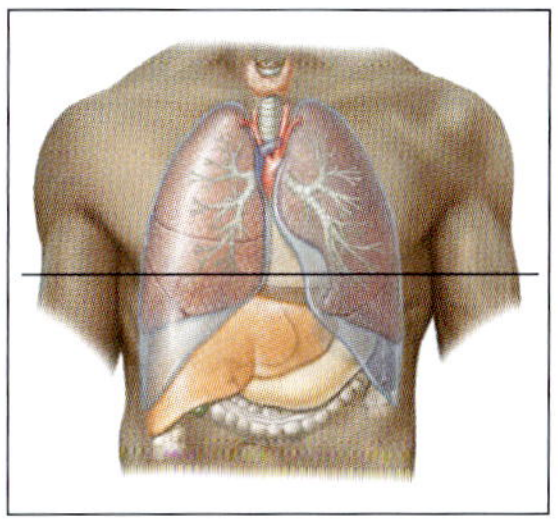

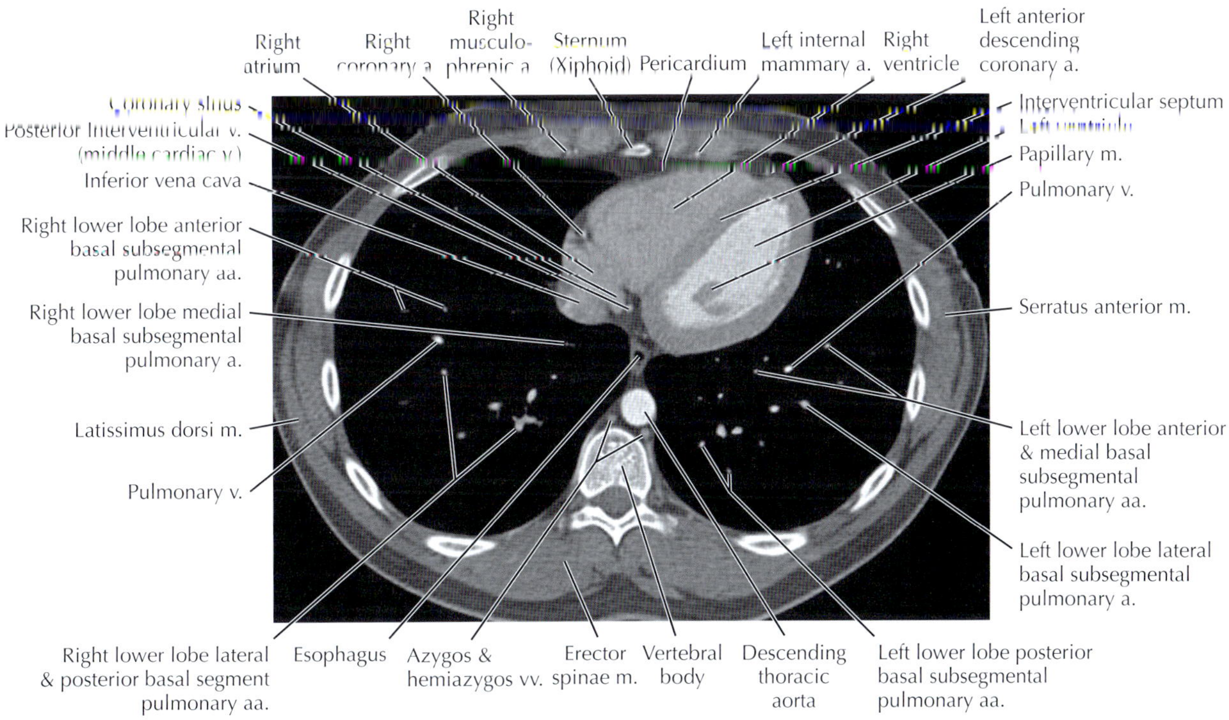

Right atrium
Right coronary a.
Right musculo-phrenic a.
Sternum (Xiphoid)
Pericardium
Left internal mammary a.
Right ventricle
Left anterior descending coronary a.
Coronary sinus
Posterior Interventricular v. (middle cardiac v.)
Inferior vena cava
Right lower lobe anterior basal subsegmental pulmonary aa.
Right lower lobe medial basal subsegmental pulmonary a.
Latissimus dorsi m.
Pulmonary v.
Interventricular septum
Papillary m.
Pulmonary v.
Serratus anterior m.
Left lower lobe anterior & medial basal subsegmental pulmonary aa.
Left lower lobe lateral basal subsegmental pulmonary a.
Right lower lobe lateral & posterior basal segment pulmonary aa.
Esophagus
Azygos & hemiazygos vv.
Erector spinae m.
Vertebral body
Descending thoracic aorta
Left lower lobe posterior basal subsegmental pulmonary aa.

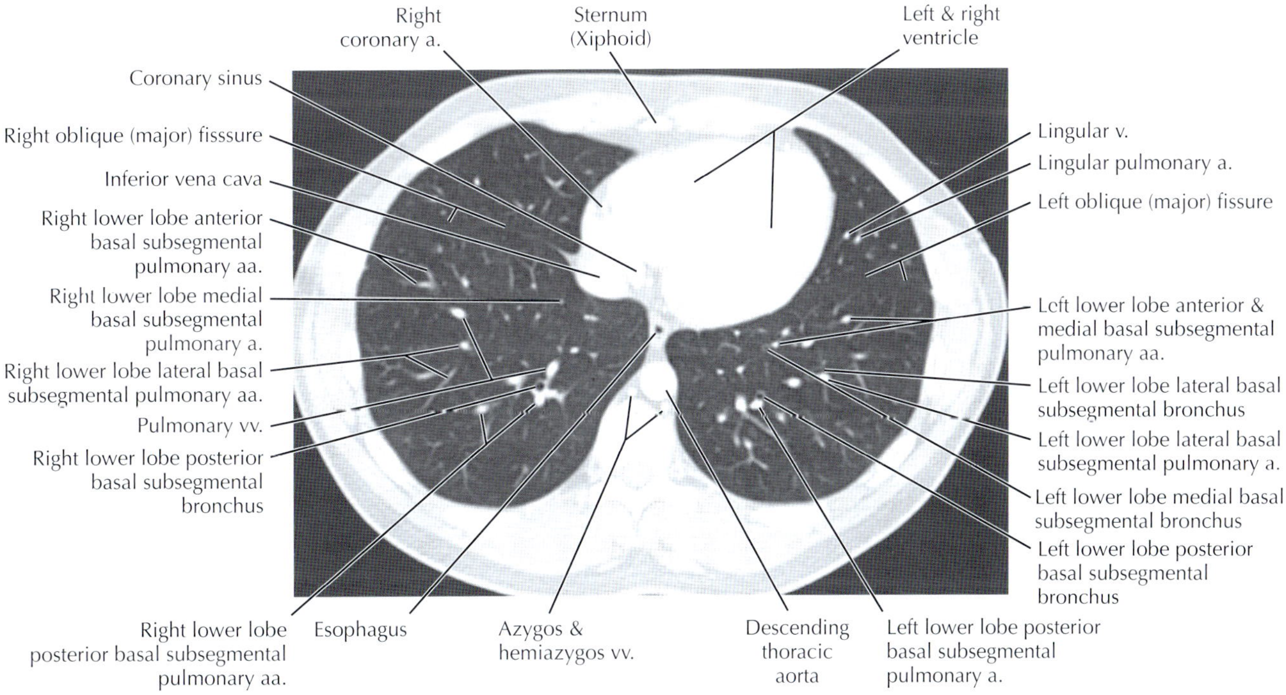

Right coronary a.
Sternum (Xiphoid)
Left & right ventricle
Coronary sinus
Right oblique (major) fisssure
Inferior vena cava
Right lower lobe anterior basal subsegmental pulmonary aa.
Right lower lobe medial basal subsegmental pulmonary a.
Right lower lobe lateral basal subsegmental pulmonary aa.
Pulmonary vv.
Right lower lobe posterior basal subsegmental bronchus
Lingular v.
Lingular pulmonary a.
Left oblique (major) fissure
Left lower lobe anterior & medial basal subsegmental pulmonary aa.
Left lower lobe lateral basal subsegmental bronchus
Left lower lobe lateral basal subsegmental pulmonary a.
Left lower lobe medial basal subsegmental bronchus
Left lower lobe posterior basal subsegmental bronchus
Right lower lobe posterior basal subsegmental pulmonary aa.
Esophagus
Azygos & hemiazygos vv.
Descending thoracic aorta
Left lower lobe posterior basal subsegmental pulmonary a.

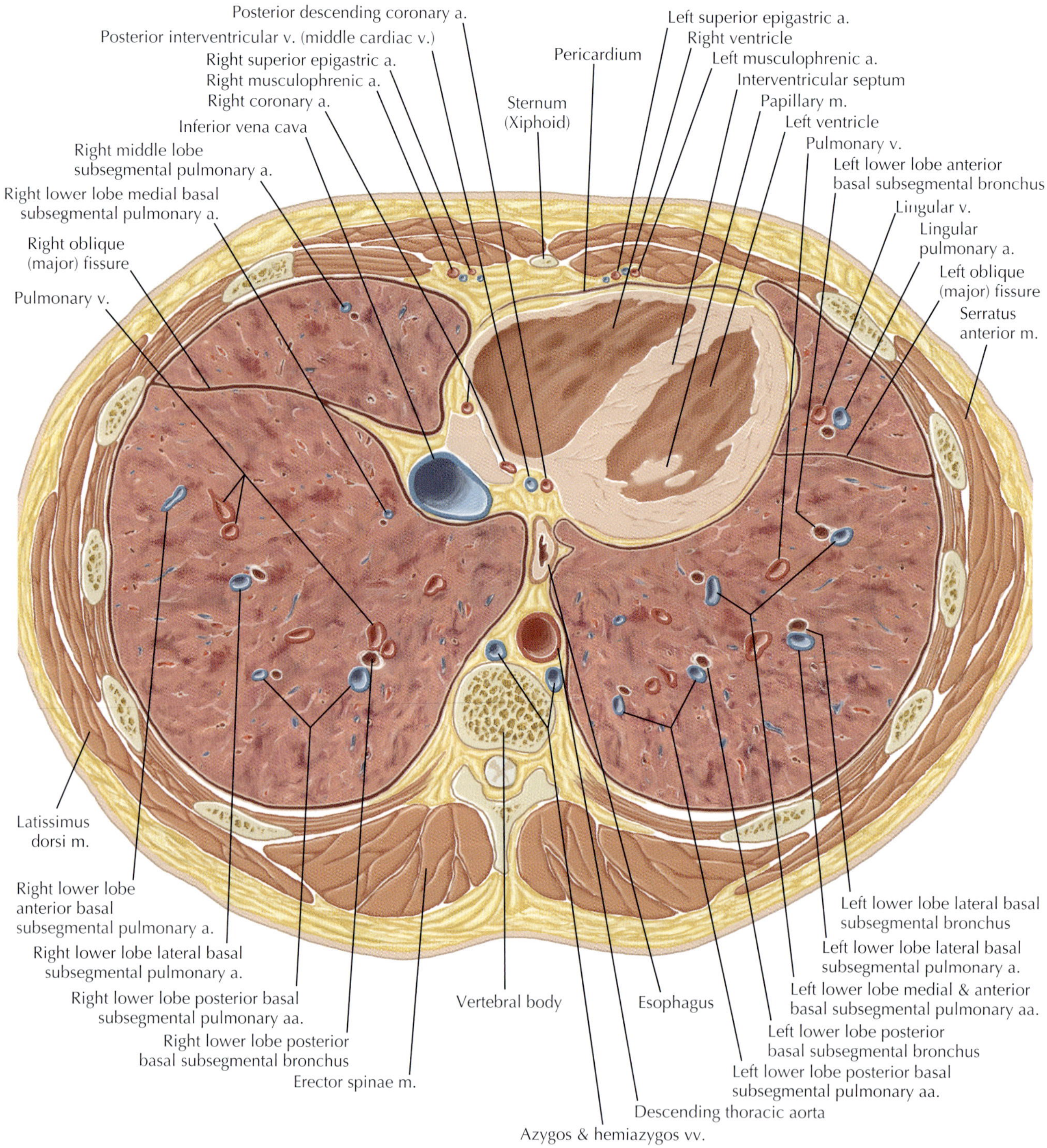
Posterior descending coronary a.
Posterior interventricular v. (middle cardiac v.)
Right superior epigastric a.
Right musculophrenic a.
Right coronary a.
Inferior vena cava
Right middle lobe subsegmental pulmonary a.
Right lower lobe medial basal subsegmental pulmonary a.
Right oblique (major) fissure
Pulmonary v.
Sternum (Xiphoid)
Pericardium
Left superior epigastric a.
Right ventricle
Left musculophrenic a.
Interventricular septum
Papillary m.
Left ventricle
Pulmonary v.
Left lower lobe anterior basal subsegmental bronchus
Lingular v.
Lingular pulmonary a.
Left oblique (major) fissure
Serratus anterior m.
Latissimus dorsi m.
Right lower lobe anterior basal subsegmental pulmonary a.
Right lower lobe lateral basal subsegmental pulmonary a.
Right lower lobe posterior basal subsegmental pulmonary aa.
Right lower lobe posterior basal subsegmental bronchus
Erector spinae m.
Vertebral body
Esophagus
Left lower lobe lateral basal subsegmental bronchus
Left lower lobe lateral basal subsegmental pulmonary a.
Left lower lobe medial & anterior basal subsegmental pulmonary aa.
Left lower lobe posterior basal subsegmental bronchus
Left lower lobe posterior basal subsegmental pulmonary aa.
Descending thoracic aorta
Azygos & hemiazygos vv.

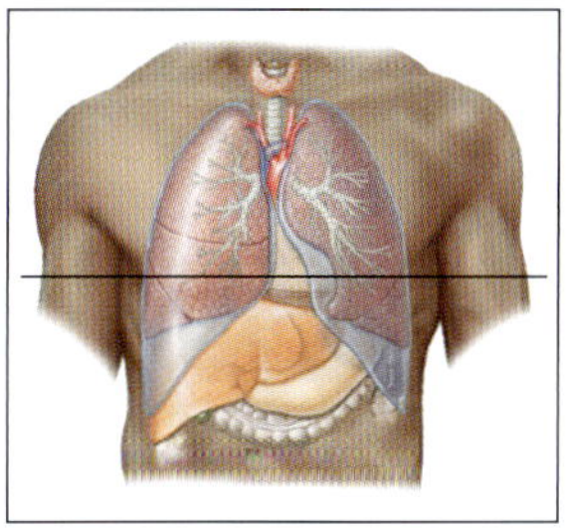

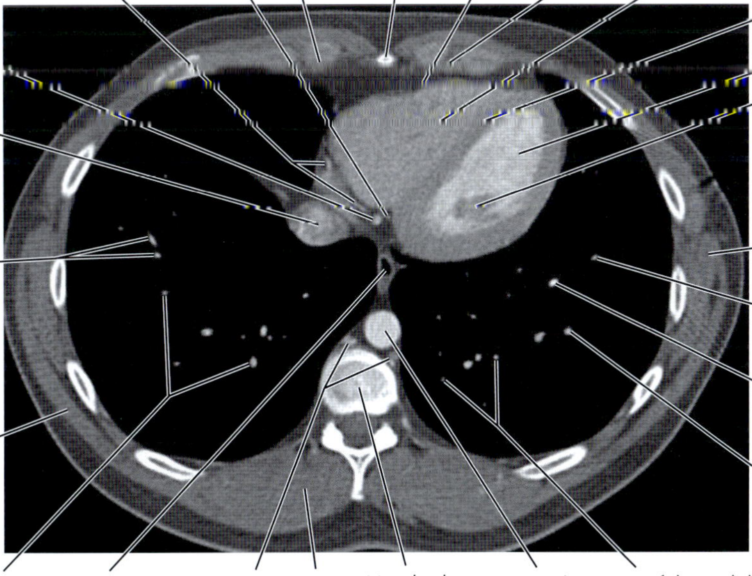
Right coronary a.
Posterior descending coronary a.
Right superior epigastric a.
Sternum (Xiphoid)
Peri- cardium
Left superior epigastric a.
Right ventricle
Posterior interventricular v. (middle cardiac v.)
Inferior vena cava
Pulmonary vv.
Latissimus dorsi m.
Interventricular septum
Left ventricle
Papillary m.
Serratus anterior m.
Left lower lobe anterior basal subsegmental pulmonary a.
Pulmonary v.
Left lower lobe lateral basal subsegmental pulmonary a.
Right lower lobe lateral & posterior basal sub- segmental pulmonary aa.
Esophagus
Azygos & hemiazygos vv.
Erector spinae m.
Vertebral body
Descending thoracic aorta
Left lower lobe posterior basal subsegmental pulmonary aa.

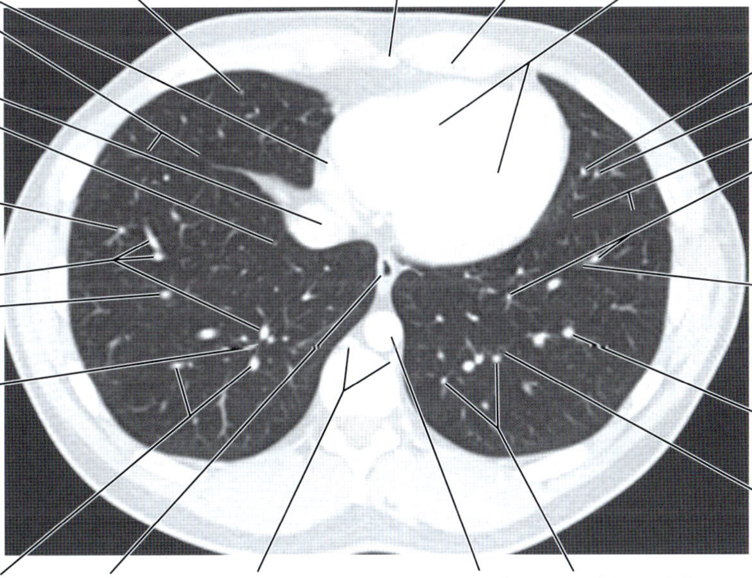
Right coronary a.
Right middle lobe subsegmental pulmonary a.
Sternum (Xiphoid)
Left superior epigastric a.
Right & left ventricle
Right oblique (major) fissure
Inferior vena cava
Right lower lobe medial basal subsegmental pulmonary a.
Right lower lobe anterior basal subsegmental pulmonary a.
Pulmonary vv.
Right lower lobe lateral basal subsegmental pulmonary a.
Right lower lobe posterior basal subsegmental bronchus
Lingular v.
Lingular pulmonary a.
Left oblique (major) fissure
Left lower lobe medial & anterior basal sub- segmental pulmonary aa.
Left lower lobe anterior basal subsegmental bronchus
Left lower lobe lateral basal subsegmental pulmonary a.
Left lower lobe posterior basal subsegmental bronchus
Right lower lobe posterior basal subsegmental pulmonary aa.
Esophagus
Azygos & hemiazygos vv.
Descending thoracic aorta
Left lower lobe posterior basal subsegmental pulmonary aa.

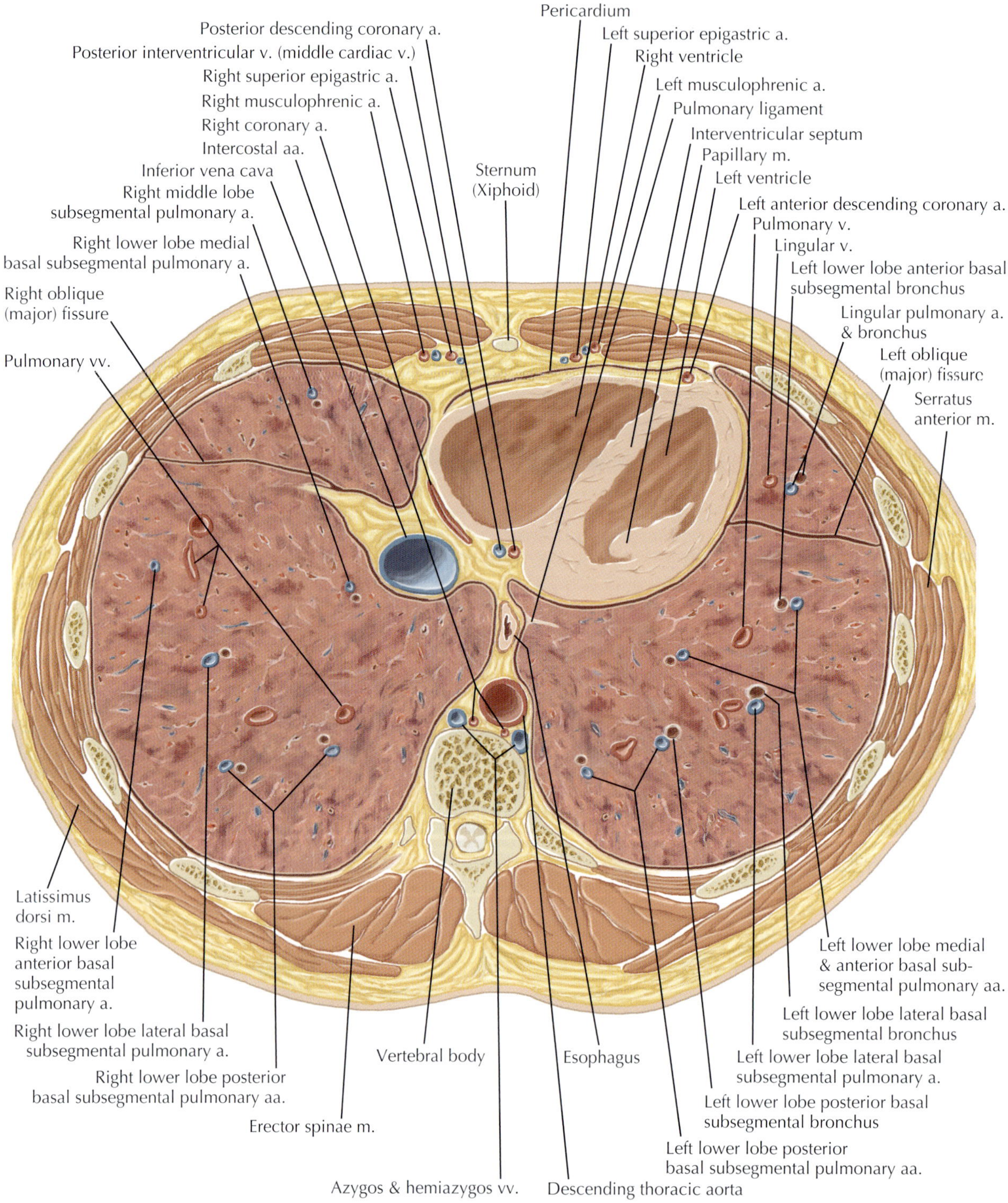

NORMAL ANATOMY

The *pulmonary ligament* is formed by the visceral pleura lining the medial lower lobes reflecting over the mediastinal pleural surface. The pulmonary ligaments extend inferiorly from the hila toward the diaphragm; occasionally the ligaments may contain systemic vessels supplying the lungs. On thoracic CT, the pulmonary ligaments are often visible as linear or triangular, narrow, short structures extending laterally from the esophagus, caudal to the inferior pulmonary veins.

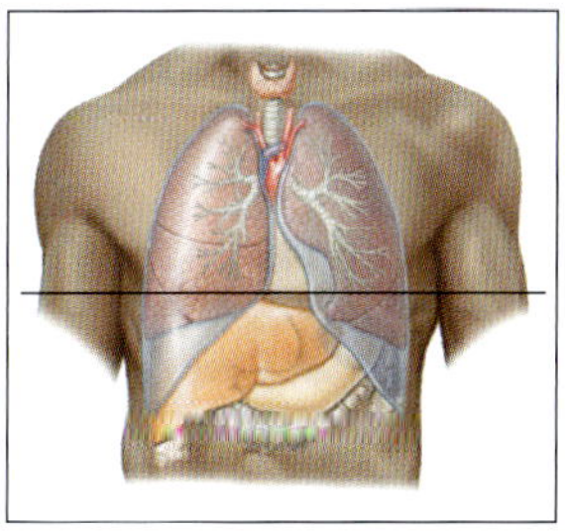

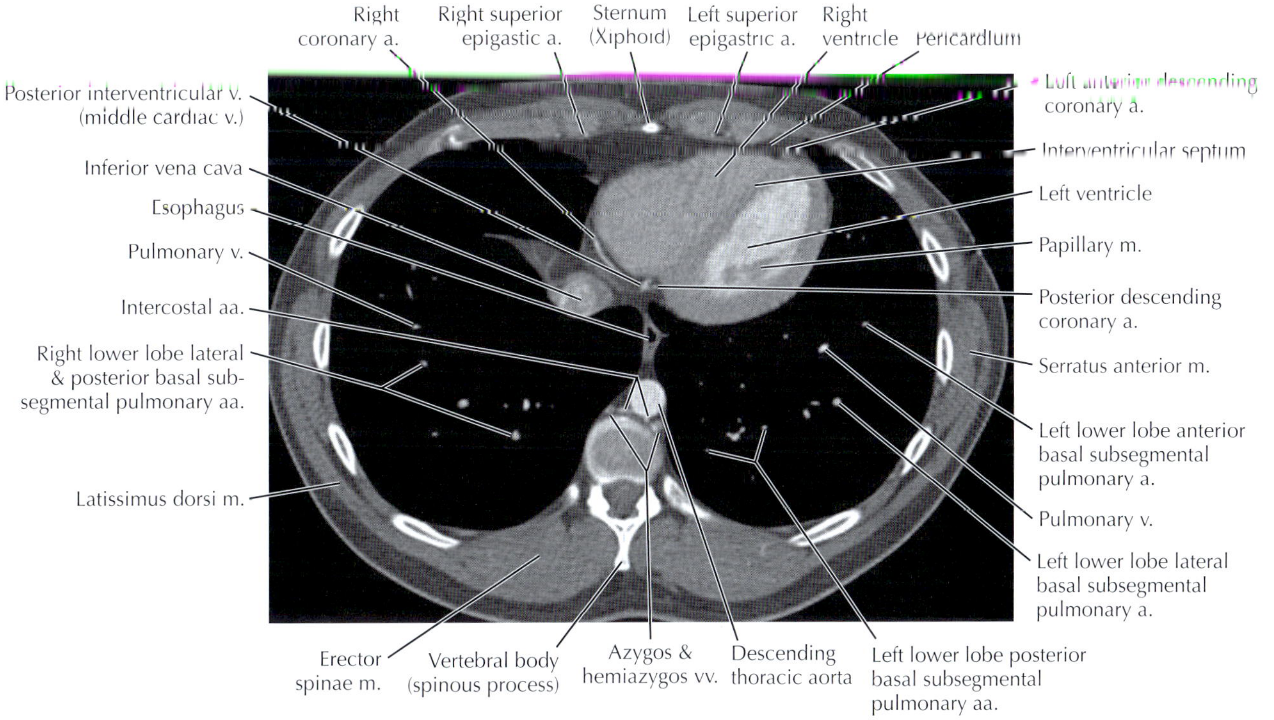
Right coronary a.
Right superior epigastic a.
Sternum (Xiphoid)
Left superior epigastric a.
Right ventricle
Pericardium
Left anterior descending coronary a.
Interventricular septum
Left ventricle
Papillary m.
Posterior descending coronary a.
Serratus anterior m.
Left lower lobe anterior basal subsegmental pulmonary a.
Pulmonary v.
Left lower lobe lateral basal subsegmental pulmonary a.
Posterior interventricular v. (middle cardiac v.)
Inferior vena cava
Esophagus
Pulmonary v.
Intercostal aa.
Right lower lobe lateral & posterior basal sub-segmental pulmonary aa.
Latissimus dorsi m.
Erector spinae m.
Vertebral body (spinous process)
Azygos & hemiazygos vv.
Descending thoracic aorta
Left lower lobe posterior basal subsegmental pulmonary aa.

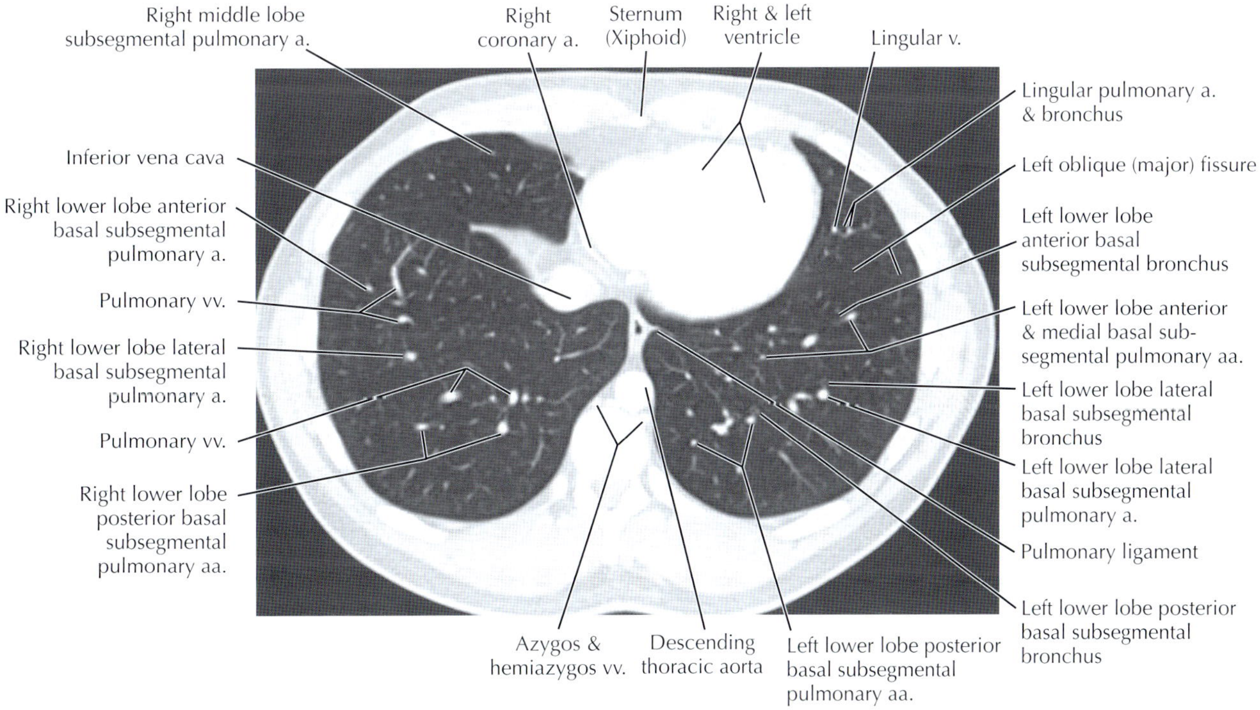
Right middle lobe subsegmental pulmonary a.
Right coronary a.
Sternum (Xiphoid)
Right & left ventricle
Lingular v.
Lingular pulmonary a. & bronchus
Left oblique (major) fissure
Left lower lobe anterior basal subsegmental bronchus
Left lower lobe anterior & medial basal sub-segmental pulmonary aa.
Left lower lobe lateral basal subsegmental bronchus
Left lower lobe lateral basal subsegmental pulmonary a.
Pulmonary ligament
Left lower lobe posterior basal subsegmental bronchus
Inferior vena cava
Right lower lobe anterior basal subsegmental pulmonary a.
Pulmonary vv.
Right lower lobe lateral basal subsegmental pulmonary a.
Pulmonary vv.
Right lower lobe posterior basal subsegmental pulmonary aa.
Azygos & hemiazygos vv.
Descending thoracic aorta
Left lower lobe posterior basal subsegmental pulmonary aa.

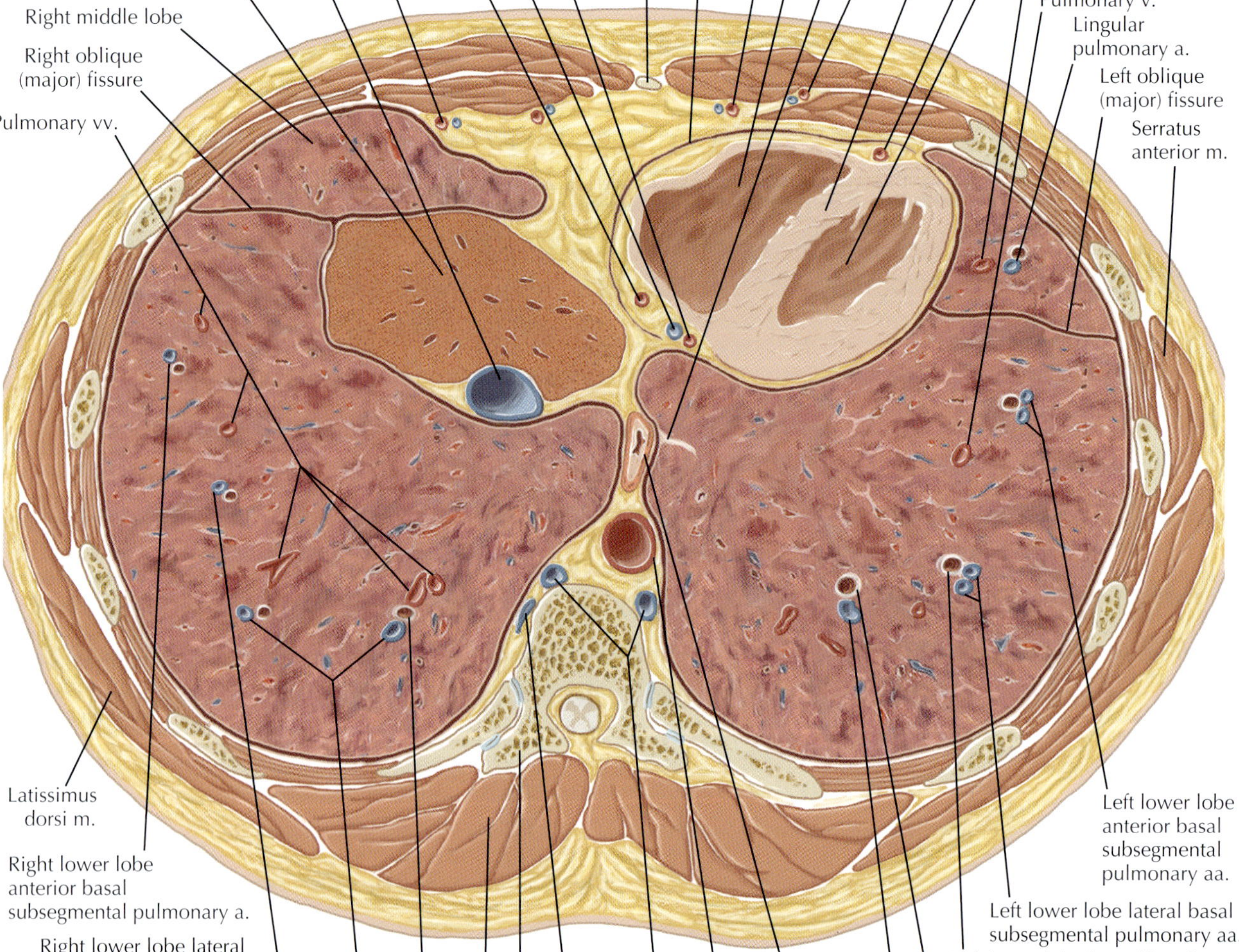

NORMAL ANATOMY

The *phrenic nerves* are occasionally seen reflecting over the diaphragm, anterior to the inferior pulmonary ligament.

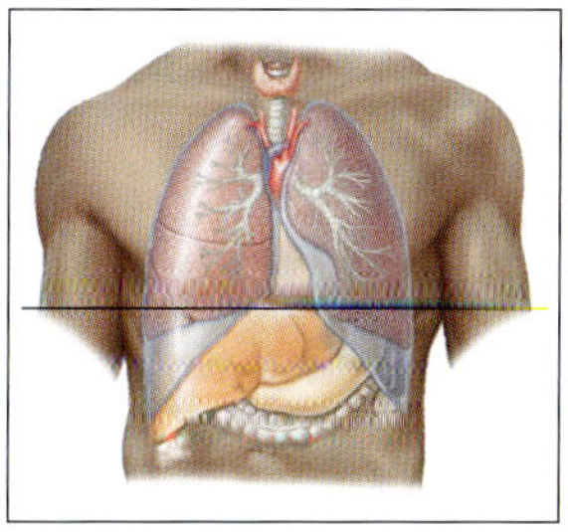

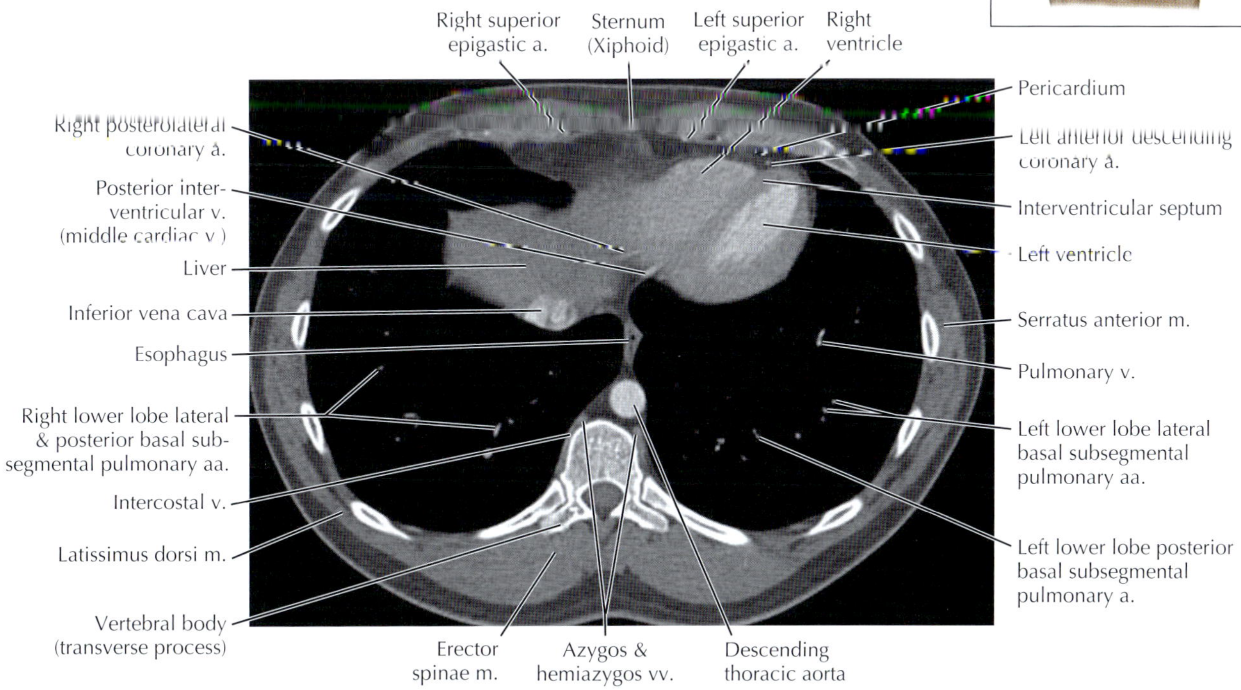
Right superior epigastic a.
Sternum (Xiphoid)
Left superior epigastic a.
Right ventricle
Pericardium
Right posterolateral coronary a.
Left anterior descending coronary a.
Posterior inter-ventricular v. (middle cardiac v.)
Interventricular septum
Left ventricle
Liver
Inferior vena cava
Serratus anterior m.
Esophagus
Pulmonary v.
Right lower lobe lateral & posterior basal sub-segmental pulmonary aa.
Left lower lobe lateral basal subsegmental pulmonary aa.
Intercostal v.
Latissimus dorsi m.
Left lower lobe posterior basal subsegmental pulmonary a.
Vertebral body (transverse process)
Erector spinae m.
Azygos & hemiazygos vv.
Descending thoracic aorta

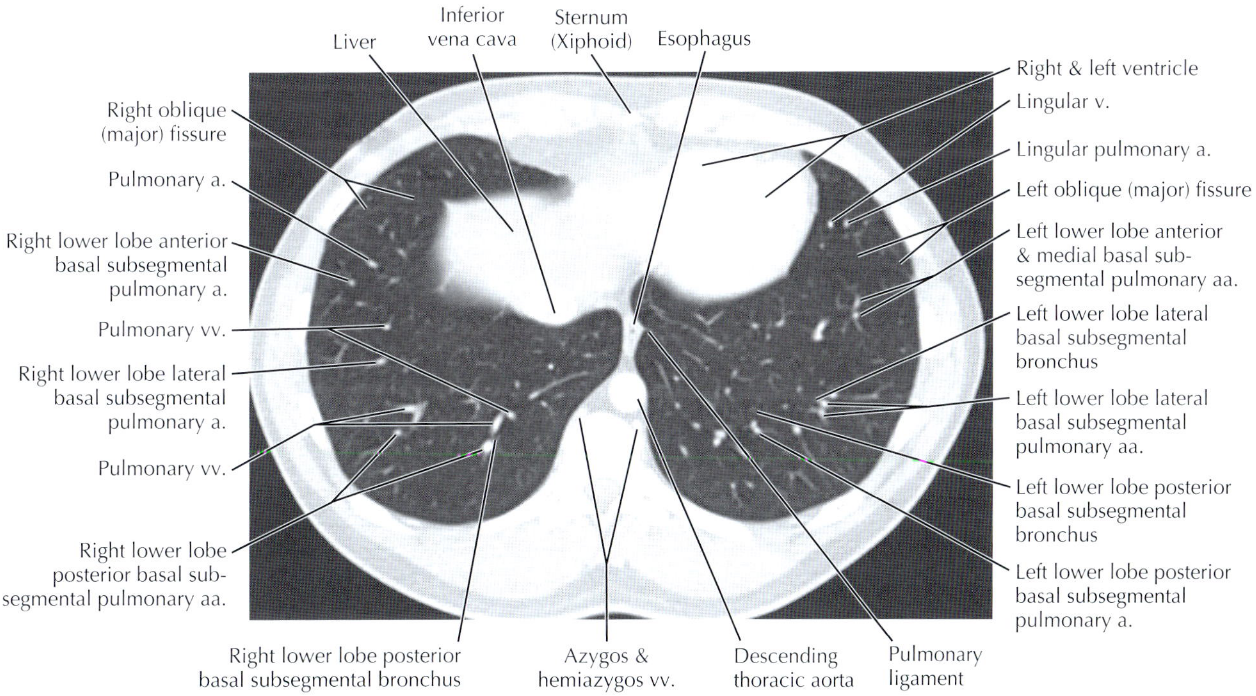
Liver
Inferior vena cava
Sternum (Xiphoid)
Esophagus
Right & left ventricle
Right oblique (major) fissure
Lingular v.
Lingular pulmonary a.
Pulmonary a.
Left oblique (major) fissure
Right lower lobe anterior basal subsegmental pulmonary a.
Left lower lobe anterior & medial basal sub-segmental pulmonary aa.
Pulmonary vv.
Left lower lobe lateral basal subsegmental bronchus
Right lower lobe lateral basal subsegmental pulmonary a.
Left lower lobe lateral basal subsegmental pulmonary aa.
Pulmonary vv.
Left lower lobe posterior basal subsegmental bronchus
Right lower lobe posterior basal sub-segmental pulmonary aa.
Left lower lobe posterior basal subsegmental pulmonary a.
Right lower lobe posterior basal subsegmental bronchus
Azygos & hemiazygos vv.
Descending thoracic aorta
Pulmonary ligament

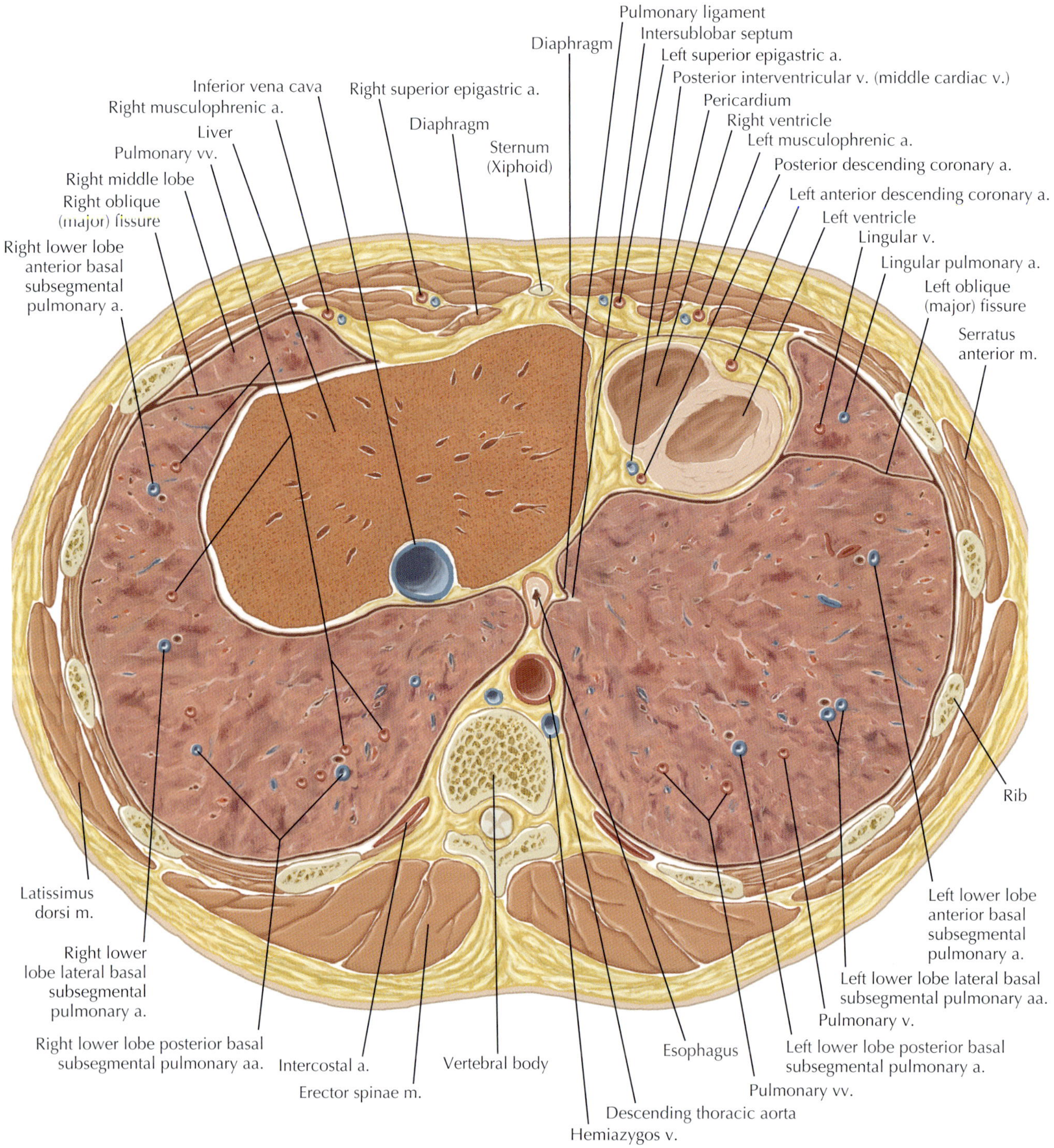
Pulmonary ligament
Intersublobar septum
Diaphragm
Left superior epigastric a.
Posterior interventricular v. (middle cardiac v.)
Inferior vena cava
Right superior epigastric a.
Pericardium
Right musculophrenic a.
Right ventricle
Diaphragm
Liver
Left musculophrenic a.
Sternum
(Xiphoid)
Pulmonary vv.
Posterior descending coronary a.
Right middle lobe
Left anterior descending coronary a.
Right oblique
(major) fissure
Left ventricle
Lingular v.
Right lower lobe
anterior basal
subsegmental
pulmonary a.
Lingular pulmonary a.
Left oblique
(major) fissure
Serratus
anterior m.
Rib
Latissimus
dorsi m.
Left lower lobe
anterior basal
subsegmental
pulmonary a.
Right lower
lobe lateral basal
subsegmental
pulmonary a.
Left lower lobe lateral basal
subsegmental pulmonary aa.
Pulmonary v.
Right lower lobe posterior basal
subsegmental pulmonary aa.
Intercostal a.
Vertebral body
Esophagus
Left lower lobe posterior basal
subsegmental pulmonary a.
Erector spinae m.
Pulmonary vv.
Descending thoracic aorta
Hemiazygos v.

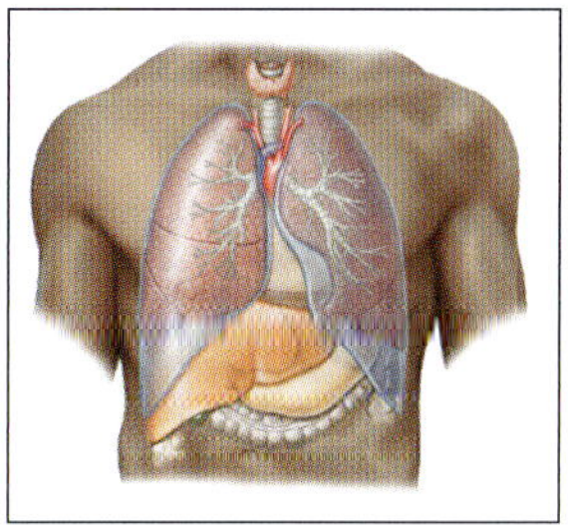

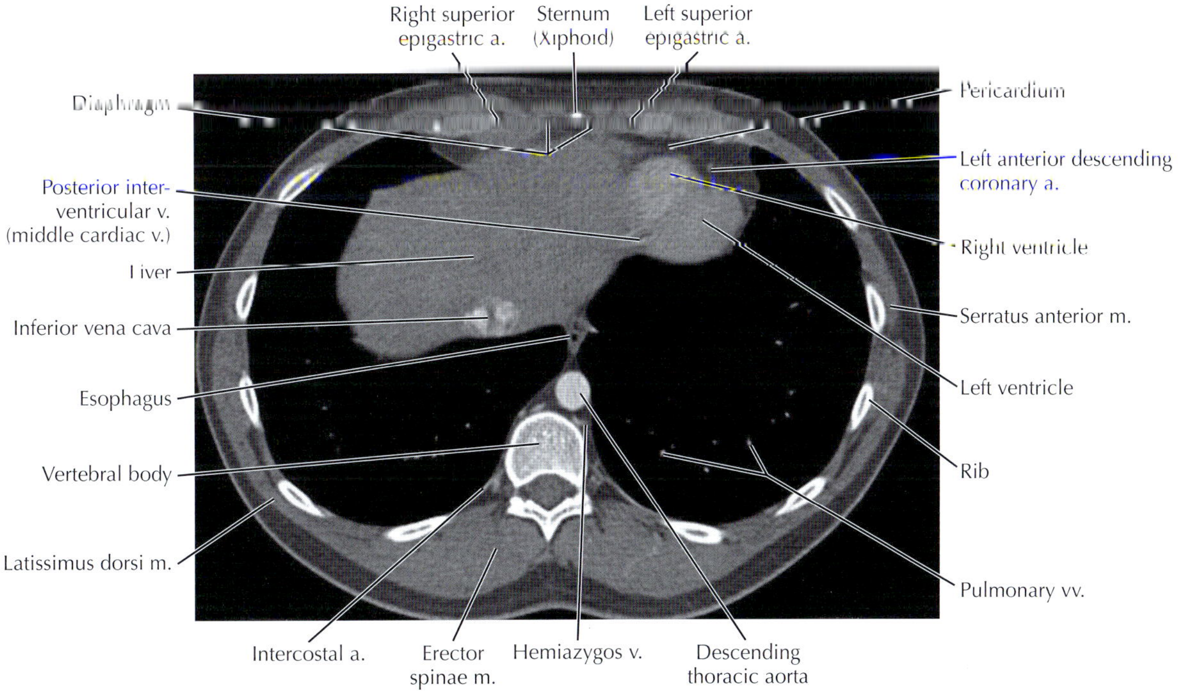
Right superior epigastric a.
Sternum (Xiphoid)
Left superior epigastric a.
Diaphragm
Pericardium
Left anterior descending coronary a.
Posterior interventricular v. (middle cardiac v.)
Right ventricle
Liver
Serratus anterior m.
Inferior vena cava
Left ventricle
Esophagus
Rib
Vertebral body
Latissimus dorsi m.
Pulmonary vv.
Intercostal a.
Erector spinae m.
Hemiazygos v.
Descending thoracic aorta

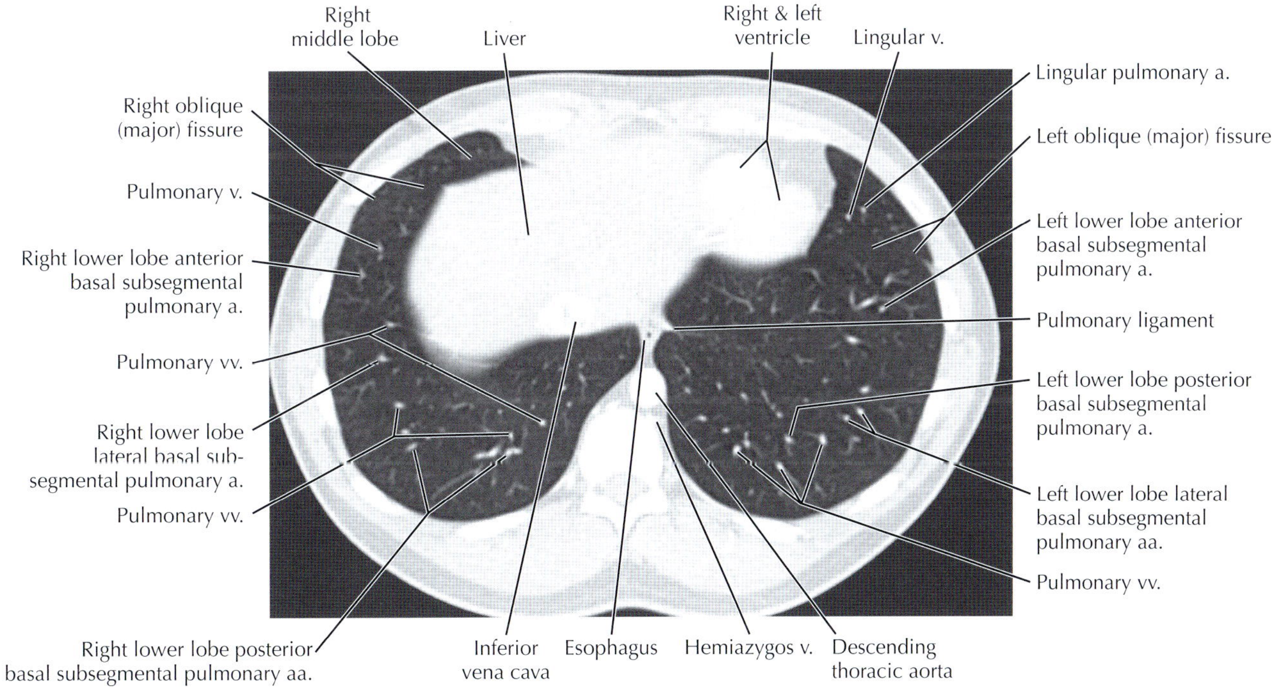
Right middle lobe
Liver
Right & left ventricle
Lingular v.
Lingular pulmonary a.
Right oblique (major) fissure
Left oblique (major) fissure
Pulmonary v.
Left lower lobe anterior basal subsegmental pulmonary a.
Right lower lobe anterior basal subsegmental pulmonary a.
Pulmonary ligament
Pulmonary vv.
Left lower lobe posterior basal subsegmental pulmonary a.
Right lower lobe lateral basal subsegmental pulmonary a.
Pulmonary vv.
Left lower lobe lateral basal subsegmental pulmonary aa.
Pulmonary vv.
Right lower lobe posterior basal subsegmental pulmonary aa.
Inferior vena cava
Esophagus
Hemiazygos v.
Descending thoracic aorta

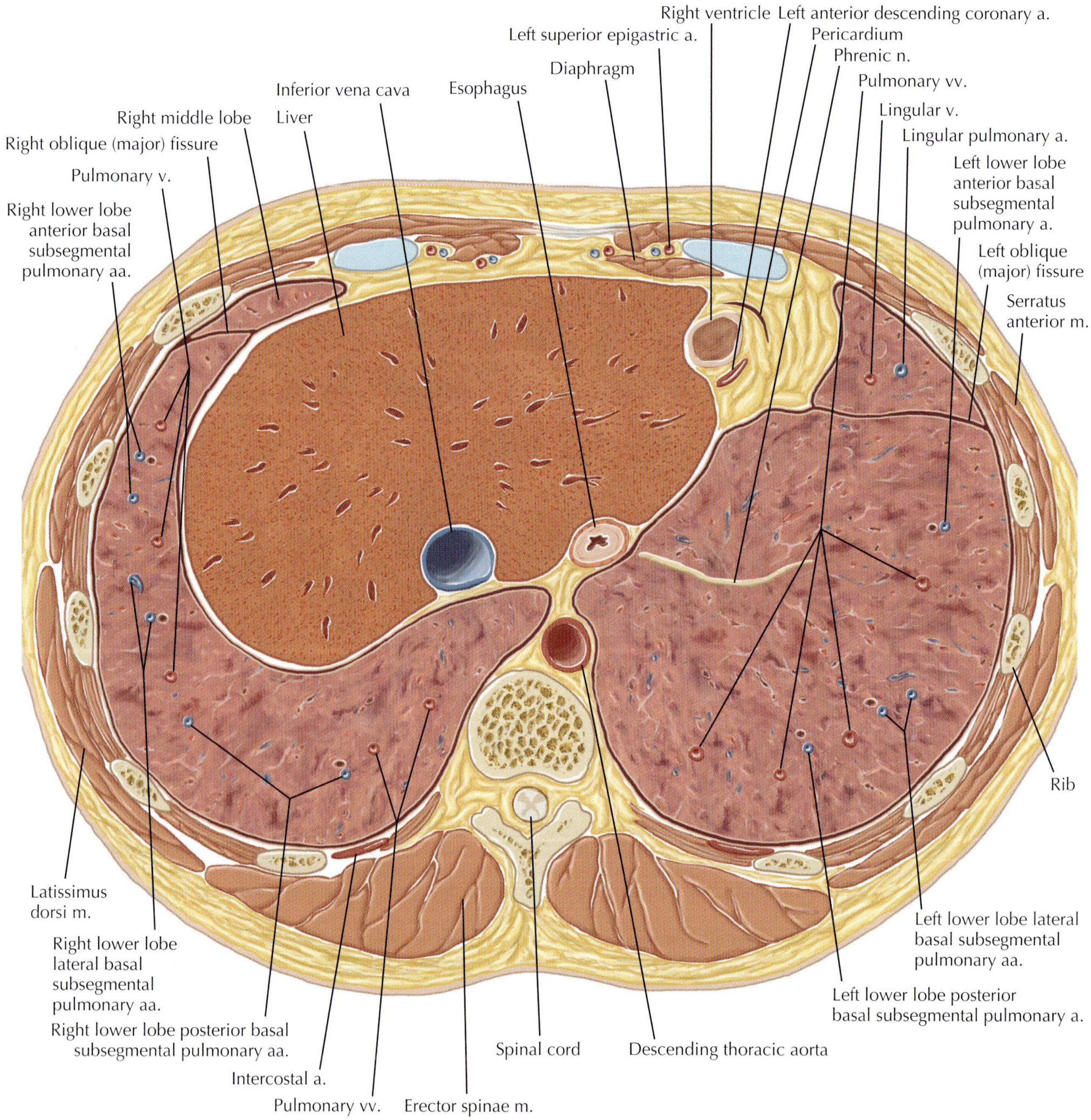

Right ventricle
Left anterior descending coronary a.
Left superior epigastric a.
Pericardium
Phrenic n.
Diaphragm
Pulmonary vv.
Inferior vena cava
Esophagus
Lingular v.
Right middle lobe
Liver
Lingular pulmonary a.
Right oblique (major) fissure
Left lower lobe anterior basal subsegmental pulmonary a.
Pulmonary v.
Right lower lobe anterior basal subsegmental pulmonary aa.
Left oblique (major) fissure
Serratus anterior m.
Rib
Latissimus dorsi m.
Left lower lobe lateral basal subsegmental pulmonary aa.
Right lower lobe lateral basal subsegmental pulmonary aa.
Left lower lobe posterior basal subsegmental pulmonary a.
Right lower lobe posterior basal subsegmental pulmonary aa.
Spinal cord
Descending thoracic aorta
Intercostal a.
Pulmonary vv.
Erector spinae m.

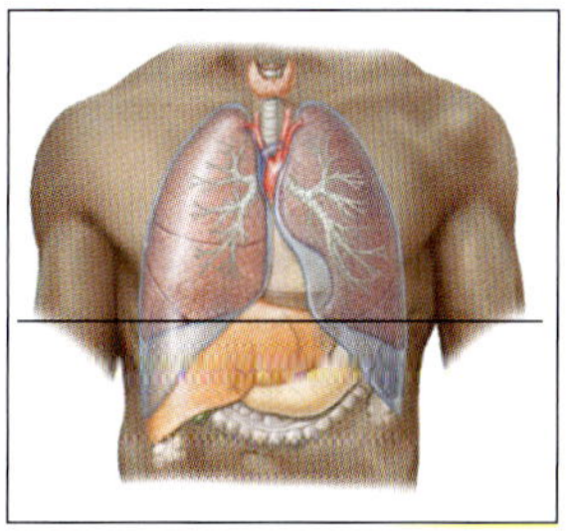

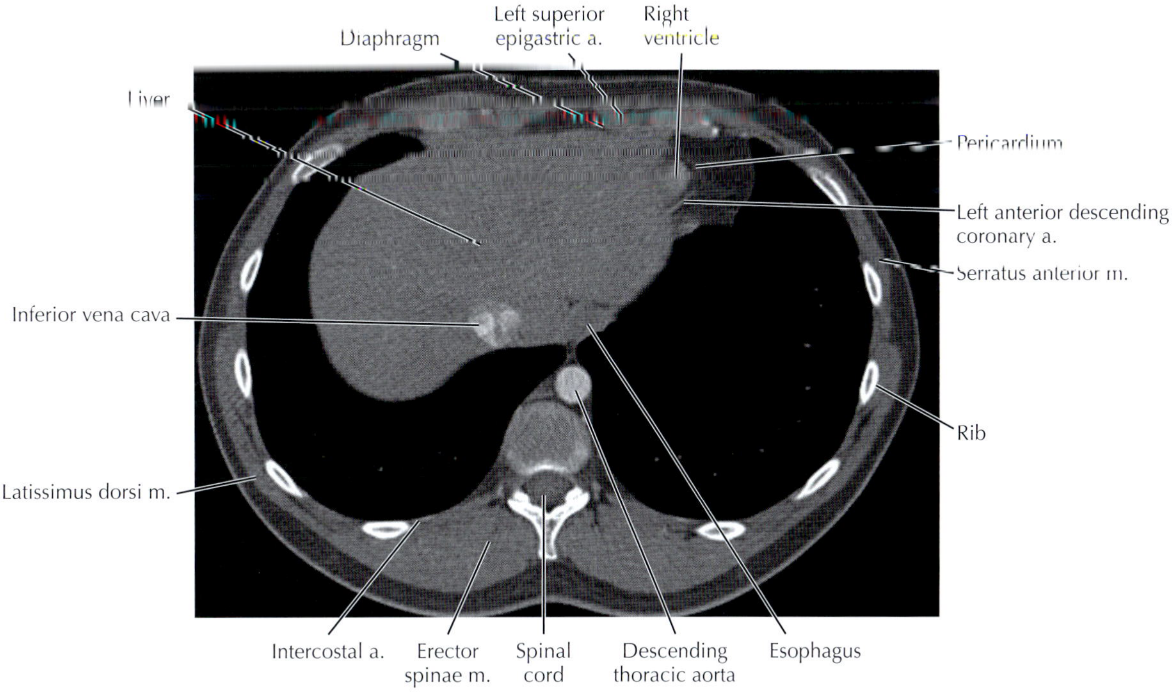
Diaphragm
Left superior epigastric a.
Right ventricle
Liver
Pericardium
Left anterior descending coronary a.
Serratus anterior m.
Inferior vena cava
Rib
Latissimus dorsi m.
Intercostal a.
Erector spinae m.
Spinal cord
Descending thoracic aorta
Esophagus

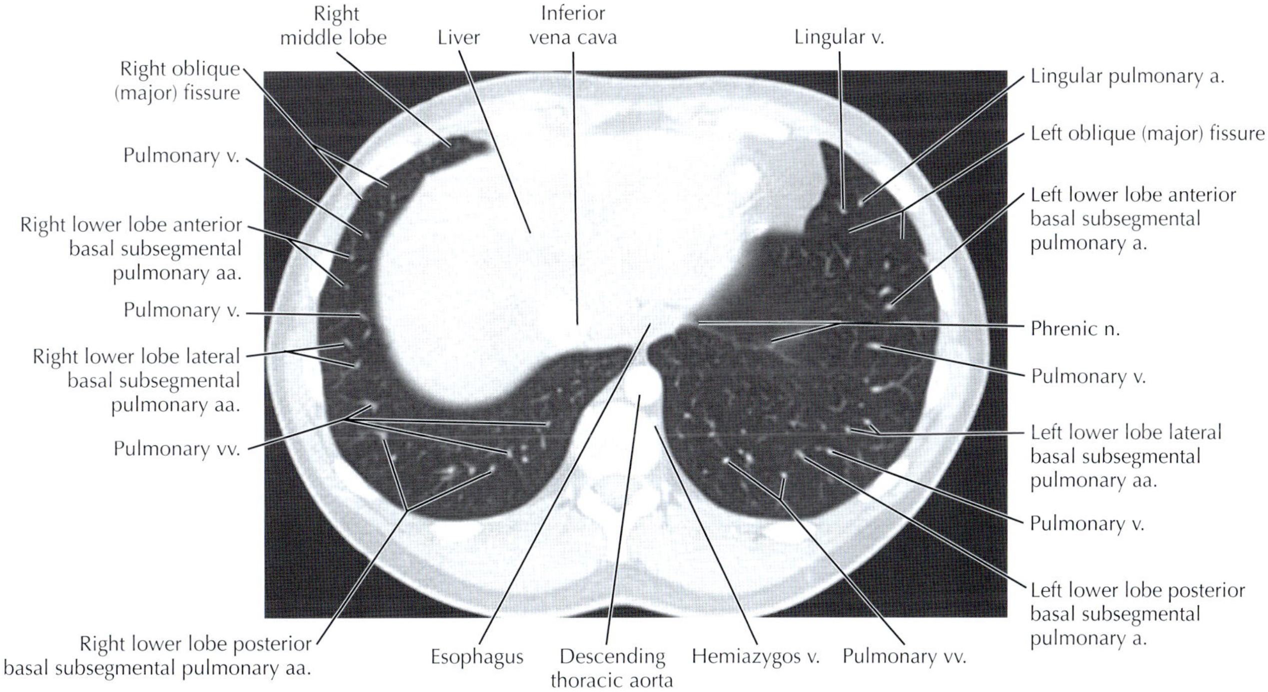
Right middle lobe
Liver
Inferior vena cava
Lingular v.
Right oblique (major) fissure
Lingular pulmonary a.
Left oblique (major) fissure
Pulmonary v.
Left lower lobe anterior basal subsegmental pulmonary a.
Right lower lobe anterior basal subsegmental pulmonary aa.
Pulmonary v.
Phrenic n.
Right lower lobe lateral basal subsegmental pulmonary aa.
Pulmonary v.
Pulmonary vv.
Left lower lobe lateral basal subsegmental pulmonary aa.
Pulmonary v.
Left lower lobe posterior basal subsegmental pulmonary a.
Right lower lobe posterior basal subsegmental pulmonary aa.
Esophagus
Descending thoracic aorta
Hemiazygos v.
Pulmonary vv.

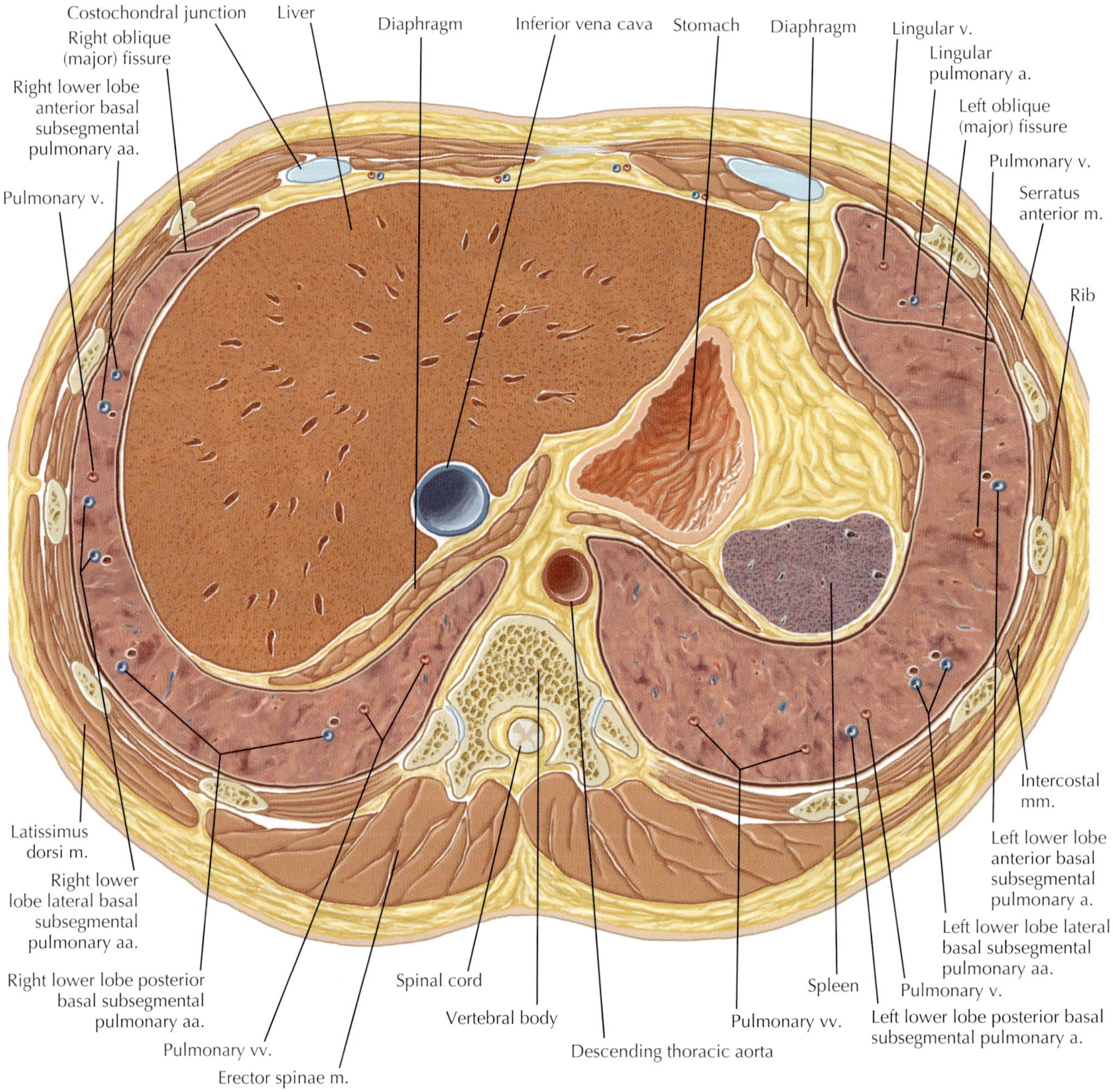

Costochondral junction
Liver
Diaphragm
Inferior vena cava
Stomach
Diaphragm
Lingular v.
Right oblique (major) fissure
Lingular pulmonary a.
Right lower lobe anterior basal subsegmental pulmonary aa.
Left oblique (major) fissure
Pulmonary v.
Pulmonary v.
Serratus anterior m.
Rib
Intercostal mm.
Latissimus dorsi m.
Left lower lobe anterior basal subsegmental pulmonary a.
Right lower lobe lateral basal subsegmental pulmonary aa.
Left lower lobe lateral basal subsegmental pulmonary aa.
Right lower lobe posterior basal subsegmental pulmonary aa.
Spinal cord
Spleen
Pulmonary v.
Vertebral body
Pulmonary vv.
Left lower lobe posterior basal subsegmental pulmonary a.
Pulmonary vv.
Descending thoracic aorta
Erector spinae m.

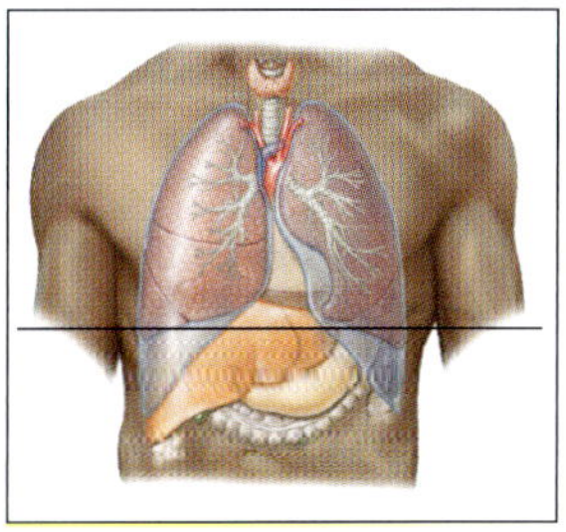

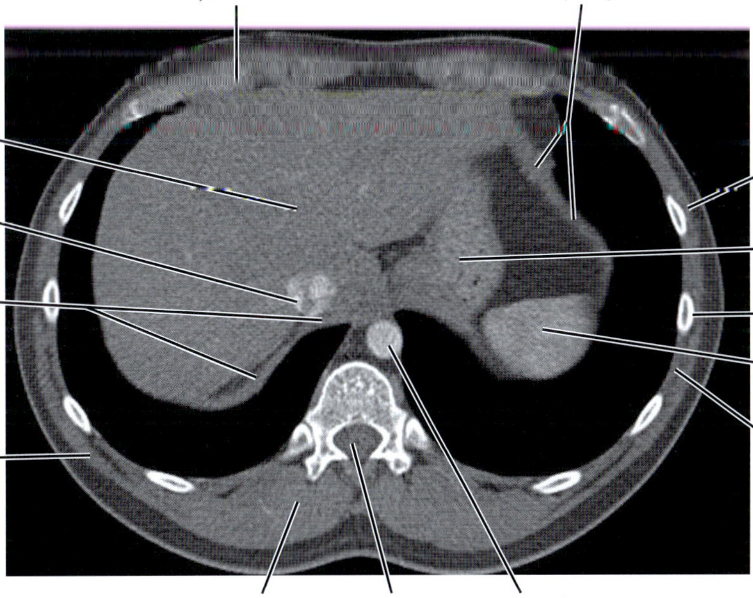

Costochondral junction
Diaphragm
Liver
Serratus anterior m.
Inferior vena cava
Stomach
Diaphragm
Rib
Spleen
Intercostal mm.
Latissimus dorsi m.
Erector spinae m.
Spinal cord
Descending thoracic aorta

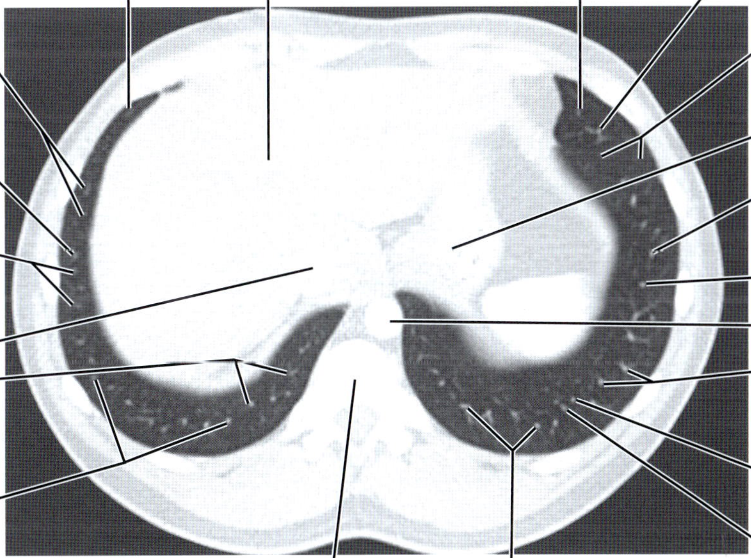

Right oblique (major) fissure
Liver
Lingular v.
Lingular pulmonary a.
Right lower lobe anterior basal subsegmental pulmonary aa.
Left oblique (major) fissure
Stomach
Pulmonary v.
Left lower lobe anterior basal subsegmental pulmonary a.
Right lower lobe lateral basal subsegmental pulmonary aa.
Pulmonary v.
Descending thoracic aorta
Inferior vena cava
Pulmonary vv.
Left lower lobe lateral basal subsegmental pulmonary aa.
Pulmonary v.
Right lower lobe posterior basal subsegmental pulmonary aa.
Left lower lobe posterior basal subsegmental pulmonary a.
Vertebral body
Pulmonary vv.

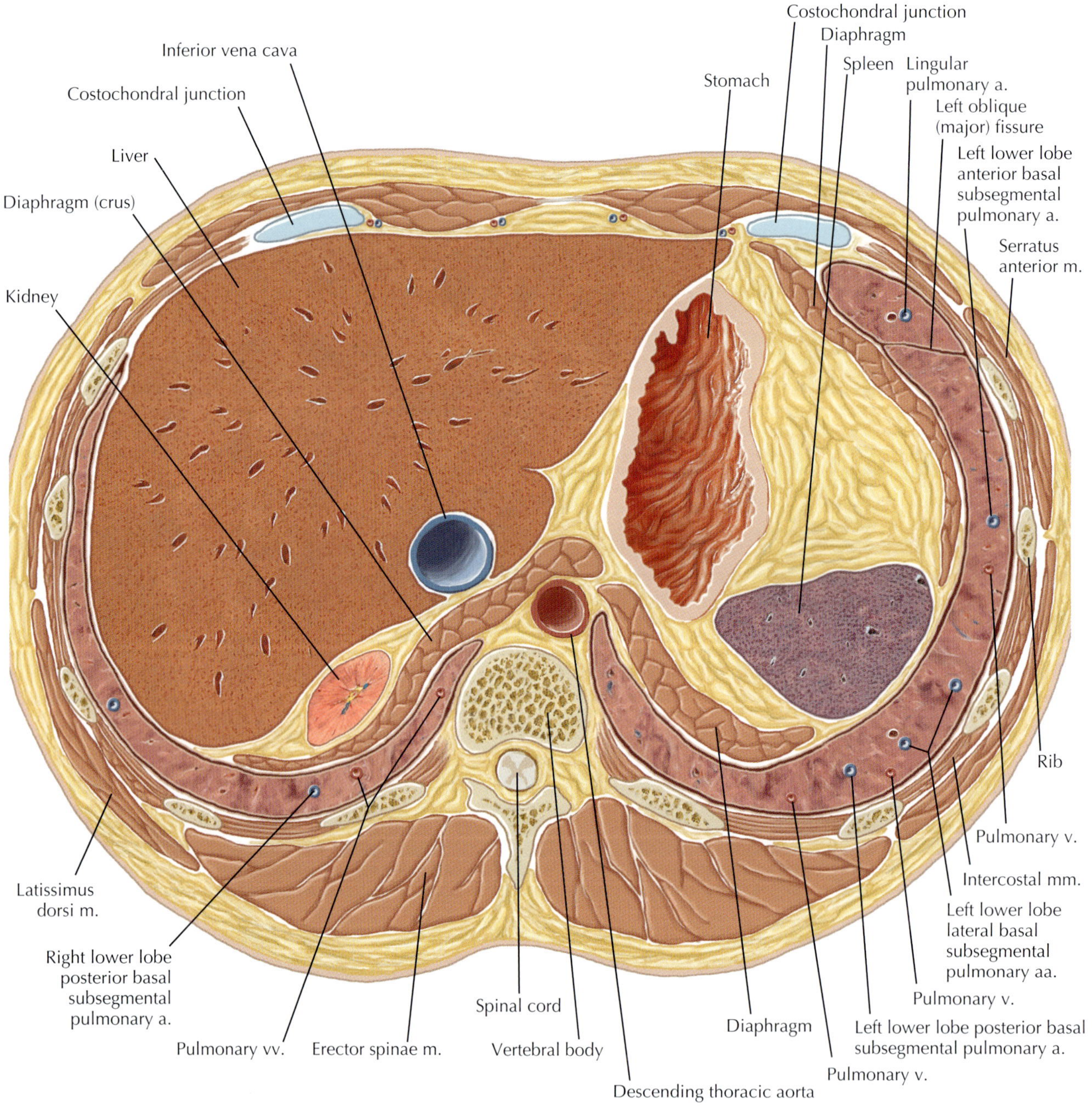
Costochondral junction
Diaphragm
Inferior vena cava
Spleen
Lingular pulmonary a.
Stomach
Costochondral junction
Left oblique (major) fissure
Liver
Left lower lobe anterior basal subsegmental pulmonary a.
Diaphragm (crus)
Serratus anterior m.
Kidney
Rib
Pulmonary v.
Intercostal mm.
Latissimus dorsi m.
Left lower lobe lateral basal subsegmental pulmonary aa.
Right lower lobe posterior basal subsegmental pulmonary a.
Pulmonary v.
Spinal cord
Diaphragm
Left lower lobe posterior basal subsegmental pulmonary a.
Pulmonary vv.
Erector spinae m.
Vertebral body
Pulmonary v.
Descending thoracic aorta

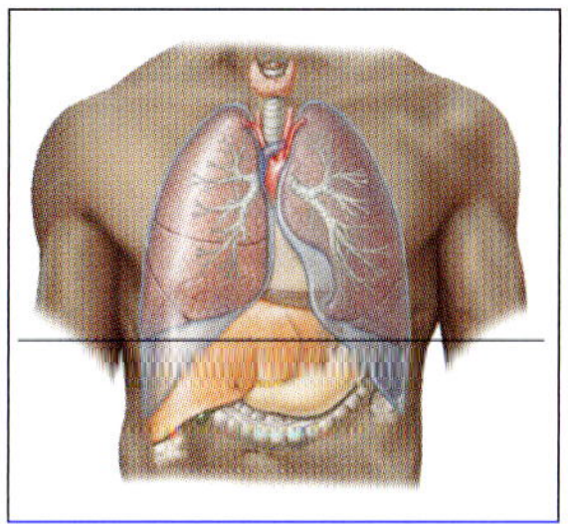

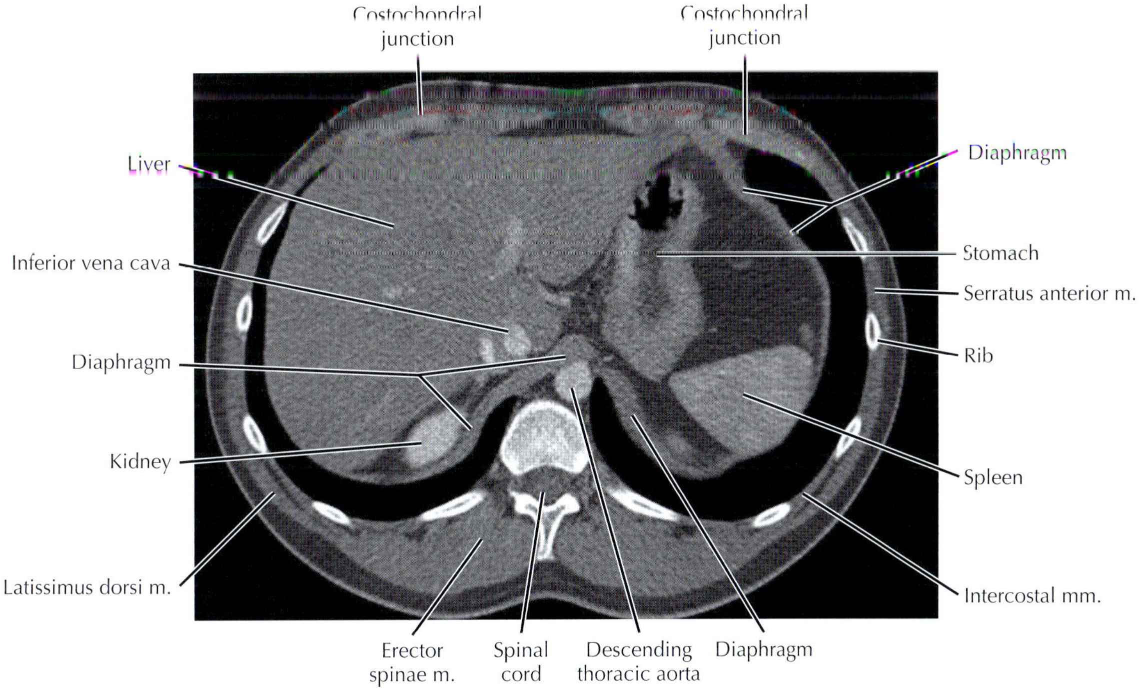
Costochondral junction
Costochondral junction
Liver
Diaphragm
Inferior vena cava
Stomach
Serratus anterior m.
Diaphragm
Rib
Kidney
Spleen
Latissimus dorsi m.
Intercostal mm.
Erector spinae m.
Spinal cord
Descending thoracic aorta
Diaphragm

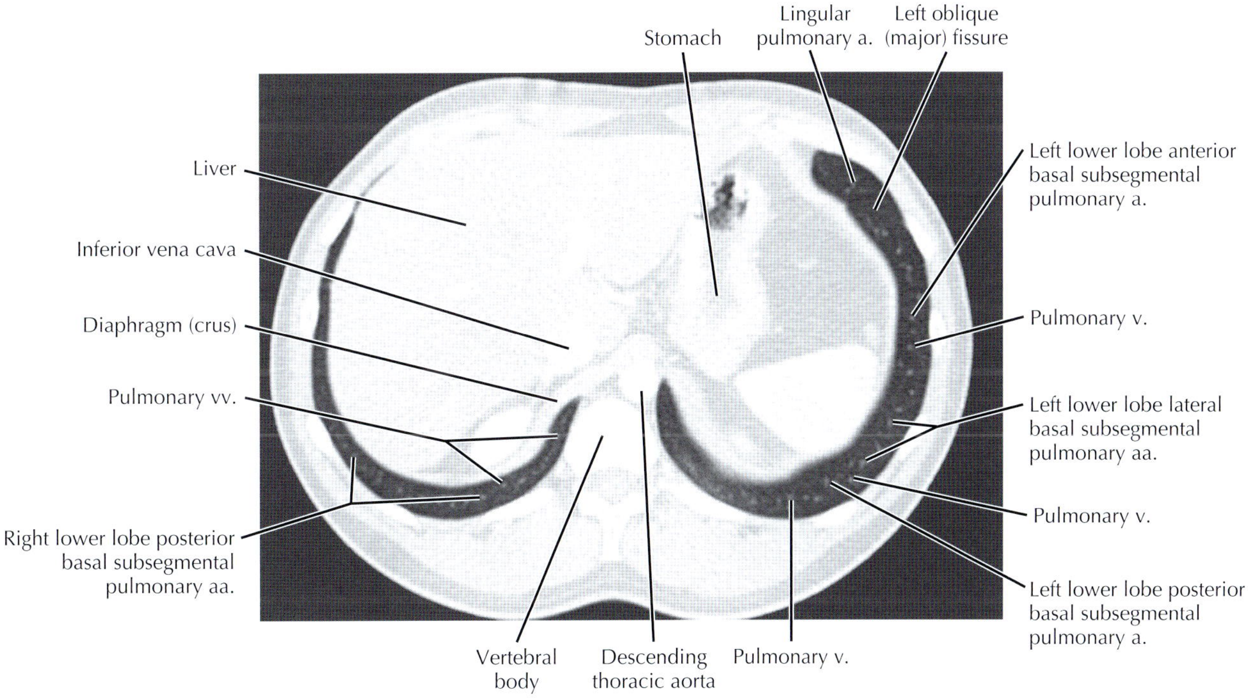
Stomach
Lingular pulmonary a.
Left oblique (major) fissure
Liver
Left lower lobe anterior basal subsegmental pulmonary a.
Inferior vena cava
Diaphragm (crus)
Pulmonary v.
Pulmonary vv.
Left lower lobe lateral basal subsegmental pulmonary aa.
Pulmonary v.
Right lower lobe posterior basal subsegmental pulmonary aa.
Left lower lobe posterior basal subsegmental pulmonary a.
Vertebral body
Descending thoracic aorta
Pulmonary v.

Soft Tissue and Lung Coronal 1

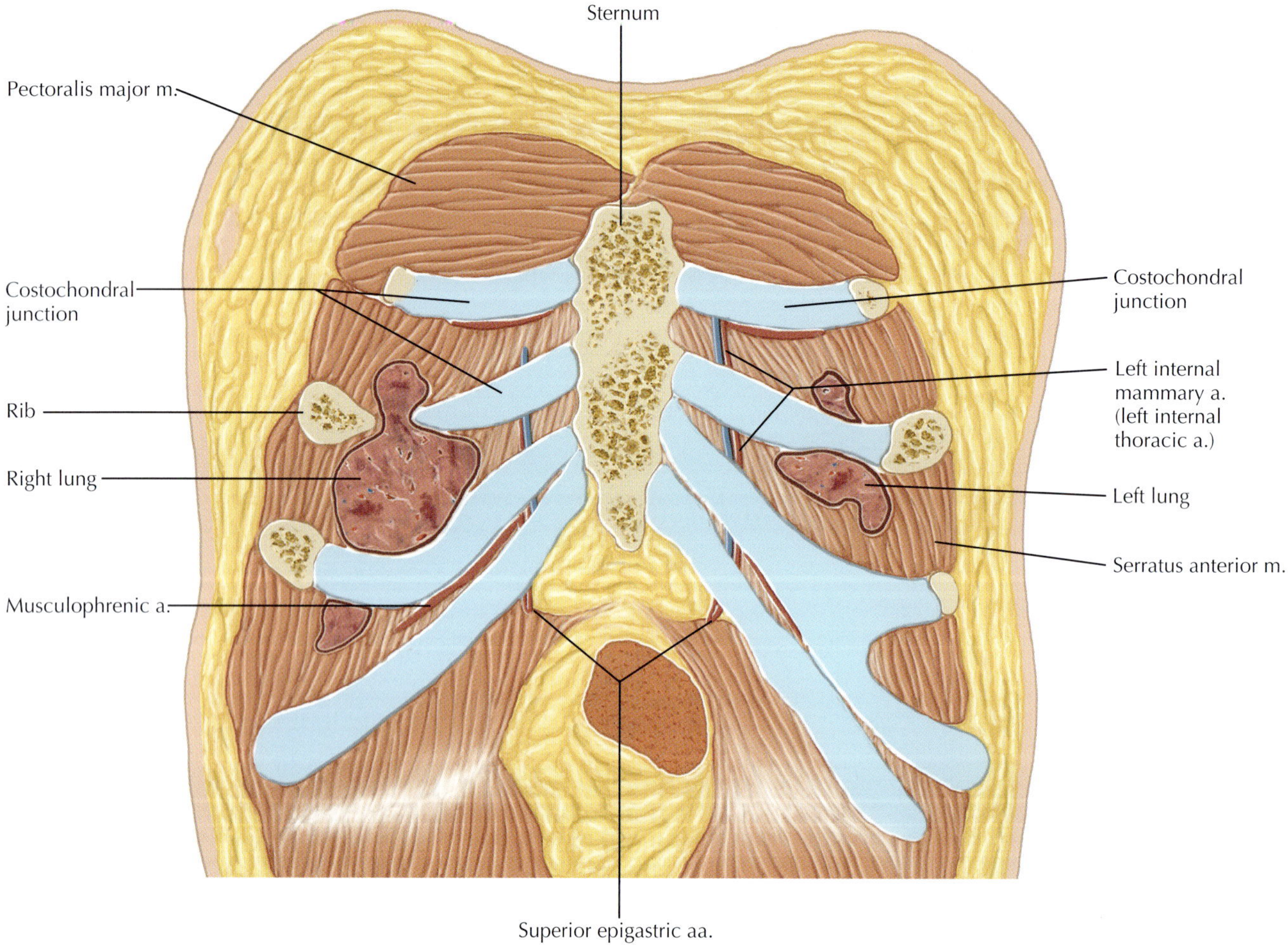

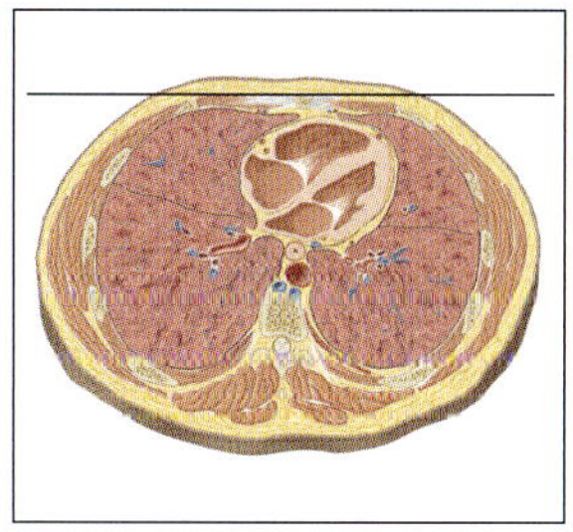

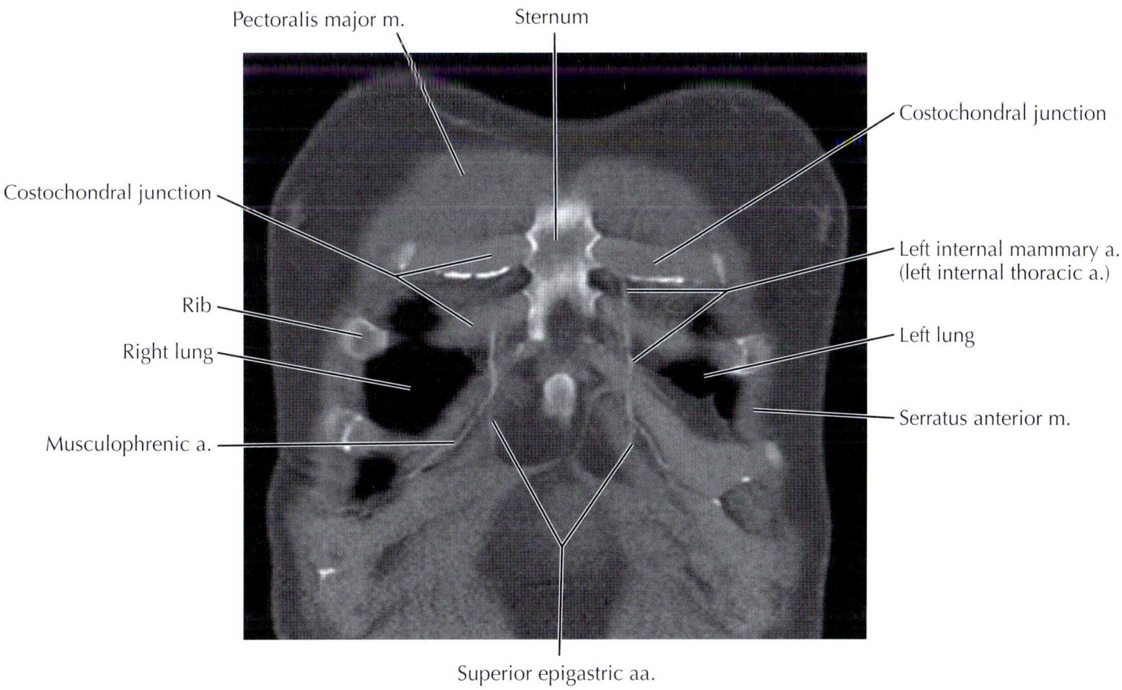
Pectoralis major m.
Sternum
Costochondral junction
Costochondral junction
Left internal mammary a.
(left internal thoracic a.)
Rib
Left lung
Right lung
Serratus anterior m.
Musculophrenic a.
Superior epigastric aa.

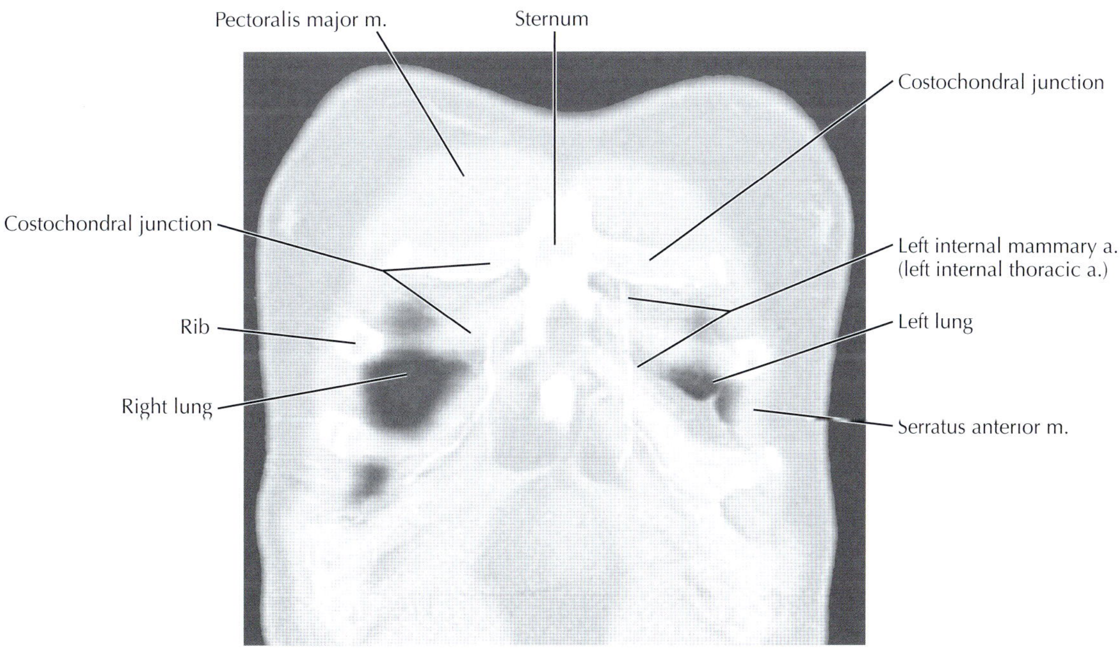
Pectoralis major m.
Sternum
Costochondral junction
Costochondral junction
Left internal mammary a.
(left internal thoracic a.)
Rib
Left lung
Right lung
Serratus anterior m.

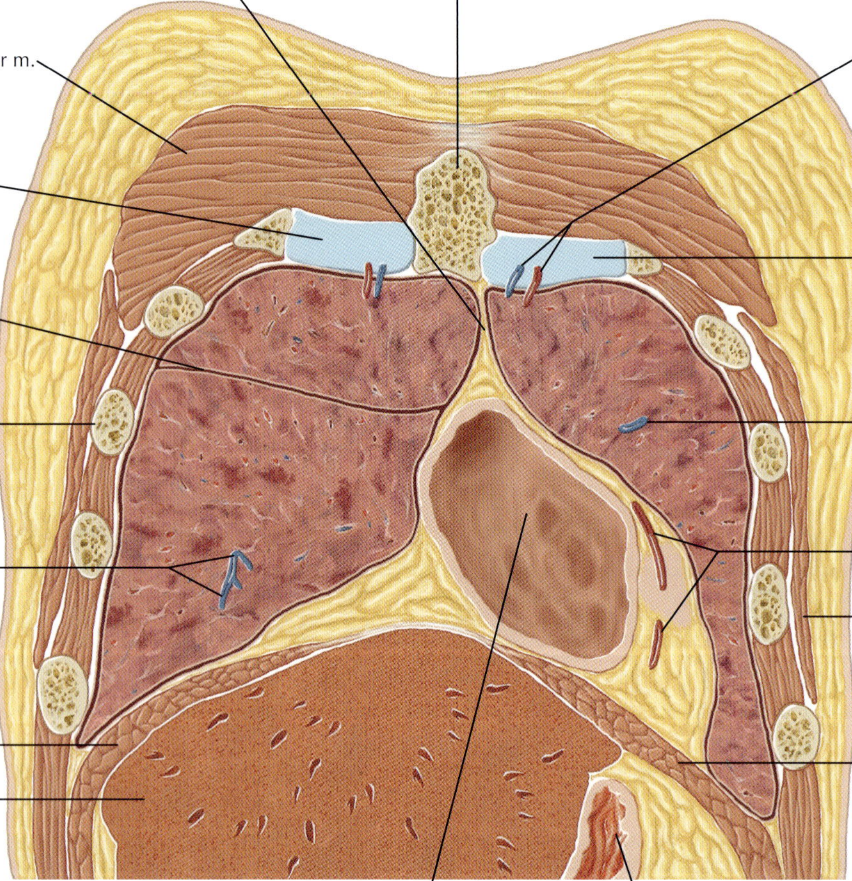

NORMAL ANATOMY

The *anterior junction line* is a linear region of contact between the anterior aspects of the right and left lungs, just posterior to the sternum. The anterior junction line consists of 4 layers of pleura with a variable amount of mediastinal fat interposed between the layers of pleura. The anterior junction line may become widened when pathological processes occur within the anterior mediastinum.

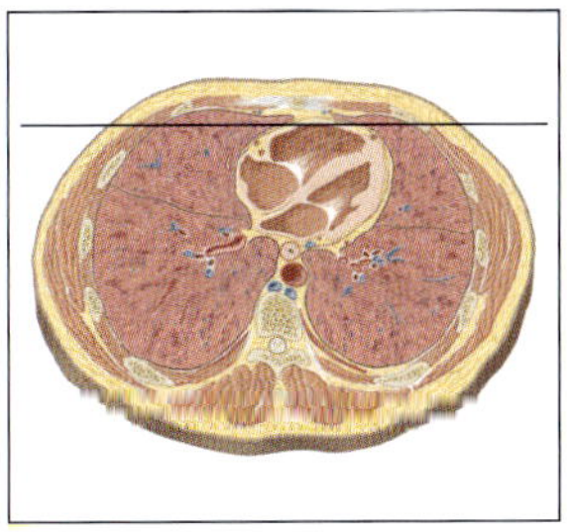

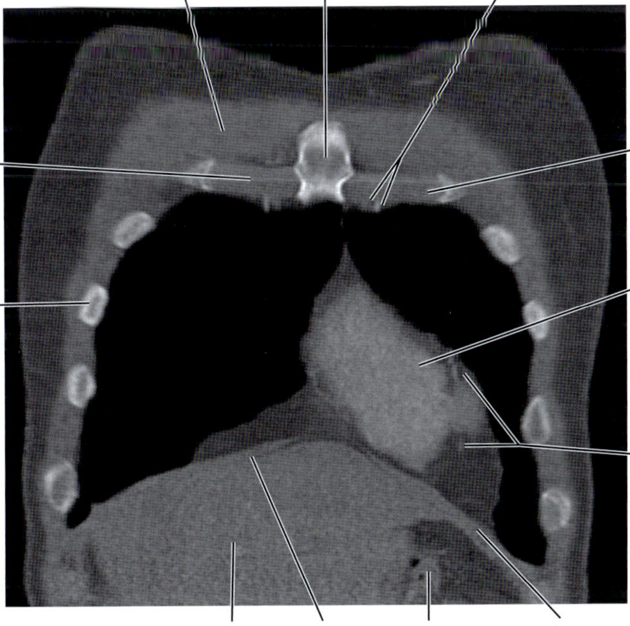
Sternum
(body)
Pectoralis major m.
Left internal mammary v. & a.
Costochondral junction
Costochondral junction
Rib
Right ventricular outflow tract
(infundibulum)
Left anterior descending
coronary a.
Liver
Diaphragm
Stomach
Diaphragm

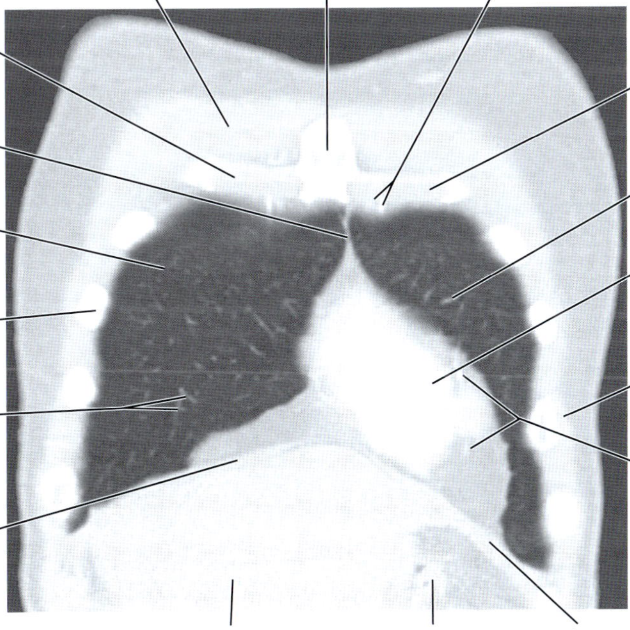
Sternum
(body)
Pectoralis major m.
Left internal mammary v. & a.
Costochondral junction
Costochondral junction
Anterior junction line
Left upper lobe anterior
subsegmental pulmonary a.
Right horizontal (minor) fissure
Right ventricular outflow tract
(infundibulum)
Rib
Serratus anterior m.
Right middle lobe medial
subsegmental pulmonary aa.
Left anterior descending
coronary a.
Diaphragm
Liver
Stomach
Diaphragm

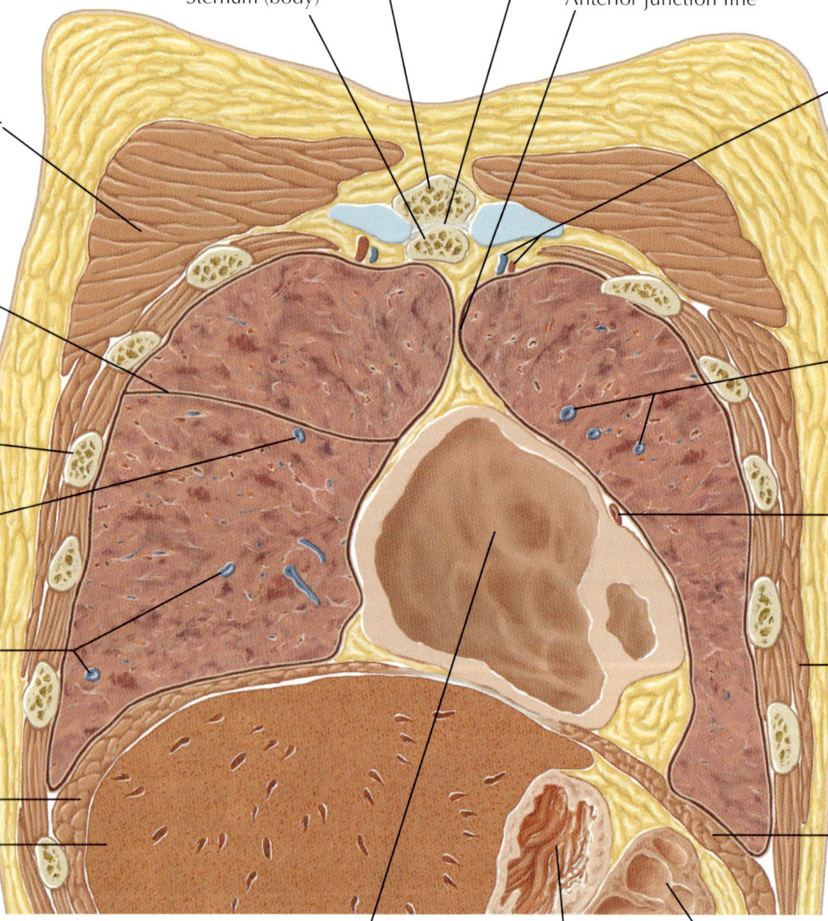

NORMAL ANATOMY

The *diaphragm* is a curved, muscular structure. Because the portion of the diaphragm located centrally between the inferior pleural space and upper abdomen is very thin and primarily oriented in the axial plane, it is difficult to visualize in the axial plane on CT. However, coronal imaging is very effective in demonstrating the curved surface of the diaphragm, as can be appreciated on this and subsequent images.

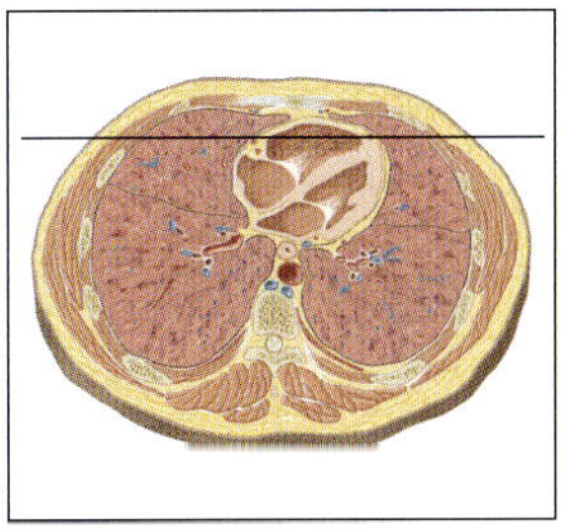

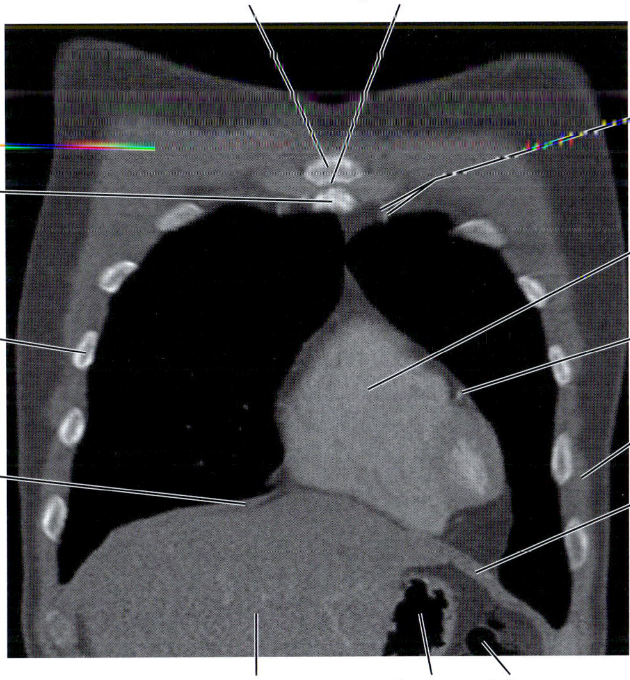
Sternum (manubrium)
Sternal-manubrial junction
Pectoralis major m.
Sternum (body)
Rib
Diaphragm
Left internal mammary v. & a.
Right ventricular outflow tract (infundibulum)
Left anterior descending coronary a.
Serratus anterior m.
Diaphragm
Liver
Stomach
Colon

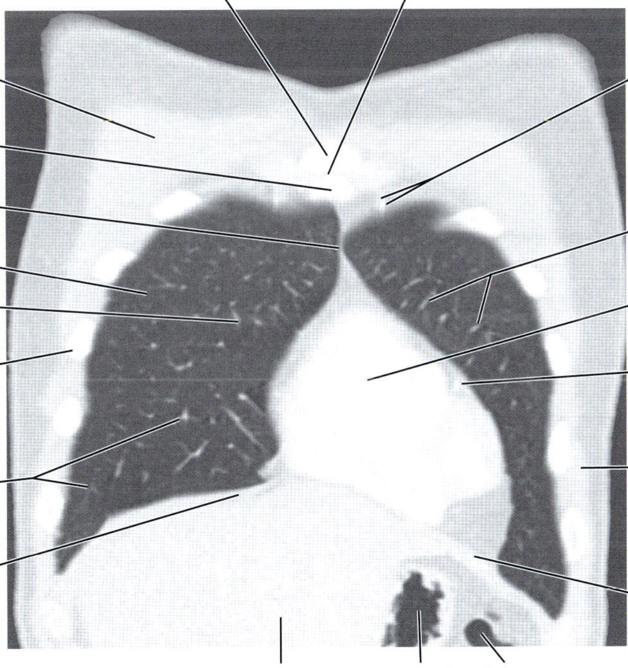
Sternum (manubrium)
Sternal-manubrial junction
Pectoralis major m.
Sternum (body)
Anterior junction line
Right horizontal (minor) fissure
Right upper lobe anterior subsegmental pulmonary a.
Rib
Right middle lobe lateral & medial subsegmental pulmonary aa.
Diaphragm
Left internal mammary v. & a.
Left upper lobe anterior subsegmental pulmonary aa.
Right ventricular outflow tract (infundibulum)
Left anterior descending coronary a.
Serratus anterior m.
Diaphragm
Liver
Stomach
Colon

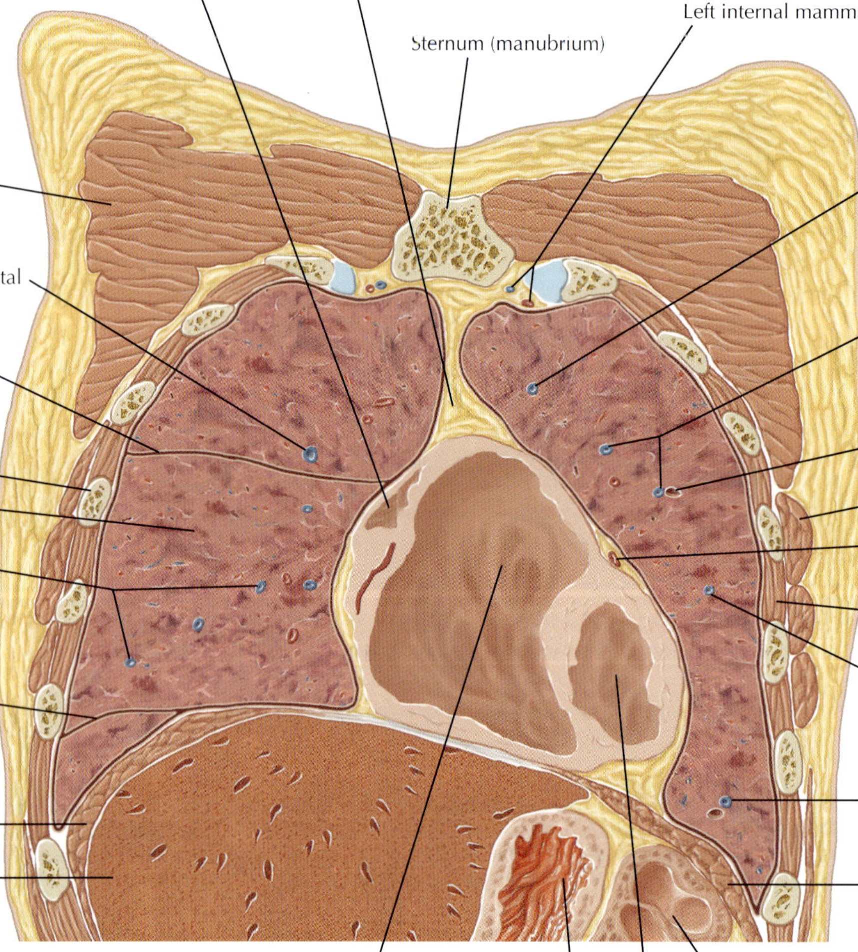
Anterior mediastinum
Right atrial appendage
Left internal mammary v. & a.
Sternum (manubrium)
Pectoralis major m.
Right upper lobe anterior subsegmental pulmonary a.
Right horizontal (minor) fissure
Rib
Right middle lobe
Right middle lobe lateral & medial subsegmental pulmonary aa.
Right oblique (major) fissure
Diaphragm
Liver
Left upper lobe apical-posterior subsegmental pulmonary a.
Left upper lobe anterior subsegmental pulmonary aa.
Left upper lobe anterior subsegmental bronchus
Serratus anterior m.
Left anterior descending coronary a.
Intercostal m.
Lingular superior subsegmental pulmonary a.
Lingular inferior subsegmental pulmonary a.
Diaphragm
Right ventricular outflow tract (infundibulum)
Stomach
Colon
Left ventricle

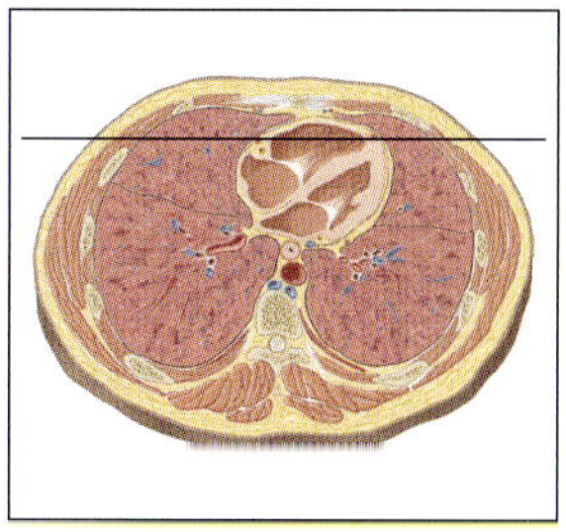

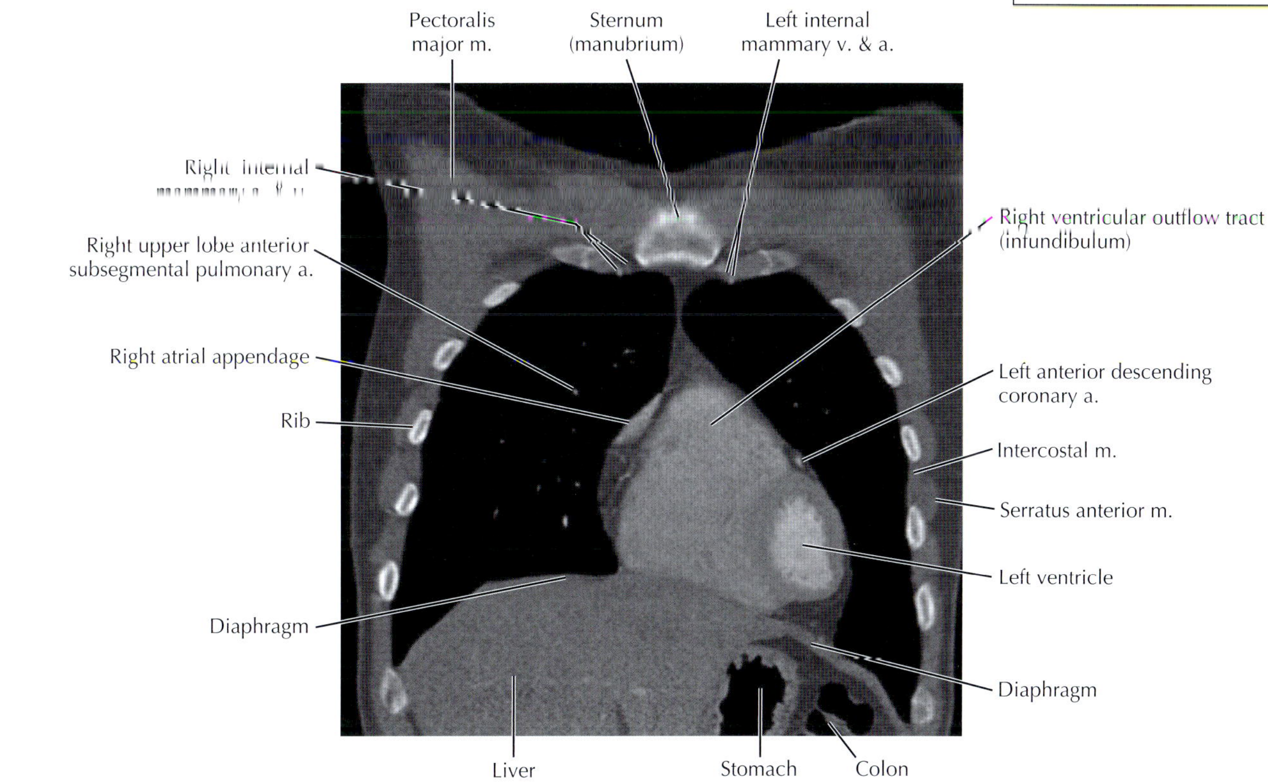
Pectoralis major m.
Sternum (manubrium)
Left internal mammary v. & a.
Right internal
Right upper lobe anterior subsegmental pulmonary a.
Right atrial appendage
Rib
Diaphragm
Liver
Stomach
Colon
Right ventricular outflow tract (infundibulum)
Left anterior descending coronary a.
Intercostal m.
Serratus anterior m.
Left ventricle
Diaphragm

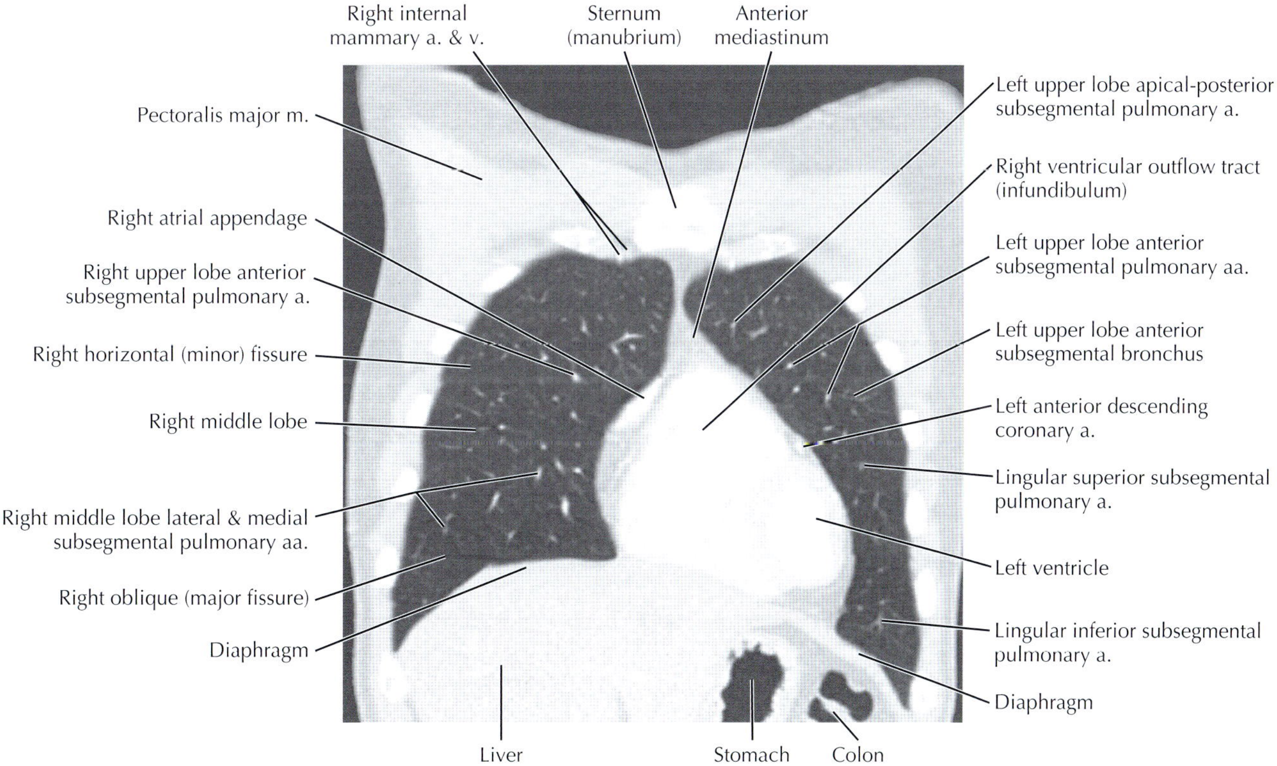
Right internal mammary a. & v.
Sternum (manubrium)
Anterior mediastinum
Pectoralis major m.
Right atrial appendage
Right upper lobe anterior subsegmental pulmonary a.
Right horizontal (minor) fissure
Right middle lobe
Right middle lobe lateral & medial subsegmental pulmonary aa.
Right oblique (major fissure)
Diaphragm
Liver
Stomach
Colon
Left upper lobe apical-posterior subsegmental pulmonary a.
Right ventricular outflow tract (infundibulum)
Left upper lobe anterior subsegmental pulmonary aa.
Left upper lobe anterior subsegmental bronchus
Left anterior descending coronary a.
Lingular superior subsegmental pulmonary a.
Left ventricle
Lingular inferior subsegmental pulmonary a.
Diaphragm

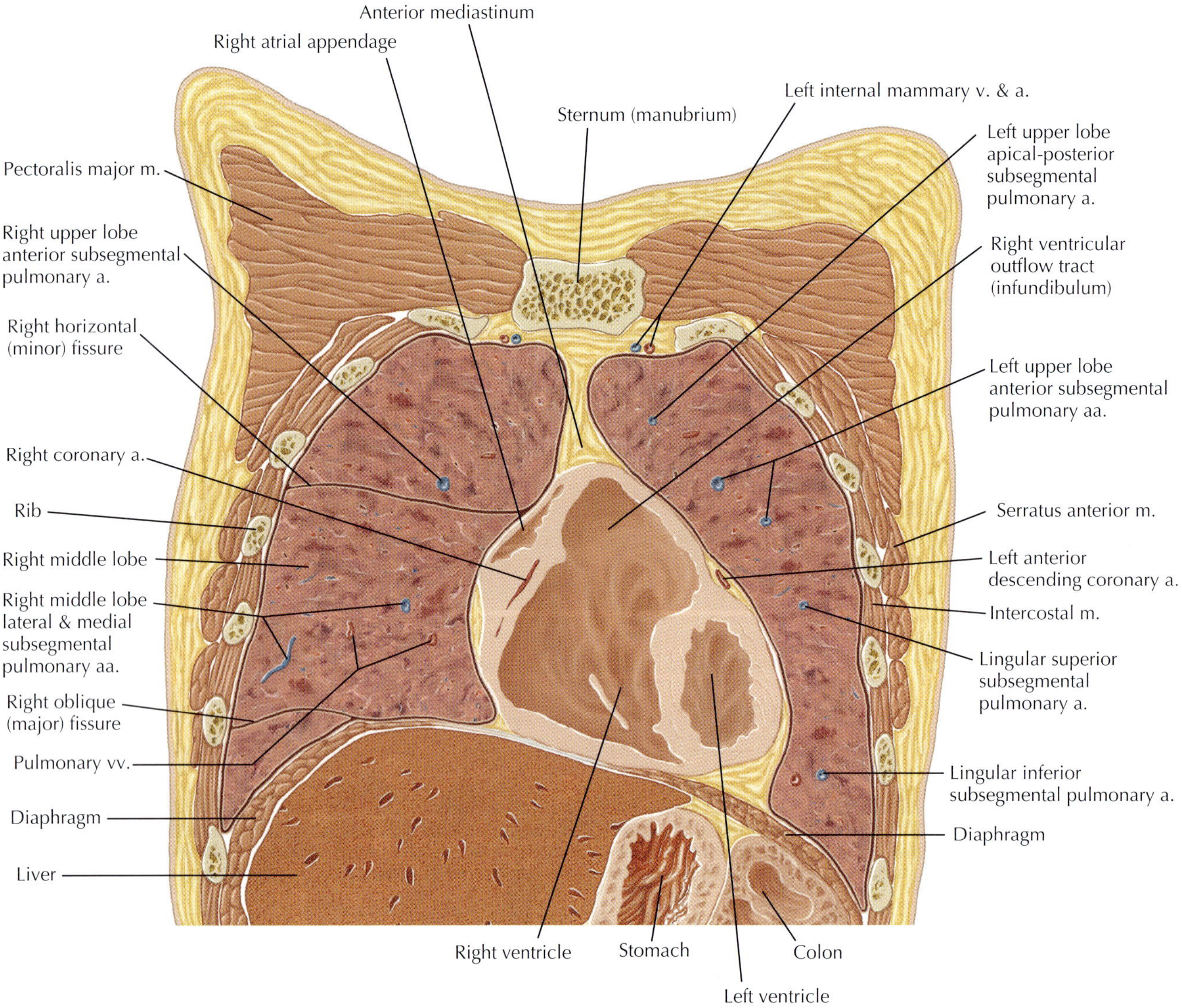
Anterior mediastinum
Right atrial appendage
Left internal mammary v. & a.
Sternum (manubrium)
Left upper lobe apical-posterior subsegmental pulmonary a.
Pectoralis major m.
Right upper lobe anterior subsegmental pulmonary a.
Right ventricular outflow tract (infundibulum)
Right horizontal (minor) fissure
Left upper lobe anterior subsegmental pulmonary aa.
Right coronary a.
Rib
Serratus anterior m.
Right middle lobe
Left anterior descending coronary a.
Right middle lobe lateral & medial subsegmental pulmonary aa.
Intercostal m.
Lingular superior subsegmental pulmonary a.
Right oblique (major) fissure
Pulmonary vv.
Lingular inferior subsegmental pulmonary a.
Diaphragm
Diaphragm
Liver
Right ventricle
Stomach
Colon
Left ventricle

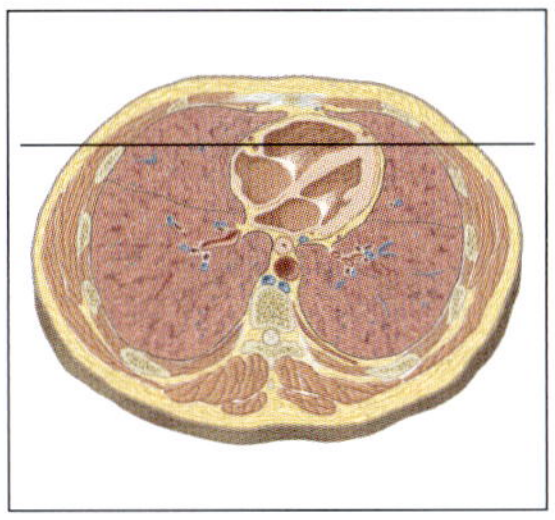

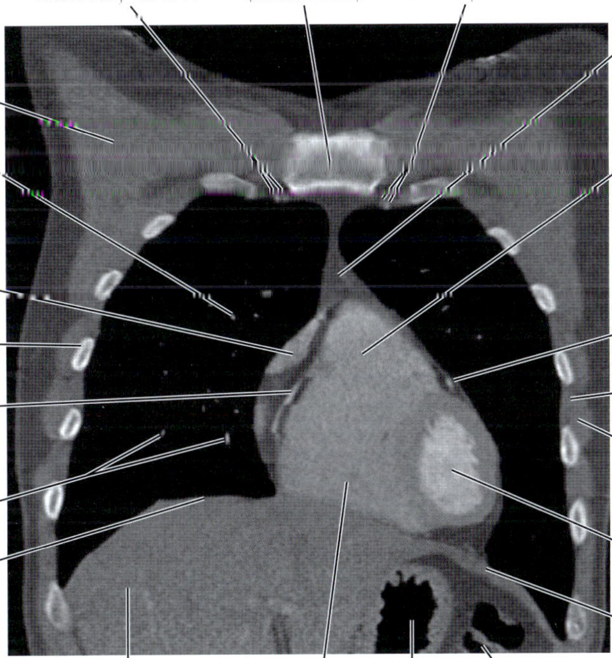
Right internal mammary a. & v.
Sternum (manubrium)
Left internal mammary v. & a.
Anterior mediastinum
Pectoralis major m.
Right upper lobe anterior subsegmental pulmonary a.
Right ventricular outflow tract (infundibulum)
Right atrial appendage
Rib
Left anterior descending coronary a.
Right coronary a.
Intercostal m.
Serratus anterior m.
Right middle lobe lateral & medial subsegmental pulmonary aa.
Left ventricle
Diaphragm
Diaphragm
Liver
Right ventricle
Stomach
Colon

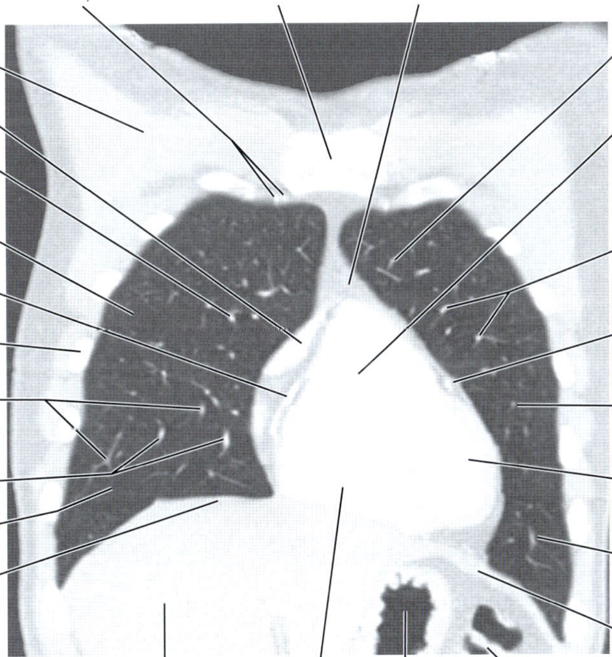
Right internal mammary a. & v.
Sternum (manubrium)
Anterior mediastinum
Pectoralis major m.
Left upper lobe apical-posterior subsegmental pulmonary a.
Right atrial appendage
Right ventricular outflow tract (infundibulum)
Right upper lobe anterior subsegmental pulmonary a.
Right horizontal (minor) fissure
Left upper lobe anterior subsegmental pulmonary aa.
Right coronary a.
Left anterior descending coronary a.
Rib
Right middle lobe lateral & medial subsegmental pulmonary aa.
Lingular superior subsegmental pulmonary a.
Pulmonary vv.
Left ventricle
Right oblique (major fissure)
Lingular inferior subsegmental pulmonary a.
Diaphragm
Diaphragm
Liver
Right ventricle
Stomach
Colon

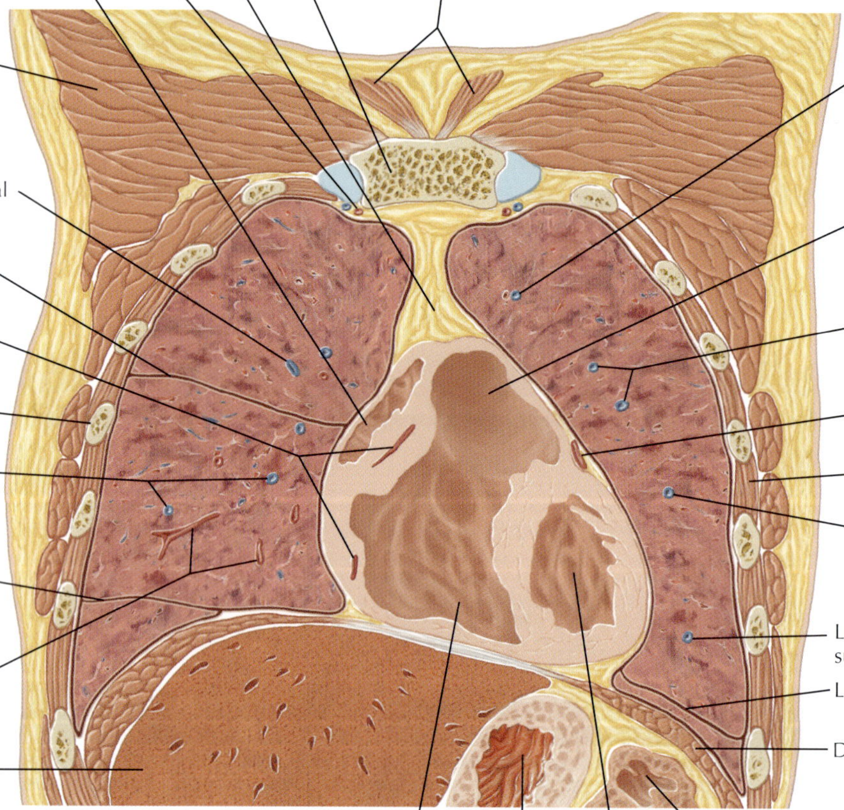
Sternum (manubrium)
Anterior mediastinum
Right internal mammary a.
Right atrial appendage
Sternocleidomastoid mm.
Pectoralis major m.
Right upper lobe anterior subsegmental pulmonary a.
Right horizontal (minor) fissure
Right coronary a.
Rib
Right middle lobe lateral & medial subsegmental pulmonary aa.
Right oblique (major) fissure
Pulmonary vv.
Liver
Left upper lobe apical-posterior subsegmental pulmonary a.
Right ventricular outflow tract (infundibulum)
Left upper lobe anterior subsegmental pulmonary aa.
Left anterior descending coronary a.
Intercostal m.
Lingular superior subsegmental pulmonary a.
Lingular inferior subsegmental pulmonary a.
Left oblique (major) fissure
Diaphragm
Right ventricle
Stomach
Colon
Left ventricle

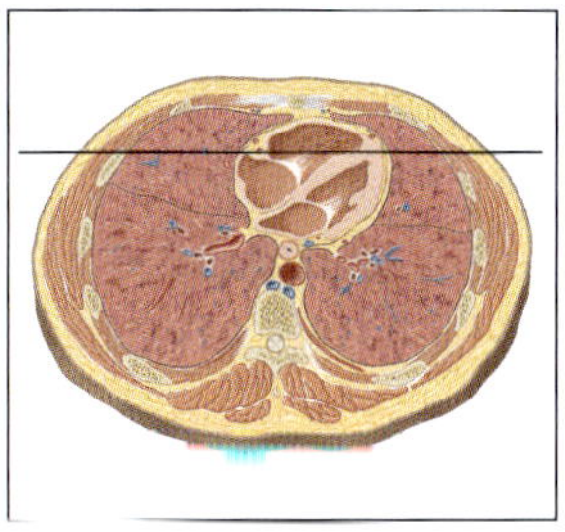

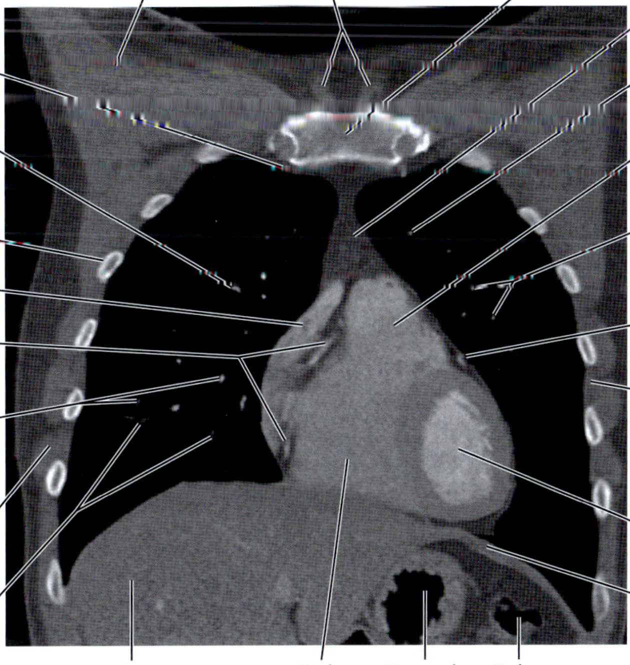
Pectoralis major m.
Sternocleidomastoid mm.
Sternum (manubrium)
Right internal mammary a.
Right upper lobe anterior subsegmental pulmonary a.
Rib
Right atrial appendage
Right coronary a.
Right middle lobe lateral & medial subsegmental pulmonary aa.
Serratus anterior m.
Pulmonary vv.
Anterior mediastinum
Left upper lobe apical posterior subsegmental pulmonary a.
Right ventricular outflow tract (infundibulum)
Left upper lobe anterior subsegmental pulmonary aa.
Left anterior descending coronary a.
Intercostal m.
Left ventricle
Diaphragm
Liver
Right ventricle
Stomach
Colon

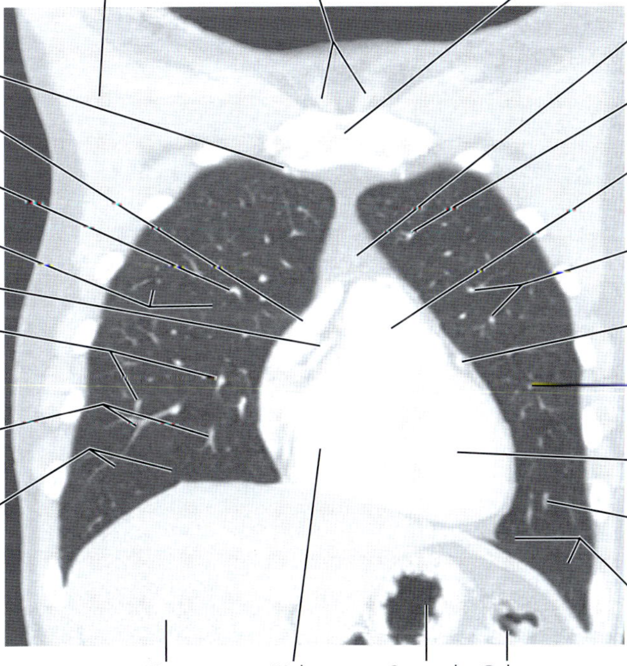
Pectoralis major m.
Sternocleidomastoid m.
Sternum (manubrium)
Right internal mammary a.
Right atrial appendage
Right upper lobe anterior subsegmental pulmonary a.
Right horizontal (minor) fissure
Right coronary a.
Right middle lobe lateral & medial subsegmental pulmonary aa.
Pulmonary vv.
Right oblique (major fissure)
Anterior mediastinum
Left upper lobe apical-posterior subsegmental pulmonary a.
Right ventricular outflow tract (infundibulum)
Left upper lobe anterior subsegmental pulmonary aa.
Left anterior descending coronary a.
Lingular superior subsegmental pulmonary a.
Left ventricle
Lingular inferior subsegmental pulmonary a.
Left oblique (major) fissure
Liver
Right ventricle
Stomach
Colon

Soft Tissue and Lung Coronal 7

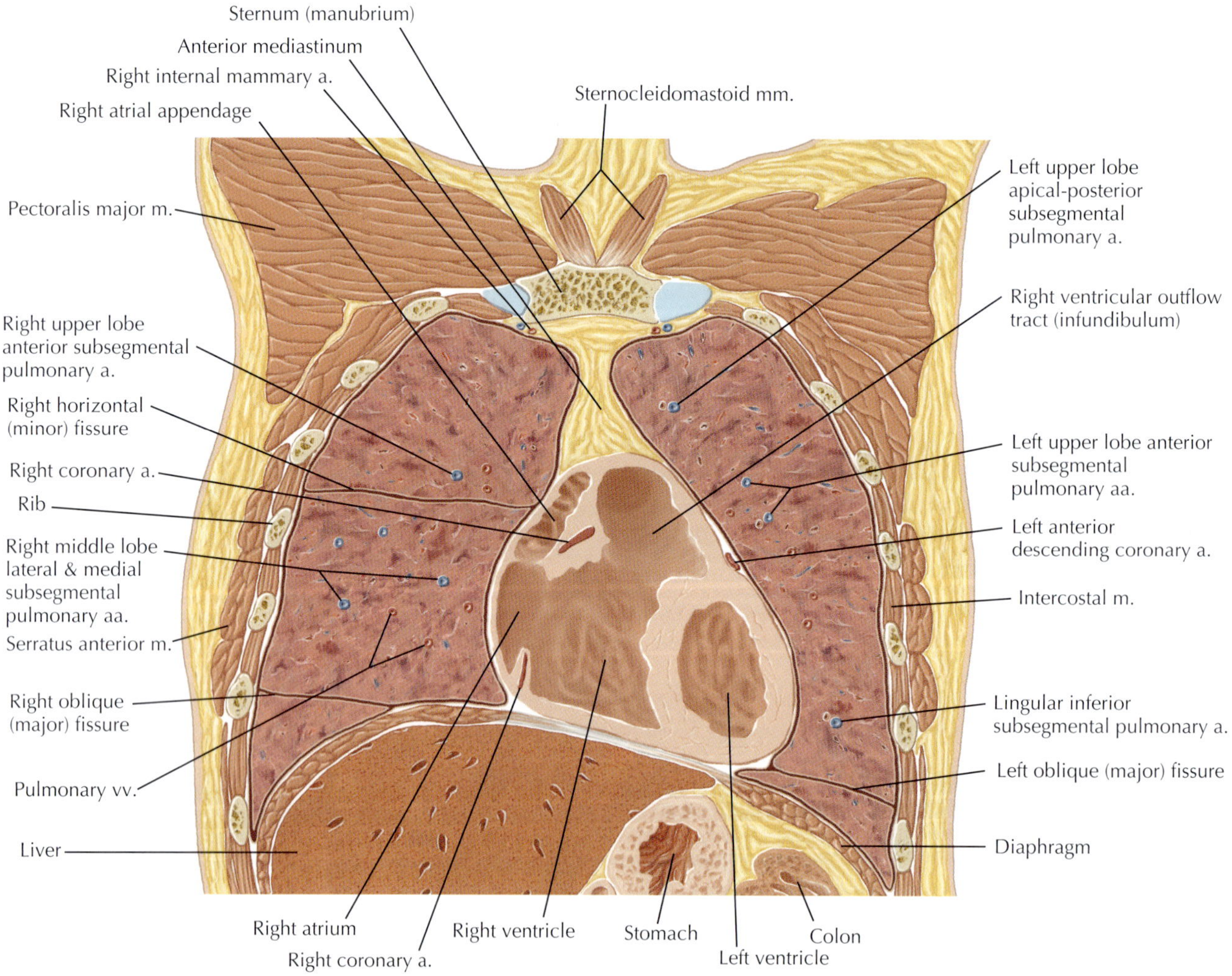

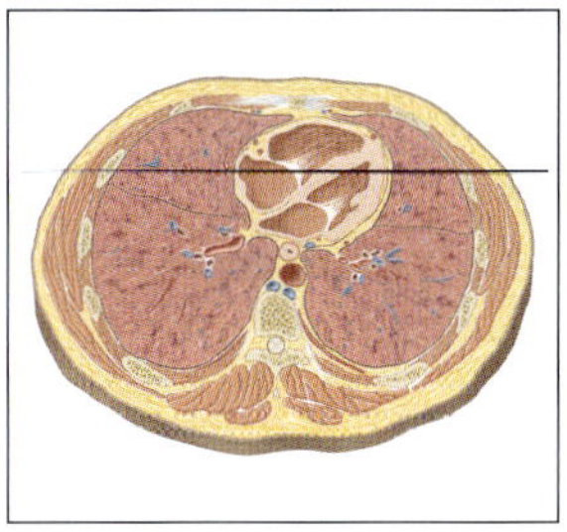

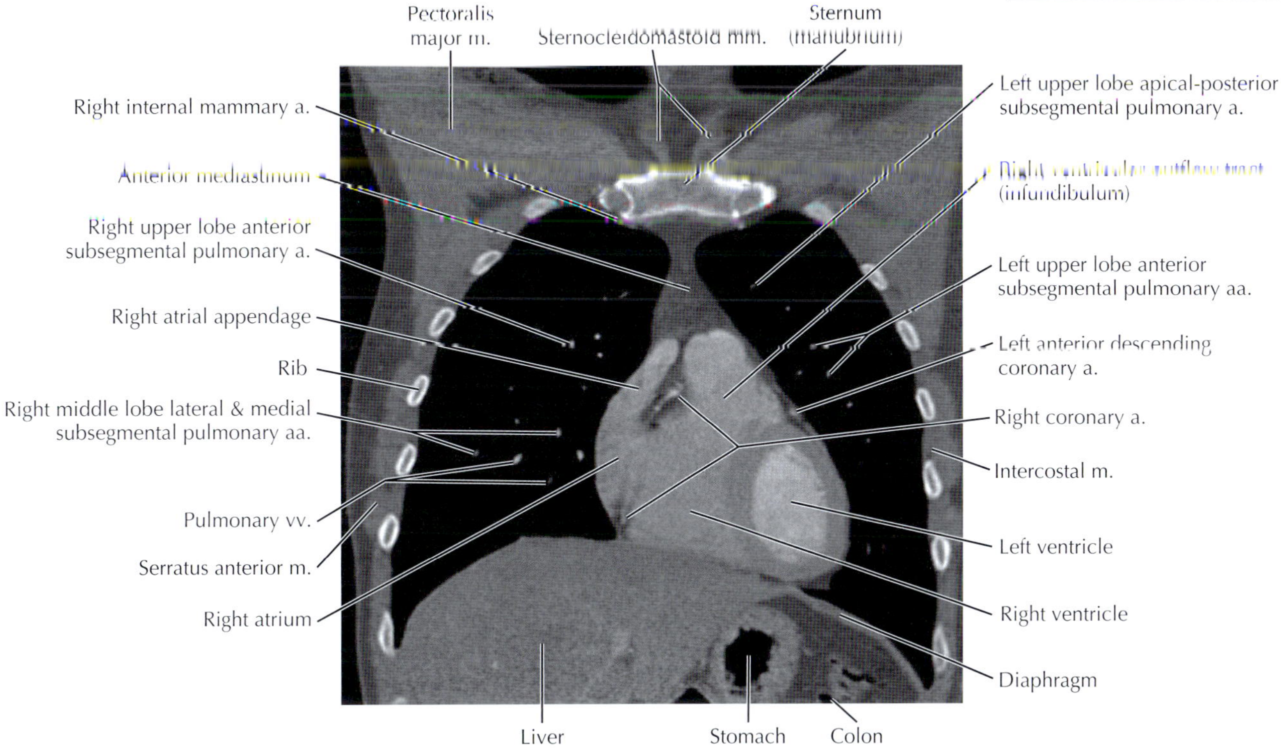
Pectoralis major m.
Sternocleidomastoid mm.
Sternum (manubrium)
Right internal mammary a.
Anterior mediastinum
Right upper lobe anterior subsegmental pulmonary a.
Right atrial appendage
Rib
Right middle lobe lateral & medial subsegmental pulmonary aa.
Pulmonary vv.
Serratus anterior m.
Right atrium
Left upper lobe apical-posterior subsegmental pulmonary a.
(infundibulum)
Left upper lobe anterior subsegmental pulmonary aa.
Left anterior descending coronary a.
Right coronary a.
Intercostal m.
Left ventricle
Right ventricle
Diaphragm
Liver
Stomach
Colon

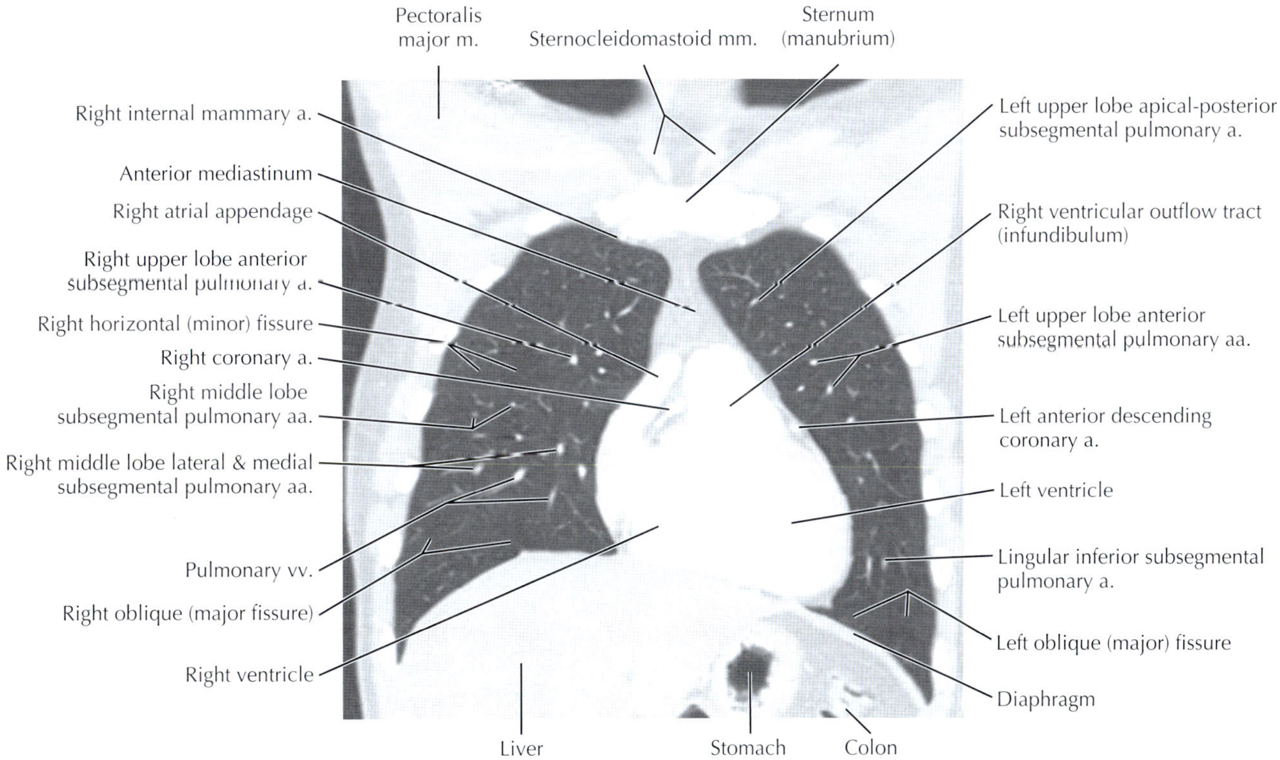
Pectoralis major m.
Sternocleidomastoid mm.
Sternum (manubrium)
Right internal mammary a.
Anterior mediastinum
Right atrial appendage
Right upper lobe anterior subsegmental pulmonary a.
Right horizontal (minor) fissure
Right coronary a.
Right middle lobe subsegmental pulmonary aa.
Right middle lobe lateral & medial subsegmental pulmonary aa.
Pulmonary vv.
Right oblique (major fissure)
Right ventricle
Left upper lobe apical-posterior subsegmental pulmonary a.
Right ventricular outflow tract (infundibulum)
Left upper lobe anterior subsegmental pulmonary aa.
Left anterior descending coronary a.
Left ventricle
Lingular inferior subsegmental pulmonary a.
Left oblique (major) fissure
Diaphragm
Liver
Stomach
Colon

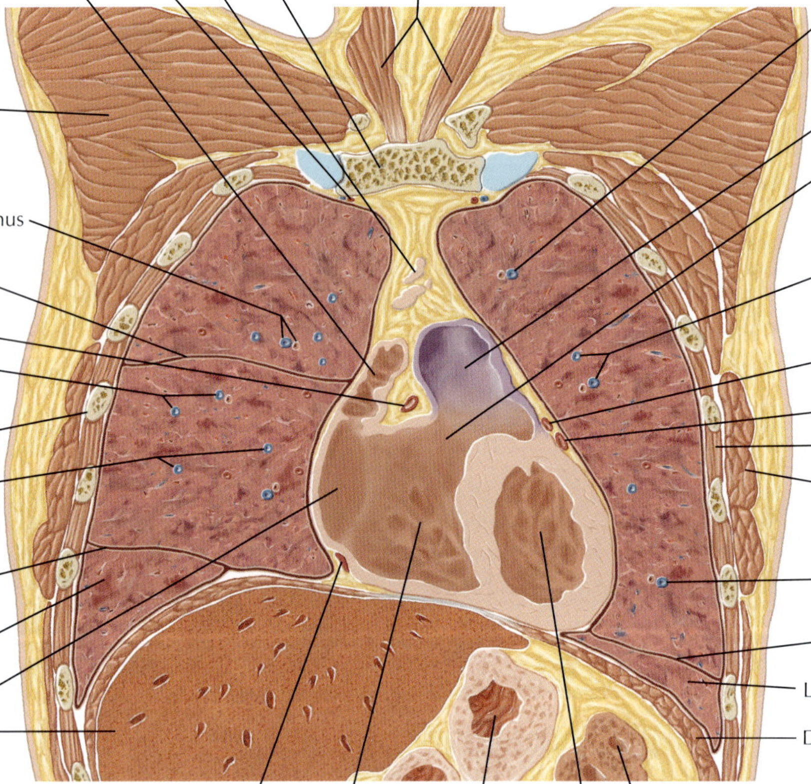

NORMAL ANATOMY

The tissue composition of the anterior mediastinum varies with age. In younger patients (particularly infants and children), abundant soft tissue, representing thymic tissue, is found residing within anterior mediastinal fat. As individuals age, the thymus normally involutes and becomes more fatty replaced, and progressively less soft tissue is visible within the anterior mediastinal fat. The pace at which thymic involution occurs is variable, and a fairly wide variation in the appearance of "normal thymus" at various ages is recognized. In young adults, such as this patient, residual thymus is often visualized as small nodular areas of soft tissue interspersed within lower-attenuation anterior mediastinal fat.

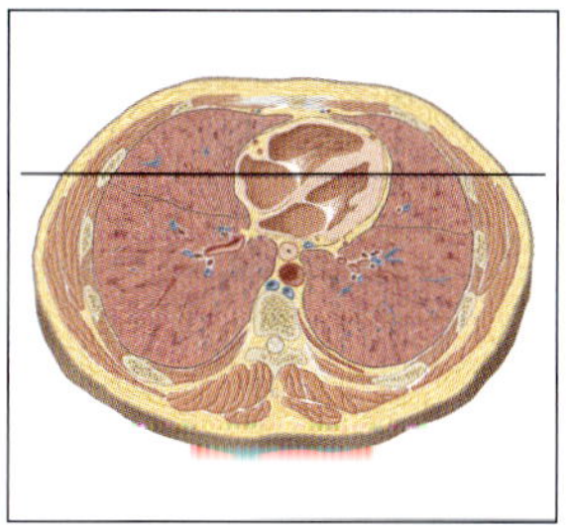

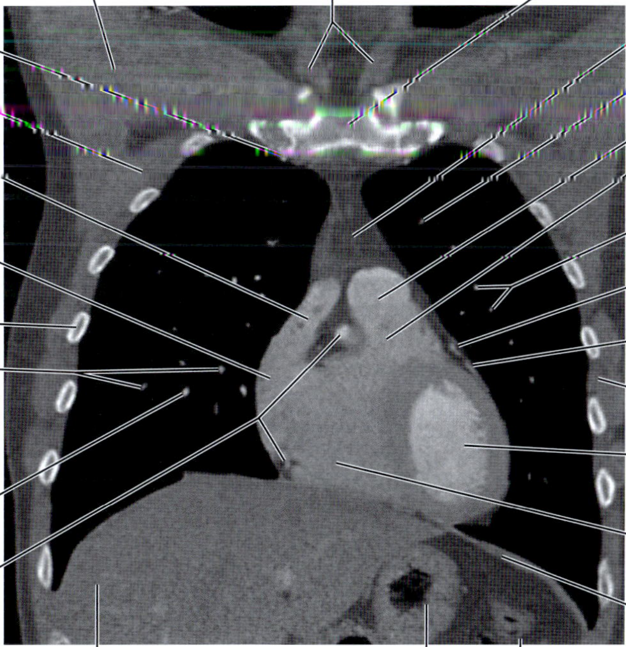
Pectoralis major m.
Sternocleidomastoid mm.
Sternum (manubrium)
Right internal mammary a.
Pectoralis minor m.
Right atrial appendage
Right atrium
Rib
Right middle lobe lateral & medial subsegmental pulmonary aa.
Right middle lobe pulmonary v.
Right coronary a.
Anterior mediastinum (residual thymus)
Left upper lobe apical-posterior subsegmental pulmonary a.
Main pulmonary a.
Right ventricular outflow tract (infundibulum)
Left upper lobe anterior subsegmental pulmonary aa.
Left anterior descending coronary a.
Diagonal coronary a.
Intercostal m.
Left ventricle
Right ventricle
Diaphragm
Liver
Stomach
Colon

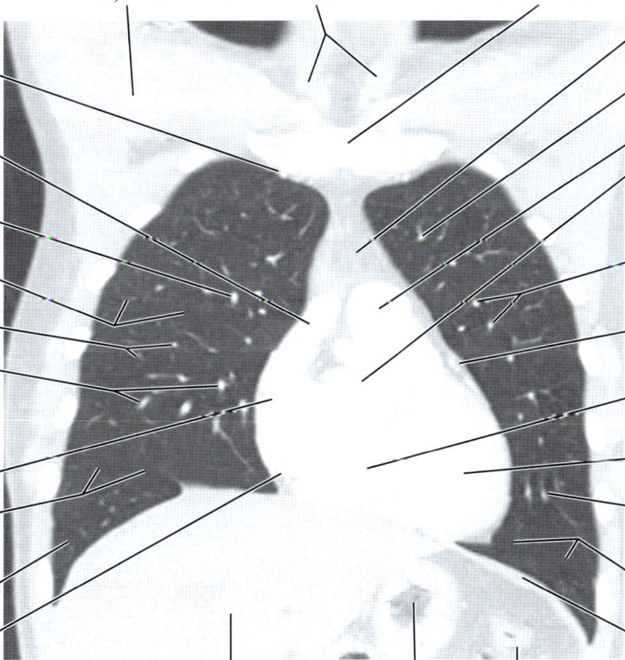
Pectoralis major m.
Sternocleidomastoid mm.
Sternum (manubrium)
Right internal mammary a.
Right atrial appendage
Right upper lobe anterior subsegmental pulmonary a.
Right horizontal (minor) fissure
Right middle lobe subsegmental pulmonary aa.
Right middle lobe lateral & medial subsegmental pulmonary aa.
Right atrium
Right oblique (major fissure)
Right lower lobe
Right coronary a.
Anterior mediastinum (residual thymus)
Left upper lobe apical-posterior subsegmental pulmonary a.
Main pulmonary a.
Right ventricular outflow tract (infundibulum)
Left upper lobe anterior subsegmental pulmonary aa.
Left anterior descending coronary a.
Right ventricle
Left ventricle
Lingular inferior subsegmental pulmonary a.
Left oblique (major) fissure
Diaphragm
Liver
Stomach
Colon

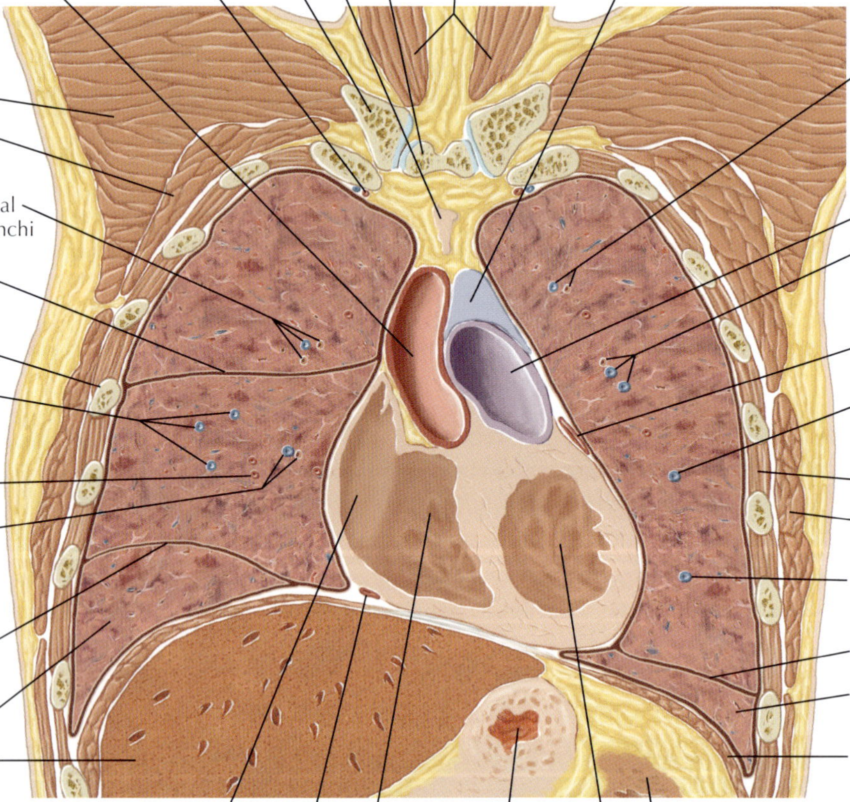

NORMAL ANATOMY

A small amount of low-attenuation fluid is visualized between the ascending aorta and main pulmonary artery; this fluid represents *pericardial fluid*. A small amount of pericardial fluid is commonly visualized in various pericardial recesses on thoracic CT studies.

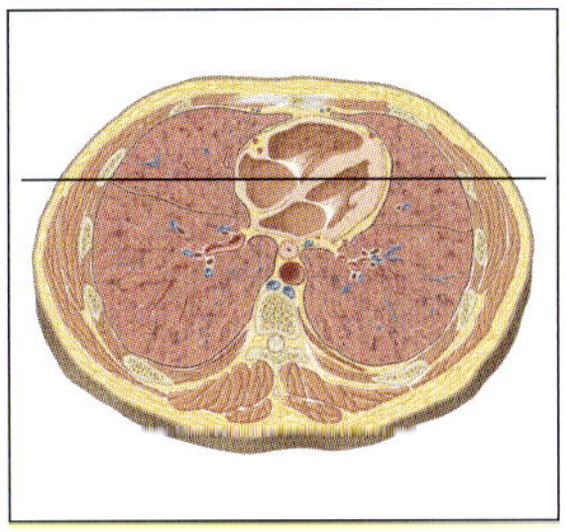

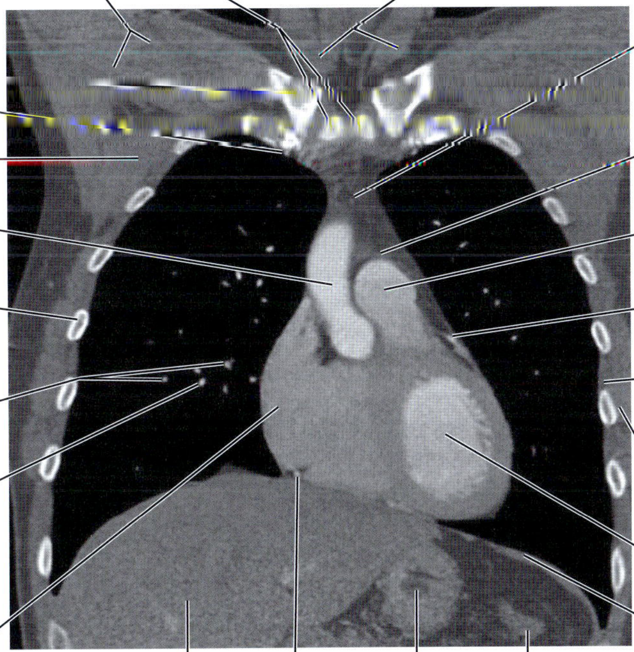
Pectoralis major m.
Sternum (manubrium)
Sternocleidomastoid mm.
Clavicle
Right internal mammary a.
Pectoralis minor m.
Ascending aorta
Rib
Right middle lobe lateral & medial subsegmental pulmonary aa.
Right middle lobe pulmonary v.
Right atrium
Liver
Right coronary a.
Stomach
Colon
Anterior mediastinum (residual thymus)
Pericardial fluid (normal)
Main pulmonary a.
Left anterior descending coronary a.
Intercostal m.
Serratus anterior m.
Left ventricle
Diaphragm

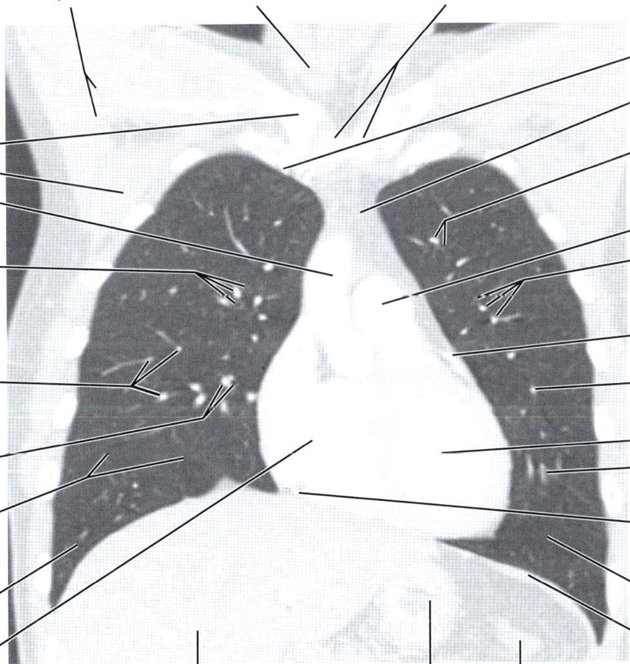
Pectoralis major m.
Sternocleidomastoid m.
Sternum (manubrium)
Clavicle
Pectoralis minor m.
Ascending aorta
Right upper lobe anterior subsegmental pulmonary a. & bronchi
Right middle lobe lateral subsegmental pulmonary aa.
Right middle lobe medial subsegmental pulmonary a. & bronchus
Right oblique (major) fissure
Right lower lobe
Right atrium
Liver
Stomach
Colon
Right internal mammary a.
Anterior mediastinum (residual thymus)
Left upper lobe apical-posterior subsegmental pulmonary a. & bronchus
Main pulmonary a.
Left upper lobe anterior subsegmental pulmonary aa. & bronchus
Left anterior descending coronary a.
Lingular superior subsegmental pulmonary a.
Left ventricle
Lingular inferior subsegmental pulmonary a.
Right coronary a.
Left oblique (major) fissure
Diaphragm

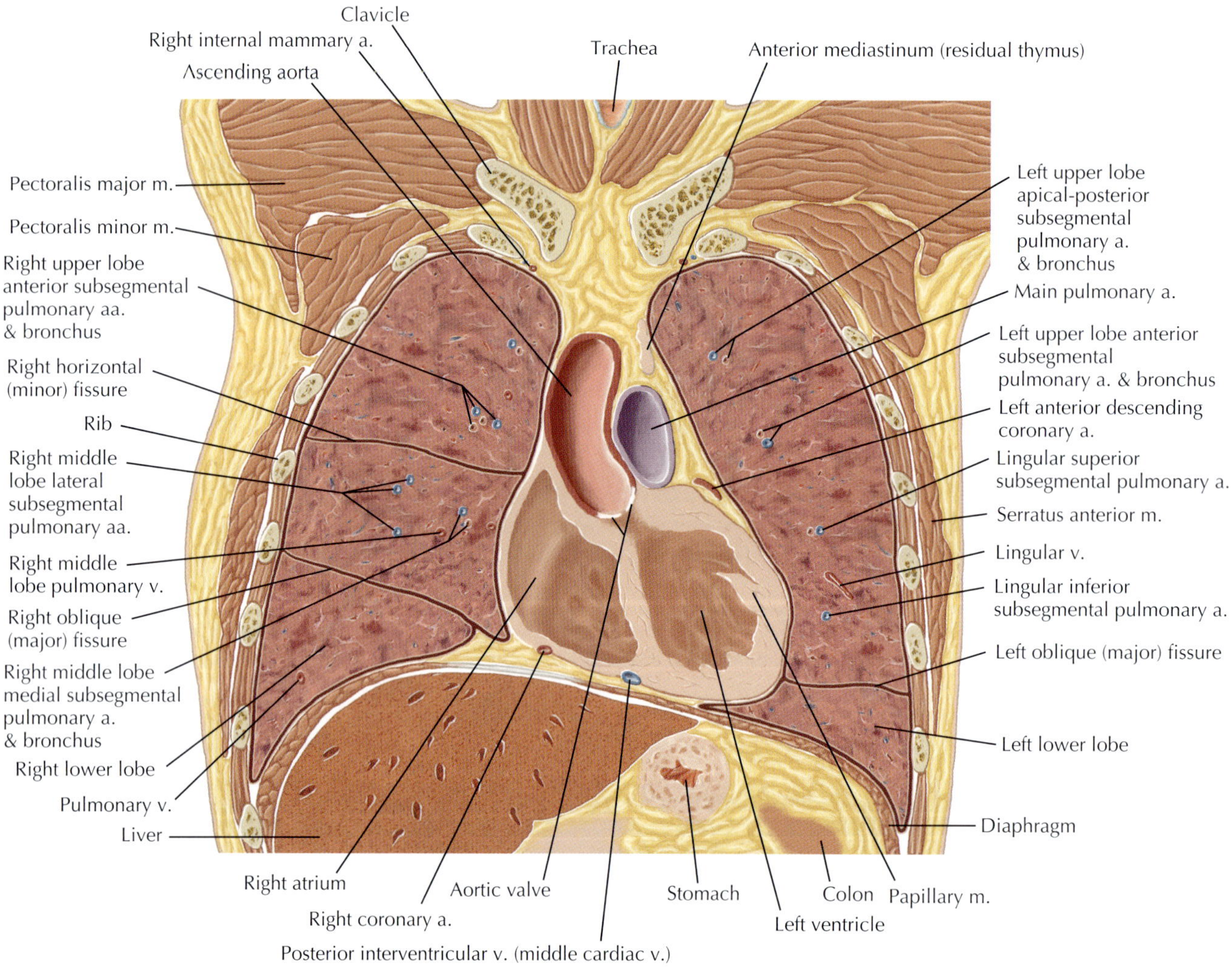

Clavicle
Right internal mammary a.
Ascending aorta
Trachea
Anterior mediastinum (residual thymus)
Pectoralis major m.
Pectoralis minor m.
Right upper lobe anterior subsegmental pulmonary aa. & bronchus
Right horizontal (minor) fissure
Rib
Right middle lobe lateral subsegmental pulmonary aa.
Right middle lobe pulmonary v.
Right oblique (major) fissure
Right middle lobe medial subsegmental pulmonary a. & bronchus
Right lower lobe
Pulmonary v.
Liver
Left upper lobe apical-posterior subsegmental pulmonary a. & bronchus
Main pulmonary a.
Left upper lobe anterior subsegmental pulmonary a. & bronchus
Left anterior descending coronary a.
Lingular superior subsegmental pulmonary a.
Serratus anterior m.
Lingular v.
Lingular inferior subsegmental pulmonary a.
Left oblique (major) fissure
Left lower lobe
Diaphragm
Right atrium
Aortic valve
Right coronary a.
Posterior interventricular v. (middle cardiac v.)
Stomach
Colon
Papillary m.
Left ventricle

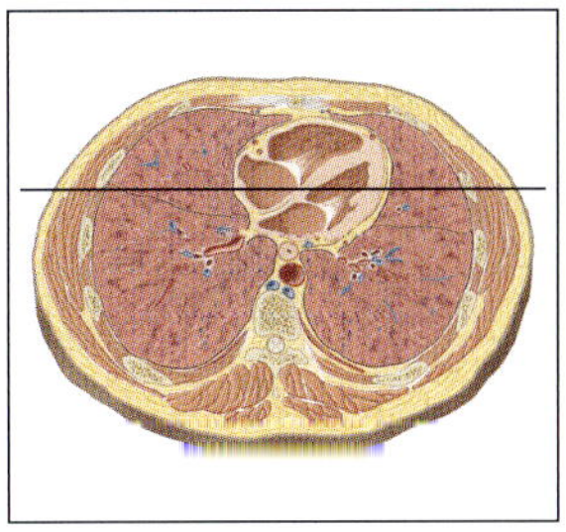

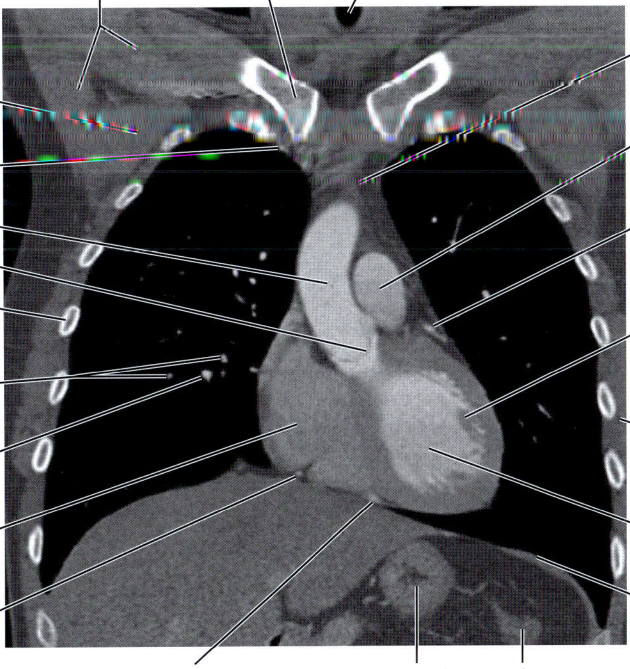
Pectoralis major m.
Clavicle
Trachea
Anterior mediastinum (residual thymus)
Pectoralis minor m.
Main pulmonary a.
Right internal mammary a.
Ascending aorta
Left anterior descending coronary a.
Aortic valve
Rib
Papillary m.
Right middle lobe lateral & medial subsegmental pulmonary aa.
Serratus anterior m.
Right middle lobe pulmonary v.
Left ventricle
Right atrium
Diaphragm
Right coronary a.
Posterior interventricular v. (middle cardiac v.)
Stomach
Colon

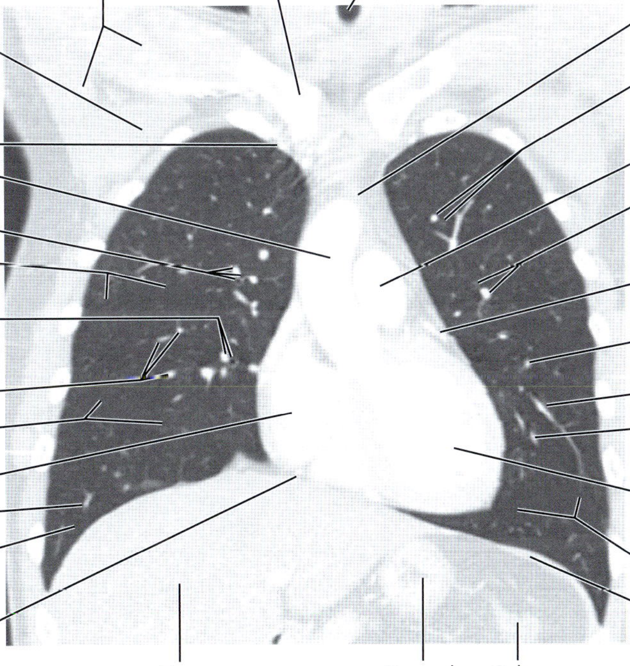
Pectoralis major m.
Clavicle
Trachea
Anterior mediastinum (residual thymus)
Pectoralis minor m.
Left upper lobe apical-posterior subsegmental pulmonary a. & bronchus
Right internal mammary a.
Main pulmonary a.
Ascending aorta
Right upper lobe anterior subsegmental pulmonary a. & bronchi
Left upper lobe anterior subsegmental pulmonary a. & bronchus
Right horizontal (minor) fissure
Right middle lobe medial subsegmental pulmonary a. & bronchus
Left anterior descending coronary a.
Lingular superior subsegmental pulmonary a.
Right middle lobe lateral subsegmental pulmonary aa.
Lingular v.
Right oblique (major fissure)
Lingular inferior subsegmental pulmonary a.
Right atrium
Left ventricle
Pulmonary a.
Right lower lobe
Left oblique (major) fissure
Diaphragm
Right coronary a.
Liver
Stomach
Colon

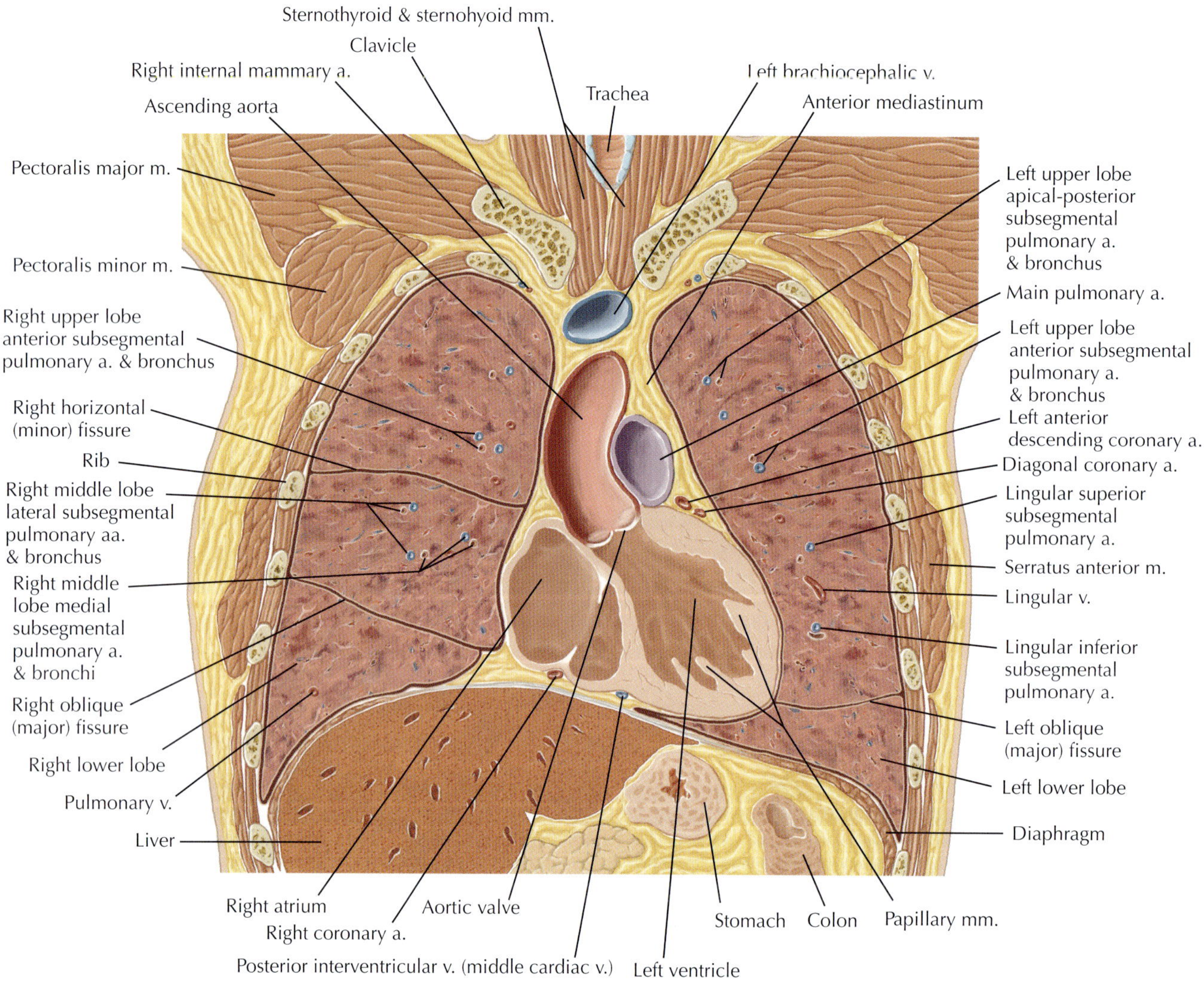
Sternothyroid & sternohyoid mm.
Clavicle
Right internal mammary a.
Ascending aorta
Trachea
Left brachiocephalic v.
Anterior mediastinum
Pectoralis major m.
Pectoralis minor m.
Right upper lobe anterior subsegmental pulmonary a. & bronchus
Right horizontal (minor) fissure
Rib
Right middle lobe lateral subsegmental pulmonary aa. & bronchus
Right middle lobe medial subsegmental pulmonary a. & bronchi
Right oblique (major) fissure
Right lower lobe
Pulmonary v.
Liver
Left upper lobe apical-posterior subsegmental pulmonary a. & bronchus
Main pulmonary a.
Left upper lobe anterior subsegmental pulmonary a. & bronchus
Left anterior descending coronary a.
Diagonal coronary a.
Lingular superior subsegmental pulmonary a.
Serratus anterior m.
Lingular v.
Lingular inferior subsegmental pulmonary a.
Left oblique (major) fissure
Left lower lobe
Diaphragm
Right atrium
Aortic valve
Right coronary a.
Posterior interventricular v. (middle cardiac v.)
Left ventricle
Stomach
Colon
Papillary mm.

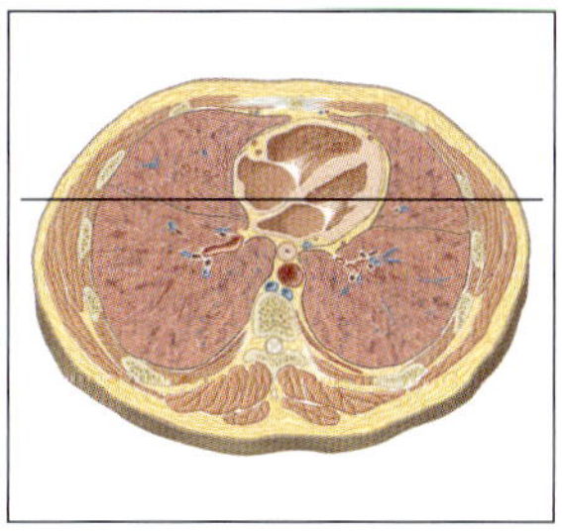

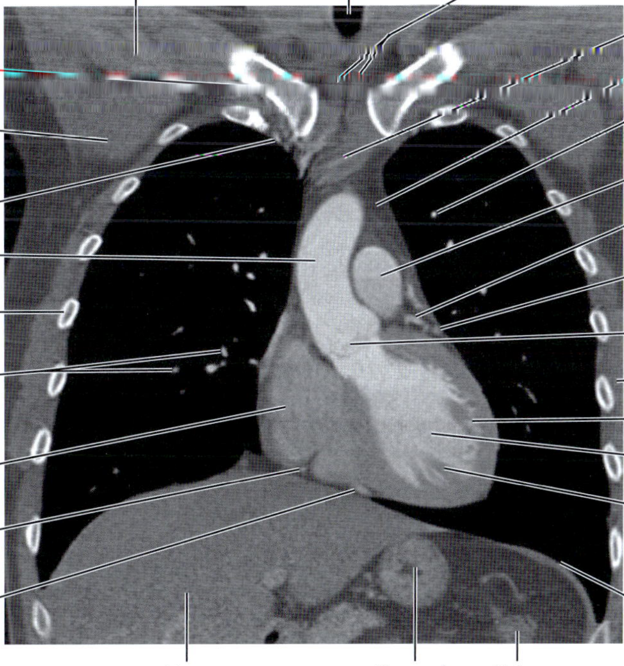
Pectoralis major m.
Trachea
Sternothyroid & sternohyoid mm.
Left brachiocephalic v.
Anterior mediastinum
Left upper lobe apical-posterior subsegmental pulmonary a.
Main pulmonary a.
Left anterior descending coronary a.
Diagonal coronary a.
Aortic valve
Serratus anterior m.
Papillary m.
Left ventricle
Papillary m.
Diaphragm
Clavicle
Pectoralis minor m.
Right internal mammary a.
Ascending aorta
Rib
Right middle lobe lateral & medial subsegmental pulmonary aa.
Right atrium
Right coronary a.
Posterior interventricular v. (middle cardiac v.)
Liver
Stomach
Colon

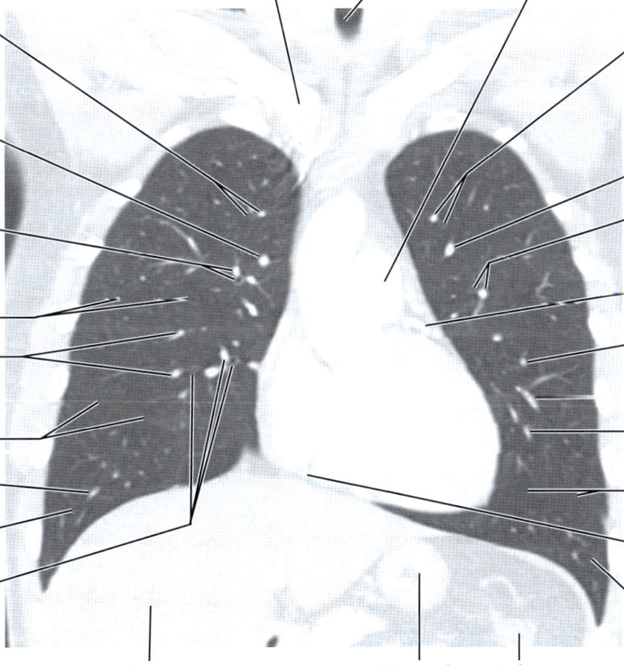
Clavicle
Trachea
Main pulmonary a.
Right upper lobe apical subsegmental pulmonary a. & bronchus
Pulmonary v.
Right upper lobe anterior subsegmental pulmonary a. & bronchus
Right horizontal (minor) fissure
Right middle lobe lateral subsegmental pulmonary aa.
Right oblique (major) fissure
Pulmonary v.
Right lower lobe
Right middle lobe medial subsegmental pulmonary a. & bronchi
Left upper lobe apical-posterior subsegmental pulmonary a. & bronchus
Pulmonary v.
Left upper lobe anterior subsegmental pulmonary a. & bronchus
Left anterior descending coronary a.
Lingular superior subsegmental pulmonary a.
Lingular v.
Lingular inferior subsegmental pulmonary a.
Left oblique (major) fissure
Right coronary a.
Left lower lobe
Liver
Stomach
Colon

Soft Tissue and Lung Coronal 12

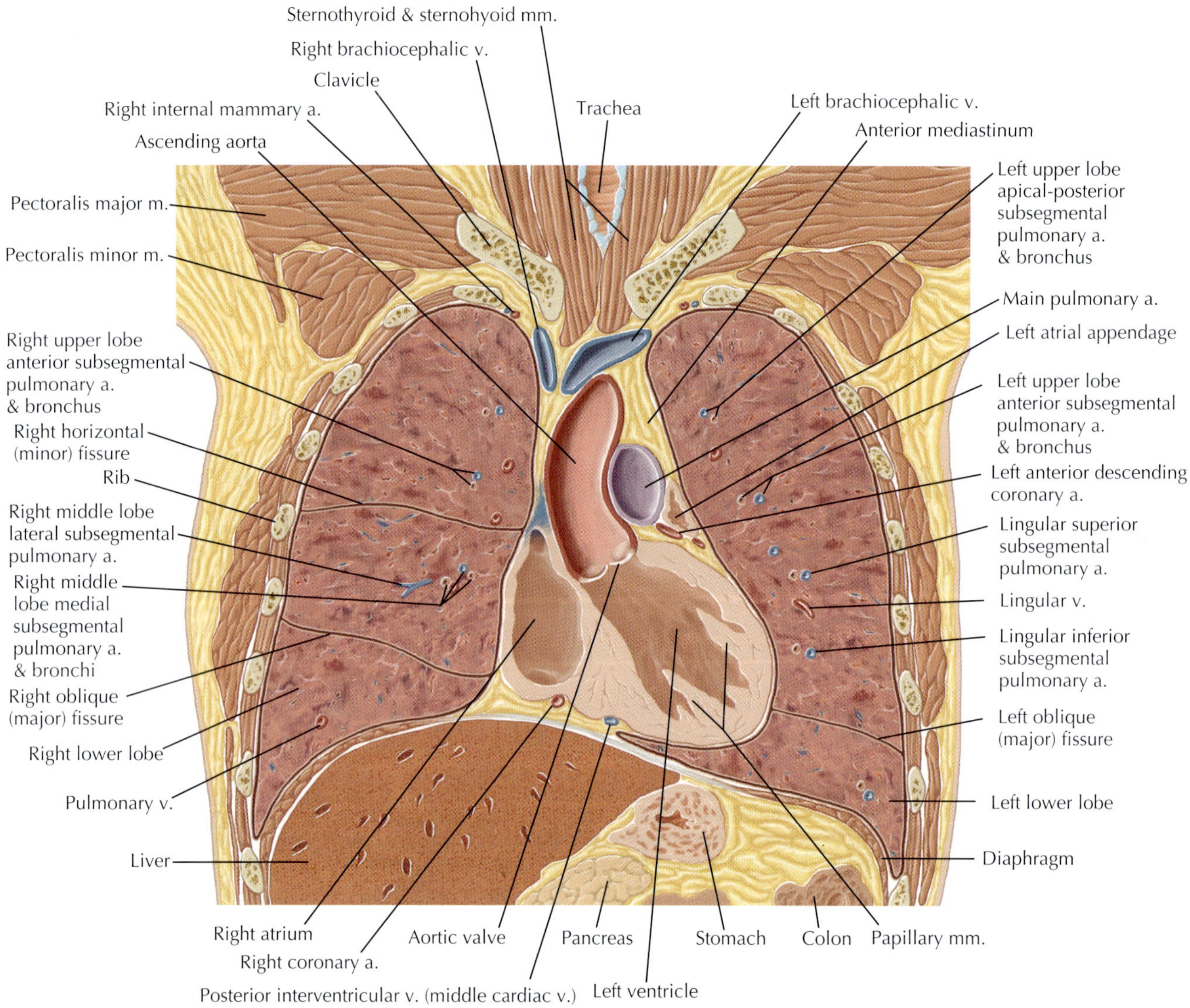

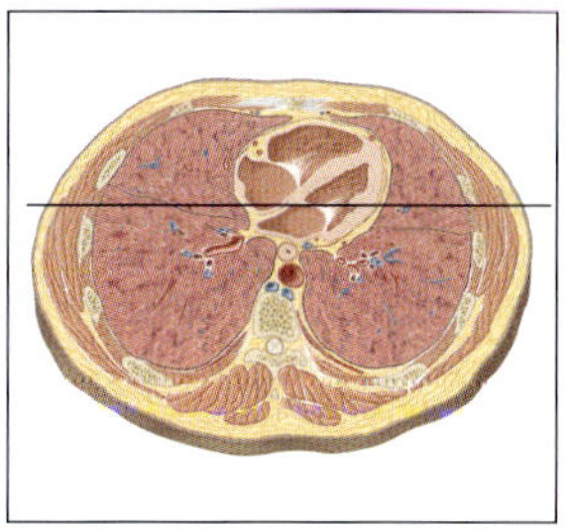

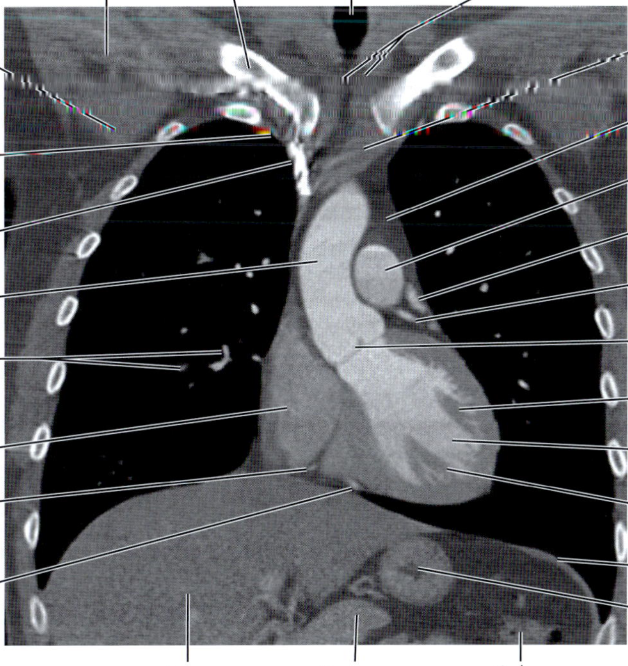
Pectoralis major m.
Clavicle
Trachea
Sternothyroid & sternohyoid mm.
Pectoralis minor m.
Left brachiocephalic v.
Anterior mediastinum
Right internal mammary a.
Main pulmonary a.
Right brachiocephalic v. (enhanced)
Left atrial appendage
Ascending aorta
Left anterior descending coronary a.
Aortic valve
Right middle lobe lateral & medial subsegmental pulmonary aa.
Papillary m.
Right atrium
Left ventricle
Right coronary a.
Papillary m.
Diaphragm
Posterior interventricular v. (middle cardiac v.)
Stomach
Liver
Pancreas
Colon

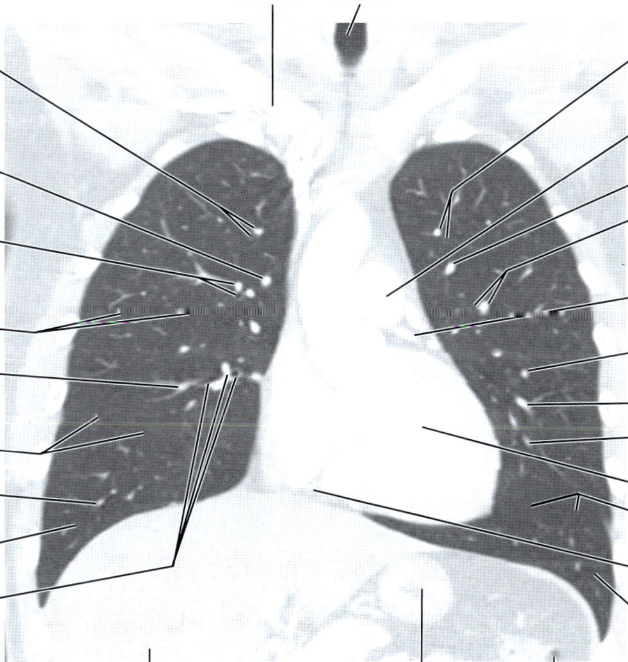
Clavicle
Trachea
Right upper lobe apical subsegmental pulmonary a. & bronchus
Left upper lobe apical-posterior subsegmental pulmonary a. & bronchus
Main pulmonary a.
Pulmonary v.
Pulmonary v.
Right upper lobe anterior subsegmental pulmonary a. & bronchus
Left upper lobe anterior subsegmental pulmonary a. & bronchus
Left anterior descending coronary a.
Right horizontal (minor) fissure
Lingular superior subsegmental pulmonary a.
Right middle lobe lateral subsegmental pulmonary a.
Lingular v.
Right oblique (major) fissure
Lingular inferior subsegmental pulmonary a.
Pulmonary v.
Left ventricle
Left oblique (major) fissure
Right lower lobe
Right coronary a.
Right middle lobe medial subsegmental pulmonary a. & bronchi
Left lower lobe
Liver
Stomach
Colon

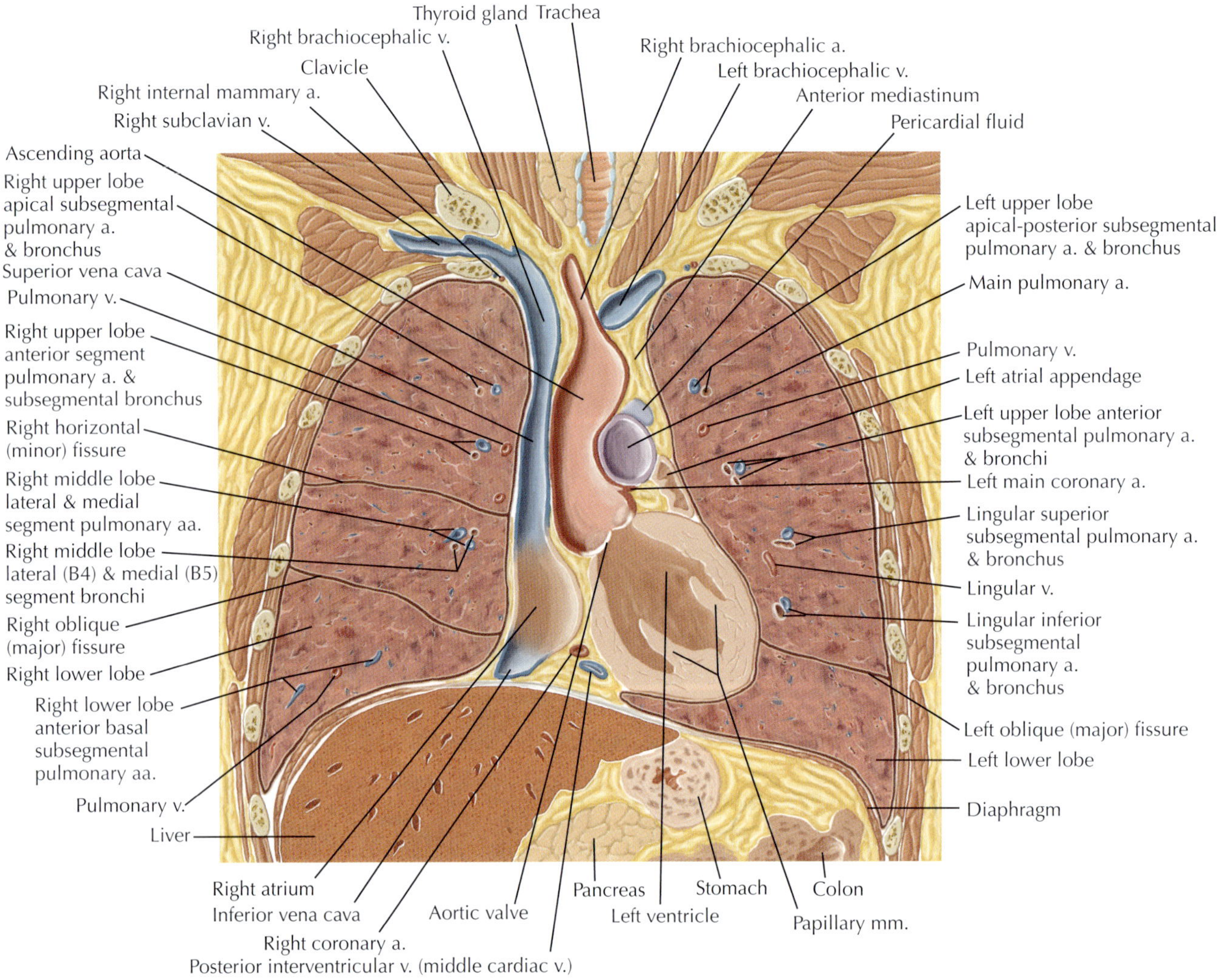

NORMAL ANATOMY

The *oblique (major)* and *horizontal (minor)* fissures are visible. The fissures appear as thin, hypovascular planes on thoracic CT. The horizontal (minor) fissure in particular is often more readily visualized on coronal imaging. Note that the right middle lobe—the region of lung inferior to the horizontal (minor) fissure and cranial to the right oblique (major) fissure—is well visualized on coronal CT imaging.

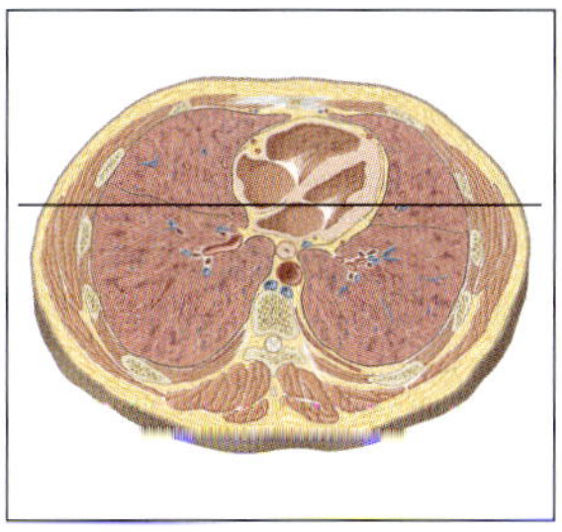

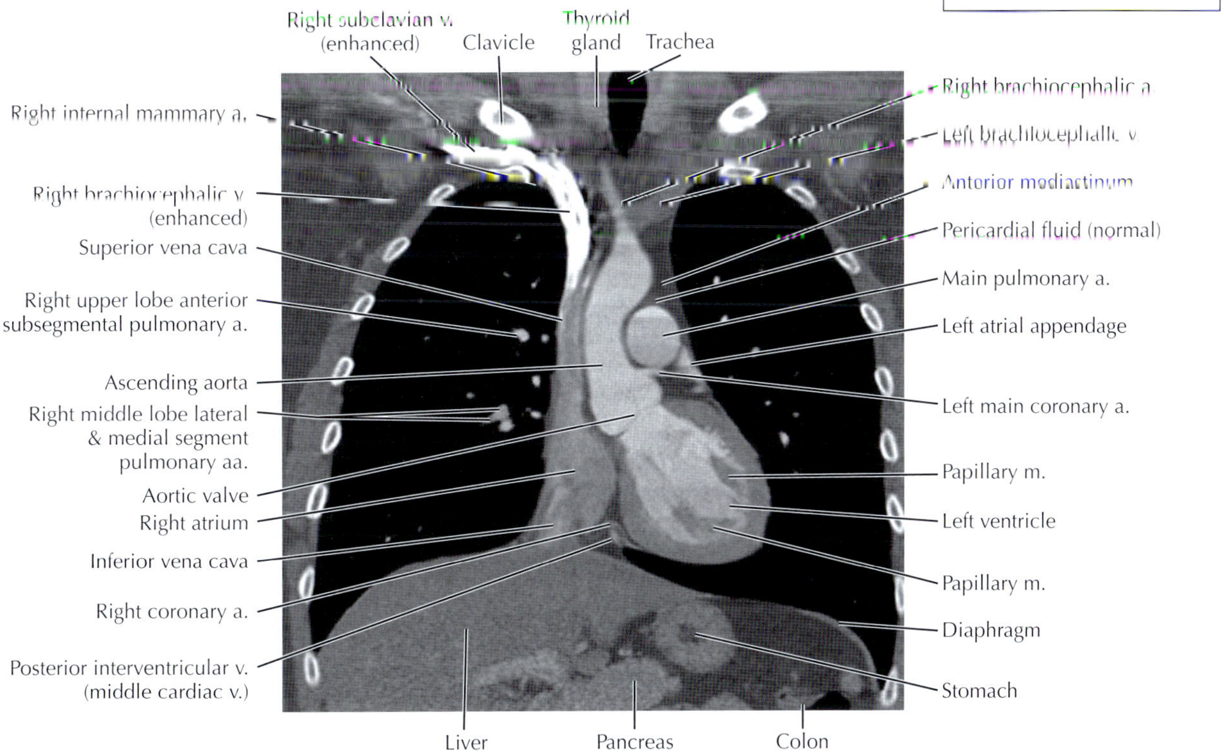
Right subclavian v. (enhanced)
Clavicle
Thyroid gland
Trachea
Right internal mammary a.
Right brachiocephalic v. (enhanced)
Superior vena cava
Right upper lobe anterior subsegmental pulmonary a.
Ascending aorta
Right middle lobe lateral & medial segment pulmonary aa.
Aortic valve
Right atrium
Inferior vena cava
Right coronary a.
Posterior interventricular v. (middle cardiac v.)
Liver
Pancreas
Colon
Right brachiocephalic a.
Left brachiocephalic v.
Anterior mediastinum
Pericardial fluid (normal)
Main pulmonary a.
Left atrial appendage
Left main coronary a.
Papillary m.
Left ventricle
Papillary m.
Diaphragm
Stomach

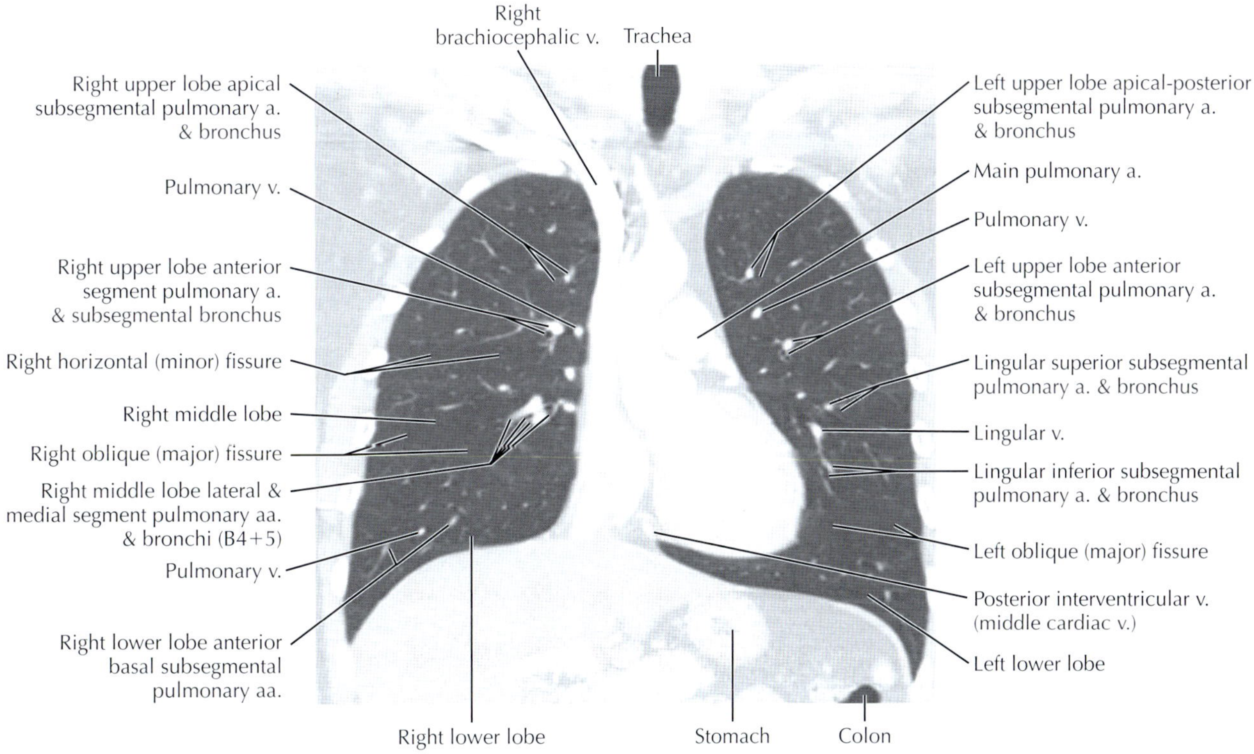
Right brachiocephalic v.
Trachea
Right upper lobe apical subsegmental pulmonary a. & bronchus
Pulmonary v.
Right upper lobe anterior segment pulmonary a. & subsegmental bronchus
Right horizontal (minor) fissure
Right middle lobe
Right oblique (major) fissure
Right middle lobe lateral & medial segment pulmonary aa. & bronchi (B4+5)
Pulmonary v.
Right lower lobe anterior basal subsegmental pulmonary aa.
Right lower lobe
Stomach
Colon
Left upper lobe apical-posterior subsegmental pulmonary a. & bronchus
Main pulmonary a.
Pulmonary v.
Left upper lobe anterior subsegmental pulmonary a. & bronchus
Lingular superior subsegmental pulmonary a. & bronchus
Lingular v.
Lingular inferior subsegmental pulmonary a. & bronchus
Left oblique (major) fissure
Posterior interventricular v. (middle cardiac v.)
Left lower lobe

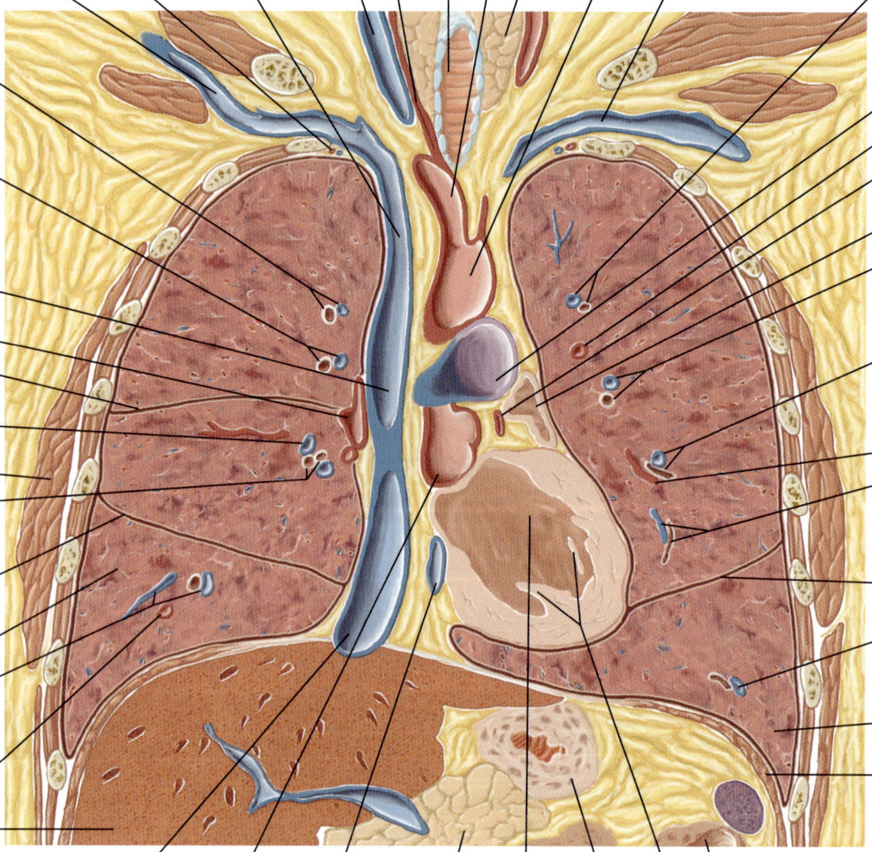
Right common carotid a.
Trachea
Right brachiocephalic a.
Right internal jugular v.
Right brachiocephalic v.
Thyroid gland
Right internal mammary a.
Aortic arch
Right subclavian v.
Left subclavian v.
Right upper lobe apical subsegmental pulmonary a. & bronchus
Right upper lobe anterior segment pulmonary a. & subsegmental bronchus
Superior vena cava
Pulmonary v.
Right horizontal (minor) fissure
Right middle lobe pulmonary a.
Serratus anterior m.
Right middle lobe lateral (B4) & medial (B5) segment bronchi
Right oblique (major) fissure
Right lower lobe
Right lower lobe anterior basal subsegmental pulmonary aa.
Pulmonary v.
Liver
Inferior vena cava
Ascending aorta
Coronary sinus
Pancreas
Left ventricle
Stomach
Papillary mm.
Colon
Left upper lobe apical-posterior subsegmental pulmonary a. & bronchus
Main pulmonary a.
Pulmonary v.
Left circumflex coronary a.
Left atrial appendage
Left upper lobe anterior subsegmental pulmonary a. & bronchus
Lingular superior subsegmental pulmonary a. & bronchus
Lingular v.
Lingular inferior subsegmental pulmonary a. & bronchus
Left oblique (major) fissure
Left lower lobe anterior basal subsegmental pulmonary a.
Left lower lobe
Diaphragm

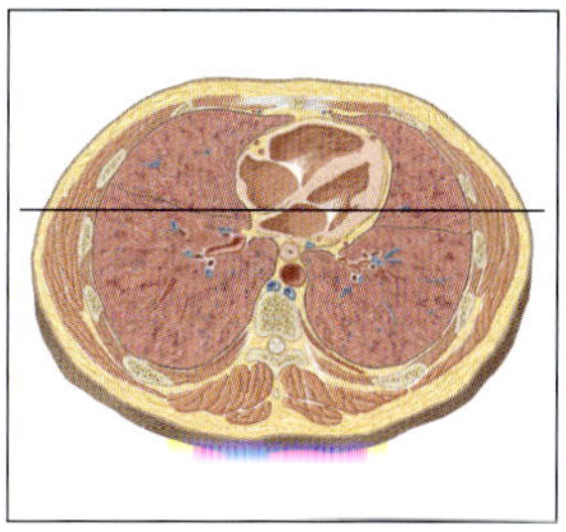

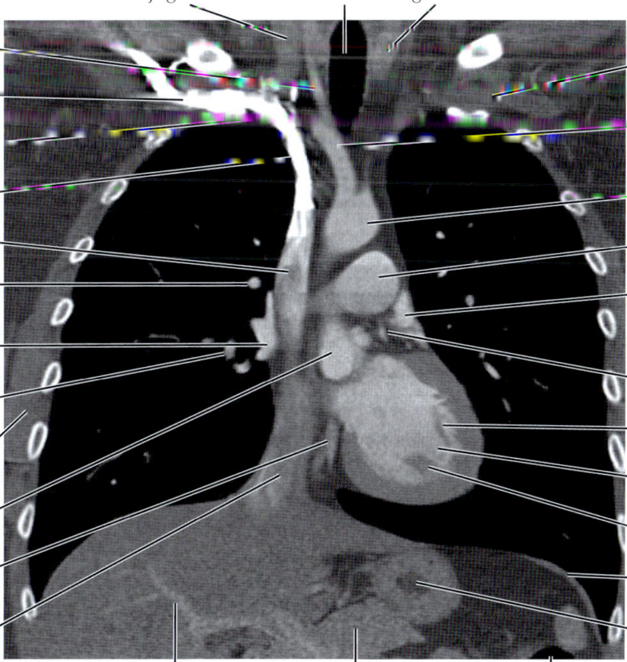
Right internal jugular v.
Trachea
Thyroid gland
Right common carotid a.
Right subclavian v. (enhanced)
Right internal mammary a.
Right brachiocephalic v. (enhanced)
Superior vena cava
Right upper lobe anterior segment pulmonary a.
Pulmonary v.
Right middle lobe pulmonary a.
Serratus anterior m.
Ascending aorta
Coronary sinus
Inferior vena cava
Left subclavian v.
Right brachiocephalic a.
Aortic arch
Main pulmonary a.
Left atrial appendage
Left circumflex coronary a.
Papillary m.
Left ventricle
Papillary m.
Diaphragm
Stomach
Liver
Pancreas
Colon

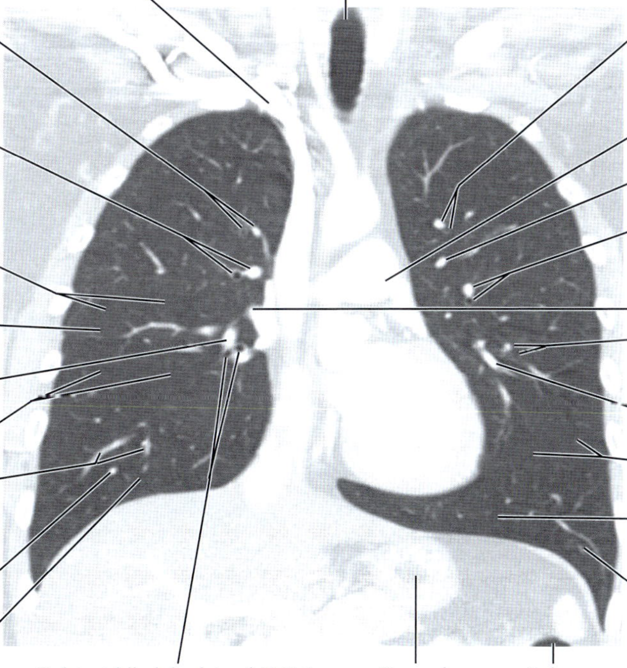
Right brachiocephalic v.
Trachea
Right upper lobe apical subsegmental pulmonary a. & bronchus
Right upper lobe anterior segment pulmonary a. & subsegmental bronchus
Right horizontal (minor) fissure
Right middle lobe
Right middle lobe pulmonary a.
Right oblique (major) fissure
Right lower lobe anterior basal subsegmental pulmonary aa.
Pulmonary v.
Right lower lobe
Left upper lobe apical-posterior subsegmental pulmonary a. & bronchus
Main pulmonary a.
Pulmonary v.
Left upper lobe anterior subsegmental pulmonary a. & bronchus
Pulmonary v.
Lingular superior subsegmental pulmonary a. & bronchus
Lingular v.
Left oblique (major) fissure
Left lower lobe
Left lower lobe anterior basal subsegmental pulmonary a.
Right middle lobe lateral (B4) & medial (B5) segment bronchi
Stomach
Colon

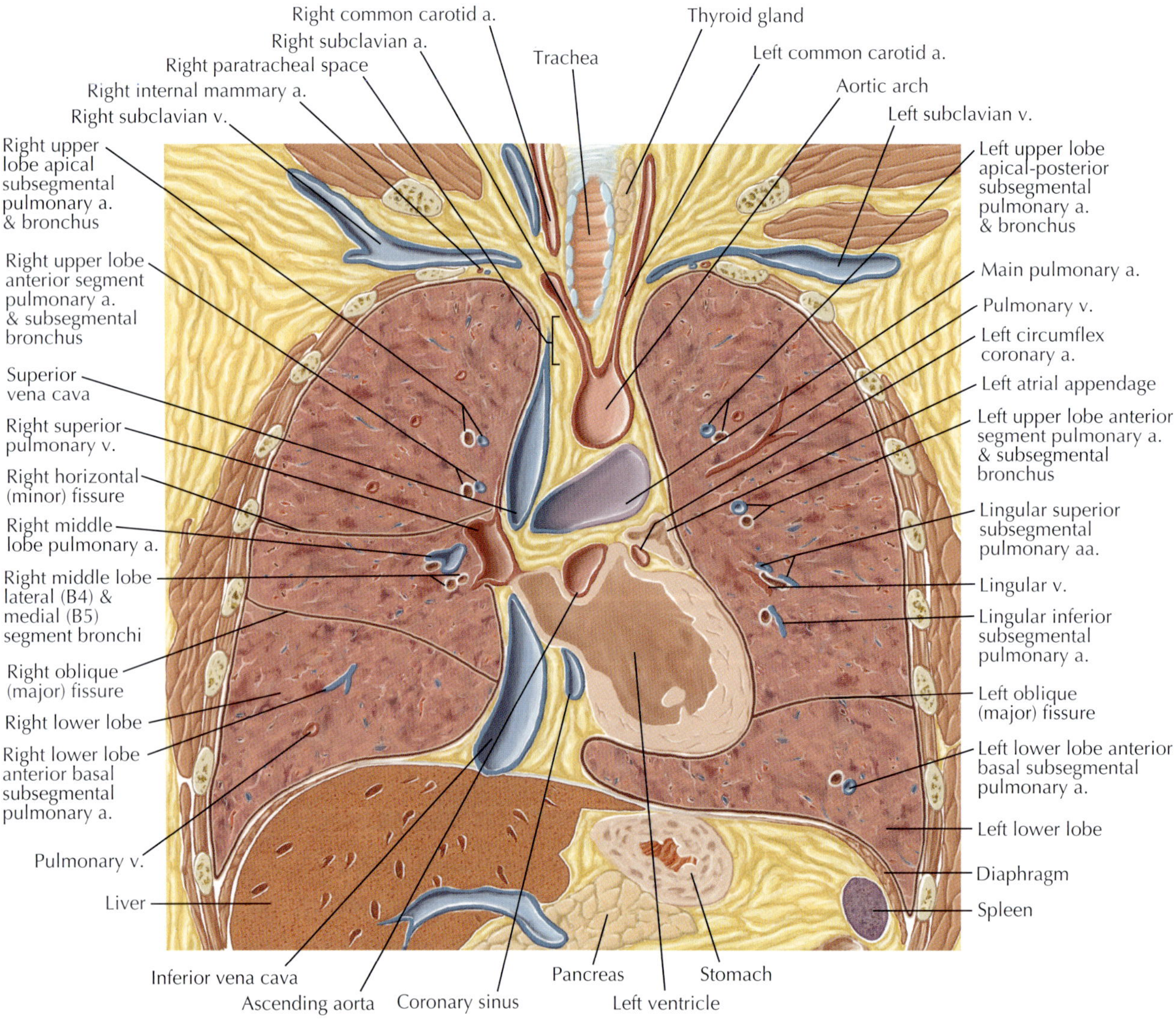

Right common carotid a.
Right subclavian a.
Right paratracheal space
Right internal mammary a.
Right subclavian v.
Right upper lobe apical subsegmental pulmonary a. & bronchus
Right upper lobe anterior segment pulmonary a. & subsegmental bronchus
Superior vena cava
Right superior pulmonary v.
Right horizontal (minor) fissure
Right middle lobe pulmonary a.
Right middle lobe lateral (B4) & medial (B5) segment bronchi
Right oblique (major) fissure
Right lower lobe
Right lower lobe anterior basal subsegmental pulmonary a.
Pulmonary v.
Liver
Inferior vena cava
Ascending aorta
Coronary sinus
Pancreas
Left ventricle
Stomach
Trachea
Thyroid gland
Left common carotid a.
Aortic arch
Left subclavian v.
Left upper lobe apical-posterior subsegmental pulmonary a. & bronchus
Main pulmonary a.
Pulmonary v.
Left circumflex coronary a.
Left atrial appendage
Left upper lobe anterior segment pulmonary a. & subsegmental bronchus
Lingular superior subsegmental pulmonary aa.
Lingular v.
Lingular inferior subsegmental pulmonary a.
Left oblique (major) fissure
Left lower lobe anterior basal subsegmental pulmonary a.
Left lower lobe
Diaphragm
Spleen

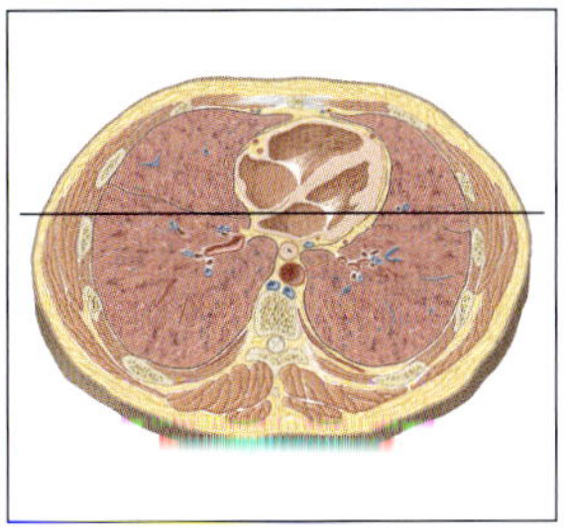

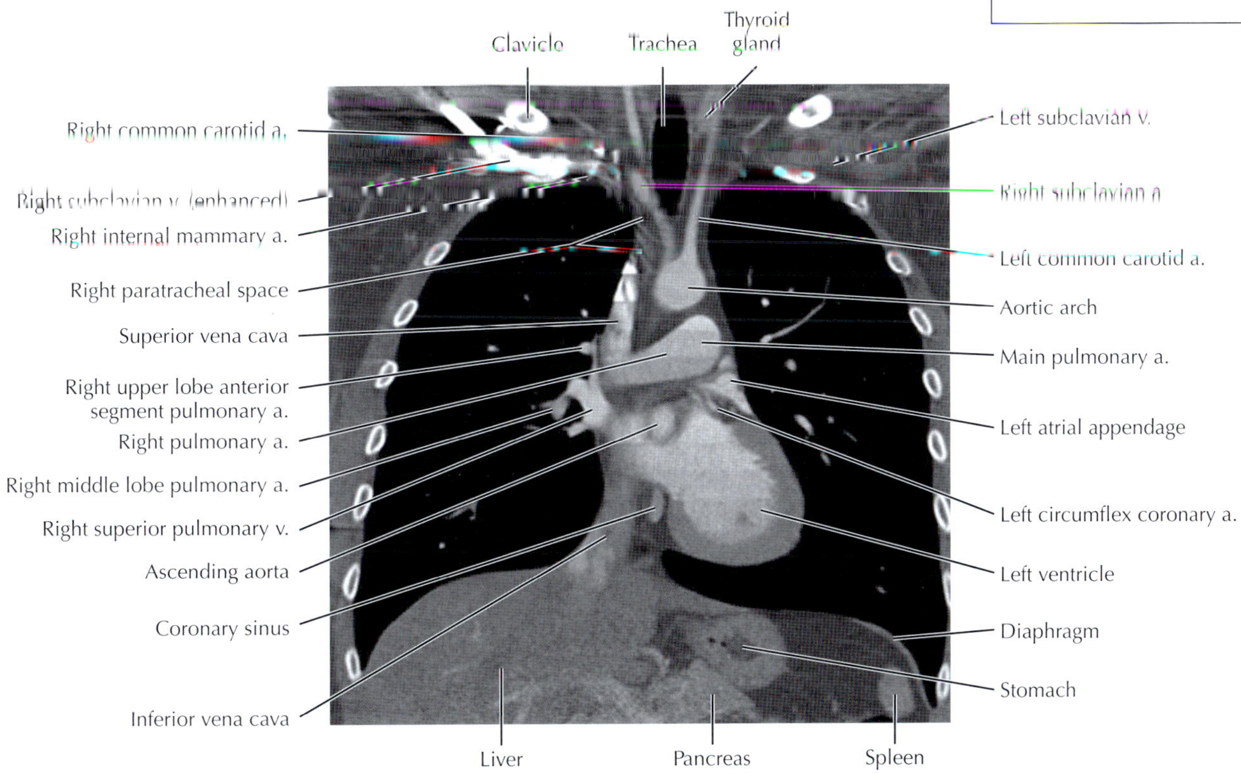
Clavicle
Trachea
Thyroid gland
Right common carotid a.
Right subclavian v. (enhanced)
Right internal mammary a.
Right paratracheal space
Superior vena cava
Right upper lobe anterior segment pulmonary a.
Right pulmonary a.
Right middle lobe pulmonary a.
Right superior pulmonary v.
Ascending aorta
Coronary sinus
Inferior vena cava
Left subclavian v.
Right subclavian a.
Left common carotid a.
Aortic arch
Main pulmonary a.
Left atrial appendage
Left circumflex coronary a.
Left ventricle
Diaphragm
Stomach
Liver
Pancreas
Spleen

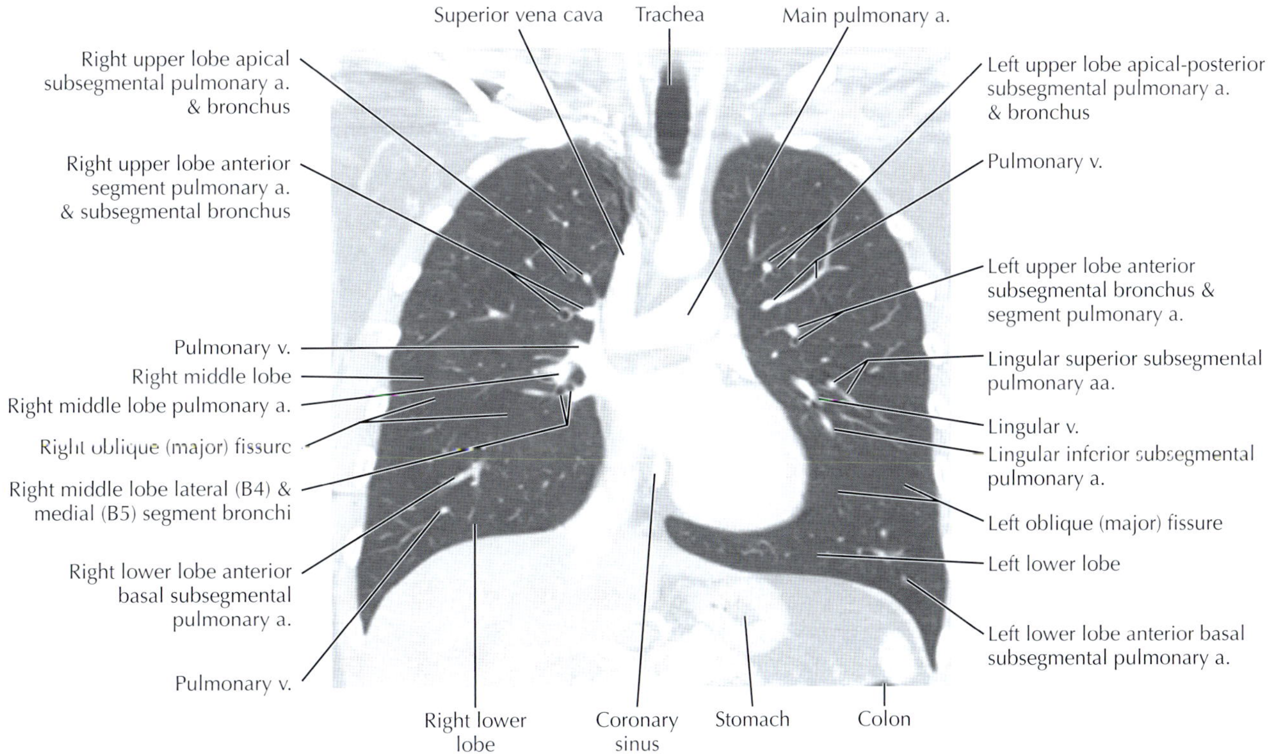
Superior vena cava
Trachea
Main pulmonary a.
Right upper lobe apical subsegmental pulmonary a. & bronchus
Right upper lobe anterior segment pulmonary a. & subsegmental bronchus
Pulmonary v.
Right middle lobe
Right middle lobe pulmonary a.
Right oblique (major) fissure
Right middle lobe lateral (B4) & medial (B5) segment bronchi
Right lower lobe anterior basal subsegmental pulmonary a.
Pulmonary v.
Left upper lobe apical-posterior subsegmental pulmonary a. & bronchus
Pulmonary v.
Left upper lobe anterior subsegmental bronchus & segment pulmonary a.
Lingular superior subsegmental pulmonary aa.
Lingular v.
Lingular inferior subsegmental pulmonary a.
Left oblique (major) fissure
Left lower lobe
Left lower lobe anterior basal subsegmental pulmonary a.
Right lower lobe
Coronary sinus
Stomach
Colon

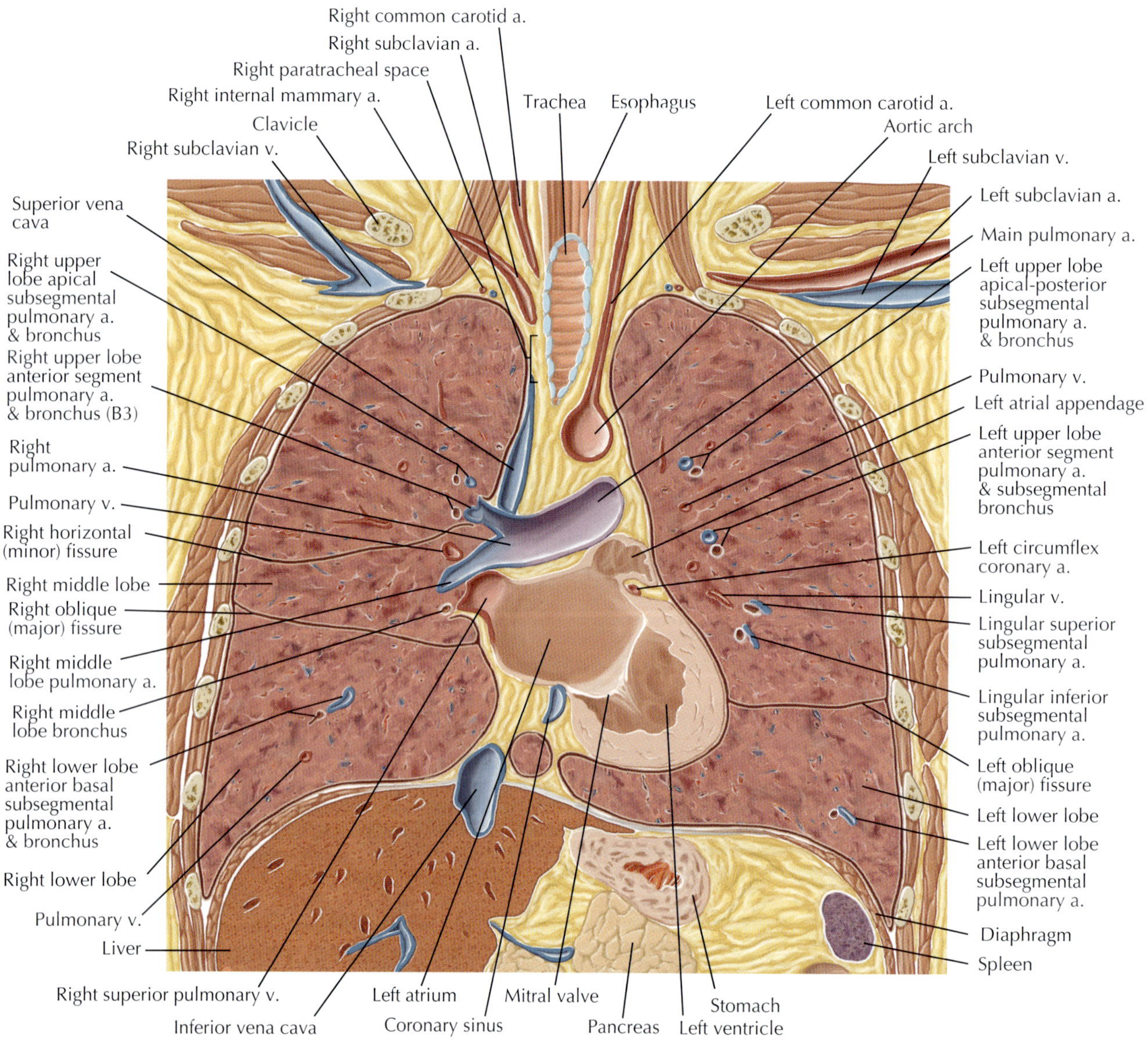
Right common carotid a.
Right subclavian a.
Right paratracheal space
Right internal mammary a.
Clavicle
Right subclavian v.
Trachea
Esophagus
Left common carotid a.
Aortic arch
Left subclavian v.
Superior vena cava
Right upper lobe apical subsegmental pulmonary a. & bronchus
Right upper lobe anterior segment pulmonary a. & bronchus (B3)
Right pulmonary a.
Pulmonary v.
Right horizontal (minor) fissure
Right middle lobe
Right oblique (major) fissure
Right middle lobe pulmonary a.
Right middle lobe bronchus
Right lower lobe anterior basal subsegmental pulmonary a. & bronchus
Right lower lobe
Pulmonary v.
Liver
Left subclavian a.
Main pulmonary a.
Left upper lobe apical-posterior subsegmental pulmonary a. & bronchus
Pulmonary v.
Left atrial appendage
Left upper lobe anterior segment pulmonary a. & subsegmental bronchus
Left circumflex coronary a.
Lingular v.
Lingular superior subsegmental pulmonary a.
Lingular inferior subsegmental pulmonary a.
Left oblique (major) fissure
Left lower lobe
Left lower lobe anterior basal subsegmental pulmonary a.
Diaphragm
Spleen
Right superior pulmonary v.
Inferior vena cava
Left atrium
Coronary sinus
Mitral valve
Pancreas
Stomach
Left ventricle

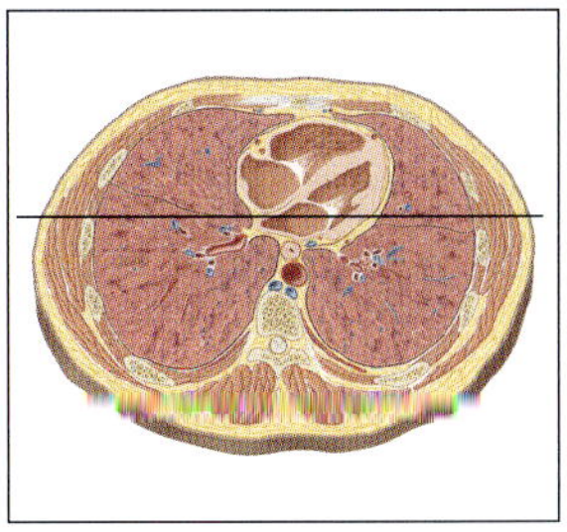

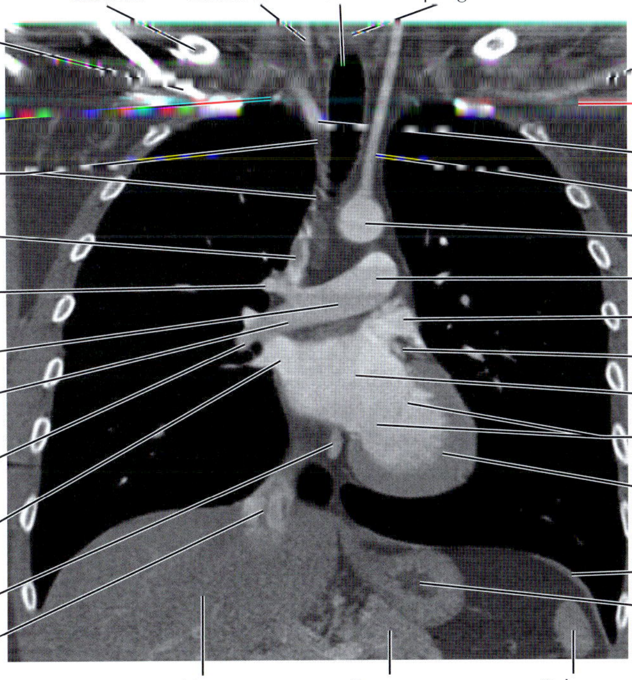
Clavicle
Right common carotid a.
Trachea
Esophagus
Right subclavian v. (enhanced)
Right internal mammary a.
Right paratracheal space
Superior vena cava
Right upper lobe anterior segment pulmonary a.
Right pulmonary a.
Right interlobar pulmonary a.
Right middle lobe pulmonary a.
Right superior pulmonary v.
Coronary sinus
Inferior vena cava
Left subclavian a.
Left subclavian v.
Right subclavian a.
Left common carotid a.
Aortic arch
Main pulmonary a.
Left atrial appendage
Left circumflex coronary a.
Left atrium
Mitral valve
Left ventricle
Diaphragm
Stomach
Liver
Pancreas
Spleen

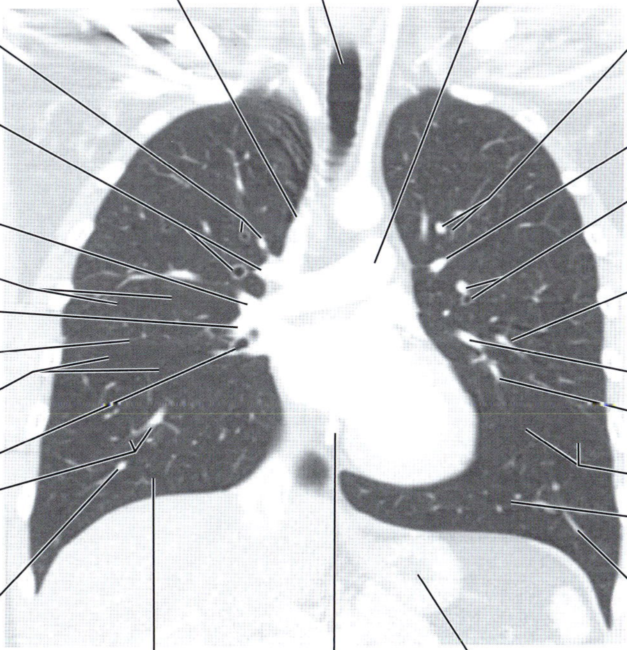
Superior vena cava
Trachea
Main pulmonary a.
Right upper lobe apical subsegmental pulmonary a. & bronchus
Right upper lobe anterior segment pulmonary a. and bronchus (B3)
Pulmonary v.
Right horizontal (minor) fissure
Right middle lobe pulmonary a.
Right middle lobe
Right oblique (major) fissure
Right middle lobe bronchus
Right lower lobe anterior basal subsegmental pulmonary a. & bronchus
Pulmonary v.
Left upper lobe apical-posterior subsegmental pulmonary a. & bronchus
Pulmonary v.
Left upper lobe anterior subsegmental bronchus & segment pulmonary a.
Lingular superior subsegmental pulmonary a.
Lingular v.
Lingular inferior subsegmental pulmonary a.
Left oblique (major) fissure
Left lower lobe
Left lower lobe anterior basal subsegmental pulmonary a.
Right lower lobe
Coronary sinus
Stomach

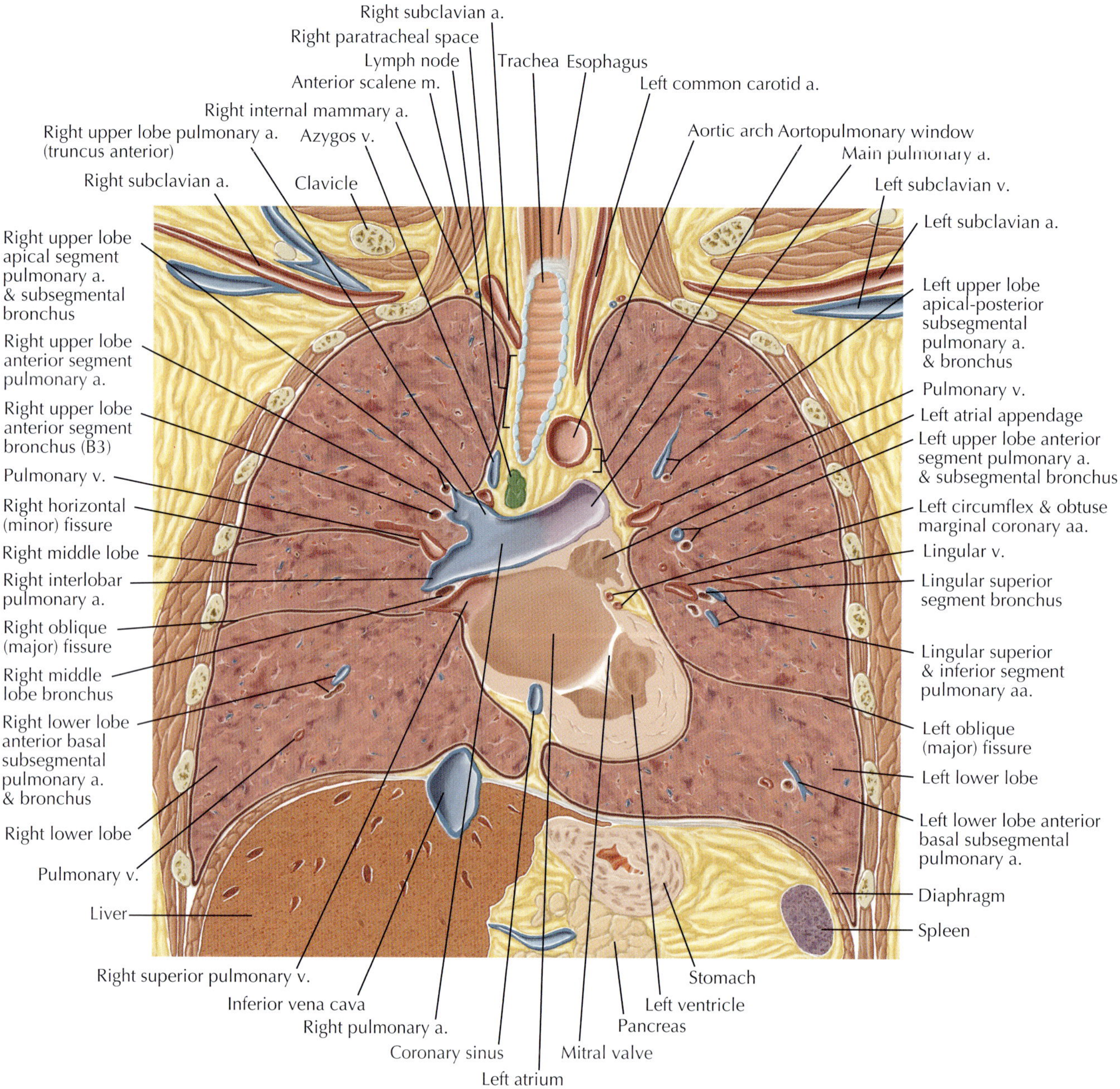
Right subclavian a.
Right paratracheal space
Lymph node
Anterior scalene m.
Right internal mammary a.
Right upper lobe pulmonary a. (truncus anterior)
Azygos v.
Right subclavian a.
Clavicle
Trachea
Esophagus
Left common carotid a.
Aortic arch
Aortopulmonary window
Main pulmonary a.
Left subclavian v.
Left subclavian a.
Right upper lobe apical segment pulmonary a. & subsegmental bronchus
Right upper lobe anterior segment pulmonary a.
Right upper lobe anterior segment bronchus (B3)
Pulmonary v.
Right horizontal (minor) fissure
Right middle lobe
Right interlobar pulmonary a.
Right oblique (major) fissure
Right middle lobe bronchus
Right lower lobe anterior basal subsegmental pulmonary a. & bronchus
Right lower lobe
Pulmonary v.
Liver
Left upper lobe apical-posterior subsegmental pulmonary a. & bronchus
Pulmonary v.
Left atrial appendage
Left upper lobe anterior segment pulmonary a. & subsegmental bronchus
Left circumflex & obtuse marginal coronary aa.
Lingular v.
Lingular superior segment bronchus
Lingular superior & inferior segment pulmonary aa.
Left oblique (major) fissure
Left lower lobe
Left lower lobe anterior basal subsegmental pulmonary a.
Diaphragm
Spleen
Right superior pulmonary v.
Inferior vena cava
Right pulmonary a.
Coronary sinus
Left atrium
Mitral valve
Pancreas
Left ventricle
Stomach

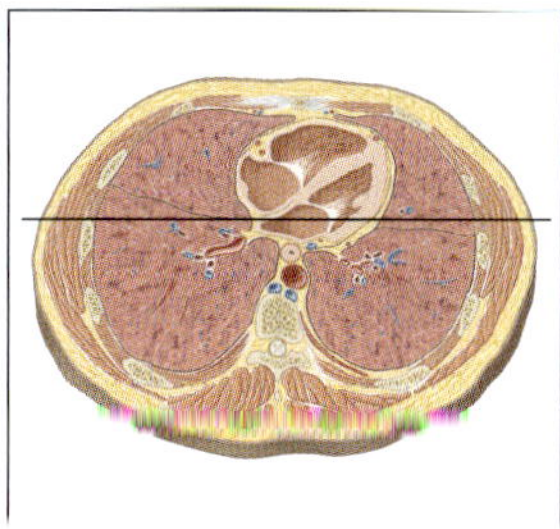

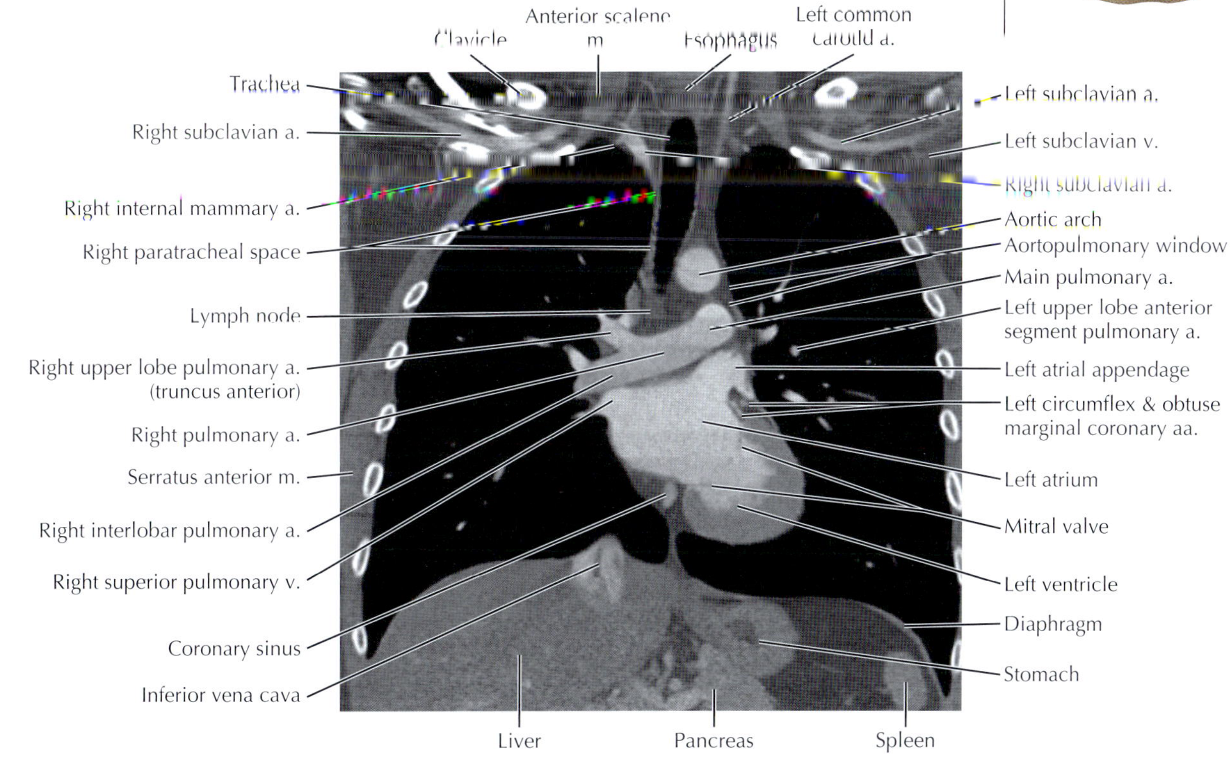
Clavicle
Anterior scalene m.
Esophagus
Left common carotid a.
Trachea
Right subclavian a.
Right internal mammary a.
Right paratracheal space
Lymph node
Right upper lobe pulmonary a. (truncus anterior)
Right pulmonary a.
Serratus anterior m.
Right interlobar pulmonary a.
Right superior pulmonary v.
Coronary sinus
Inferior vena cava
Left subclavian a.
Left subclavian v.
Right subclavian a.
Aortic arch
Aortopulmonary window
Main pulmonary a.
Left upper lobe anterior segment pulmonary a.
Left atrial appendage
Left circumflex & obtuse marginal coronary aa.
Left atrium
Mitral valve
Left ventricle
Diaphragm
Stomach
Liver
Pancreas
Spleen

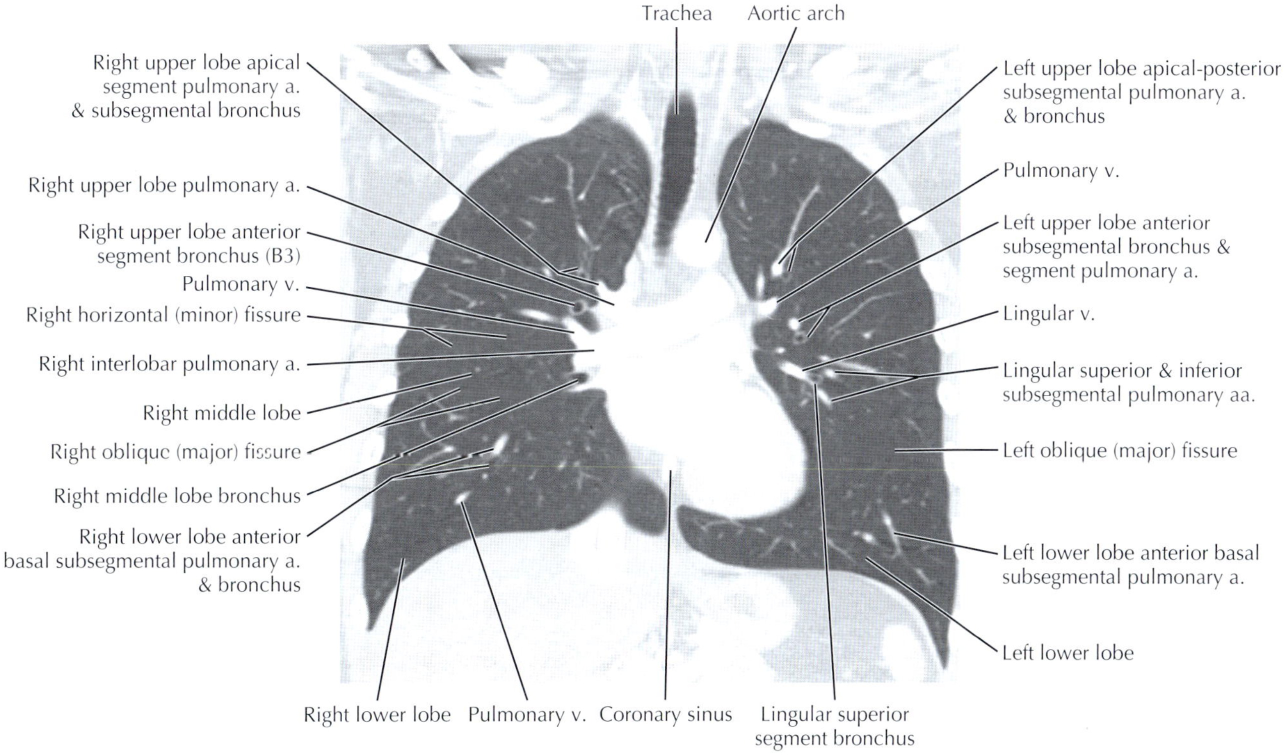
Trachea
Aortic arch
Right upper lobe apical segment pulmonary a. & subsegmental bronchus
Right upper lobe pulmonary a.
Right upper lobe anterior segment bronchus (B3)
Pulmonary v.
Right horizontal (minor) fissure
Right interlobar pulmonary a.
Right middle lobe
Right oblique (major) fissure
Right middle lobe bronchus
Right lower lobe anterior basal subsegmental pulmonary a. & bronchus
Left upper lobe apical-posterior subsegmental pulmonary a. & bronchus
Pulmonary v.
Left upper lobe anterior subsegmental bronchus & segment pulmonary a.
Lingular v.
Lingular superior & inferior subsegmental pulmonary aa.
Left oblique (major) fissure
Left lower lobe anterior basal subsegmental pulmonary a.
Left lower lobe
Right lower lobe
Pulmonary v.
Coronary sinus
Lingular superior segment bronchus

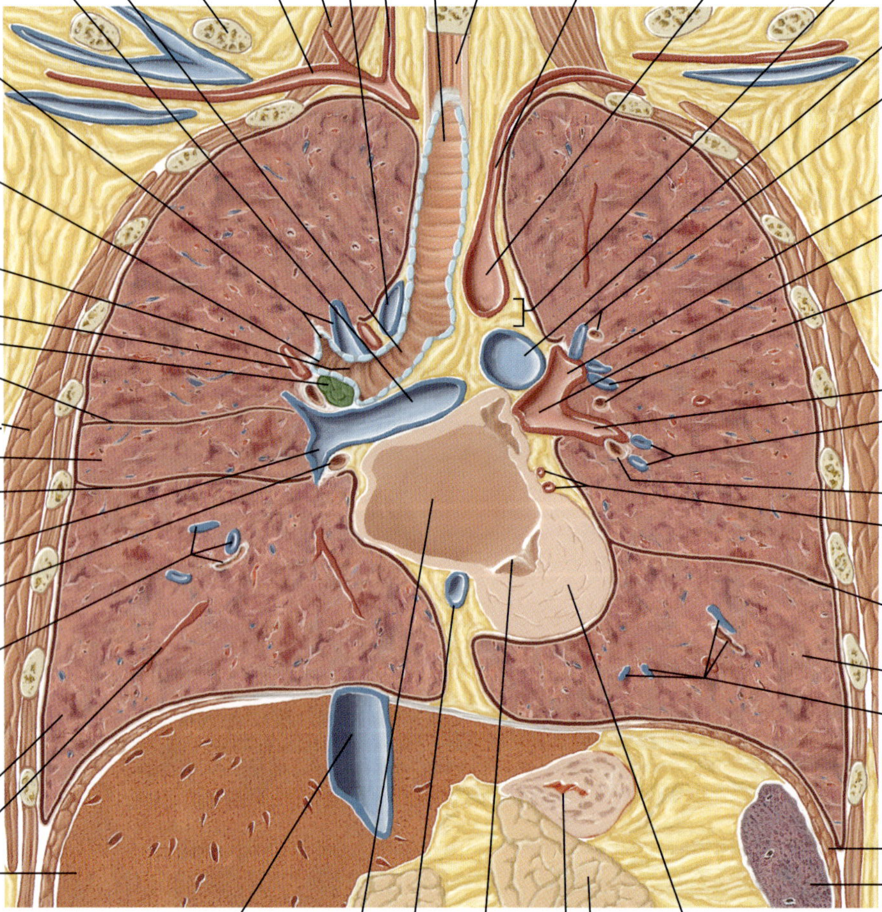
Right vertebral a.
Azygos v.
Trachea
Anterior scalene m.
Right mainstem bronchus
Right subclavian a.
Esophagus
Left subclavian a.
Right pulmonary a.
Clavicle
Aortic arch
Aortopulmonary window
Left pulmonary a.
Right upper lobe apical segment pulmonary a. & bronchus (B1)
Left upper lobe apical-posterior segment pulmonary a. & subsegmental bronchus
Right upper lobe anterior segment bronchus (B3)
Pulmonary v.
Left superior pulmonary v.
Right upper lobe bronchus
Left upper lobe anterior segment pulmonary a. & subsegmental bronchus
Pulmonary v.
Lymph node
Right horizontal (minor) fissure
Pulmonary v.
Serratus anterior m.
Lingular superior & inferior segment pulmonary aa.
Right middle lobe
Right oblique (major) fissure
Lingular bronchus
Right lower lobe pulmonary a.
Left circumflex and obtuse marginal coronary aa.
Right middle lobe bronchus
Left oblique (major) fissure
Right lower lobe anterior basal subsegmental pulmonary aa. & segment bronchus (B8)
Left lower lobe
Left lower lobe anterior & medial basal subsegmental pulmonary aa. & bronchus
Right lower lobe
Pulmonary v.
Diaphragm
Liver
Spleen
Inferior vena cava
Left atrium
Pancreas
Left ventricle
Coronary sinus
Mitral valve
Stomach

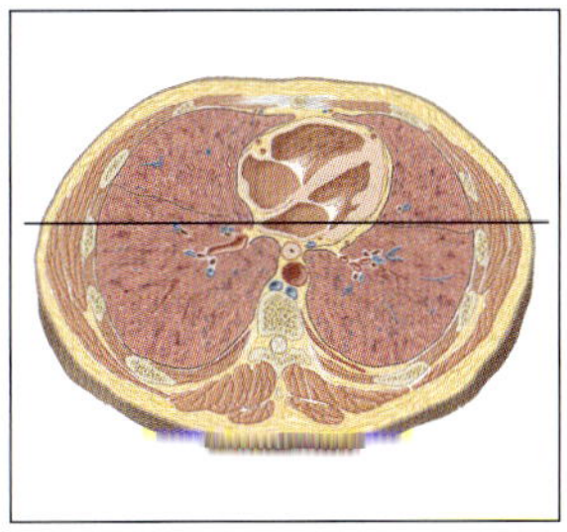

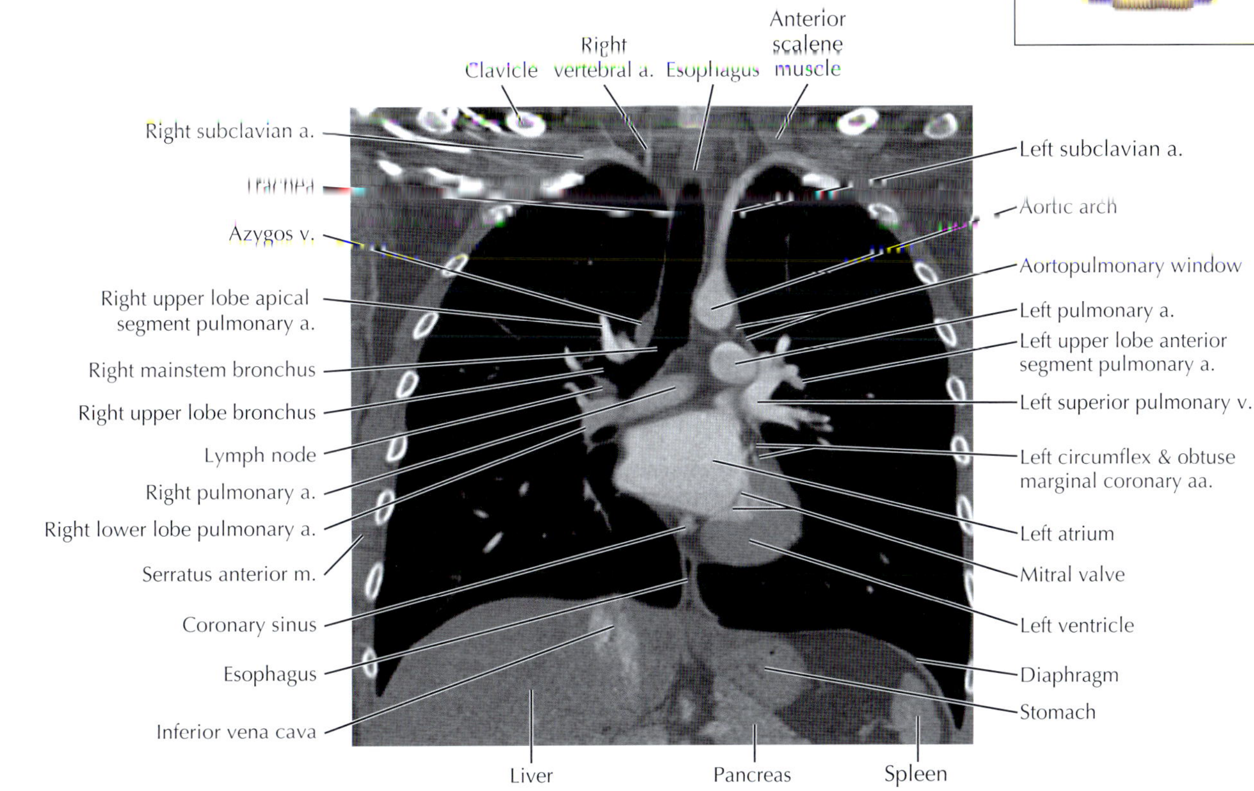
Anterior scalene muscle
Right vertebral a.
Clavicle
Esophagus
Right subclavian a.
Trachea
Azygos v.
Right upper lobe apical segment pulmonary a.
Right mainstem bronchus
Right upper lobe bronchus
Lymph node
Right pulmonary a.
Right lower lobe pulmonary a.
Serratus anterior m.
Coronary sinus
Esophagus
Inferior vena cava
Left subclavian a.
Aortic arch
Aortopulmonary window
Left pulmonary a.
Left upper lobe anterior segment pulmonary a.
Left superior pulmonary v.
Left circumflex & obtuse marginal coronary aa.
Left atrium
Mitral valve
Left ventricle
Diaphragm
Stomach
Liver
Pancreas
Spleen

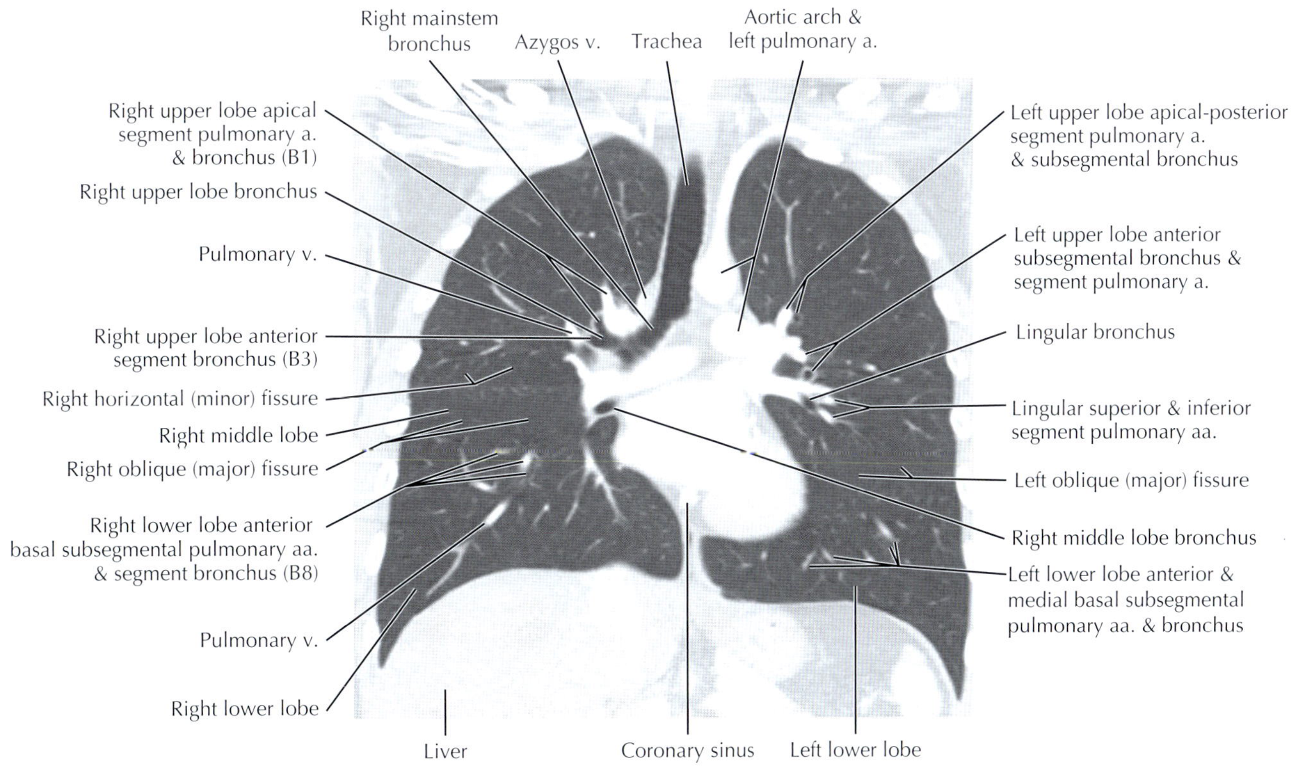
Right mainstem bronchus
Azygos v.
Trachea
Aortic arch & left pulmonary a.
Right upper lobe apical segment pulmonary a. & bronchus (B1)
Right upper lobe bronchus
Pulmonary v.
Right upper lobe anterior segment bronchus (B3)
Right horizontal (minor) fissure
Right middle lobe
Right oblique (major) fissure
Right lower lobe anterior basal subsegmental pulmonary aa. & segment bronchus (B8)
Pulmonary v.
Right lower lobe
Left upper lobe apical-posterior segment pulmonary a. & subsegmental bronchus
Left upper lobe anterior subsegmental bronchus & segment pulmonary a.
Lingular bronchus
Lingular superior & inferior segment pulmonary aa.
Left oblique (major) fissure
Right middle lobe bronchus
Left lower lobe anterior & medial basal subsegmental pulmonary aa. & bronchus
Liver
Coronary sinus
Left lower lobe

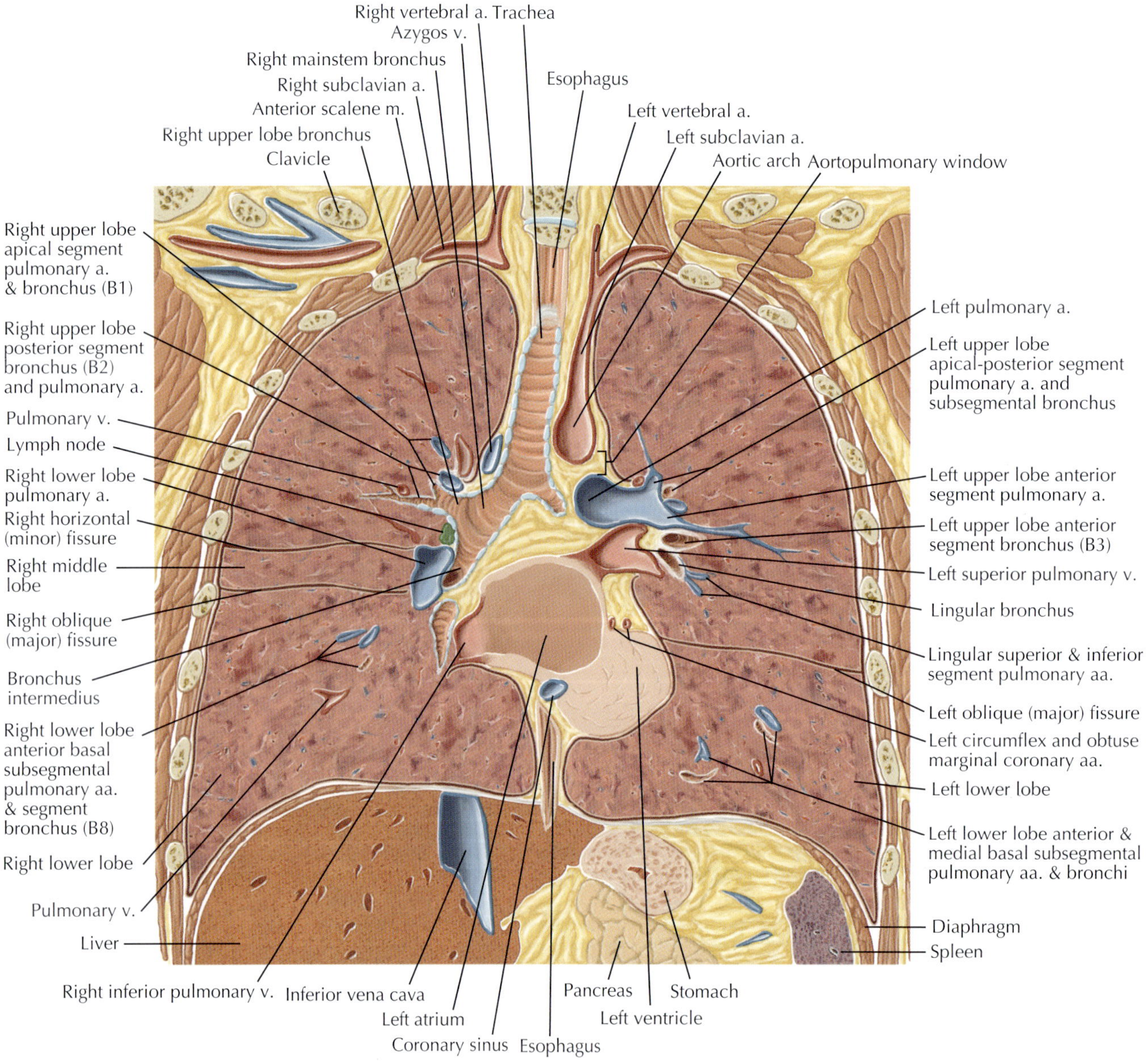

Right vertebral a.
Trachea
Azygos v.
Right mainstem bronchus
Right subclavian a.
Esophagus
Anterior scalene m.
Left vertebral a.
Right upper lobe bronchus
Left subclavian a.
Clavicle
Aortic arch
Aortopulmonary window
Right upper lobe apical segment pulmonary a. & bronchus (B1)
Right upper lobe posterior segment bronchus (B2) and pulmonary a.
Pulmonary v.
Lymph node
Right lower lobe pulmonary a.
Right horizontal (minor) fissure
Right middle lobe
Right oblique (major) fissure
Bronchus intermedius
Right lower lobe anterior basal subsegmental pulmonary aa. & segment bronchus (B8)
Right lower lobe
Pulmonary v.
Liver
Right inferior pulmonary v.
Inferior vena cava
Left atrium
Coronary sinus
Esophagus
Pancreas
Left ventricle
Stomach
Left pulmonary a.
Left upper lobe apical-posterior segment pulmonary a. and subsegmental bronchus
Left upper lobe anterior segment pulmonary a.
Left upper lobe anterior segment bronchus (B3)
Left superior pulmonary v.
Lingular bronchus
Lingular superior & inferior segment pulmonary aa.
Left oblique (major) fissure
Left circumflex and obtuse marginal coronary aa.
Left lower lobe
Left lower lobe anterior & medial basal subsegmental pulmonary aa. & bronchi
Diaphragm
Spleen

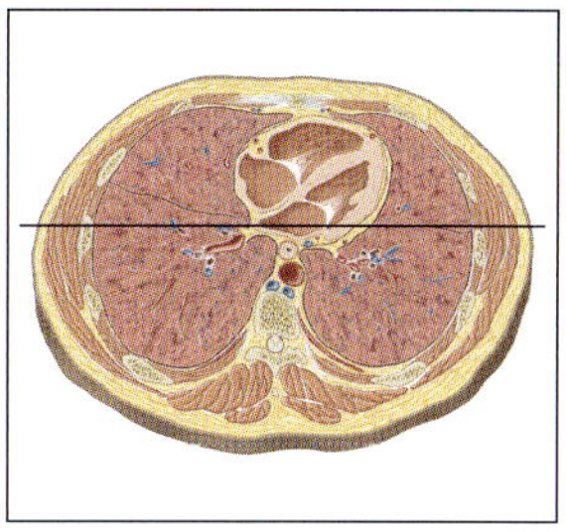

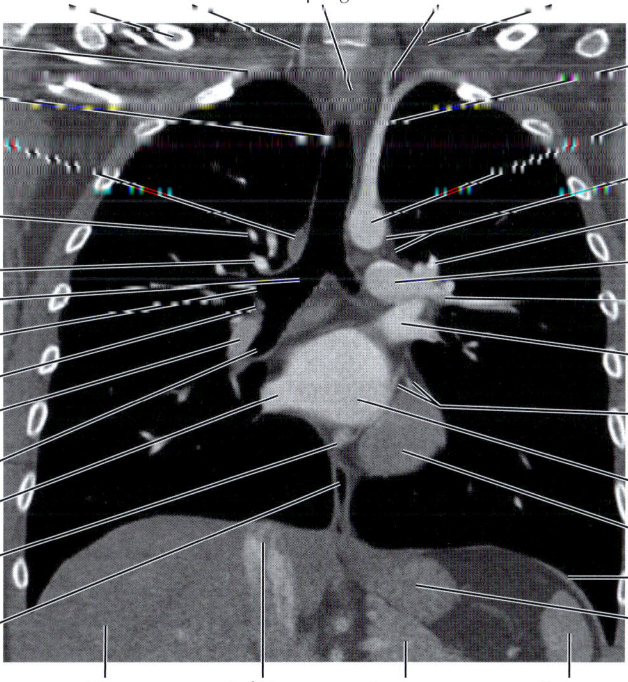
Clavicle
Right vertebral a.
Esophagus
Left vertebral a.
Anterior scalene muscle
Right subclavian a.
Trachea
Azygos v.
Right upper lobe apical segment pulmonary a.
Right upper lobe posterior segment pulmonary a.
Right mainstem bronchus
Right upper lobe bronchus
Lymph node
Right lower lobe pulmonary a.
Bronchus intermedius
Right inferior pulmonary v.
Coronary sinus
Esophagus
Left subclavian a.
Aortic arch
Aortopulmonary window
Left upper lobe apical-posterior segment pulmonary
Left pulmonary a.
Left upper lobe anterior segment pulmonary a.
Left superior pulmonary v.
Left circumflex & obtuse marginal coronary aa.
Left atrium
Left ventricle
Diaphragm
Stomach
Liver
Inferior vena cava
Pancreas
Spleen

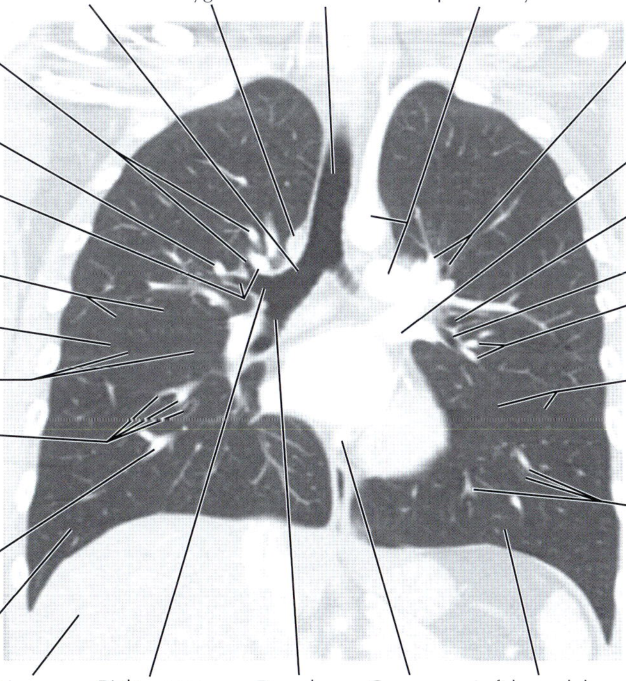
Right mainstem bronchus
Azygos v.
Trachea
Aortic arch & left pulmonary a.
Right upper lobe apical segment pulmonary a. & bronchus (B1)
Pulmonary v.
Right upper lobe posterior segment bronchus (B2) & pulmonary a.
Right horizontal (minor) fissure
Right middle lobe
Right oblique (major) fissure
Right lower lobe anterior basal subsegmental pulmonary aa. & segment bronchus (B8)
Pulmonary v.
Right lower lobe
Left upper lobe apical-posterior segment pulmonary a. & subsegmental bronchus
Left superior pulmonary v.
Left upper lobe anterior segment bronchus (B3)
Lingular bronchus
Lingular superior & inferior segment pulmonary aa.
Left oblique (major) fissure
Left lower lobe anterior & medial basal subsegmental pulmonary aa. & bronchus
Liver
Right upper lobe bronchus
Bronchus intermedius
Coronary sinus
Left lower lobe

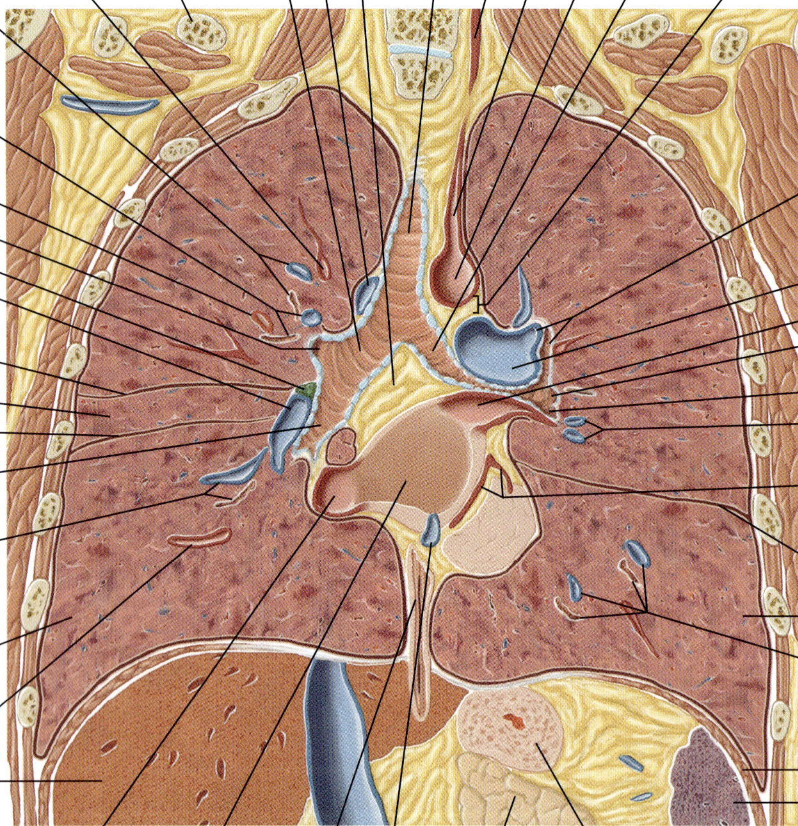

NORMAL ANATOMY

The *subcarinal space* is illustrated on this and subsequent images. The subcarinal space is the region of the mediastinum just inferior to the carina, and often contains lymph nodes. The subcarinal space is occasionally involved with a number of pathological processes, notably lymphadenopathy.

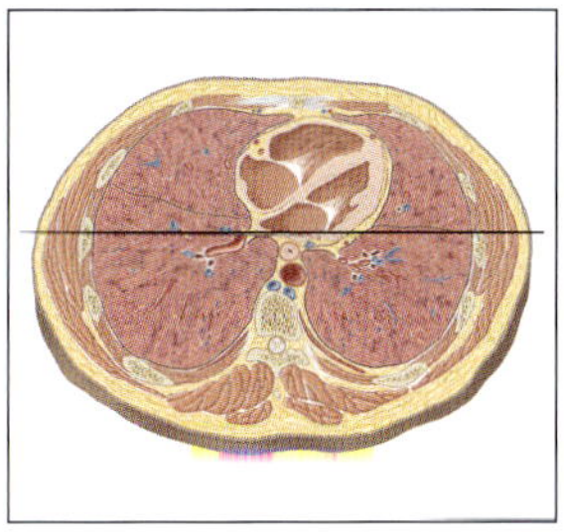

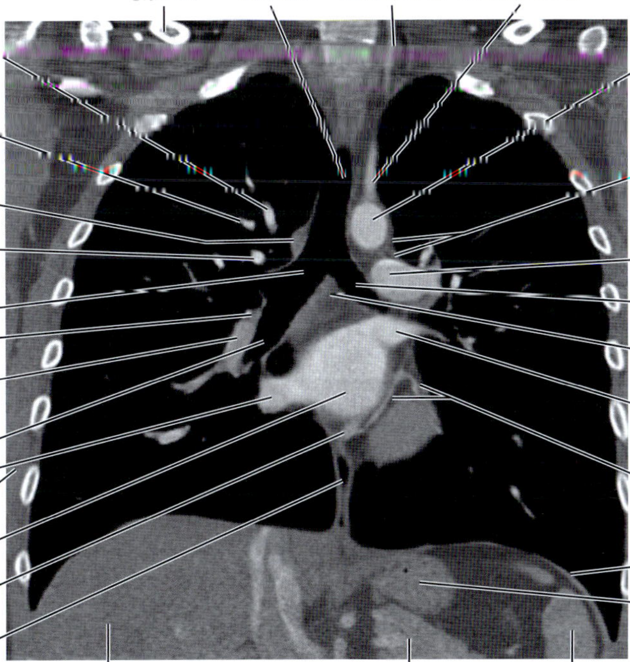
Clavicle
Trachea
Left vertebral a.
Left subclavian a.
Pulmonary v.
Descending thoracic aorta
Right upper lobe apical segment pulmonary a.
Aortopulmonary window
Azygos v.
Right upper lobe posterior segment pulmonary a.
Left interlobar pulmonary a.
Right mainstem bronchus
Left mainstem bronchus
Lymph node
Subcarinal space
Right lower lobe basal trunk pulmonary a.
Left superior pulmonary v.
Bronchus intermedius
Right inferior pulmonary v.
Serratus anterior m.
Left circumflex & obtuse marginal coronary aa.
Left atrium
Diaphragm
Coronary sinus
Stomach
Esophagus
Liver
Pancreas
Spleen

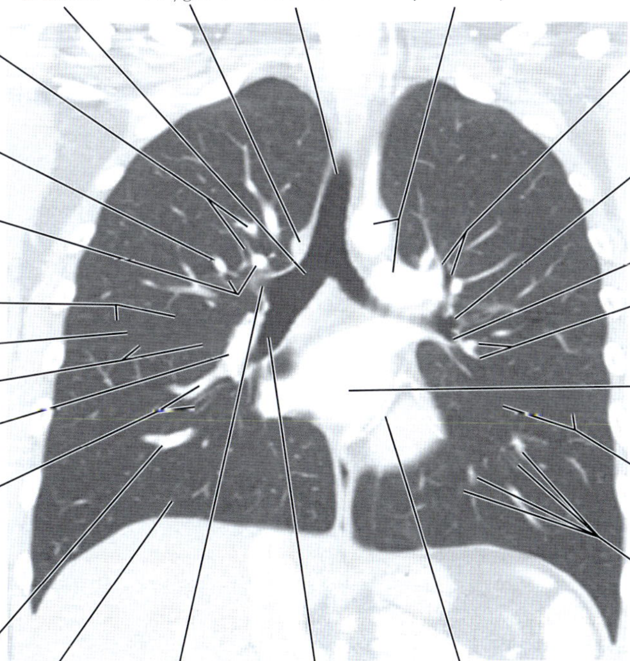
Right mainstem bronchus
Azygos v.
Trachea
Descending thoracic aorta & left pulmonary a.
Right upper lobe apical subsegmental pulmonary a. & segment bronchus (B1)
Left upper lobe apical-posterior segment pulmonary a. & bronchus (B1+2)
Pulmonary v.
Left upper lobe anterior segment bronchus (B3)
Right upper lobe posterior segment bronchus (B2) & pulmonary a.
Lingular bronchus
Right horizontal (minor) fissure
Lingular superior & inferior segment pulmonary aa.
Right middle lobe
Right oblique (major) fissure
Left atrium
Right lower lobe basal trunk pulmonary a.
Right lower lobe anterior basal segment pulmonary a. & bronchus (B8)
Left oblique (major) fissure
Left lower lobe anterior & medial basal subsegmental pulmonary aa. & bronchi
Pulmonary v.
Right lower lobe
Right upper lobe bronchus
Bronchus intermedius
Left circumflex coronary a.

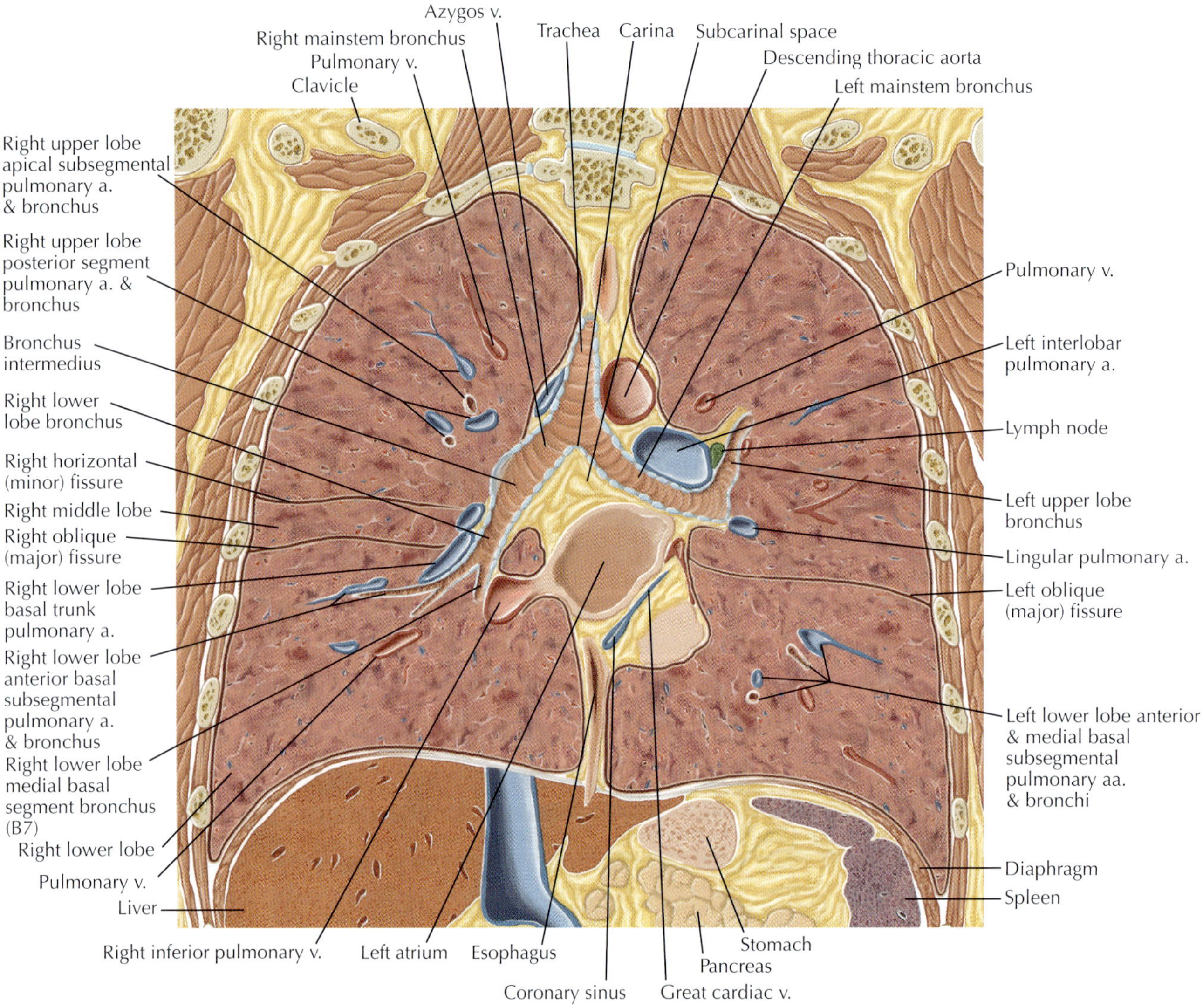
Azygos v.
Right mainstem bronchus
Pulmonary v.
Clavicle
Trachea
Carina
Subcarinal space
Descending thoracic aorta
Left mainstem bronchus
Right upper lobe apical subsegmental pulmonary a. & bronchus
Right upper lobe posterior segment pulmonary a. & bronchus
Bronchus intermedius
Right lower lobe bronchus
Right horizontal (minor) fissure
Right middle lobe
Right oblique (major) fissure
Right lower lobe basal trunk pulmonary a.
Right lower lobe anterior basal subsegmental pulmonary a. & bronchus
Right lower lobe medial basal segment bronchus (B7)
Right lower lobe
Pulmonary v.
Liver
Pulmonary v.
Left interlobar pulmonary a.
Lymph node
Left upper lobe bronchus
Lingular pulmonary a.
Left oblique (major) fissure
Left lower lobe anterior & medial basal subsegmental pulmonary aa. & bronchi
Diaphragm
Spleen
Right inferior pulmonary v.
Left atrium
Esophagus
Coronary sinus
Stomach
Pancreas
Great cardiac v.

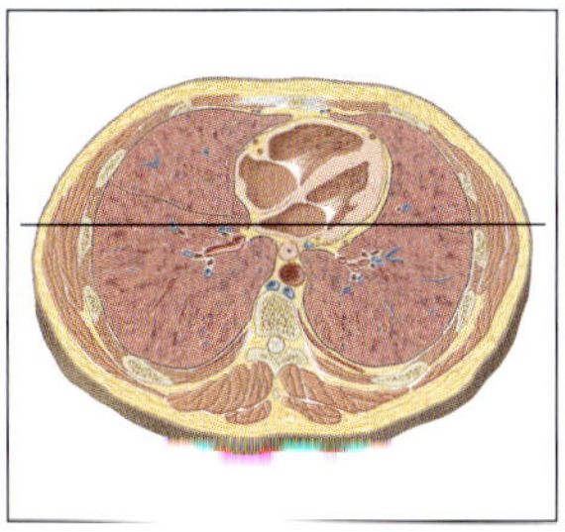

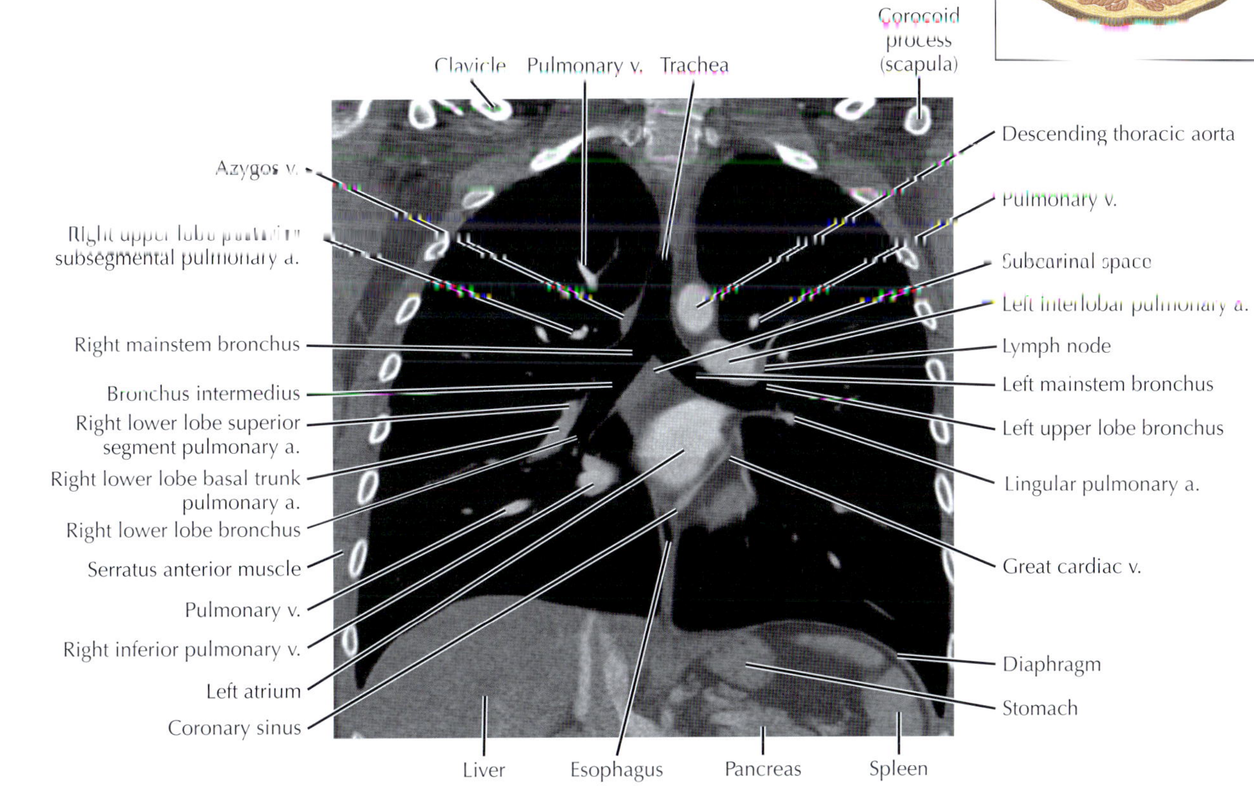
Clavicle
Pulmonary v.
Trachea
Coracoid process (scapula)
Azygos v.
Right upper lobe posterior subsegmental pulmonary a.
Right mainstem bronchus
Bronchus intermedius
Right lower lobe superior segment pulmonary a.
Right lower lobe basal trunk pulmonary a.
Right lower lobe bronchus
Serratus anterior muscle
Pulmonary v.
Right inferior pulmonary v.
Left atrium
Coronary sinus
Descending thoracic aorta
Pulmonary v.
Subcarinal space
Left interlobar pulmonary a.
Lymph node
Left mainstem bronchus
Left upper lobe bronchus
Lingular pulmonary a.
Great cardiac v.
Diaphragm
Stomach
Liver
Esophagus
Pancreas
Spleen

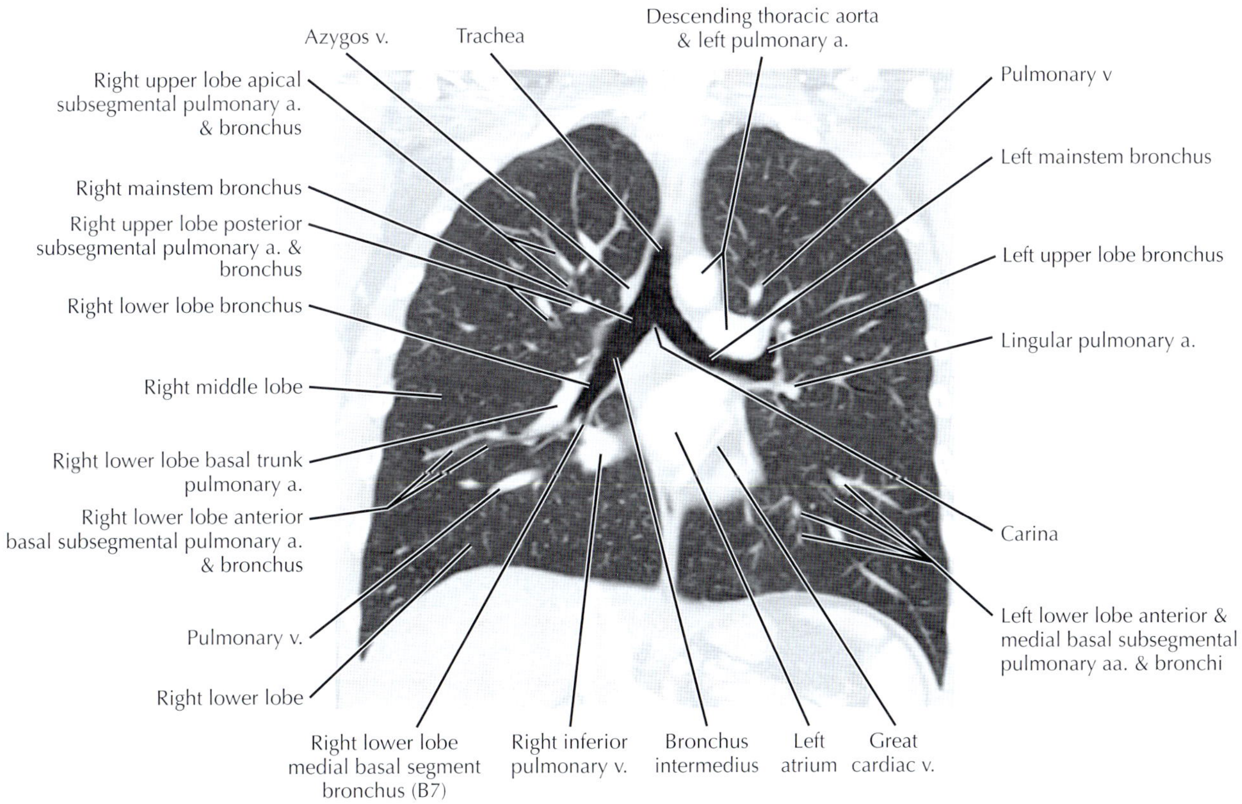
Azygos v.
Trachea
Descending thoracic aorta & left pulmonary a.
Right upper lobe apical subsegmental pulmonary a. & bronchus
Right mainstem bronchus
Right upper lobe posterior subsegmental pulmonary a. & bronchus
Right lower lobe bronchus
Right middle lobe
Right lower lobe basal trunk pulmonary a.
Right lower lobe anterior basal subsegmental pulmonary a. & bronchus
Pulmonary v.
Right lower lobe
Pulmonary v
Left mainstem bronchus
Left upper lobe bronchus
Lingular pulmonary a.
Carina
Left lower lobe anterior & medial basal subsegmental pulmonary aa. & bronchi
Right lower lobe medial basal segment bronchus (B7)
Right inferior pulmonary v.
Bronchus intermedius
Left atrium
Great cardiac v.

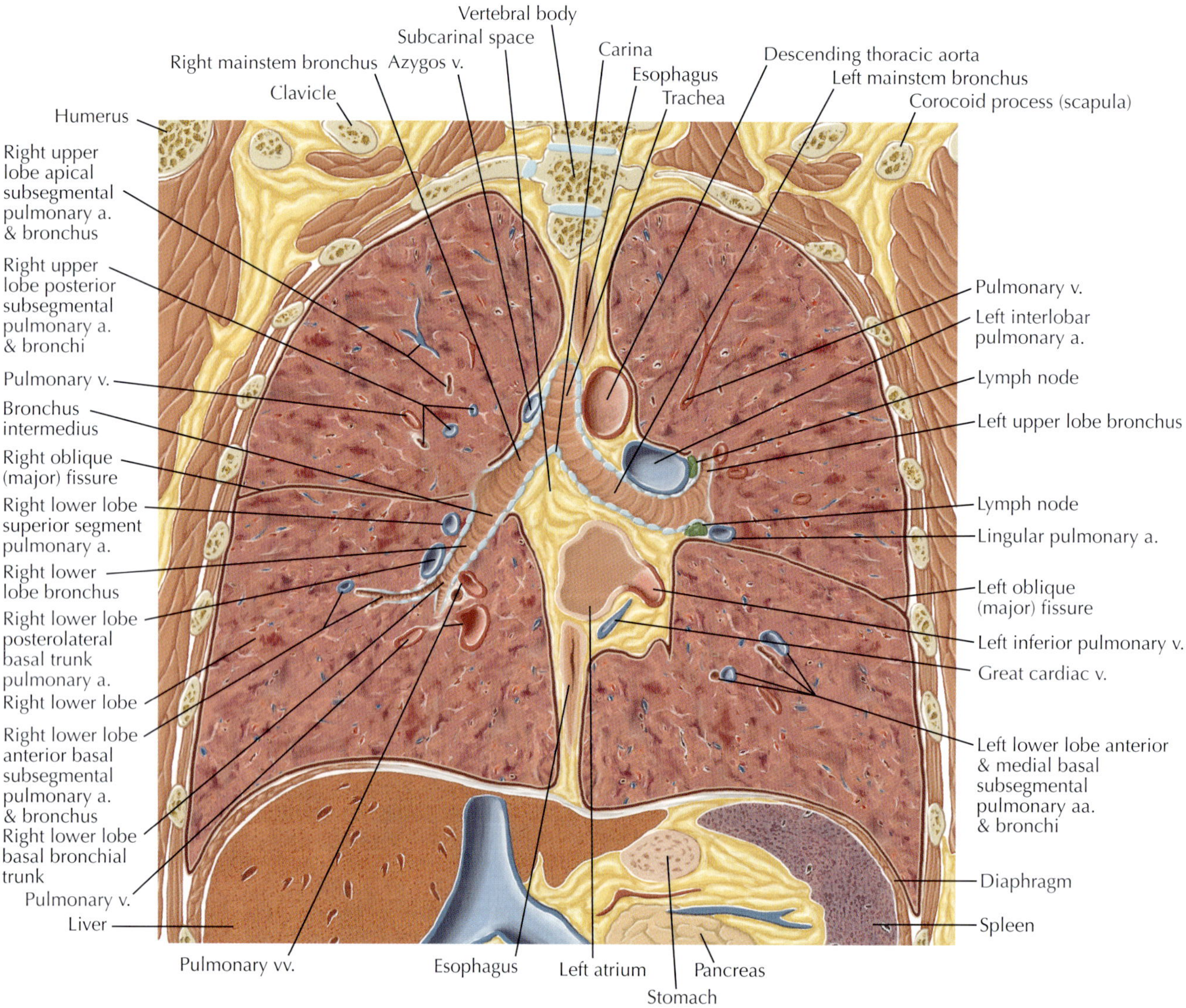

Vertebral body
Subcarinal space
Carina
Right mainstem bronchus
Azygos v.
Esophagus
Descending thoracic aorta
Left mainstem bronchus
Trachea
Clavicle
Corocoid process (scapula)
Humerus
Right upper lobe apical subsegmental pulmonary a. & bronchus
Right upper lobe posterior subsegmental pulmonary a. & bronchi
Pulmonary v.
Bronchus intermedius
Right oblique (major) fissure
Right lower lobe superior segment pulmonary a.
Right lower lobe bronchus
Right lower lobe posterolateral basal trunk pulmonary a.
Right lower lobe
Right lower lobe anterior basal subsegmental pulmonary a. & bronchus
Right lower lobe basal bronchial trunk
Pulmonary v.
Liver
Pulmonary vv.
Esophagus
Left atrium
Stomach
Pancreas
Pulmonary v.
Left interlobar pulmonary a.
Lymph node
Left upper lobe bronchus
Lymph node
Lingular pulmonary a.
Left oblique (major) fissure
Left inferior pulmonary v.
Great cardiac v.
Left lower lobe anterior & medial basal subsegmental pulmonary aa. & bronchi
Diaphragm
Spleen

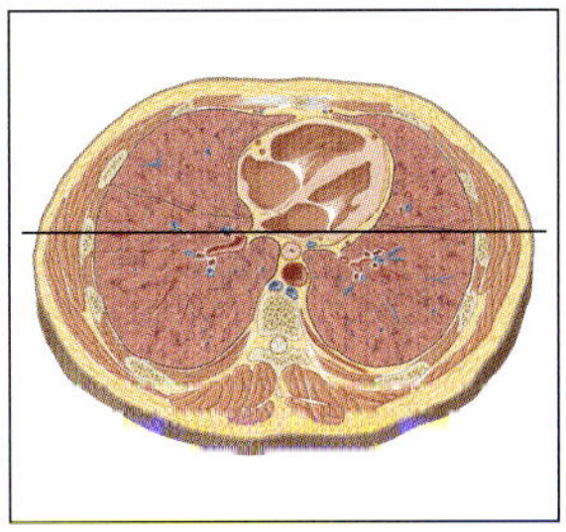

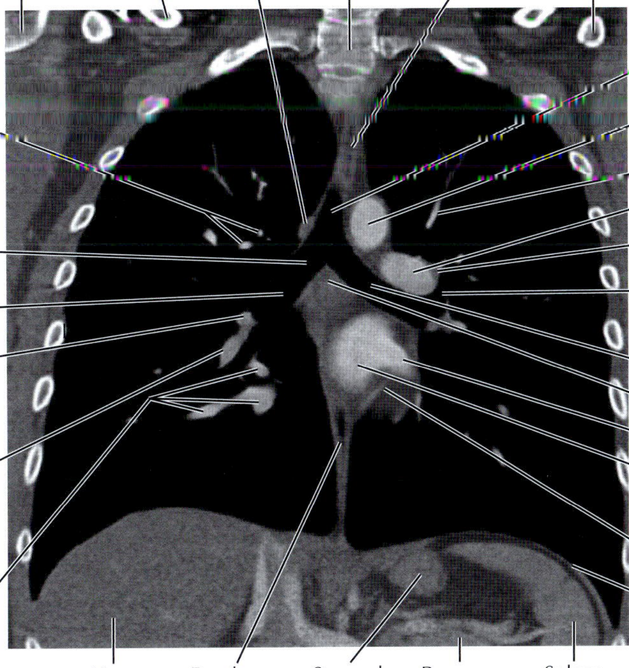
Humerus
Clavicle
Azygos v.
Vertebral body
Esophagus
Corocoid process (scapula)
Trachea
Descending thoracic aorta
Pulmonary v.
Left interlobar pulmonary a.
Lymph node
Left upper lobe bronchus
Left mainstem bronchus
Subcarinal space
Left inferior pulmonary v.
Left atrium
Great cardiac v.
Diaphragm
Right upper lobe posterior subsegmental pulmonary aa.
Right mainstem bronchus
Bronchus intermedius
Right lower lobe superior segment pulmonary a.
Right lower lobe posterolateral basal trunk pulmonary a.
Pulmonary vv.
Liver
Esophagus
Stomach
Pancreas
Spleen

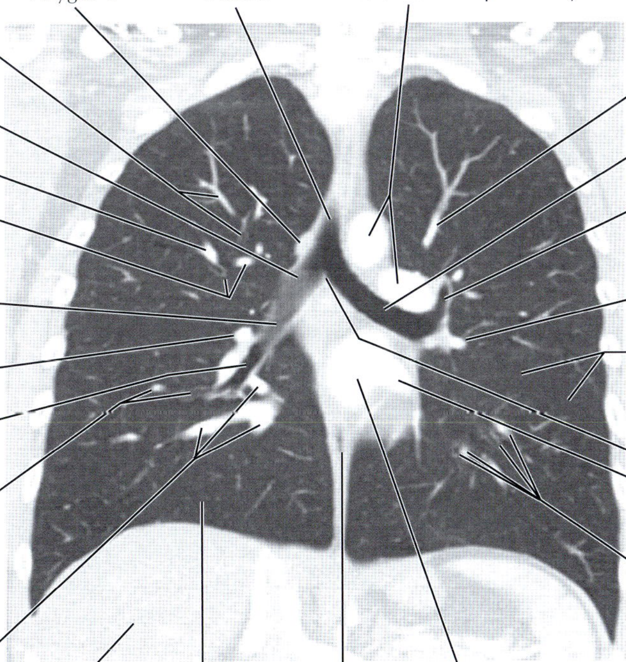
Azygos v.
Trachea
Descending thoracic aorta & left interlobar pulmonary a.
Right upper lobe apical subsegmental pulmonary a. & bronchus
Right mainstem bronchus
Pulmonary v.
Right upper lobe posterior subsegmental pulmonary a. & bronchus
Right lower lobe bronchus
Right lower lobe superior segment pulmonary a.
Right lower lobe basal bronchial trunk
Right lower lobe anterior basal subsegmental pulmonary a. & bronchus
Pulmonary vv.
Pulmonary v.
Left mainstem bronchus
Left upper lobe bronchus
Lingular pulmonary a.
Left oblique (major) fissure
Carina
Left inferior pulmonary v.
Left lower lobe anterior & medial basal subsegmental pulmonary aa. & bronchi
Liver
Right lower lobe
Esophagus
Left atrium

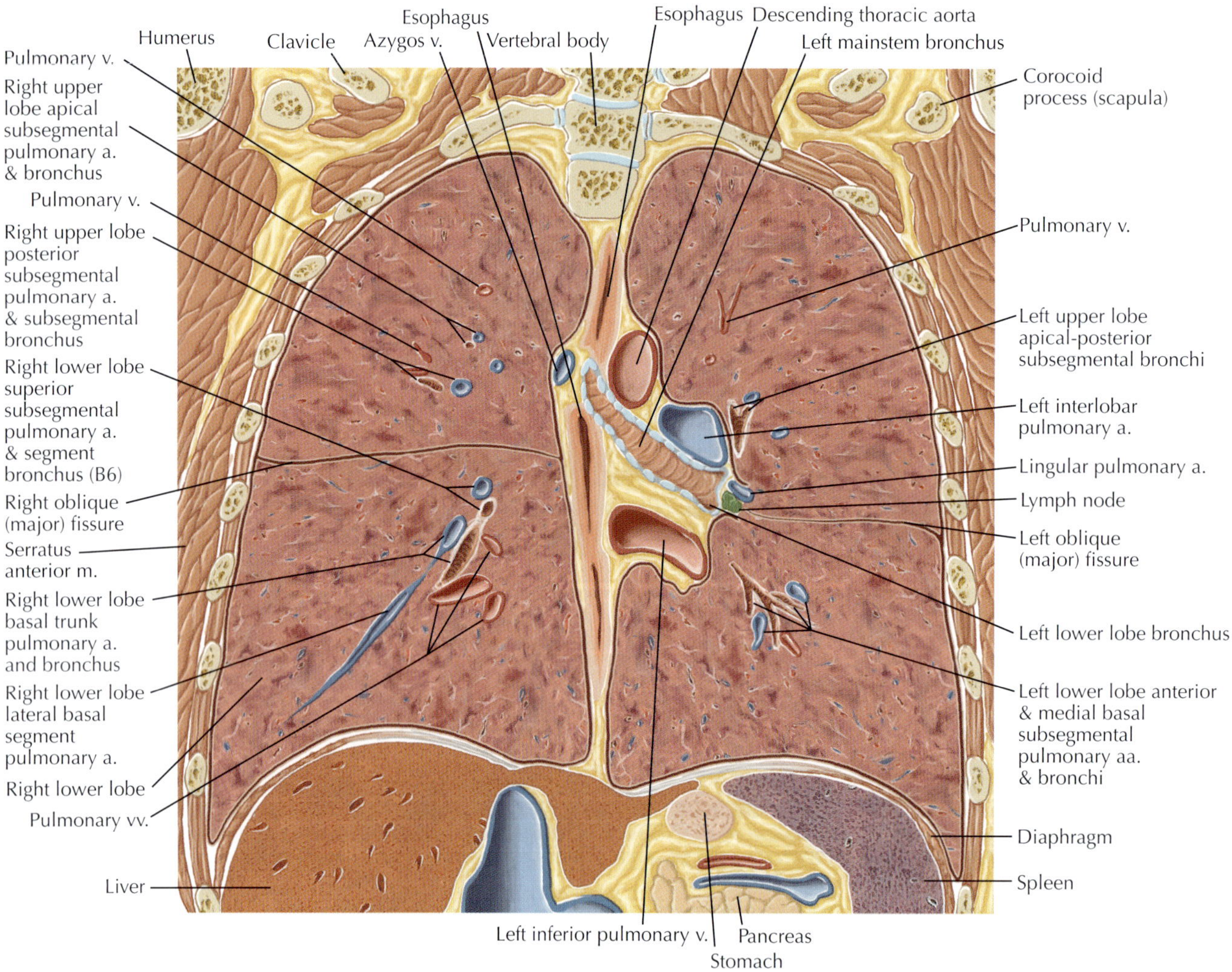
Humerus
Clavicle
Esophagus
Azygos v.
Vertebral body
Esophagus
Descending thoracic aorta
Left mainstem bronchus
Pulmonary v.
Right upper lobe apical subsegmental pulmonary a. & bronchus
Pulmonary v.
Right upper lobe posterior subsegmental pulmonary a. & subsegmental bronchus
Right lower lobe superior subsegmental pulmonary a. & segment bronchus (B6)
Right oblique (major) fissure
Serratus anterior m.
Right lower lobe basal trunk pulmonary a. and bronchus
Right lower lobe lateral basal segment pulmonary a.
Right lower lobe
Pulmonary vv.
Liver
Corocoid process (scapula)
Pulmonary v.
Left upper lobe apical-posterior subsegmental bronchi
Left interlobar pulmonary a.
Lingular pulmonary a.
Lymph node
Left oblique (major) fissure
Left lower lobe bronchus
Left lower lobe anterior & medial basal subsegmental pulmonary aa. & bronchi
Diaphragm
Spleen
Left inferior pulmonary v.
Pancreas
Stomach

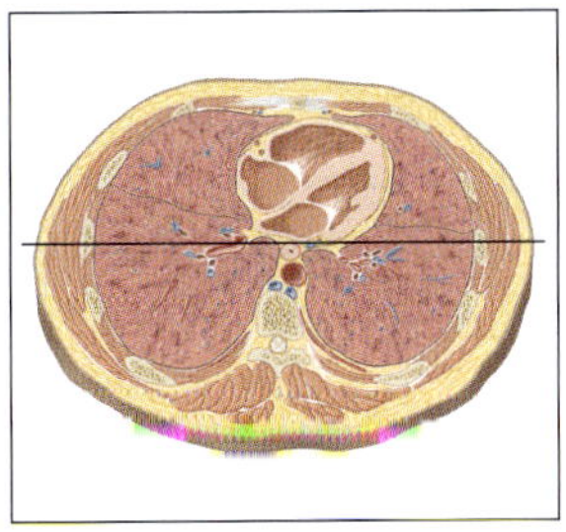

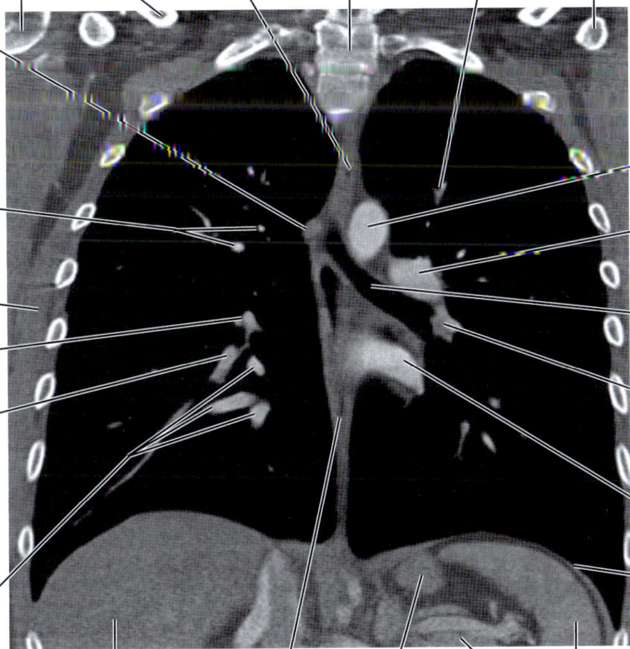

Humerus
Clavicle
Esophagus
Vertebral body
Pulmonary v.
Corocoid process (scapula)
Azygos v.
Descending thoracic aorta
Right upper lobe posterior subsegmental pulmonary aa.
Left interlobar pulmonary a.
Serratus anterior m.
Left mainstem bronchus
Right lower lobe superior subsegmental pulmonary a.
Lymph node
Right lower lobe posterolateral basal trunk pulmonary a.
Left inferior pulmonary v.
Diaphragm
Pulmonary vv.
Liver
Esophagus
Stomach
Pancreas
Spleen

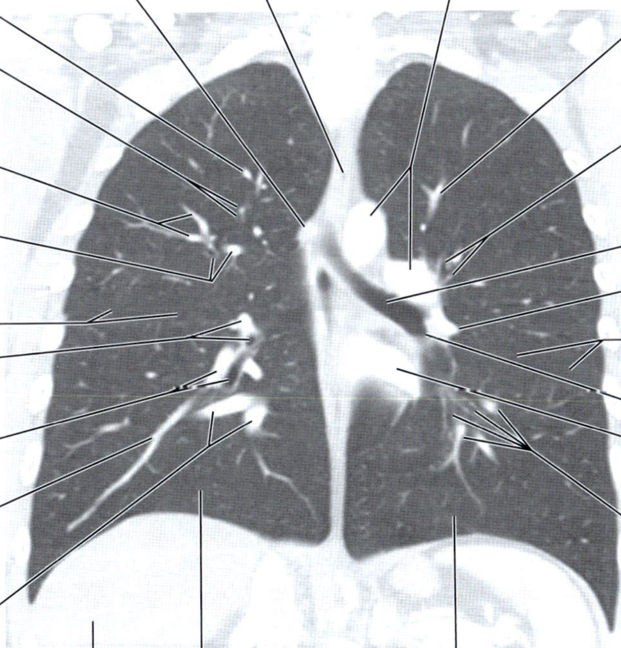

Pulmonary v.
Azygos v.
Esophagus
Descending thoracic aorta & left interlobar pulmonary a.
Pulmonary v.
Right upper lobe apical subsegmental pulmonary a. & bronchus
Left upper lobe apical-posterior subsegmental bronchi
Pulmonary vv.
Right upper lobe posterior subsegmental pulmonary a. & bronchus
Left mainstem bronchus
Lingular pulmonary a.
Right oblique (major) fissure
Left oblique (major) fissure
Right lower lobe superior subsegmental pulmonary a. & segment bronchus (B6)
Left lower lobe bronchus
Right lower lobe basal trunk bronchus & pulmonary a.
Left inferior pulmonary v.
Right lower lobe lateral basal segment pulmonary a.
Left lower lobe anterior & medial basal subsegmental pulmonary aa. & bronchi
Pulmonary v.
Liver
Right lower lobe
Left lower lobe

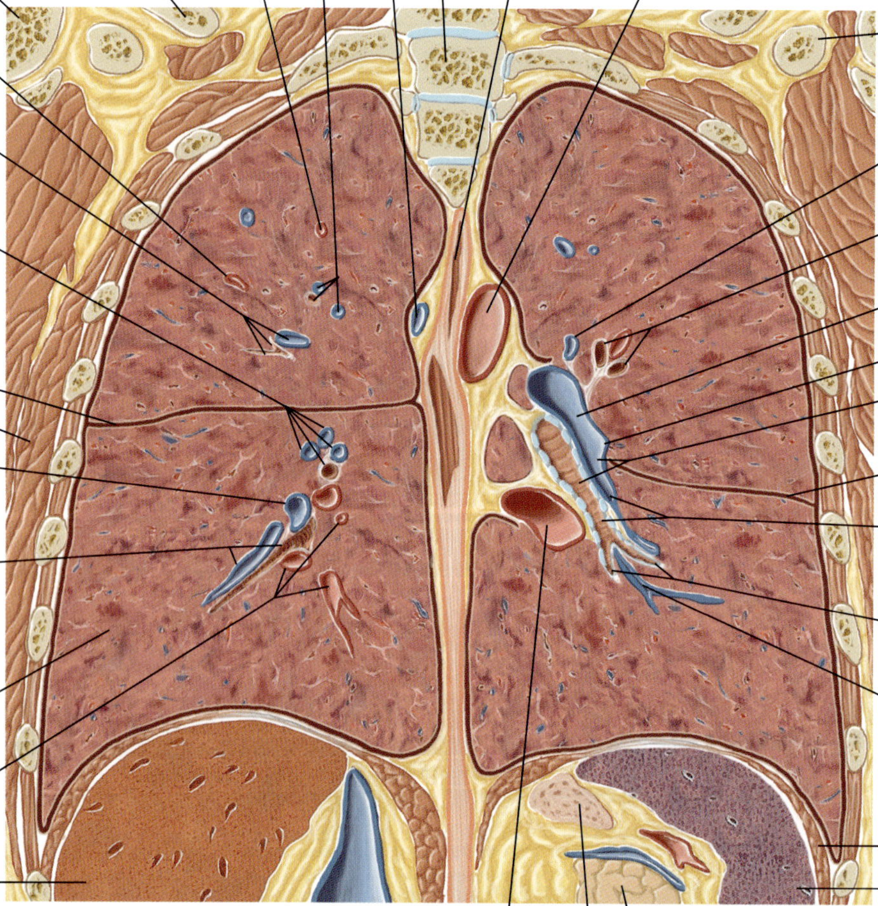

Vertebral body
Right upper lobe apical subsegmental pulmonary aa. & bronchus
Esophagus
Humerus
Clavicle
Pulmonary v.
Azygos v.
Descending thoracic aorta
Pulmonary v.
Corocoid process (scapula)
Right upper lobe posterior subsegmental pulmonary a. & bronchi
Pulmonary a.
Right lower lobe superior segment bronchus (B6) & subsegmental pulmonary aa.
Left upper lobe apical-posterior subsegmental bronchi
Left interlobar pulmonary a.
Lingular pulmonary a.
Right oblique (major) fissure
Left lower lobe bronchus & pulmonary a.
Serratus anterior m.
Right lower lobe posterior basal segment pulmonary a.
Left oblique (major) fissure
Left lower lobe anteromedial basal segment pulmonary a. & bronchus (B7+8)
Right lower lobe lateral basal segment pulmonary a. & bronchus (B9)
Left lower lobe anterior & medial basal subsegmental bronchi
Right lower lobe
Left lower lobe medial basal subsegmental pulmonary a.
Pulmonary vv.
Diaphragm
Liver
Spleen
Left inferior pulmonary v.
Pancreas
Stomach

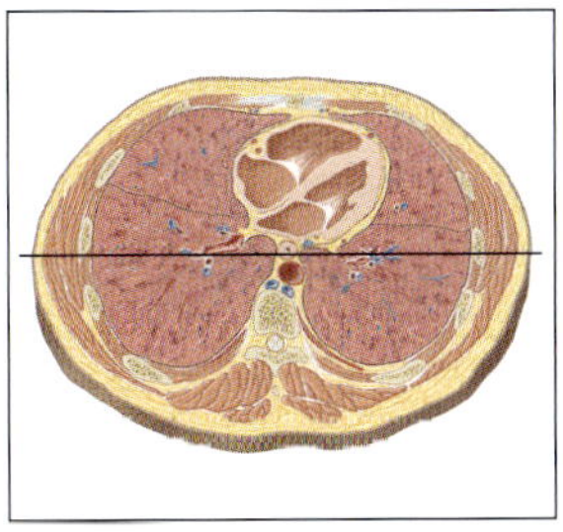

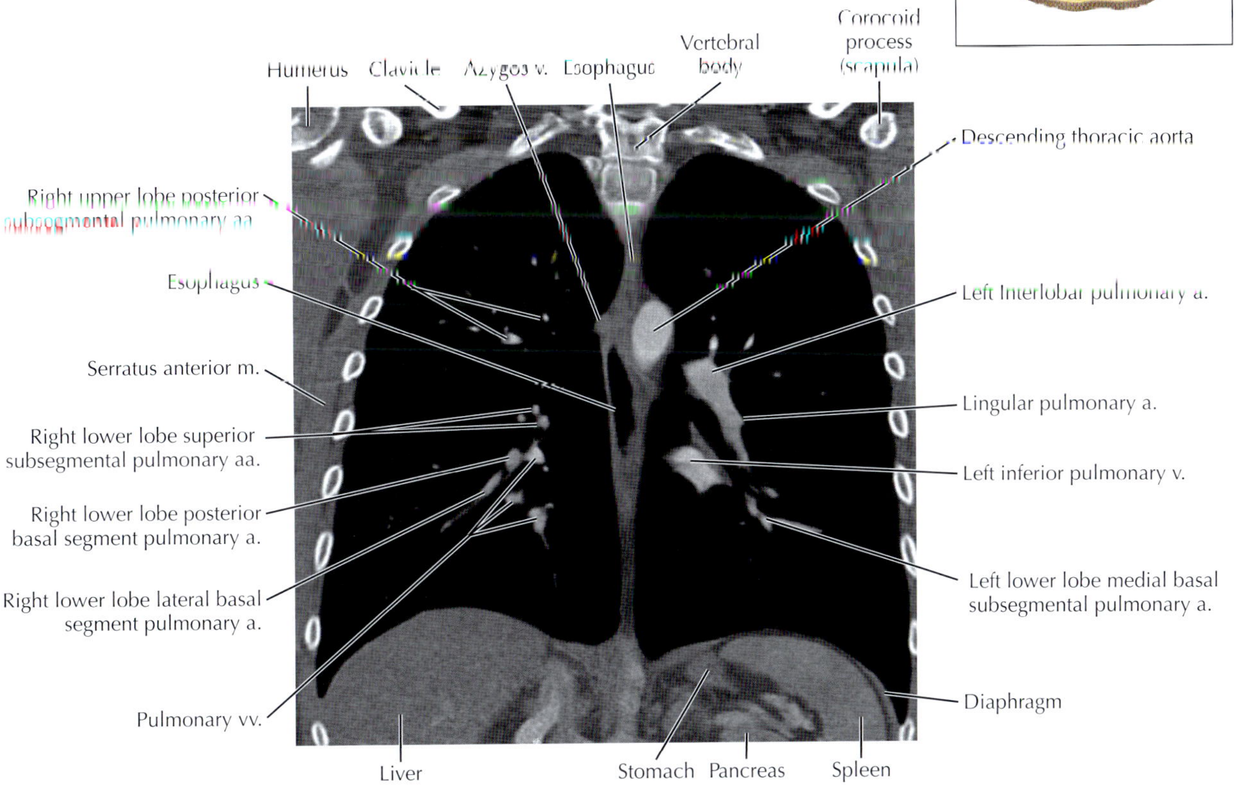
Humerus
Clavicle
Azygos v.
Esophagus
Vertebral body
Coracoid process (scapula)
Descending thoracic aorta
Right upper lobe posterior subsegmental pulmonary aa.
Esophagus
Serratus anterior m.
Right lower lobe superior subsegmental pulmonary aa.
Right lower lobe posterior basal segment pulmonary a.
Right lower lobe lateral basal segment pulmonary a.
Pulmonary vv.
Left interlobar pulmonary a.
Lingular pulmonary a.
Left inferior pulmonary v.
Left lower lobe medial basal subsegmental pulmonary a.
Diaphragm
Liver
Stomach
Pancreas
Spleen

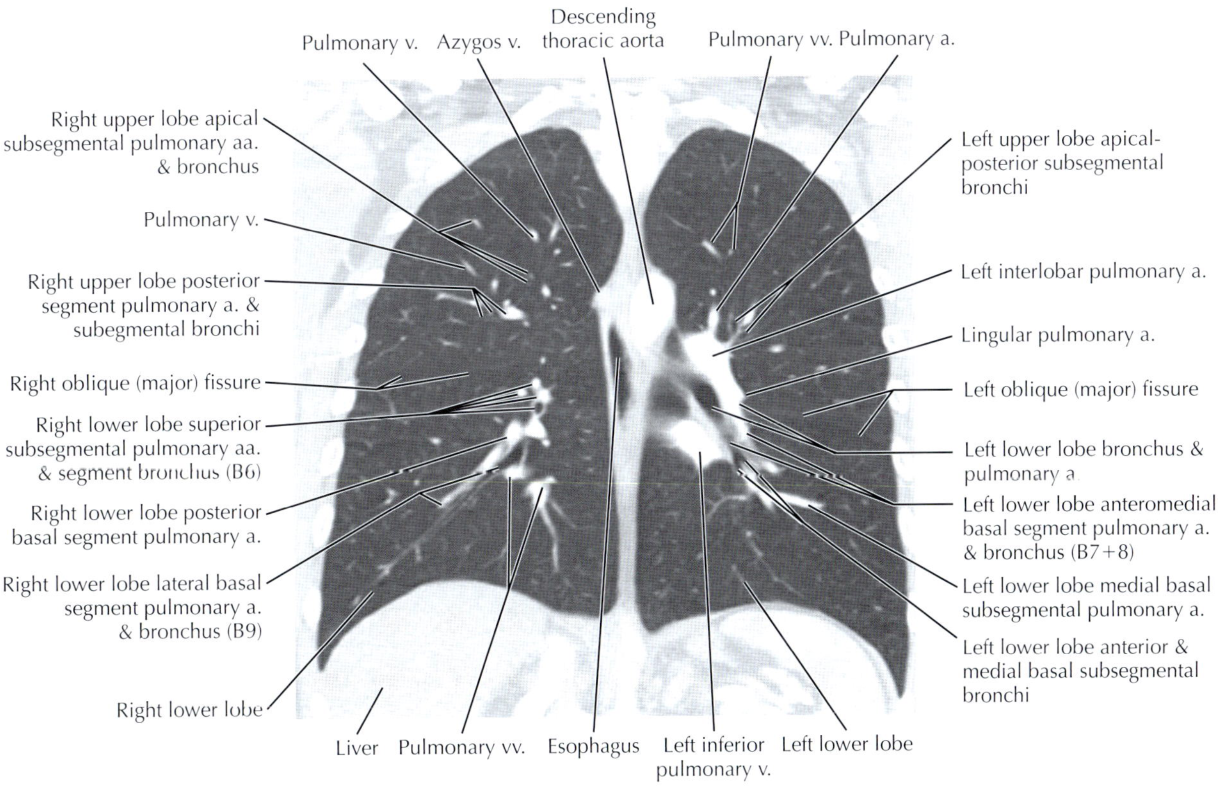
Pulmonary v.
Azygos v.
Descending thoracic aorta
Pulmonary vv.
Pulmonary a.
Right upper lobe apical subsegmental pulmonary aa. & bronchus
Pulmonary v.
Right upper lobe posterior segment pulmonary a. & subegmental bronchi
Right oblique (major) fissure
Right lower lobe superior subsegmental pulmonary aa. & segment bronchus (B6)
Right lower lobe posterior basal segment pulmonary a.
Right lower lobe lateral basal segment pulmonary a. & bronchus (B9)
Right lower lobe
Left upper lobe apical-posterior subsegmental bronchi
Left interlobar pulmonary a.
Lingular pulmonary a.
Left oblique (major) fissure
Left lower lobe bronchus & pulmonary a.
Left lower lobe anteromedial basal segment pulmonary a. & bronchus (B7+8)
Left lower lobe medial basal subsegmental pulmonary a.
Left lower lobe anterior & medial basal subsegmental bronchi
Liver
Pulmonary vv.
Esophagus
Left inferior pulmonary v.
Left lower lobe

Soft Tissue and Lung Coronal 25

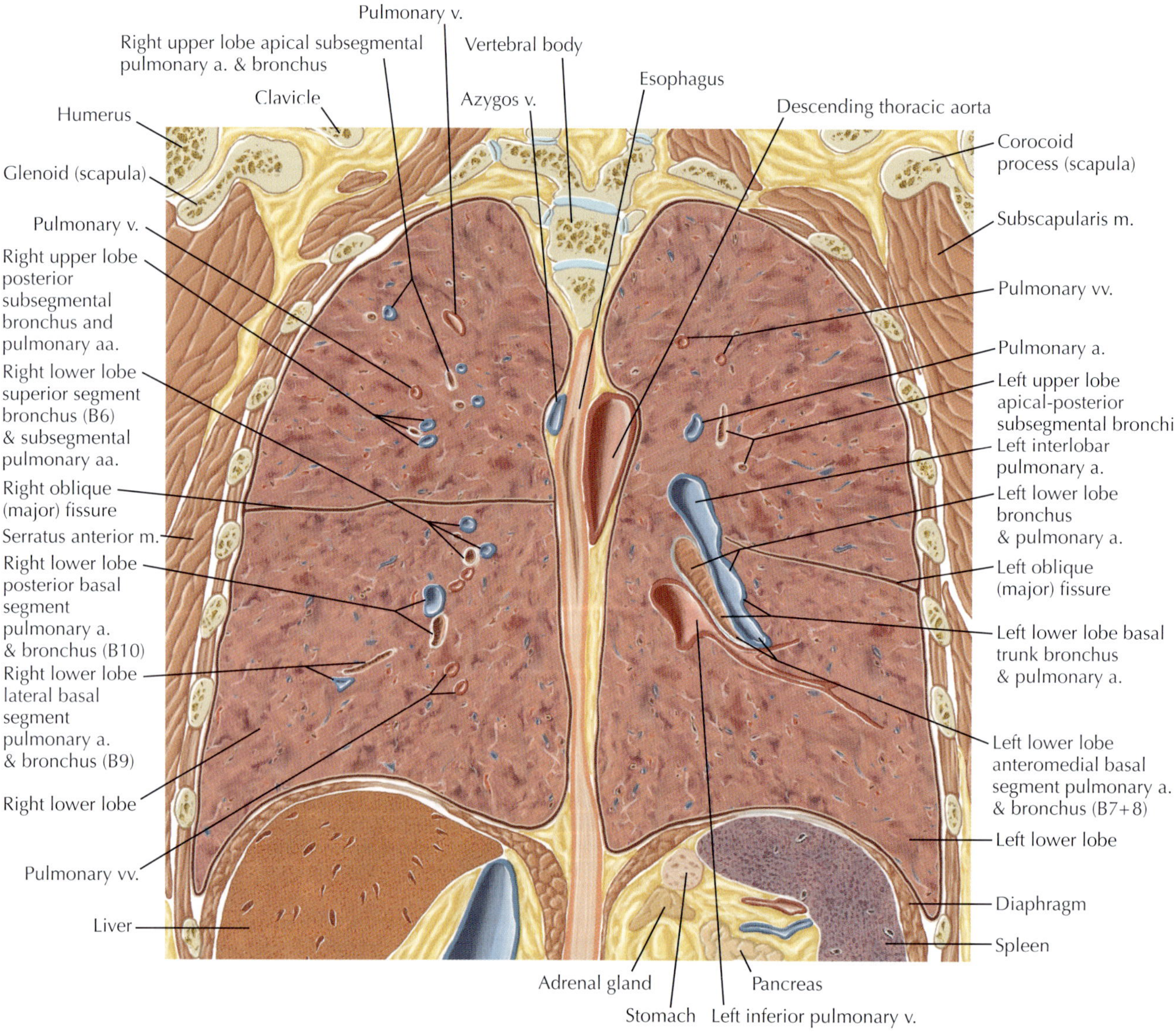

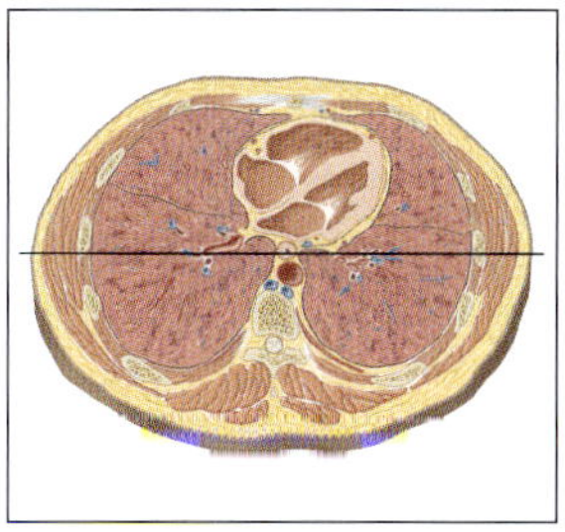

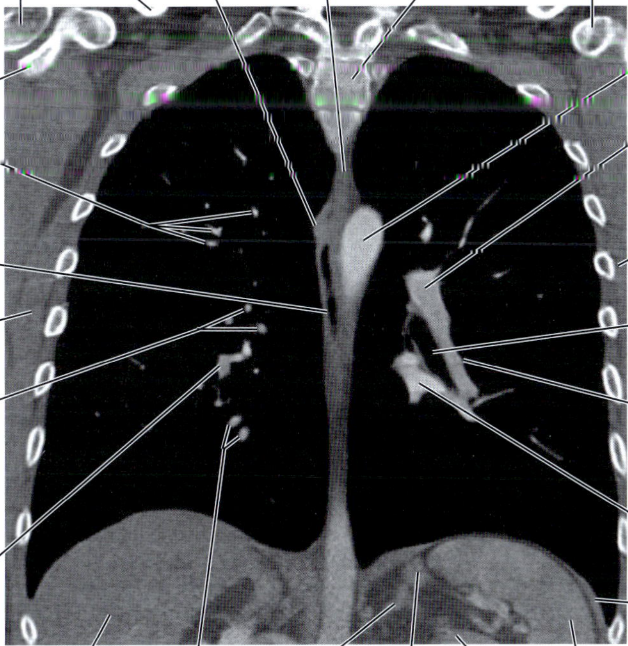
Humerus
Clavicle
Azygos v.
Esophagus
Vertebral body
Coracoid process (scapula)
Glenoid (scapula)
Right upper lobe posterior subsegmental pulmonary aa.
Esophagus
Serratus anterior m.
Right lower lobe superior subsegmental pulmonary aa.
Right lower lobe posterior basal segment pulmonary a.
Descending thoracic aorta
Left interlobar pulmonary a.
Subscapularis m.
Left lower lobe bronchus
Left lower lobe anteromedial basal segment pulmonary a.
Left inferior pulmonary v.
Diaphragm
Liver
Pulmonary vv.
Adrenal gland
Stomach
Pancreas
Spleen

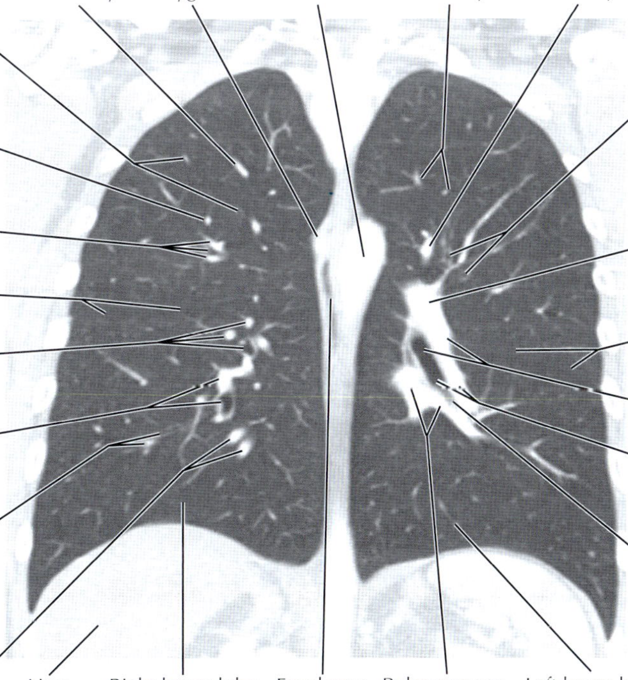
Pulmonary v.
Azygos v.
Descending thoracic aorta
Pulmonary v.
Pulmonary a.
Right upper lobe apical subsegmental pulmonary a. & bronchus
Pulmonary v.
Right upper lobe posterior subsegmental aa. & bronchus
Right oblique (major) fissure
Right lower lobe superior subsegmental pulmonary aa. & segment bronchus (B6)
Right lower lobe posterior basal segment pulmonary a. & bronchus (B10)
Right lower lobe lateral basal segment pulmonary a. & bronchus (B9)
Pulmonary vv.
Left upper lobe apical-posterior subsegmental bronchi
Left interlobar pulmonary a.
Left oblique (major) fissure
Left lower lobe bronchus & pulmonary a.
Left lower lobe basal trunk bronchus & pulmonary a.
Left lower lobe anteromedial basal segment bronchus (B7+8)
Liver
Right lower lobe
Esophagus
Pulmonary vv.
Left lower lobe

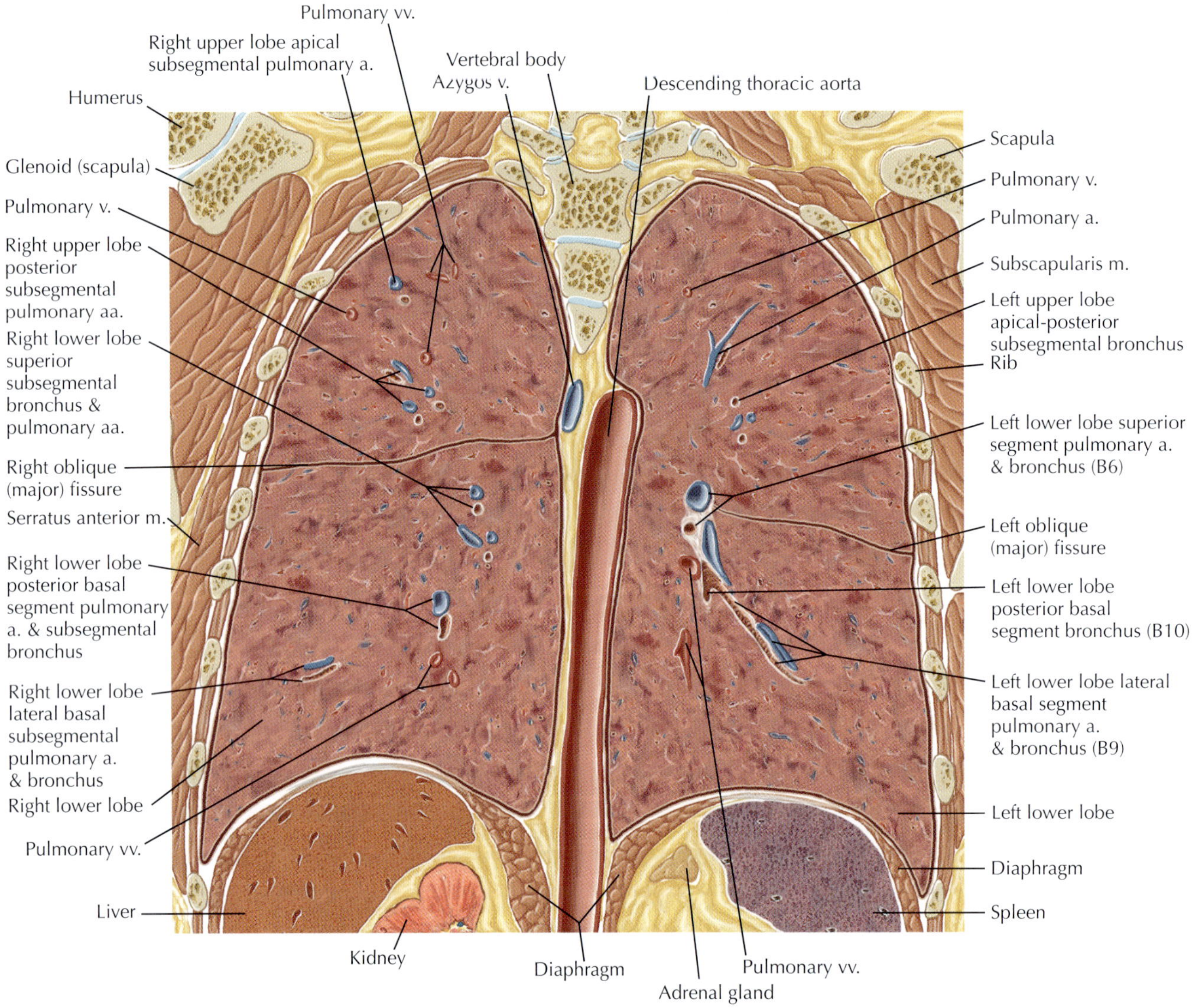
Pulmonary vv.
Right upper lobe apical subsegmental pulmonary a.
Vertebral body
Azygos v.
Descending thoracic aorta
Humerus
Glenoid (scapula)
Pulmonary v.
Right upper lobe posterior subsegmental pulmonary aa.
Right lower lobe superior subsegmental bronchus & pulmonary aa.
Right oblique (major) fissure
Serratus anterior m.
Right lower lobe posterior basal segment pulmonary a. & subsegmental bronchus
Right lower lobe lateral basal subsegmental pulmonary a. & bronchus
Right lower lobe
Pulmonary vv.
Liver
Kidney
Diaphragm
Adrenal gland
Pulmonary vv.
Scapula
Pulmonary v.
Pulmonary a.
Subscapularis m.
Left upper lobe apical-posterior subsegmental bronchus
Rib
Left lower lobe superior segment pulmonary a. & bronchus (B6)
Left oblique (major) fissure
Left lower lobe posterior basal segment bronchus (B10)
Left lower lobe lateral basal segment pulmonary a. & bronchus (B9)
Left lower lobe
Diaphragm
Spleen

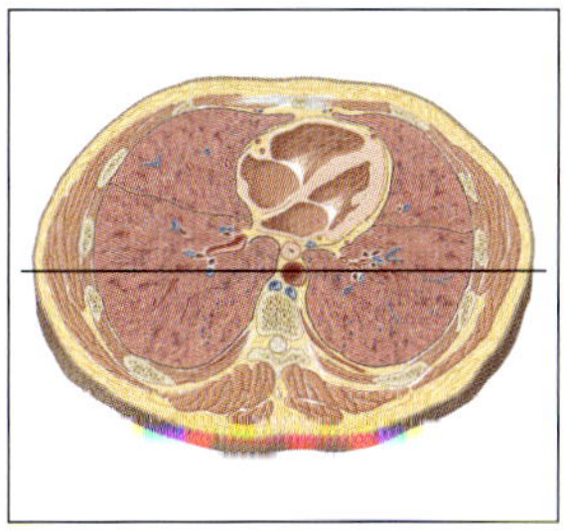

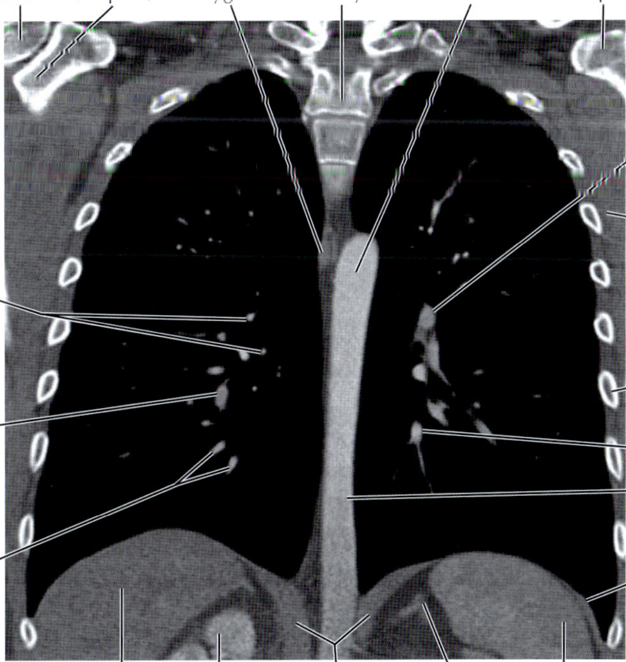
Humerus
Glenoid (scapula)
Azygos v.
Vertebral body
Descending thoracic aorta
Scapula
Left lower lobe superior segment pulmonary a.
Subscapularis m.
Right lower lobe superior subsegmental pulmonary aa.
Rib
Right lower lobe posterior basal subsegmental pulmonary a.
Pulmonary v.
Descending thoracic aorta
Pulmonary vv.
Diaphragm
Liver
Kidney
Diaphragm
Adrenal gland
Spleen

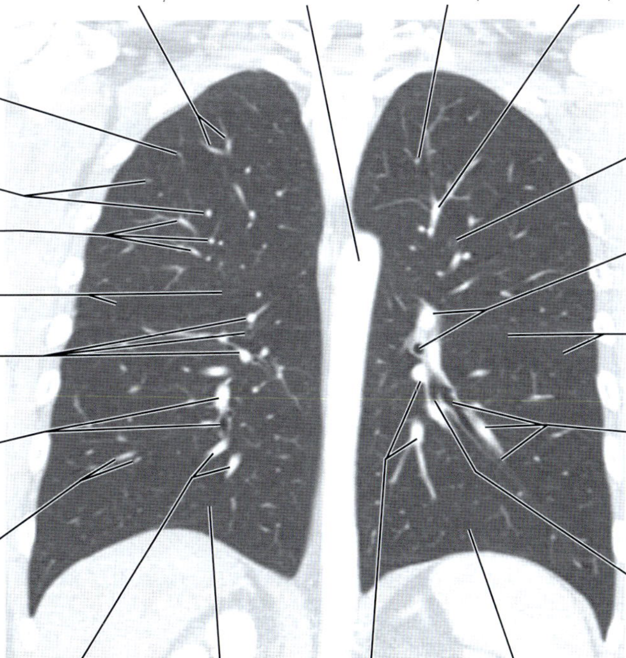
Pulmonary vv.
Descending thoracic aorta
Pulmonary v.
Pulmonary a.
Right upper lobe apical subsegmental pulmonary a.
Left upper lobe apical-posterior subsegmental bronchus
Pulmonary v.
Right upper lobe posterior subsegmental pulmonary aa.
Left lower lobe superior segment pulmonary a. & bronchus (B6)
Right oblique (major) fissure
Left oblique (major) fissure
Right lower lobe superior subsegmental pulmonary aa. & bronchus
Right lower lobe posterior basal segment pulmonary a. & subsegmental bronchus
Left lower lobe lateral basal segment pulmonary a. & bronchus (B9)
Right lower lobe lateral basal subsegmental pulmonary a. & bronchus (B9)
Left lower lobe posterior basal segment bronchus (B10)
Pulmonary vv.
Right lower lobe
Pulmonary vv.
Left lower lobe

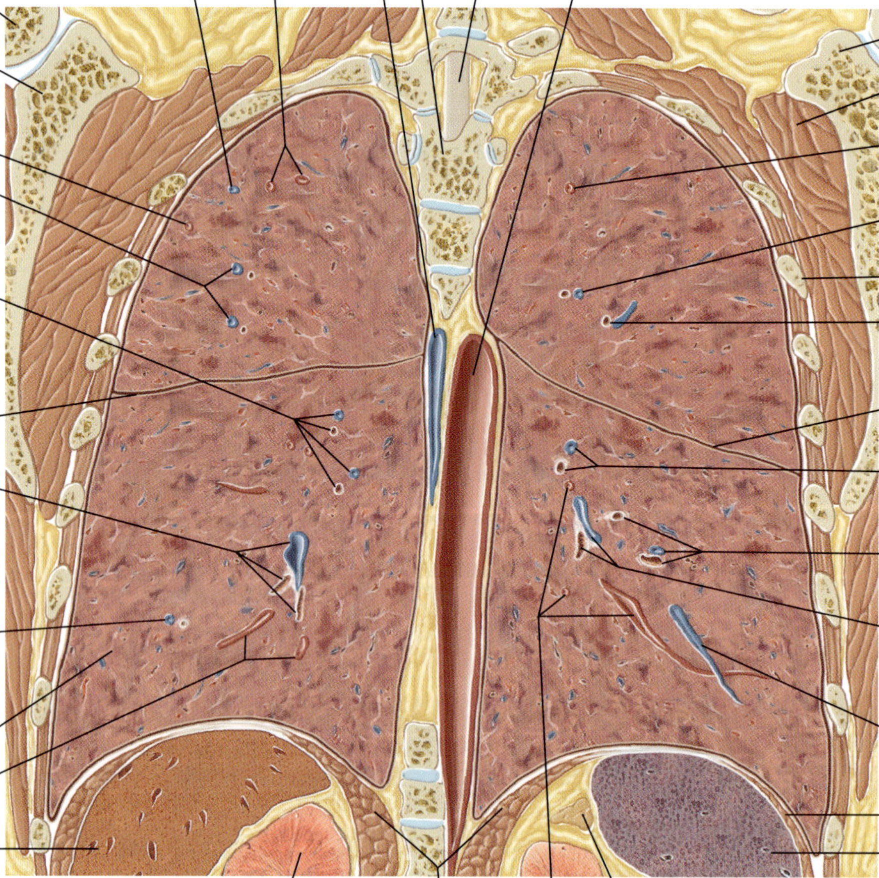

Pulmonary vv.
Right upper lobe apical subsegmental pulmonary a.
Vertebral body
Azygos v.
Spinal cord
Descending thoracic aorta
Humerus
Glenoid (scapula)
Pulmonary v.
Right upper lobe posterior subsegmental pulmonary aa.
Right lower lobe superior subsegmental bronchi & pulmonary aa.
Right oblique (major) fissure
Right lower lobe posterior basal segment pulmonary a. & subsegmental bronchi
Right lower lobe lateral basal subsegmental pulmonary a.
Right lower lobe
Pulmonary vv.
Liver
Kidney
Diaphragm
Pulmonary vv.
Adrenal gland
Scapula
Subscapularis m.
Pulmonary v.
Pulmonary a.
Rib
Left upper lobe apical-posterior subsegmental bronchus
Left oblique (major) fissure
Left lower lobe superior segment pulmonary a. & bronchus (B6)
Left lower lobe lateral basal subsegmental pulmonary a. & bronchi
Left lower lobe posterior basal segment bronchus (B10) & pulmonary a.
Left lower lobe lateral basal subsegmental pulmonary a.
Diaphragm
Spleen

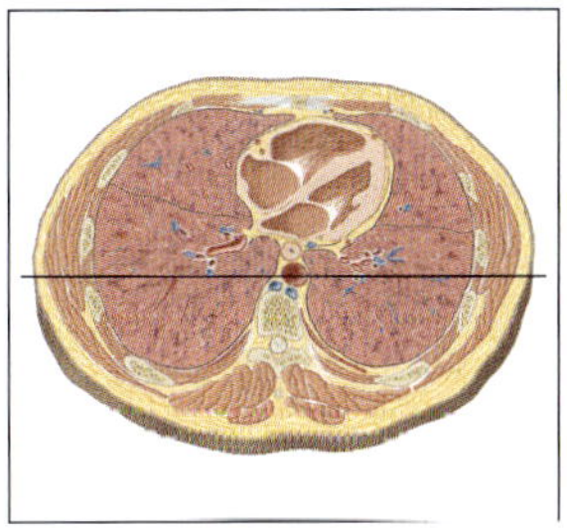

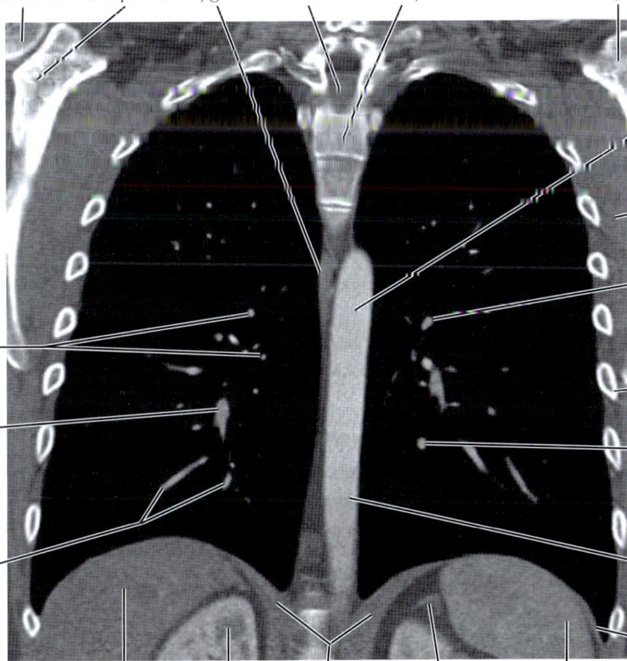
Humerus
Glenoid (scapula)
Azygos v.
Spinal cord
Vertebral body
Scapula
Descending thoracic aorta
Subscapularis m.
Left lower lobe superior segment pulmonary a.
Rib
Pulmonary v.
Descending thoracic aorta
Diaphragm
Right lower lobe superior subsegmental pulmonary aa.
Right lower lobe posterior basal subsegmental pulmonary a.
Pulmonary vv.
Liver
Kidney
Diaphragm
Adrenal gland
Spleen

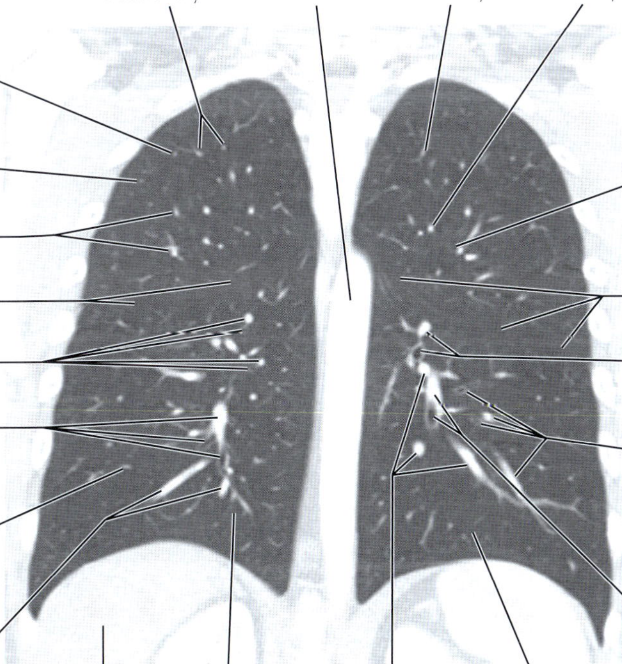
Pulmonary vv.
Descending thoracic aorta
Pulmonary v.
Pulmonary a.
Right upper lobe apical subsegmental pulmonary a.
Pulmonary v.
Right upper lobe posterior subsegmental pulmonary aa.
Right oblique (major) fissure
Right lower lobe superior subsegmental pulmonary aa. & bronchi
Right lower lobe posterior basal segment pulmonary a. & subsegmental bronchi
Right lower lobe lateral basal subsegmental pulmonary a.
Pulmonary vv.
Left upper lobe apical-posterior subsegmental bronchus
Left oblique (major) fissure
Left lower lobe superior segment pulmonary a. & bronchus (B6)
Left lower lobe lateral basal subsegmental pulmonary aa. & bronchi
Left lower lobe posterior basal segment bronchus (B10) & pulmonary a.
Liver
Right lower lobe
Pulmonary vv.
Left lower lobe

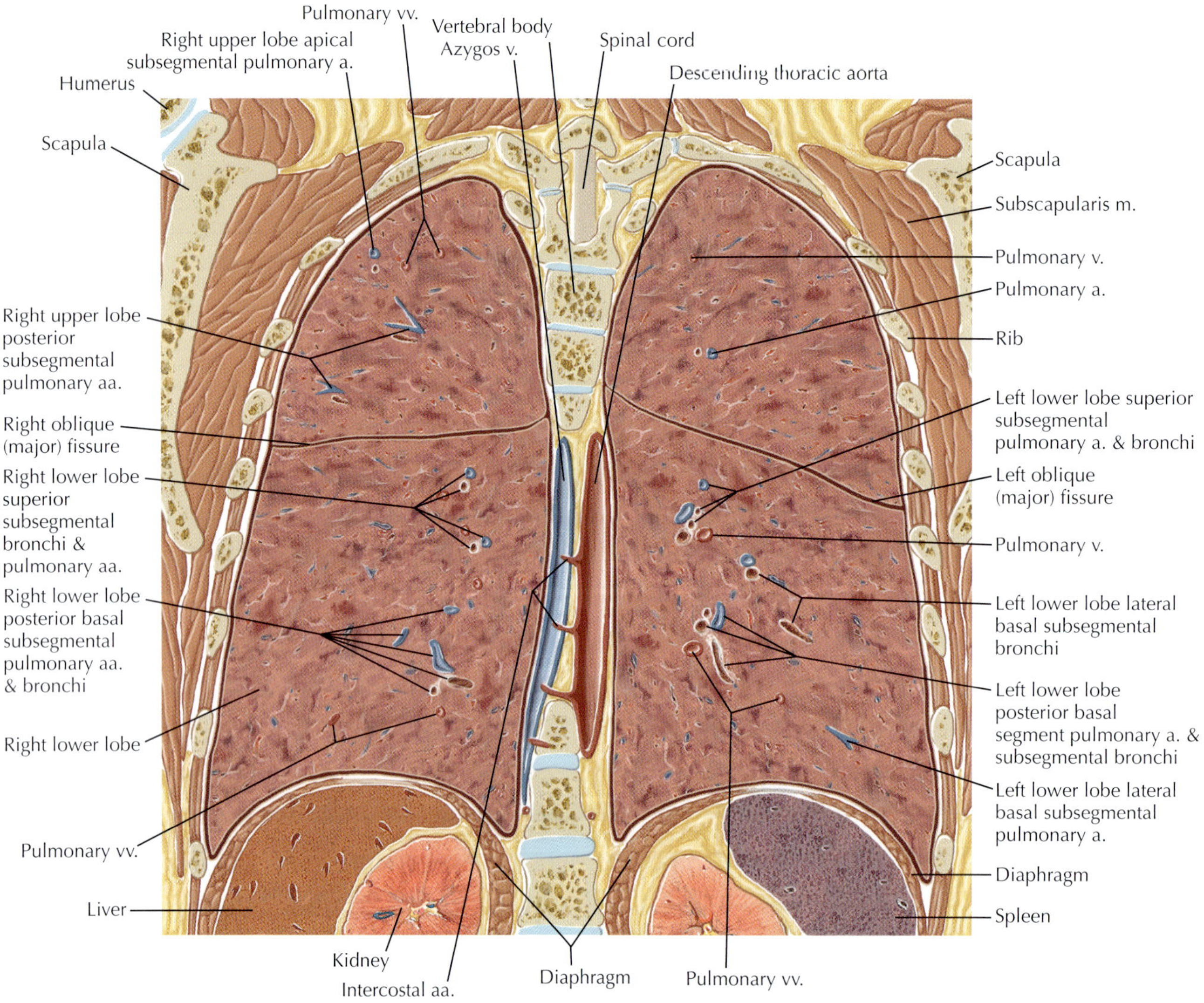

Pulmonary vv.
Right upper lobe apical subsegmental pulmonary a.
Humerus
Vertebral body
Azygos v.
Spinal cord
Descending thoracic aorta
Scapula
Subscapularis m.
Pulmonary v.
Pulmonary a.
Rib
Right upper lobe posterior subsegmental pulmonary aa.
Right oblique (major) fissure
Right lower lobe superior subsegmental bronchi & pulmonary aa.
Right lower lobe posterior basal subsegmental pulmonary aa. & bronchi
Right lower lobe
Pulmonary vv.
Liver
Kidney
Intercostal aa.
Diaphragm
Pulmonary vv.
Left lower lobe superior subsegmental pulmonary a. & bronchi
Left oblique (major) fissure
Pulmonary v.
Left lower lobe lateral basal subsegmental bronchi
Left lower lobe posterior basal segment pulmonary a. & subsegmental bronchi
Left lower lobe lateral basal subsegmental pulmonary a.
Diaphragm
Spleen

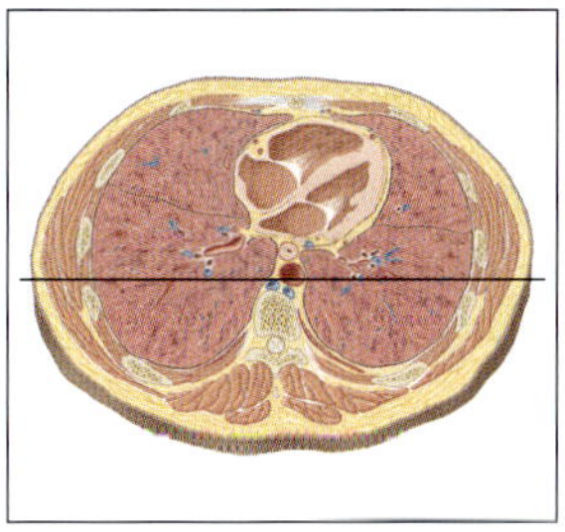

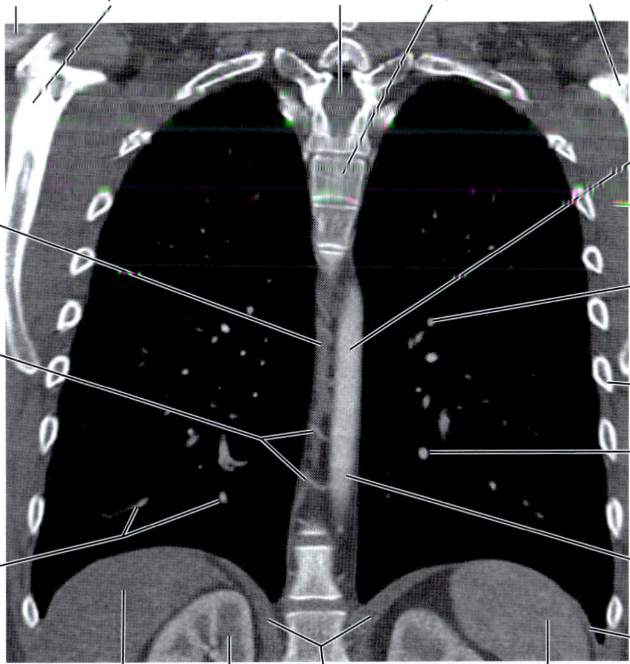
Humerus
Scapula
Spinal cord
Vertebral body
Scapula
Descending thoracic aorta
Subscapularis m.
Azygos v.
Left lower lobe superior subsegmental pulmonary a.
Intercostal aa.
Rib
Pulmonary v.
Pulmonary vv.
Descending thoracic aorta
Diaphragm
Liver
Kidney
Diaphragm
Spleen

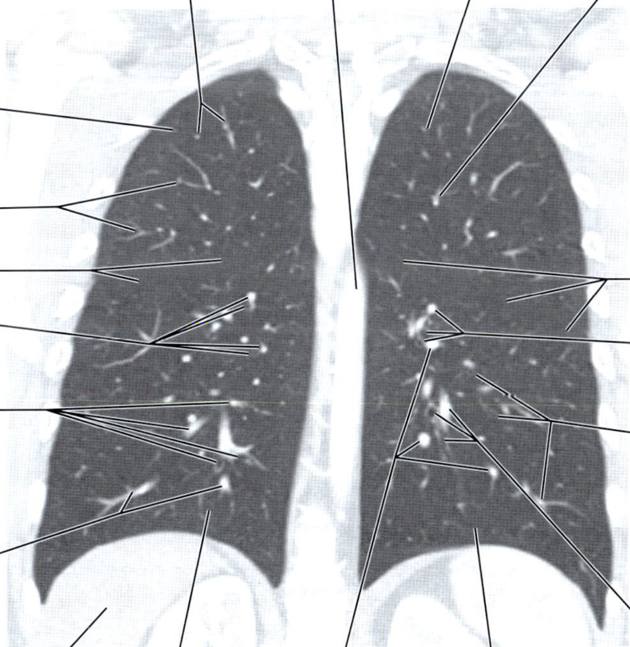
Pulmonary vv.
Descending thoracic aorta
Pulmonary v.
Pulmonary a.
Right upper lobe apical subsegmental pulmonary a.
Right upper lobe posterior subsegmental pulmonary aa.
Right oblique (major) fissure
Left oblique (major) fissure
Right lower lobe superior subsegmental pulmonary aa. & bronchi
Left lower lobe superior subsegmental pulmonary a. & bronchi
Right lower lobe posterior basal subsegmental pulmonary aa. & bronchi
Left lower lobe lateral basal subsegmental pulmonary a. & bronchi
Pulmonary vv.
Liver
Right lower lobe
Pulmonary vv.
Left lower lobe
Left lower lobe posterior basal segment pulmonary a. & subsegmental bronchi

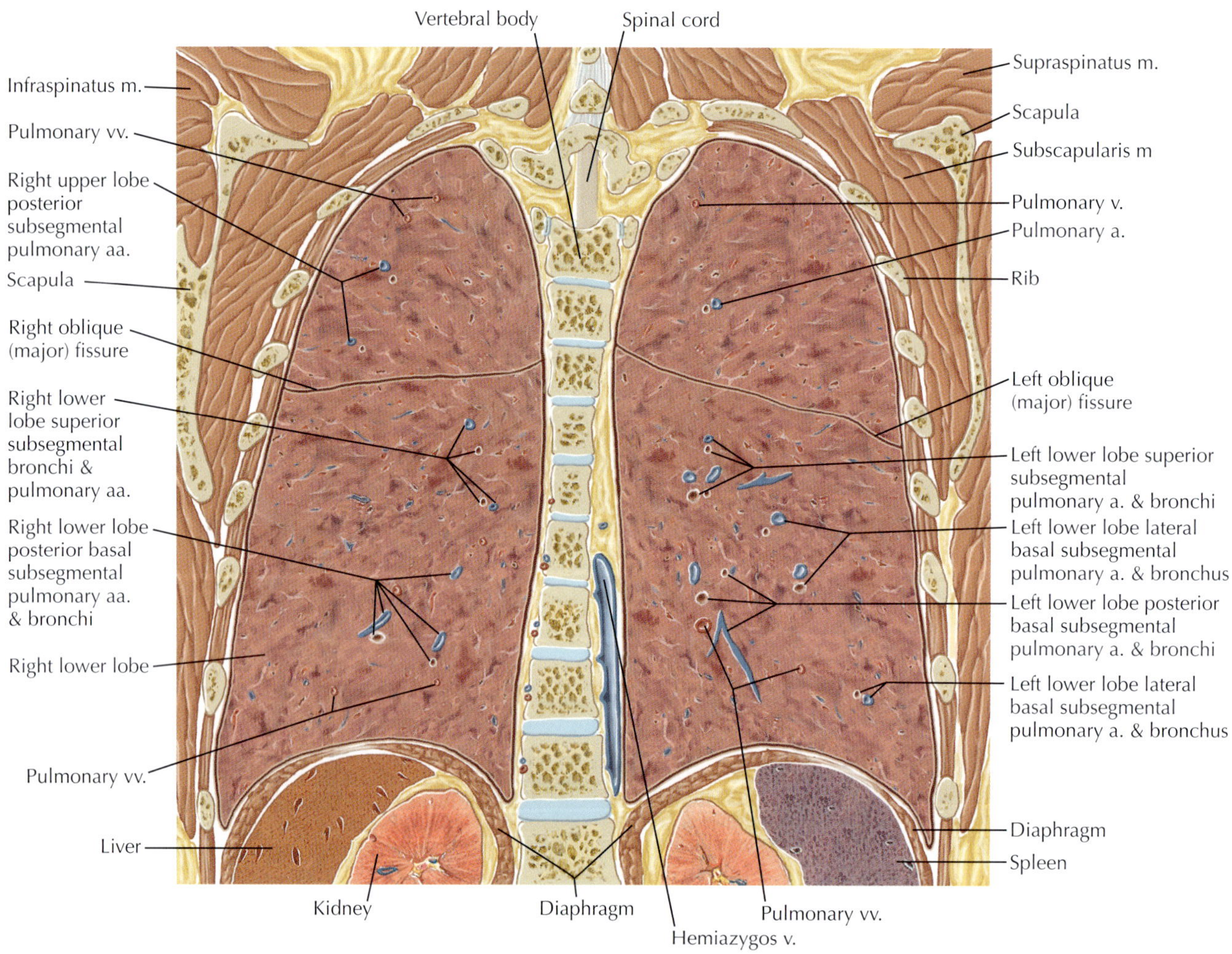
Vertebral body
Spinal cord
Infraspinatus m.
Pulmonary vv.
Right upper lobe posterior subsegmental pulmonary aa.
Scapula
Right oblique (major) fissure
Right lower lobe superior subsegmental bronchi & pulmonary aa.
Right lower lobe posterior basal subsegmental pulmonary aa. & bronchi
Right lower lobe
Pulmonary vv.
Liver
Kidney
Diaphragm
Hemiazygos v.
Pulmonary vv.
Supraspinatus m.
Scapula
Subscapularis m
Pulmonary v.
Pulmonary a.
Rib
Left oblique (major) fissure
Left lower lobe superior subsegmental pulmonary a. & bronchi
Left lower lobe lateral basal subsegmental pulmonary a. & bronchus
Left lower lobe posterior basal subsegmental pulmonary a. & bronchi
Left lower lobe lateral basal subsegmental pulmonary a. & bronchus
Diaphragm
Spleen

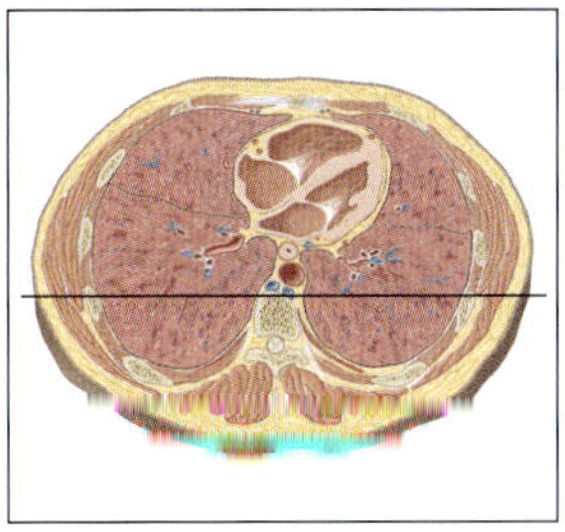

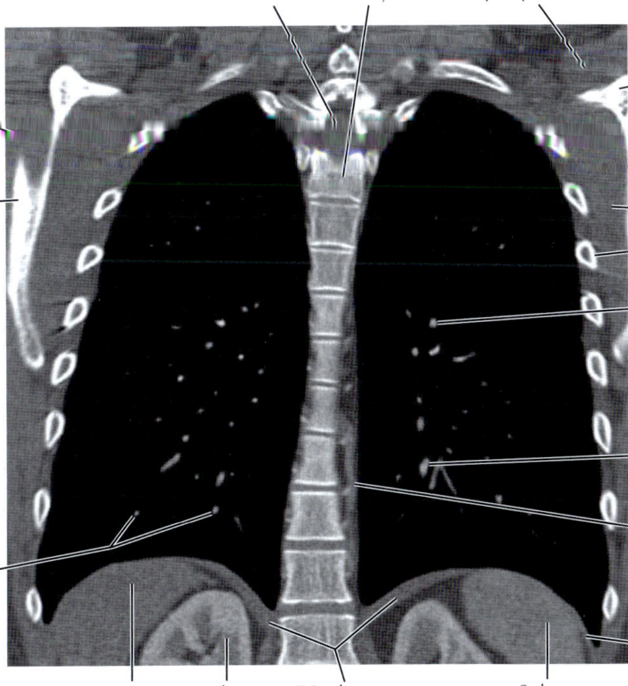
Spinal cord
Vertebral body
Supraspinatus m.
Scapula
Scapula
Subscapularis m.
Rib
Left lower lobe superior subsegmental pulmonary a.
Pulmonary v.
Hemiazygos v.
Pulmonary vv.
Diaphragm
Liver
Kidney
Diaphragm
Spleen

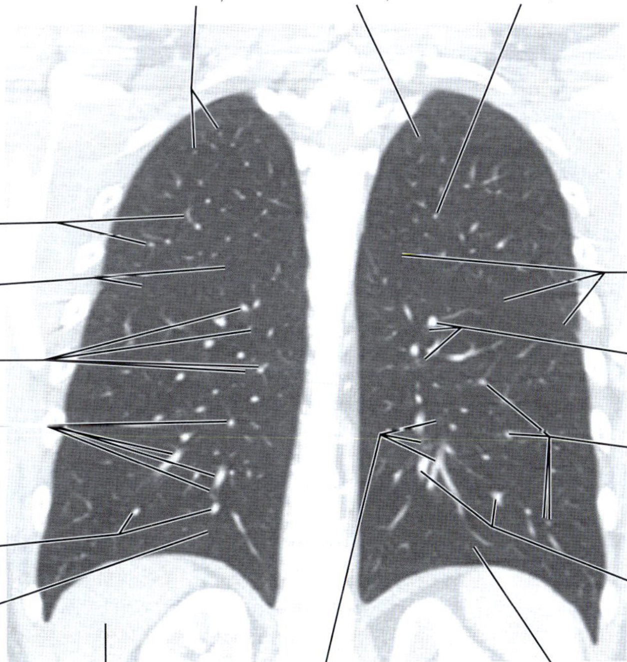
Pulmonary vv.
Pulmonary v.
Pulmonary a.
Right upper lobe posterior subsegmental pulmonary aa.
Right oblique (major) fissure
Right lower lobe superior subsegmental pulmonary aa. & bronchi
Right lower lobe posterior basal subsegmental pulmonary aa. & bronchus
Pulmonary vv.
Right lower lobe
Left oblique (major) fissure
Left lower lobe superior subsegmental pulmonary a. & bronchi
Left lower lobe lateral basal subsegmental pulmonary aa. & bronchus
Pulmonary vv.
Liver
Left lower lobe posterior basal subsegmental pulmonary a. & bronchi
Left lower lobe

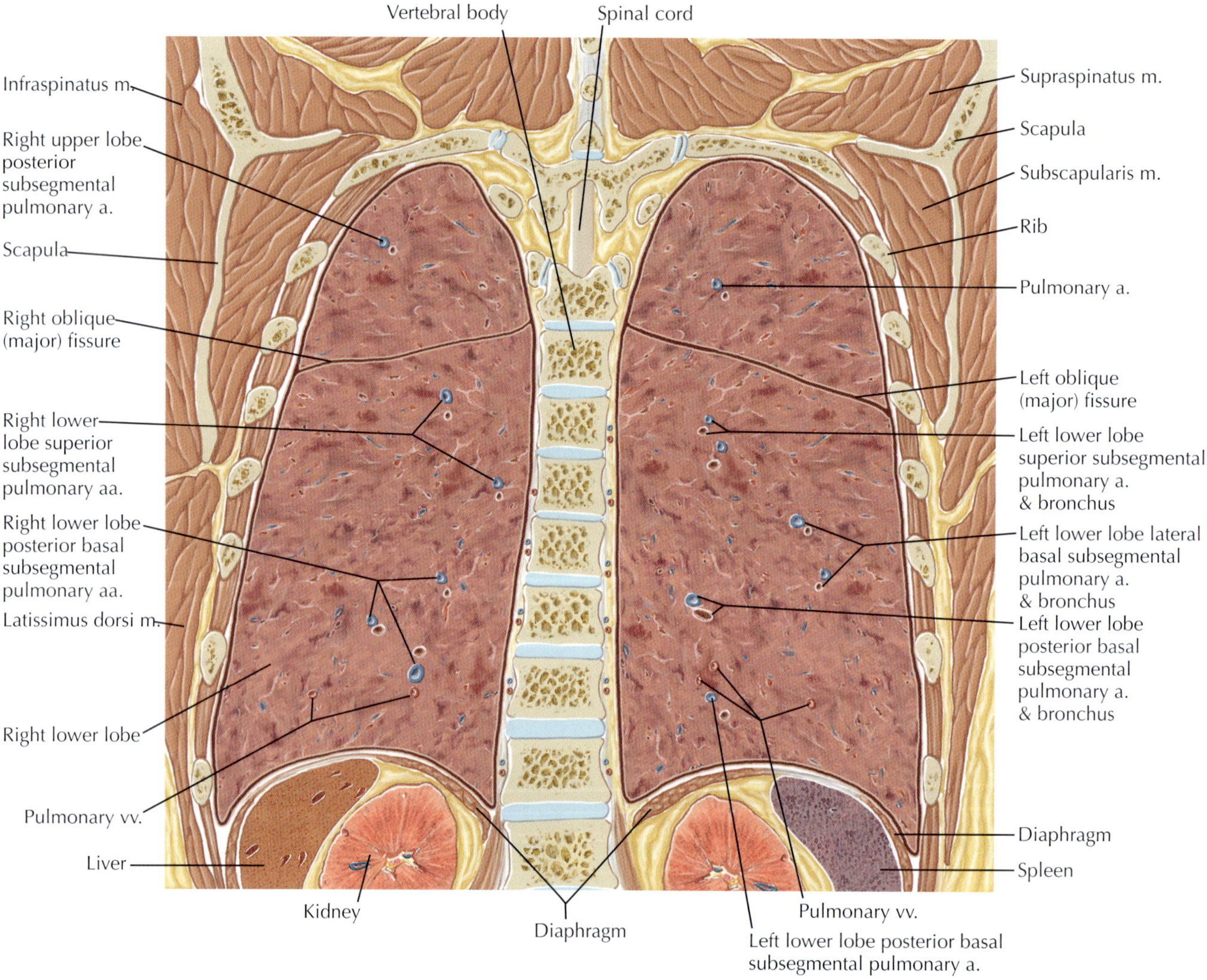

Vertebral body
Spinal cord
Infraspinatus m.
Right upper lobe posterior subsegmental pulmonary a.
Scapula
Right oblique (major) fissure
Right lower lobe superior subsegmental pulmonary aa.
Right lower lobe posterior basal subsegmental pulmonary aa.
Latissimus dorsi m.
Right lower lobe
Pulmonary vv.
Liver
Kidney
Diaphragm
Pulmonary vv.
Left lower lobe posterior basal subsegmental pulmonary a.
Supraspinatus m.
Scapula
Subscapularis m.
Rib
Pulmonary a.
Left oblique (major) fissure
Left lower lobe superior subsegmental pulmonary a. & bronchus
Left lower lobe lateral basal subsegmental pulmonary a. & bronchus
Left lower lobe posterior basal subsegmental pulmonary a. & bronchus
Diaphragm
Spleen

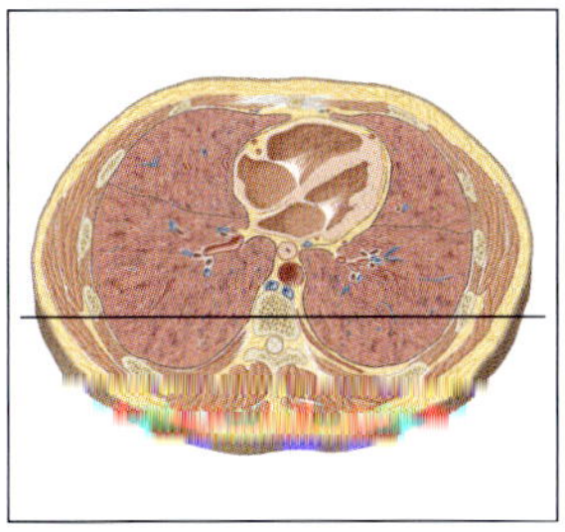

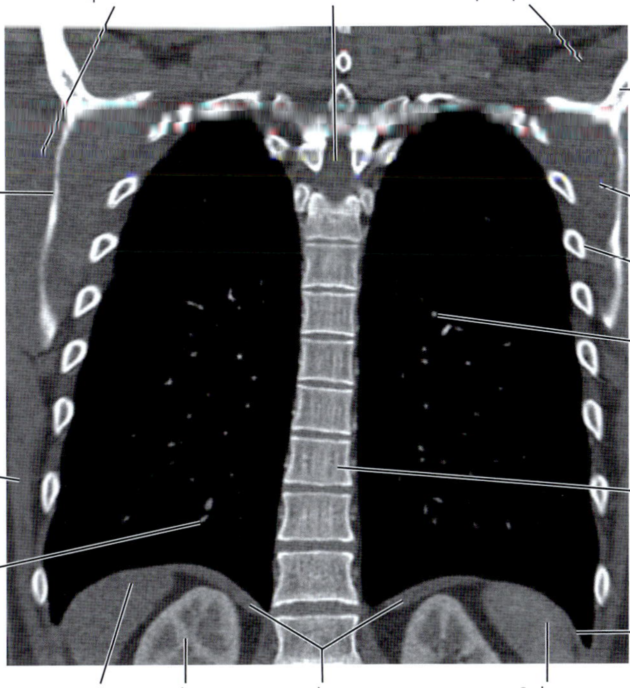
Spinal cord
Infraspinatus m.
Supraspinatus m.
Scapula
Scapula
Subscapularis m.
Rib
Left lower lobe superior subsegmental pulmonary a.
Latissimus dorsi m.
Vertebral body
Pulmonary v.
Diaphragm
Liver
Kidney
Diaphragm
Spleen

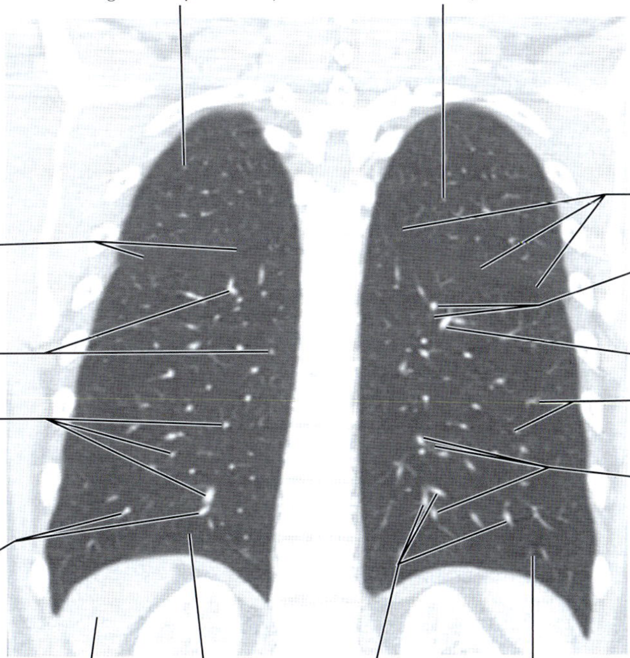
Right upper lobe posterior subsegmental pulmonary a.
Pulmonary a.
Left oblique (major) fissure
Right oblique (major) fissure
Left lower lobe superior subsegmental pulmonary a. & bronchus
Right lower lobe superior subsegmental pulmonary aa.
Pulmonary a.
Left lower lobe lateral basal subsegmental pulmonary a. & bronchus
Right lower lobe posterior basal subsegmental pulmonary aa.
Left lower lobe posterior basal subsegmental pulmonary aa. & bronchus
Pulmonary vv.
Liver
Right lower lobe
Pulmonary vv.
Left lower lobe

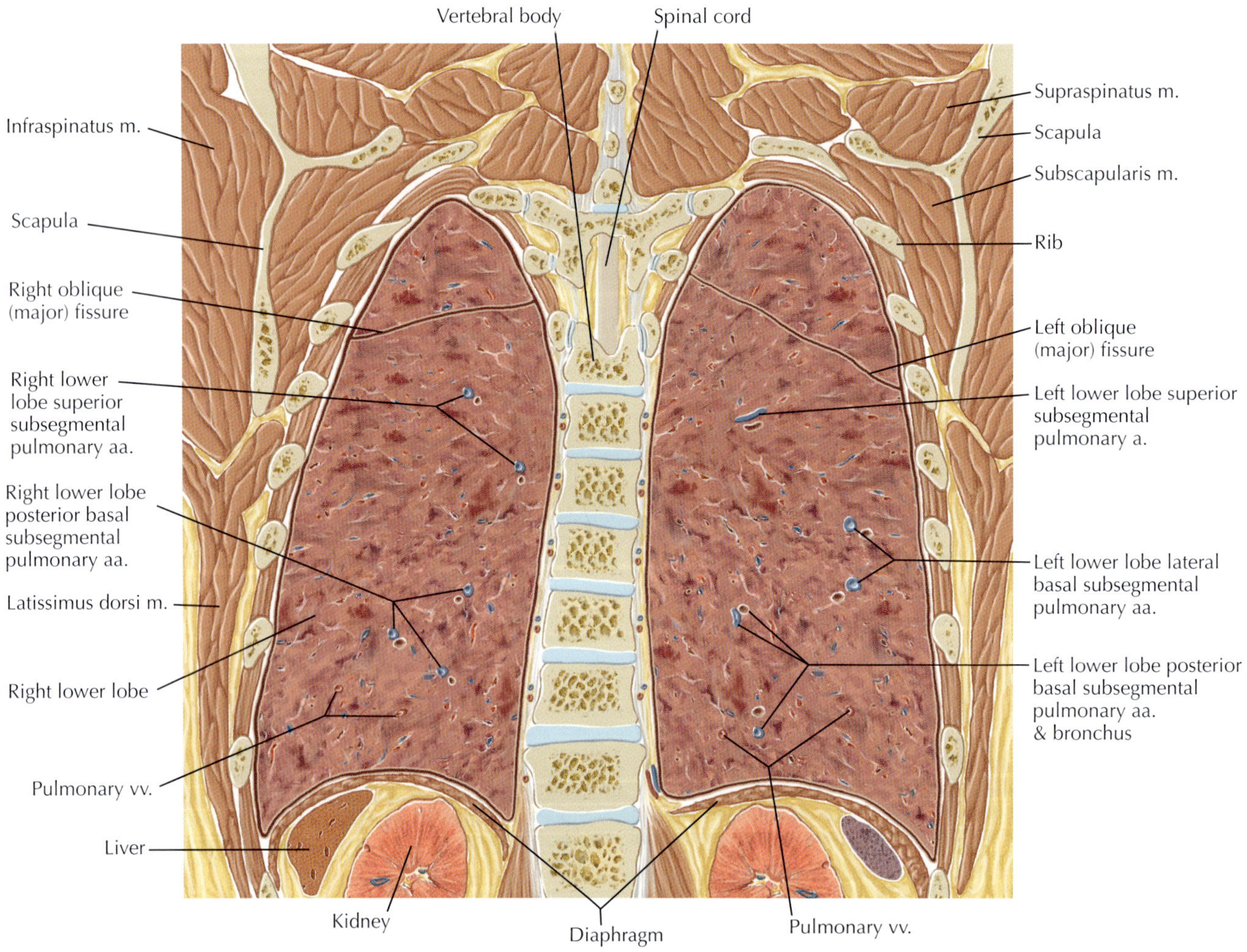

Vertebral body
Spinal cord
Infraspinatus m.
Scapula
Right oblique (major) fissure
Right lower lobe superior subsegmental pulmonary aa.
Right lower lobe posterior basal subsegmental pulmonary aa.
Latissimus dorsi m.
Right lower lobe
Pulmonary vv.
Liver
Kidney
Diaphragm
Pulmonary vv.
Supraspinatus m.
Scapula
Subscapularis m.
Rib
Left oblique (major) fissure
Left lower lobe superior subsegmental pulmonary a.
Left lower lobe lateral basal subsegmental pulmonary aa.
Left lower lobe posterior basal subsegmental pulmonary aa. & bronchus

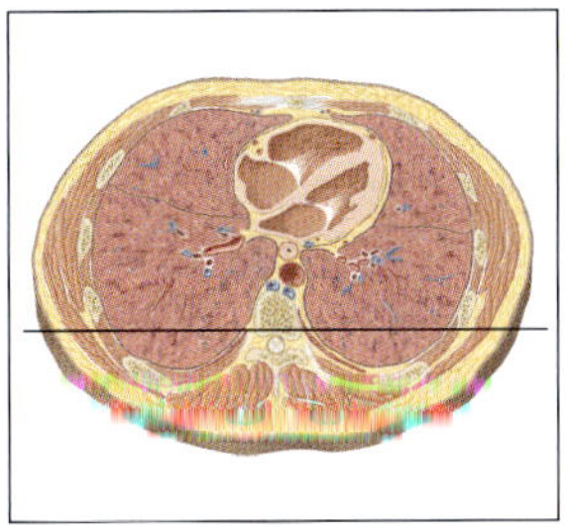

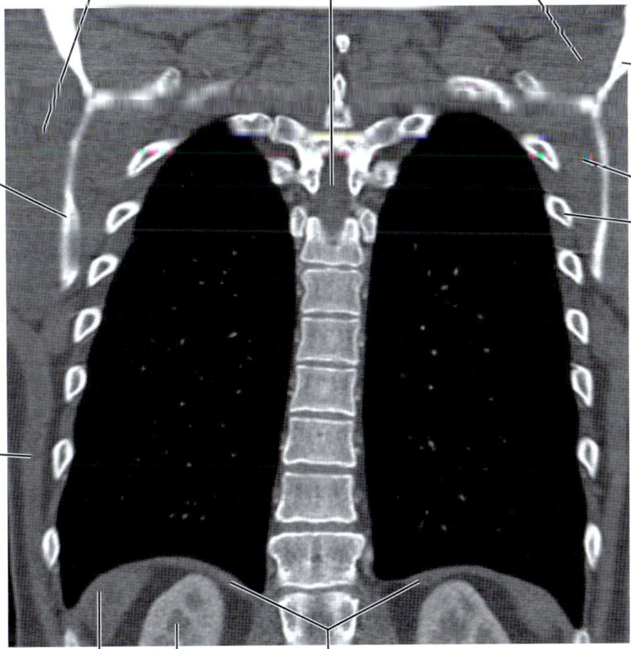
Infraspinatus m.
Spinal cord
Supraspinatus m.
Scapula
Scapula
Subscapularis m.
Rib
Latissimus dorsi m.
Liver
Kidney
Diaphragm

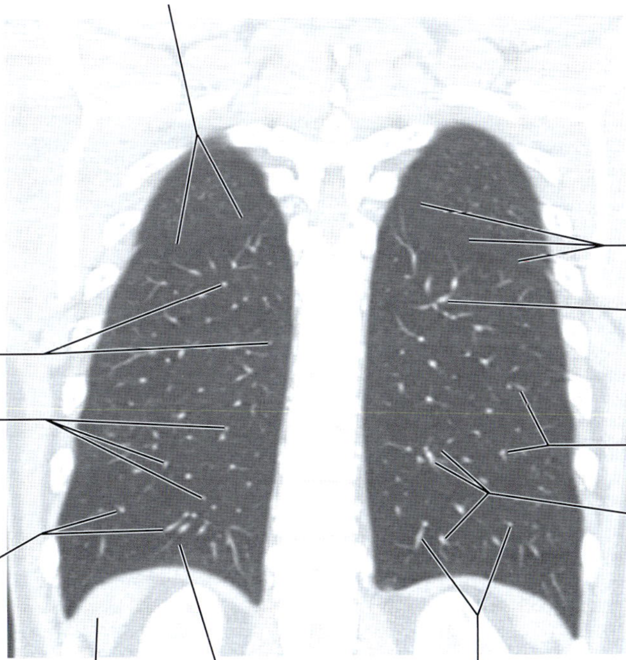
Right oblique (major) fissure
Left oblique (major) fissure
Left lower lobe superior subsegmental pulmonary a.
Right lower lobe superior subsegmental pulmonary aa.
Right lower lobe posterior basal subsegmental pulmonary aa.
Left lower lobe lateral basal subsegmental pulmonary aa.
Left lower lobe posterior basal subsegmental pulmonary aa. & bronchus
Pulmonary vv.
Liver
Right lower lobe
Pulmonary vv.

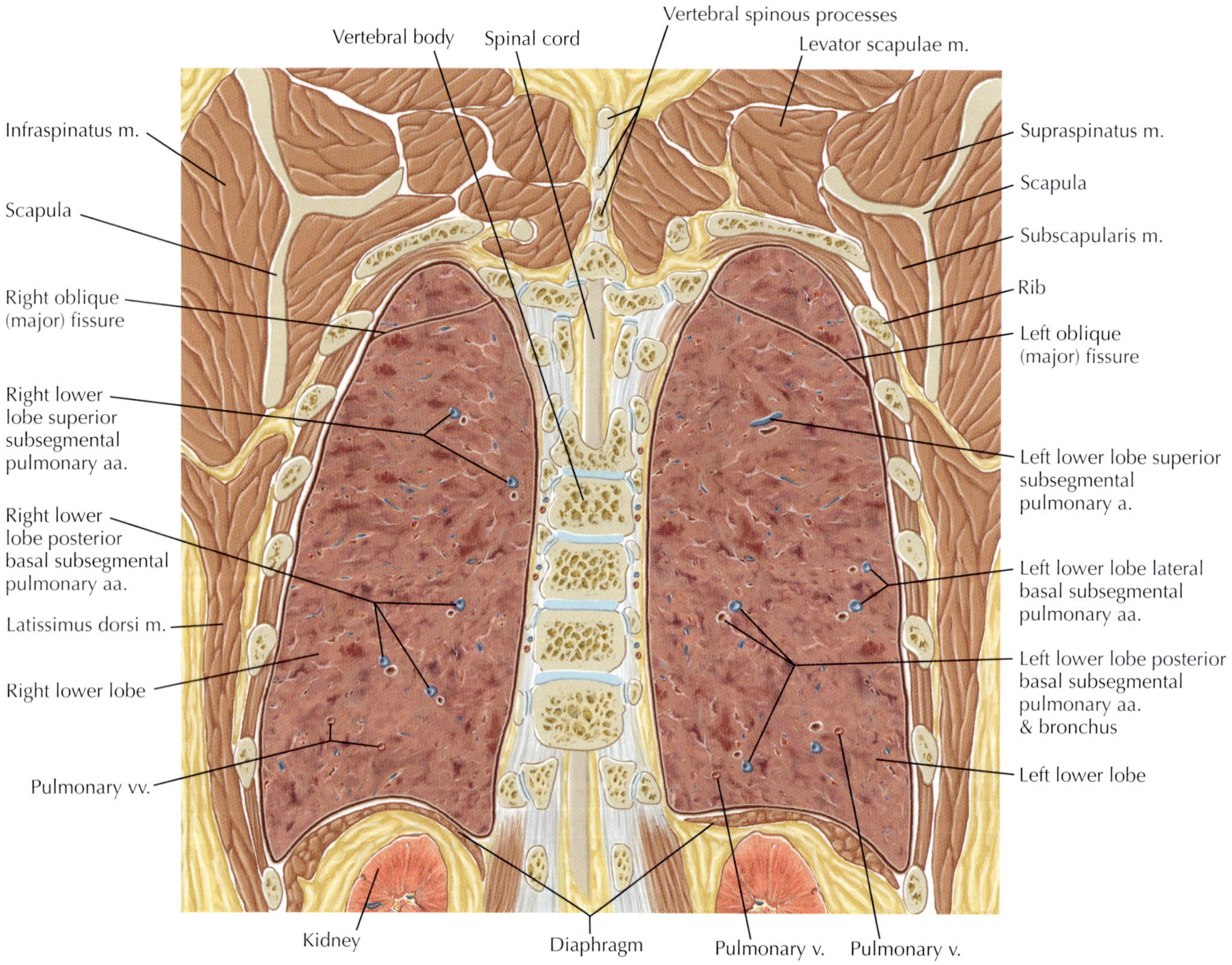

Vertebral spinous processes
Vertebral body
Spinal cord
Levator scapulae m.
Infraspinatus m.
Supraspinatus m.
Scapula
Scapula
Subscapularis m.
Rib
Right oblique (major) fissure
Left oblique (major) fissure
Right lower lobe superior subsegmental pulmonary aa.
Left lower lobe superior subsegmental pulmonary a.
Right lower lobe posterior basal subsegmental pulmonary aa.
Left lower lobe lateral basal subsegmental pulmonary aa.
Latissimus dorsi m.
Left lower lobe posterior basal subsegmental pulmonary aa. & bronchus
Right lower lobe
Left lower lobe
Pulmonary vv.
Kidney
Diaphragm
Pulmonary v.
Pulmonary v.

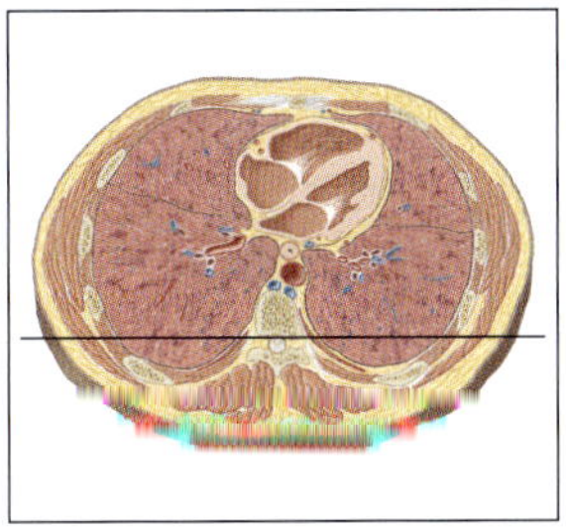

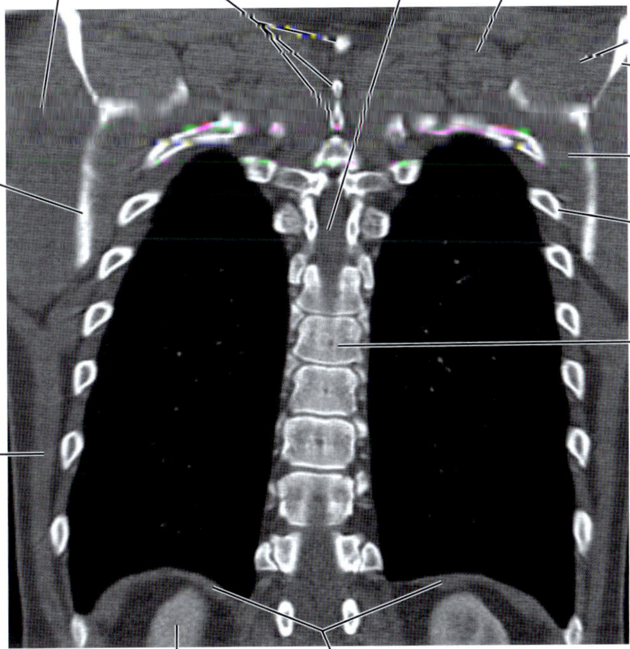
Infraspinatus m.
Vertebral spinous processes
Spinal cord
Levator scapulae m.
Supraspinatus m.
Scapula
Subscapularis m.
Rib
Vertebral body
Scapula
Latissimus dorsi m.
Kidney
Diaphragm

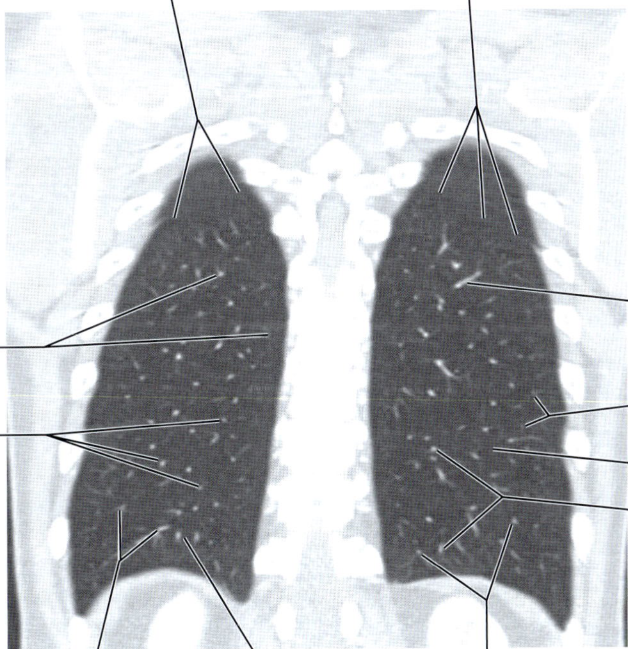
Right oblique (major) fissure
Left oblique (major) fissure
Left lower lobe superior subsegmental pulmonary a.
Right lower lobe superior subsegmental pulmonary aa.
Left lower lobe lateral basal subsegmental pulmonary aa.
Right lower lobe posterior basal subsegmental pulmonary aa.
Left lower lobe
Left lower lobe posterior basal subsegmental pulmonary aa.
Pulmonary vv.
Right lower lobe
Pulmonary vv.

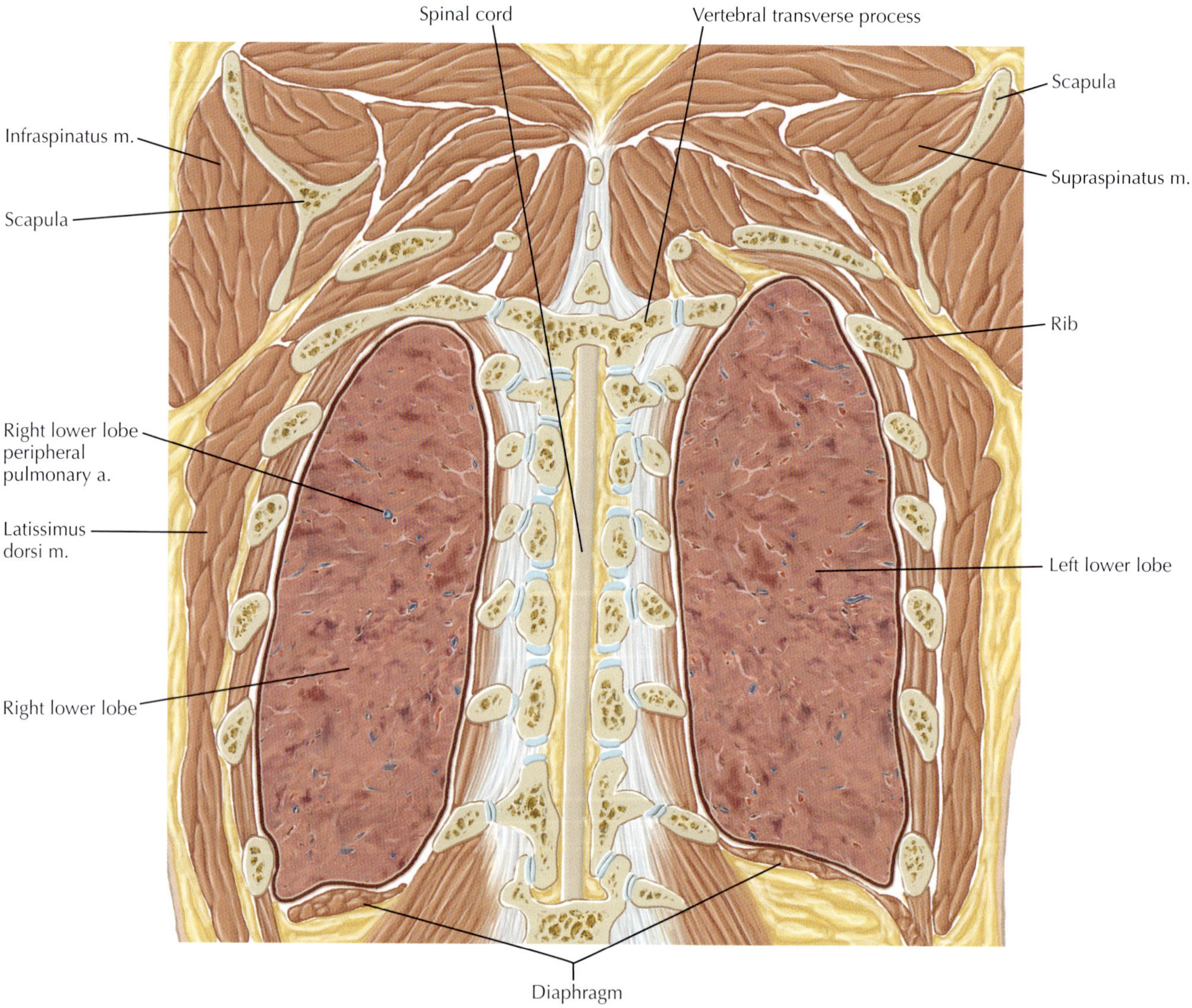
Spinal cord
Vertebral transverse process
Scapula
Infraspinatus m.
Supraspinatus m.
Scapula
Rib
Right lower lobe peripheral pulmonary a.
Latissimus dorsi m.
Left lower lobe
Right lower lobe
Diaphragm

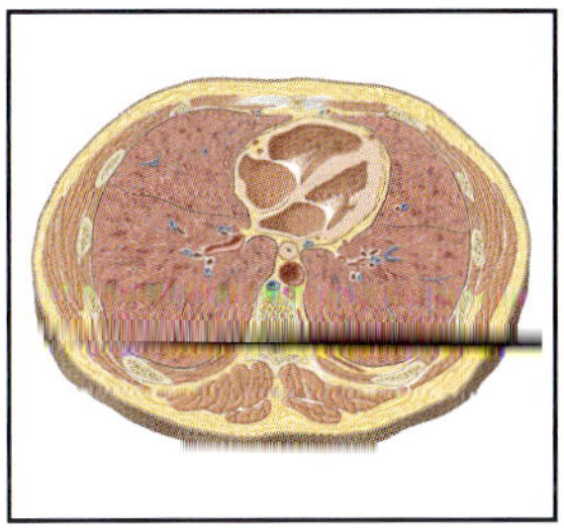

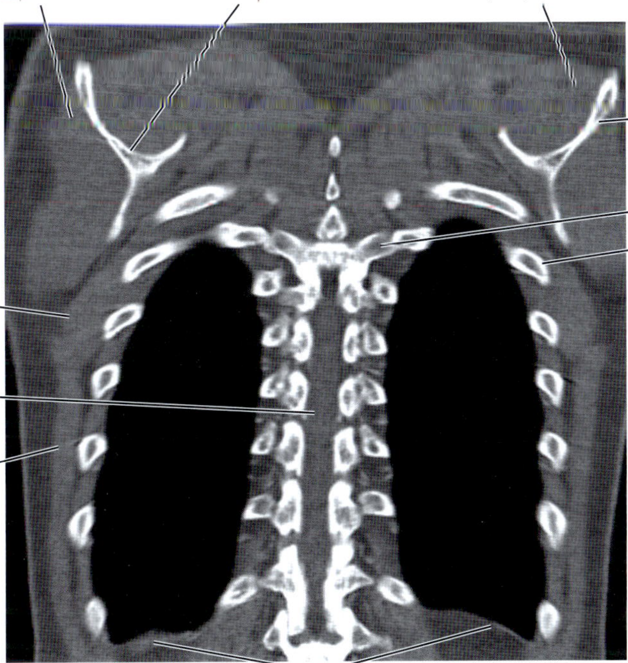
Infraspinatus m.
Scapula
Supraspinatus m.
Scapula
Vertebral transverse process
Rib
Rhomboid major m.
Spinal cord
Latissimus dorsi m.
Diaphragm

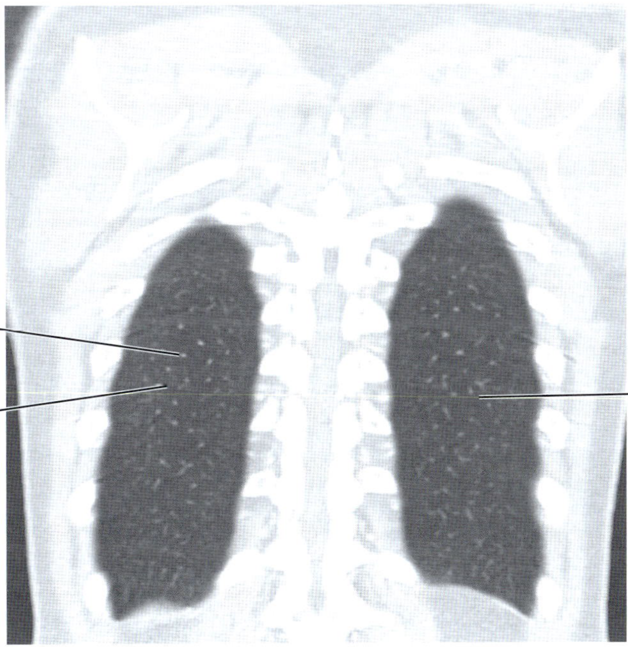
Right lower lobe peripheral pulmonary a.
Right lower lobe
Left lower lobe

Chapter 3 PULMONARY ANATOMY AND VARIANTS

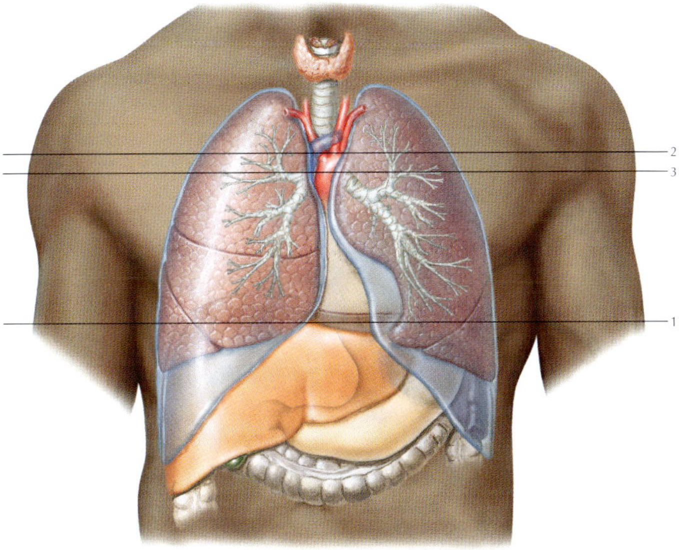

AXIAL 160

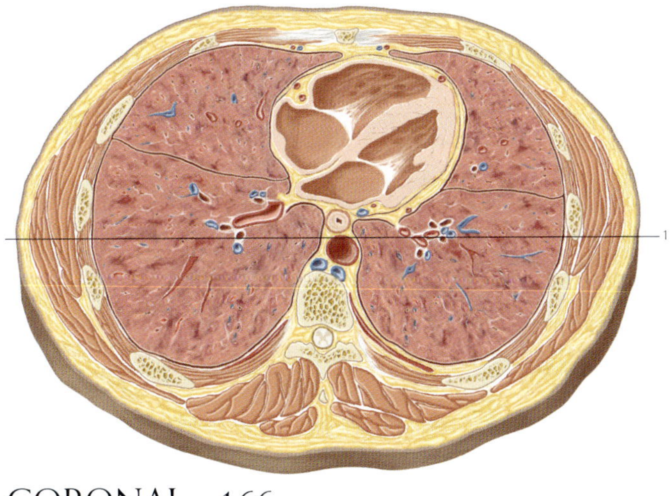

CORONAL 166

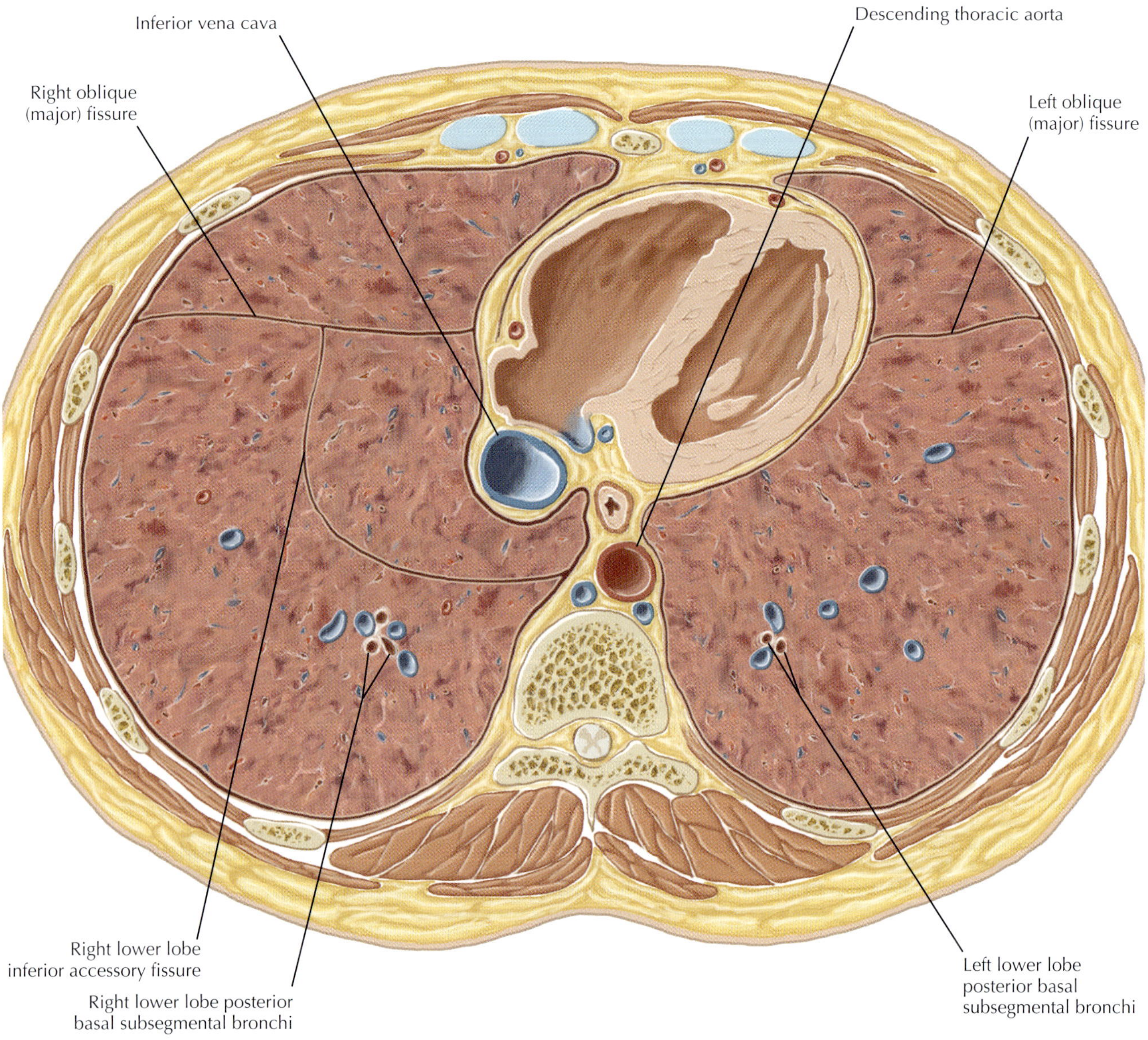

NORMAL VARIANTS

A thin, well-defined linear structure representing an *inferior accessory fissure*. An inferior accessory fissure segregates the medial basal segment of either lower lobe from the remaining basal segments. This variation is a common finding in the population and generally of no clinical significance.

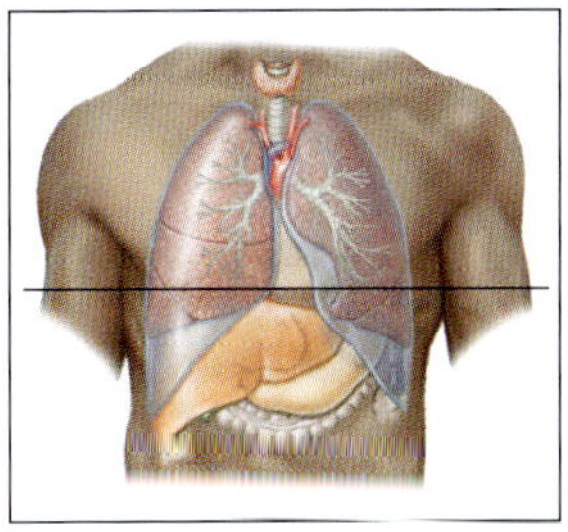

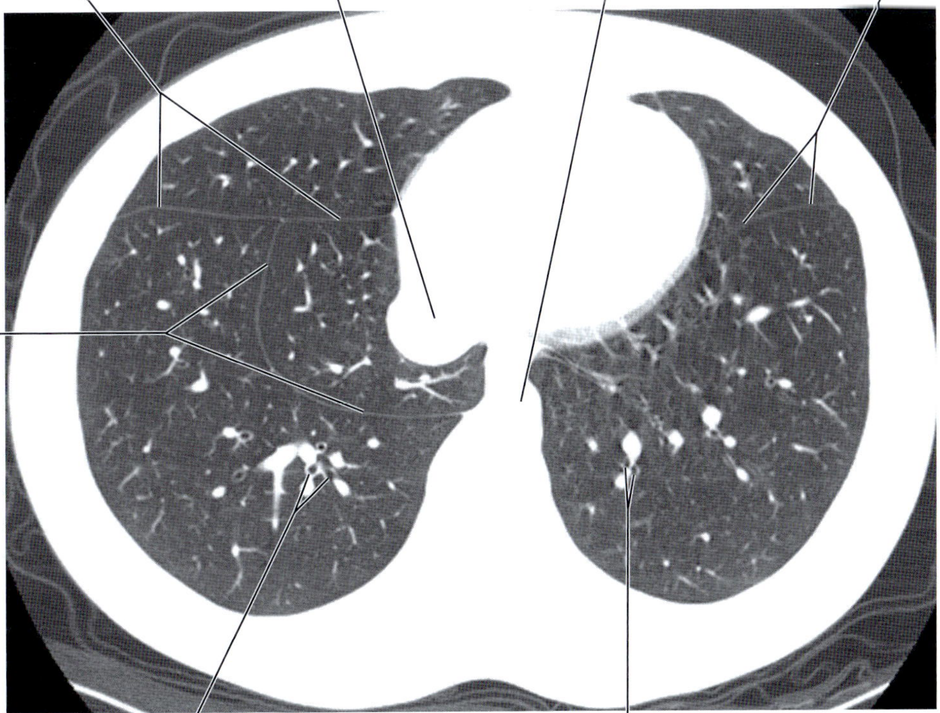
Right oblique (major) fissure
Inferior vena cava
Descending thoracic aorta
Left oblique (major) fissure
Right lower lobe inferior accessory fissure
Right lower lobe posterior basal subsegmental bronchi
Left lower lobe posterior basal subsegmental bronchi

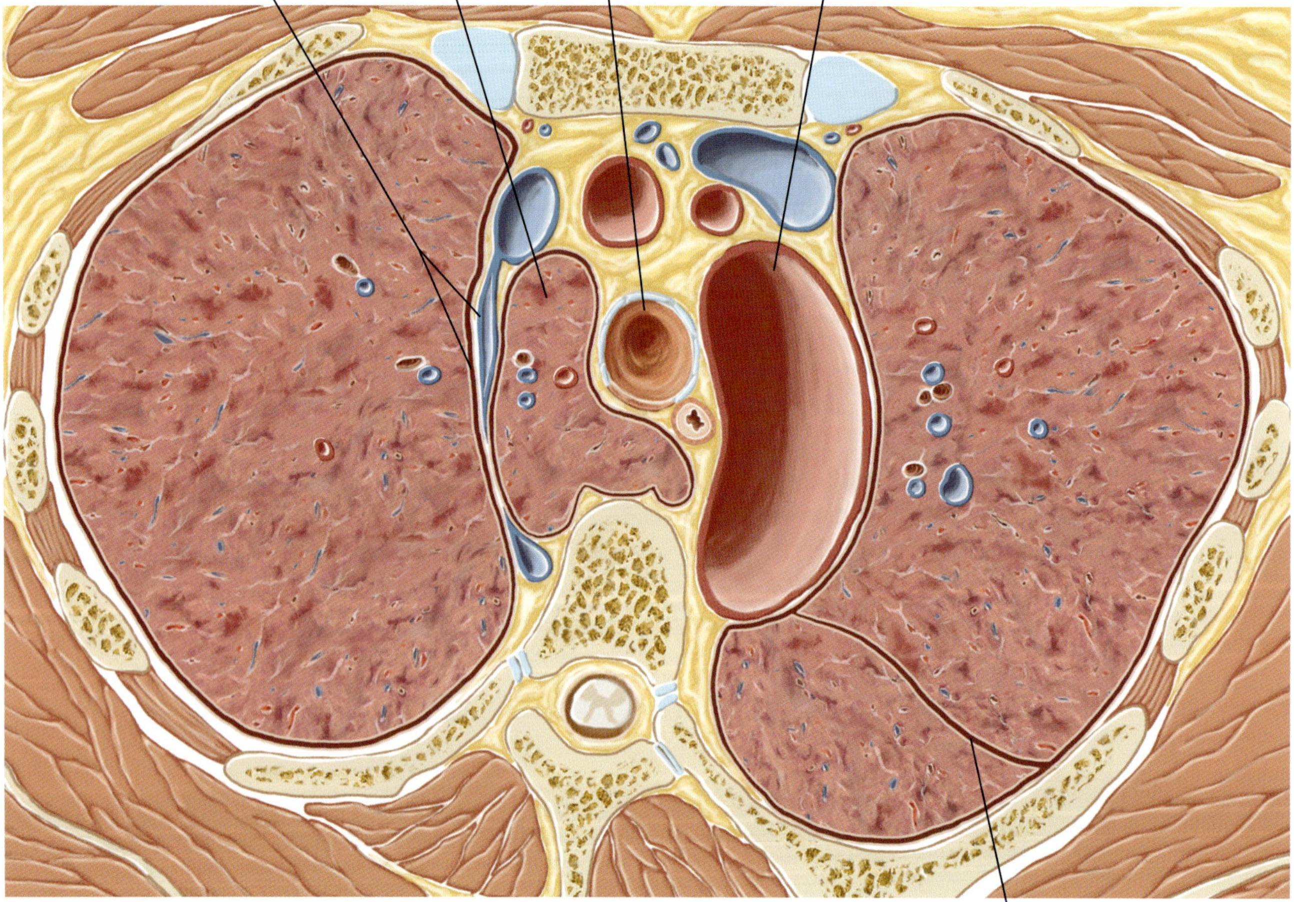

NORMAL VARIANTS

A thin, curvilinear structure extends through the medial right upper lobe, representing an *azygos fissure*—the lung subtended by the azygos fissure is referred to as the *azygos lobe*. The azygos vein courses through the azygos fissure. This anomaly is formed when the azygos vein extends into the right upper lobe during fetal development. The azygos fissure consists of 4 layers of pleura: 2 of visceral pleura and 2 of parietal pleura. This finding is a usually an incidentally detected anomaly, without clinical significance, and is found in 0.3% to 0.5% of the population.

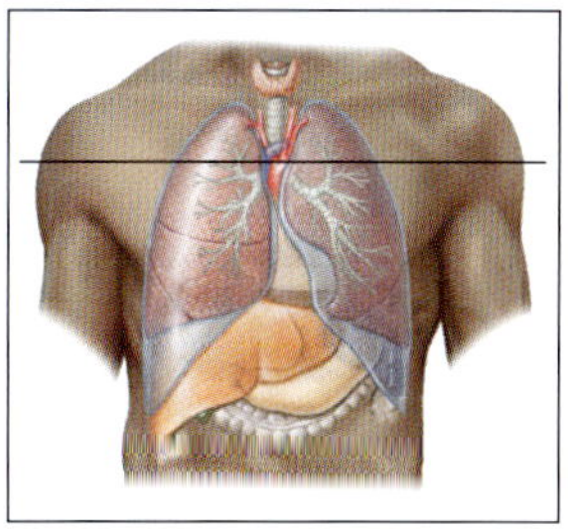

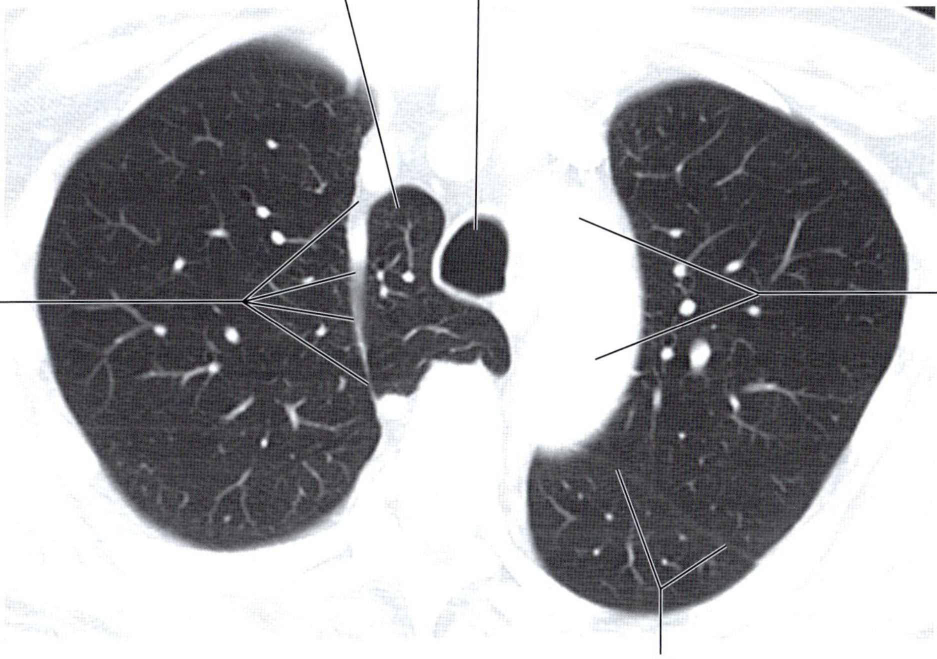
Azygos lobe
Trachea
Azygos fissure & v.
Aortic arch
Left oblique (major) fissure

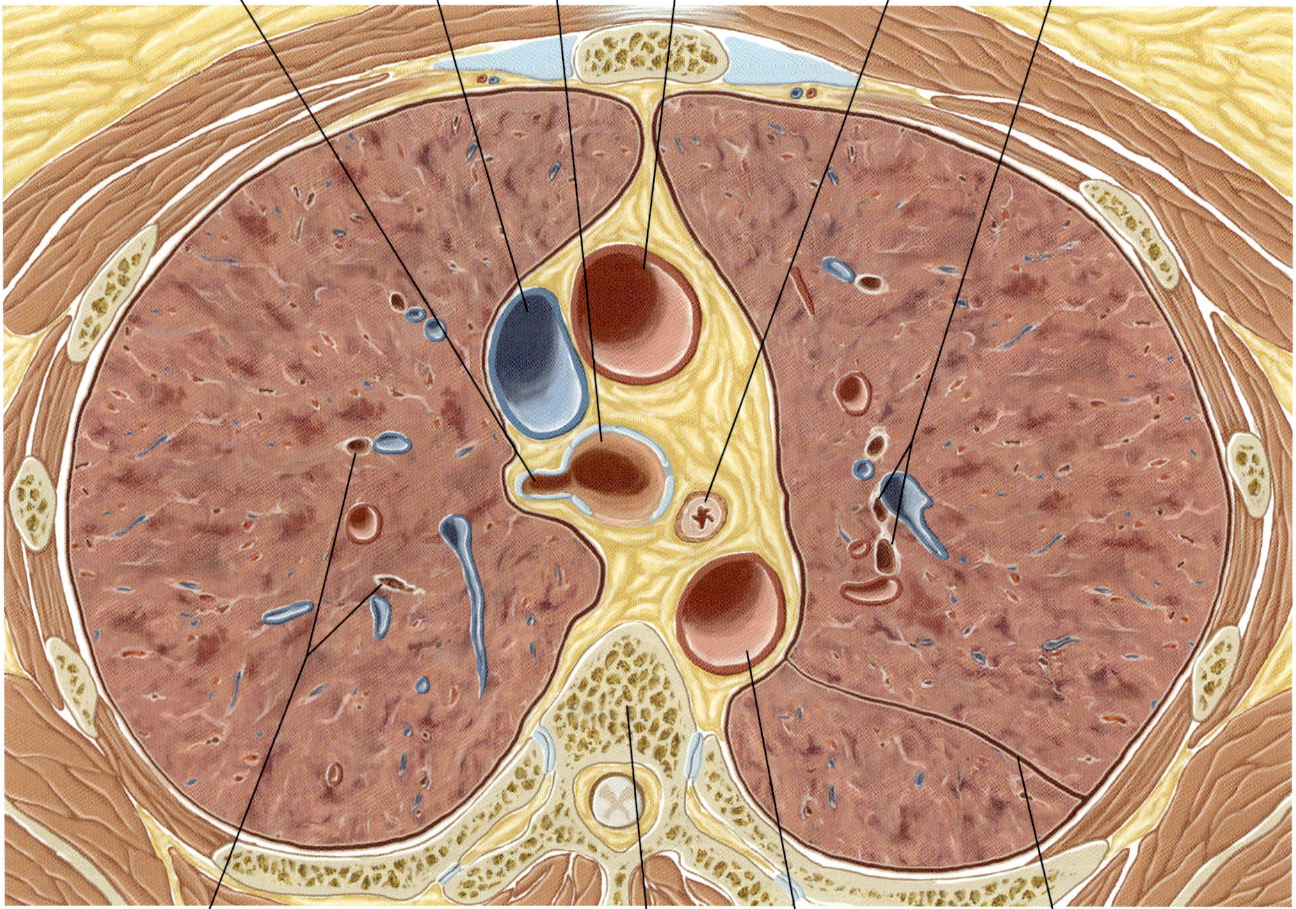

NORMAL VARIANTS

An anomalous bronchus originating directly from the right lateral trachea wall—this anomaly is known as a *tracheal bronchus*. A tracheal bronchus supplies all or a portion of the apical segment of the right upper lobe and is found in 0.1% of the population.

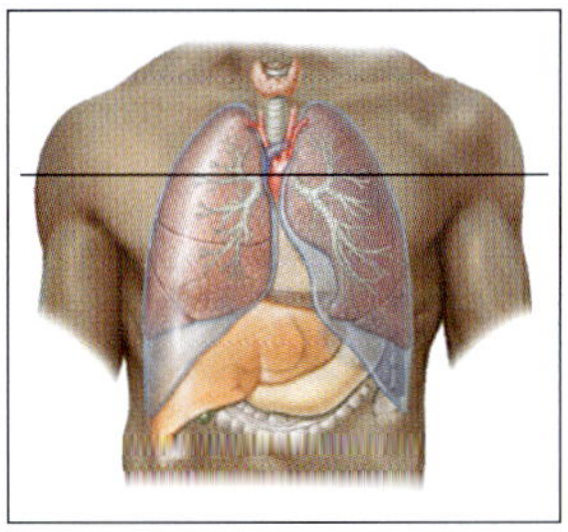

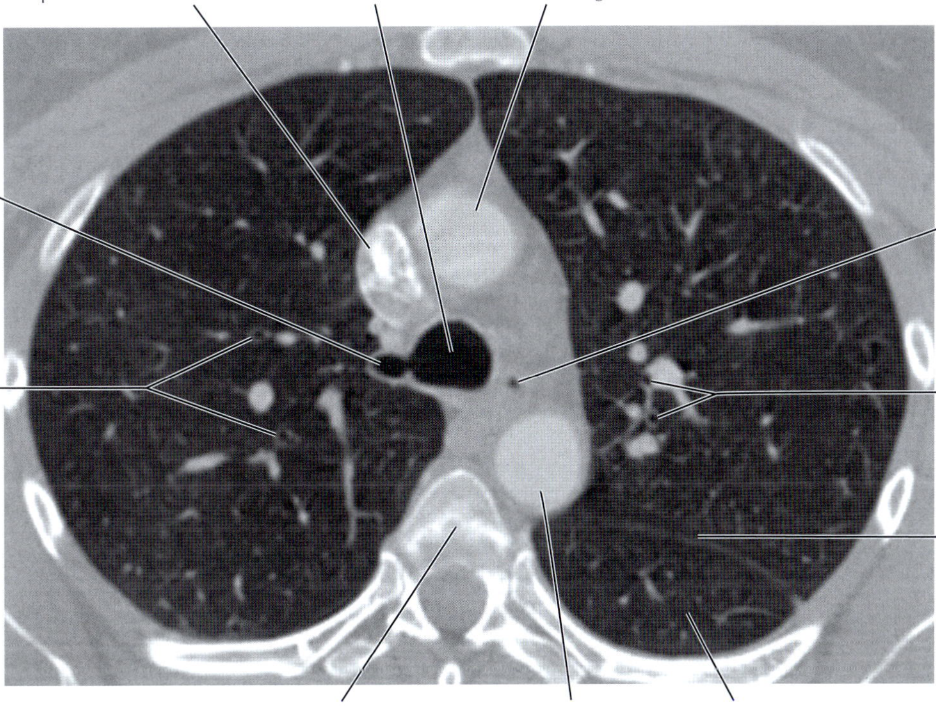

Superior vena cava
Trachea
Ascending aorta
Tracheal bronchus
Esophagus
Right upper lobe subsegmental bronchi
Left upper lobe bronchi
Left oblique (major) fissure
Spine
Descending thoracic aorta
Left lower lobe superior segment

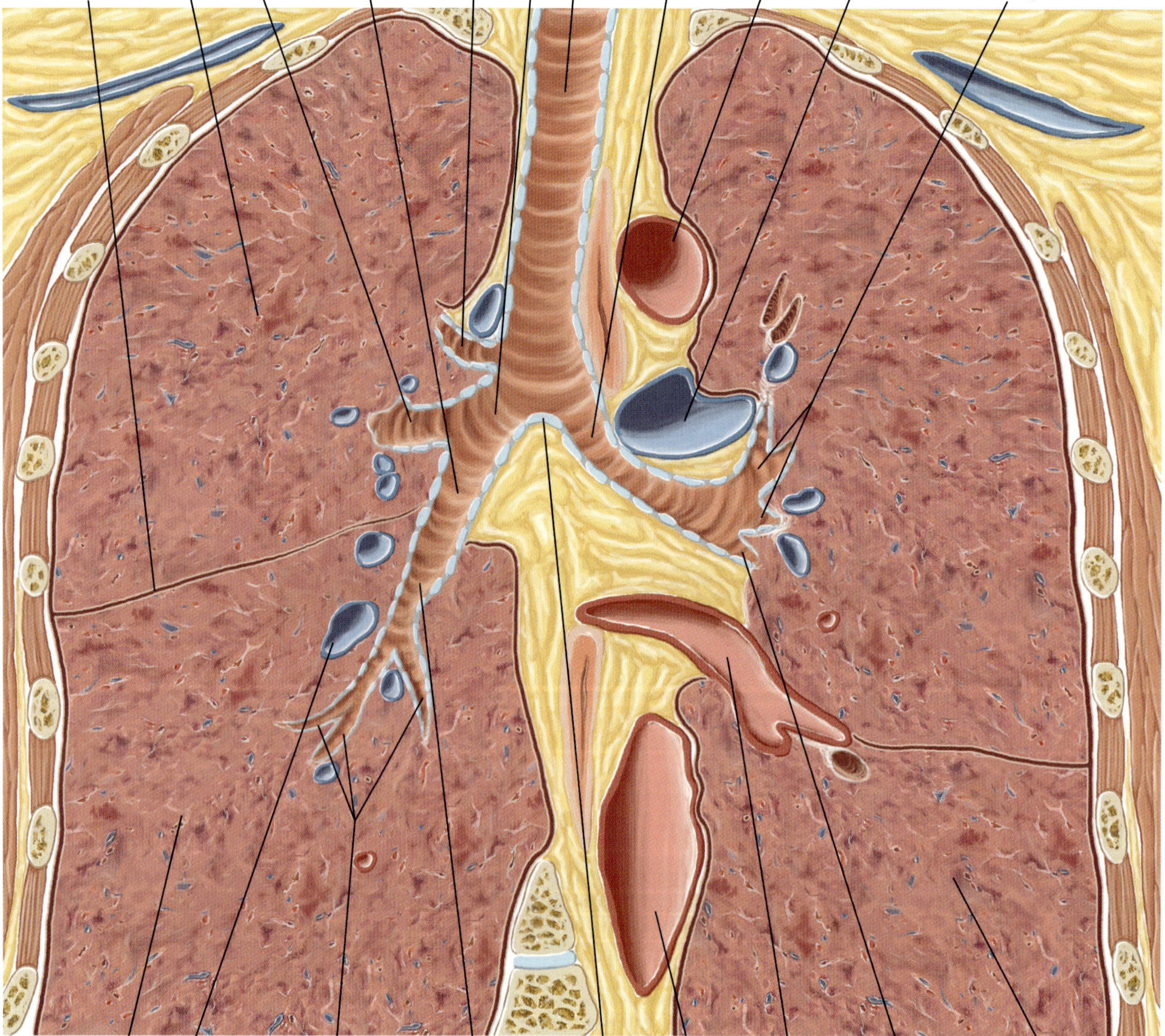

NORMAL VARIANTS

The coronal projection of the patient shown in Axial 3. The right upper lobe *tracheal bronchus* is seen to advantage.

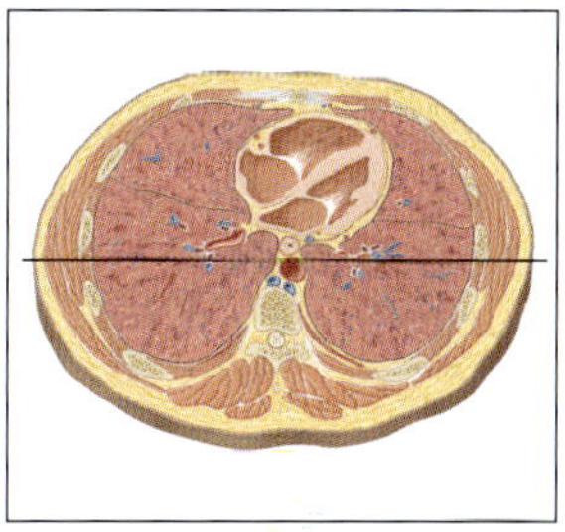

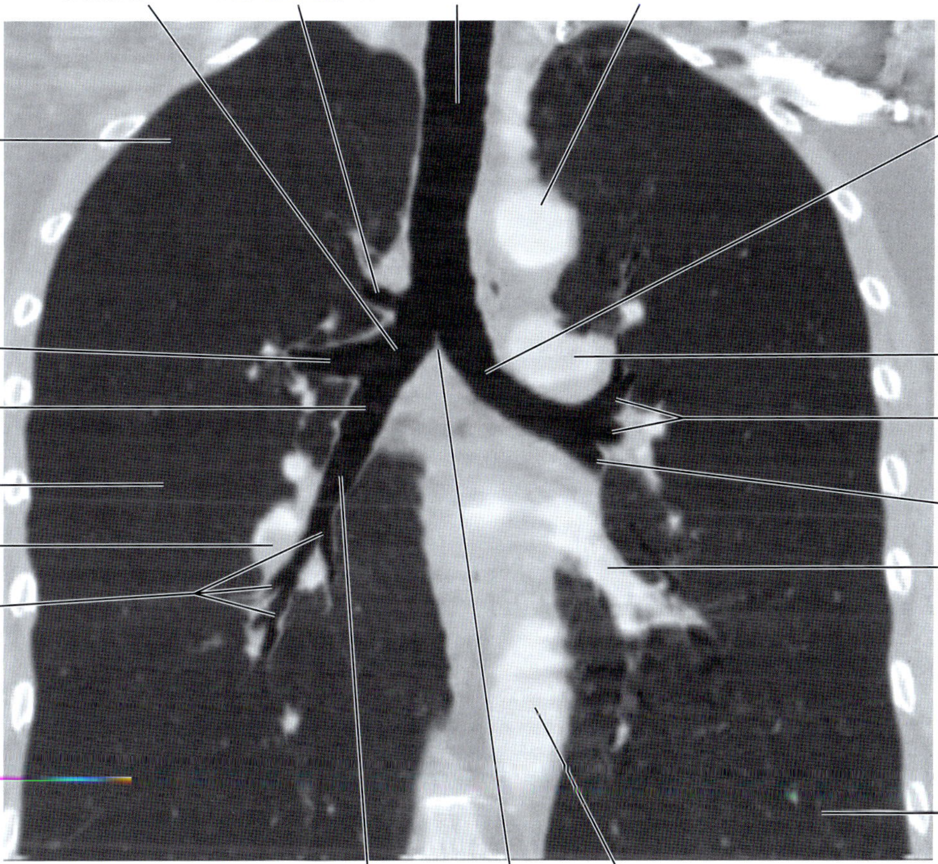
Right mainstem bronchus
Tracheal bronchus
Trachea
Aorta
Right upper lobe
Left mainstem bronchus
Right upper lobe bronchus
Pulmonary a.
Bronchus intermedius
Left upper lobe & lingular bronchus
Right oblique (major) fissure
Left lower lobe bronchus
Right lower lobe pulmonary a.
Left inferior pulmonary v.
Right lower lobe basal segment bronchi
Right lower lobe
Left lower lobe
Right lower lobe bronchus
Carina
Aorta

Chapter 4

THORACIC LYMPH NODES

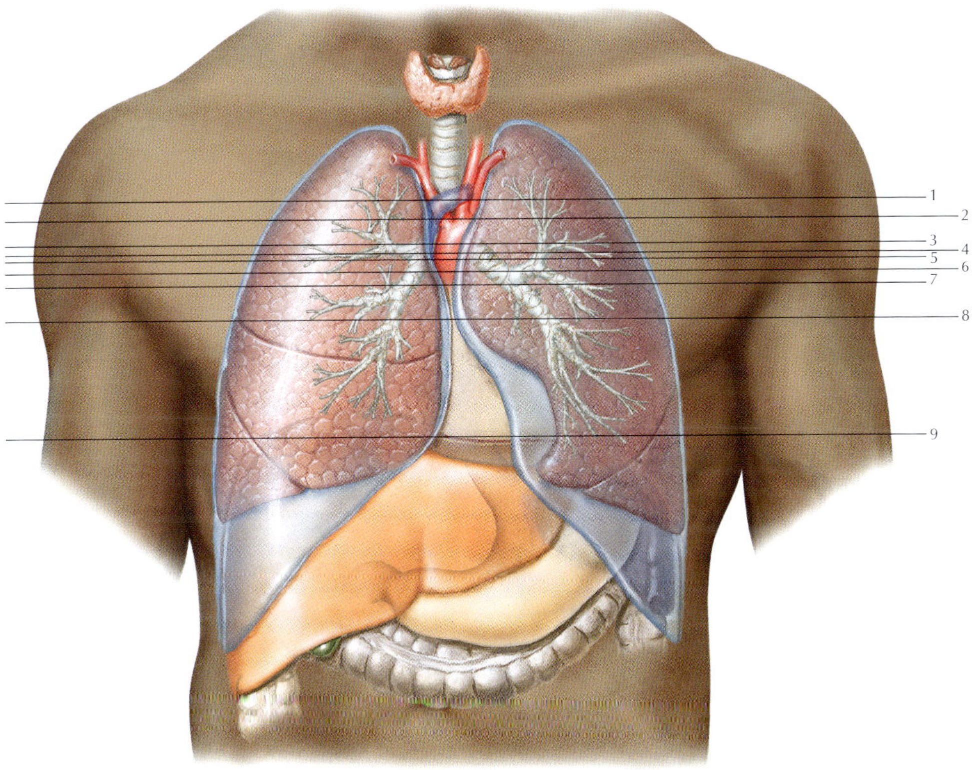

AXIAL 170

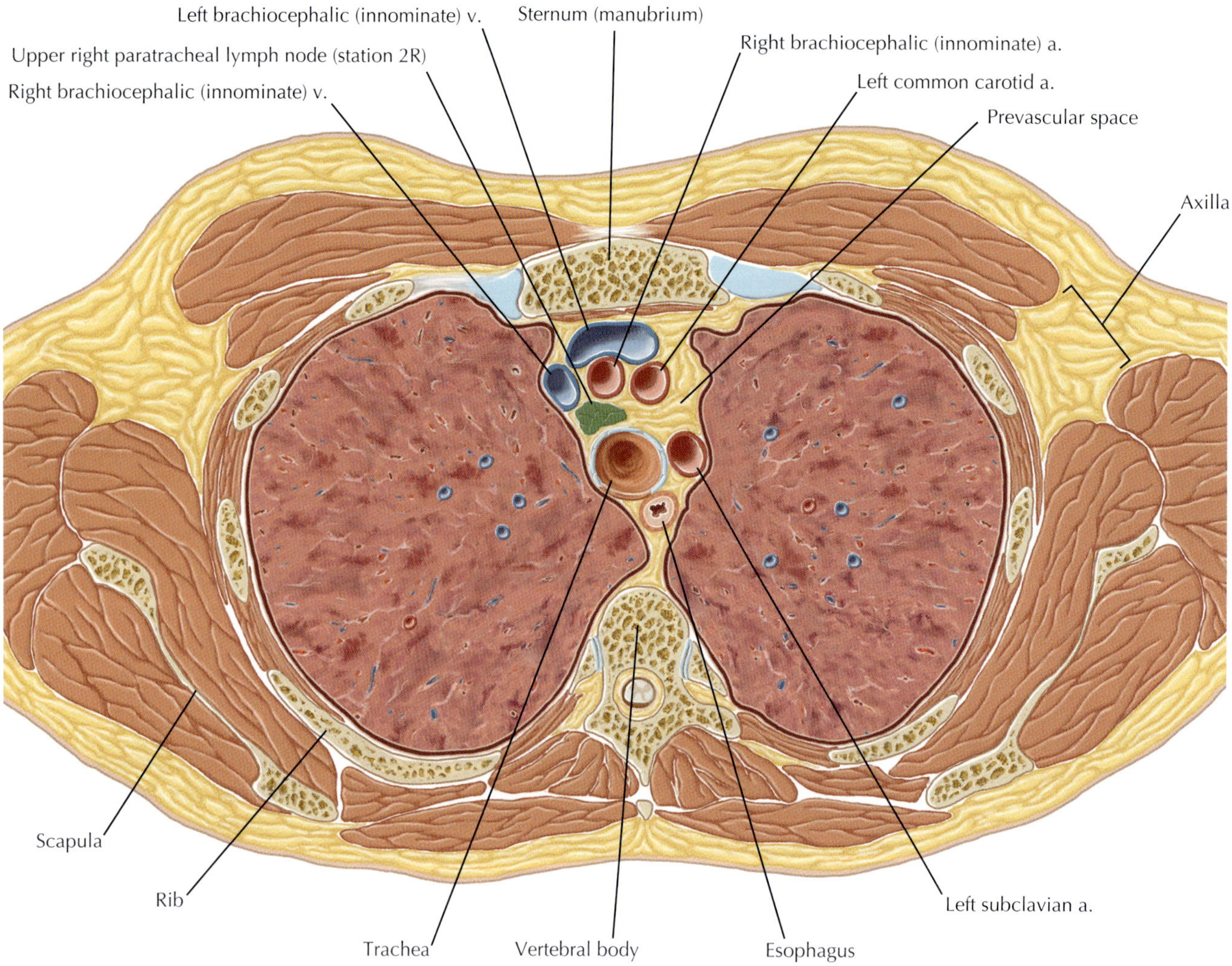

DIAGNOSTIC CONSIDERATION

Thoracic CT plays a major role in the evaluation of patients with suspected pulmonary malignancy. In particular, one major role for thoracic CT for patients with pulmonary malignancy is the depiction of hilar, mediastinal, and intrapulmonary lymph node enlargement. Correct identification and classification of lymph node locations is critical for accurate staging for lung cancer patients as well as numerous other thoracic diseases. Intrathoracic lymph nodes are commonly referred to in clinical practice using descriptive terms, although a widely accepted lymph node classification system, set forth by the American Joint Committee on Cancer (AJCC) and International Union Against Lung Cancer (UICC), is often used to standardize reporting of lymph node involvement in lung cancer patients. Although an extensive review of thoracic lymph node classifications is beyond the scope of this work, several images illustrating locations of abnormal lymph nodes in a patient with sarcoidosis will be reviewed. In this system, the designation "R" and "L" refers to "right" and "left" of midline, respectively.

Enlarged lymph nodes is seen just anterior and to the right of the trachea; this region is often referred to as the "right paratracheal space." In the AJCC classification system, lymph nodes in this location are referred to as "upper paratracheal lymph nodes" (station 2); these lymph nodes lie inferior to the cranial margin of the left brachiocephalic vein, where this vein crosses anterior to the trachea, and superior to the cranial margin of the aortic arch.

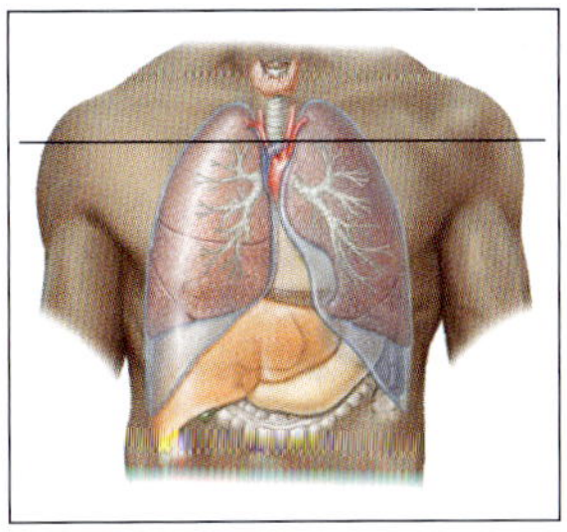

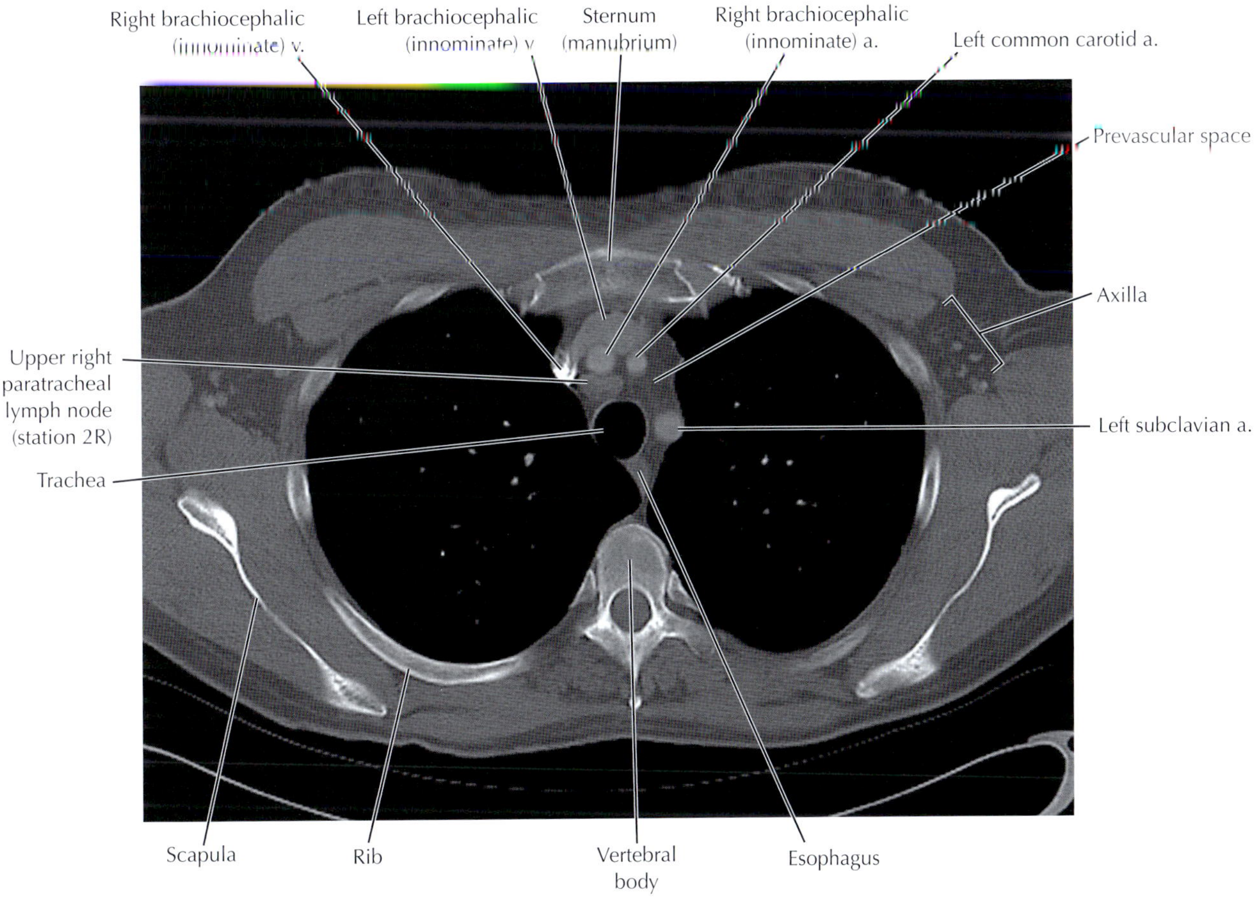
Right brachiocephalic (innominate) v.
Left brachiocephalic (innominate) v.
Sternum (manubrium)
Right brachiocephalic (innominate) a.
Left common carotid a.
Prevascular space
Axilla
Upper right paratracheal lymph node (station 2R)
Left subclavian a.
Trachea
Scapula
Rib
Vertebral body
Esophagus

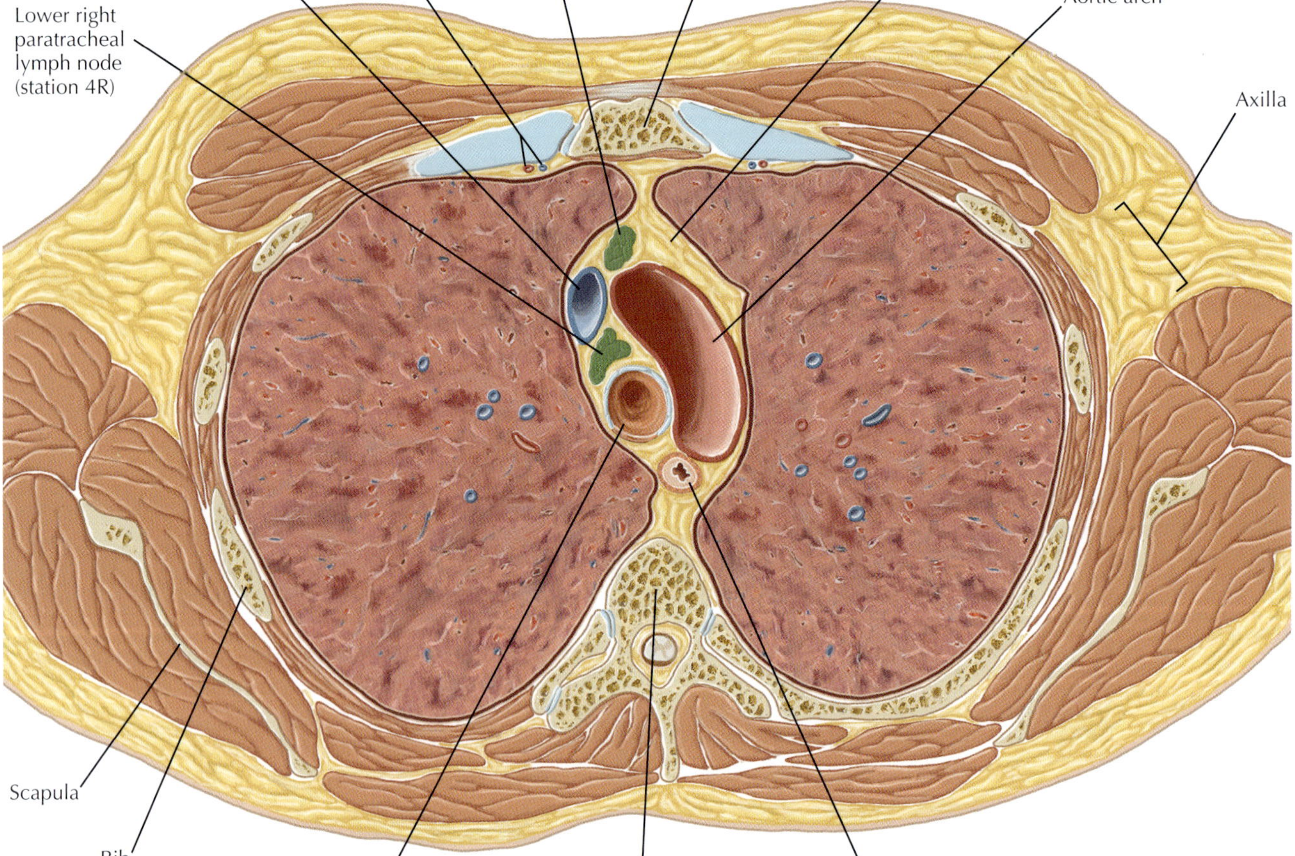

DIAGNOSTIC CONSIDERATION

A focus of high attenuation is present within the mildly enlarged right paratracheal lymph node; this high-attenuation focus represents calcification, which is a common occurrence in patients with sarcoidosis. In the AJCC lymph node classification, this lymph node is considered a "lower paratracheal lymph node (station 4)." This lymph node lies inferior to the cranial aspect of the aortic arch and cranial to the superior margin of the right upper lobe bronchus.

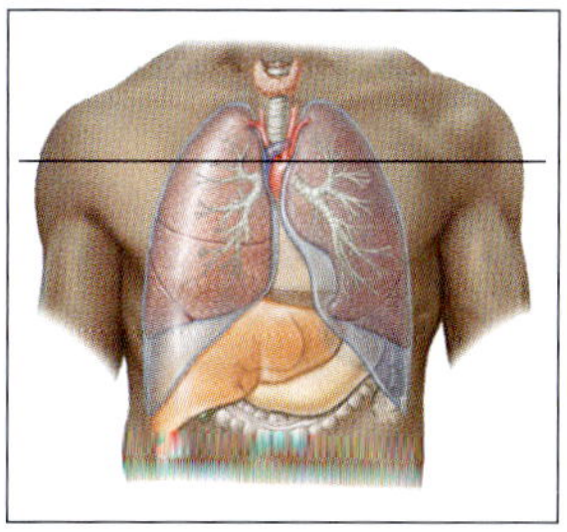

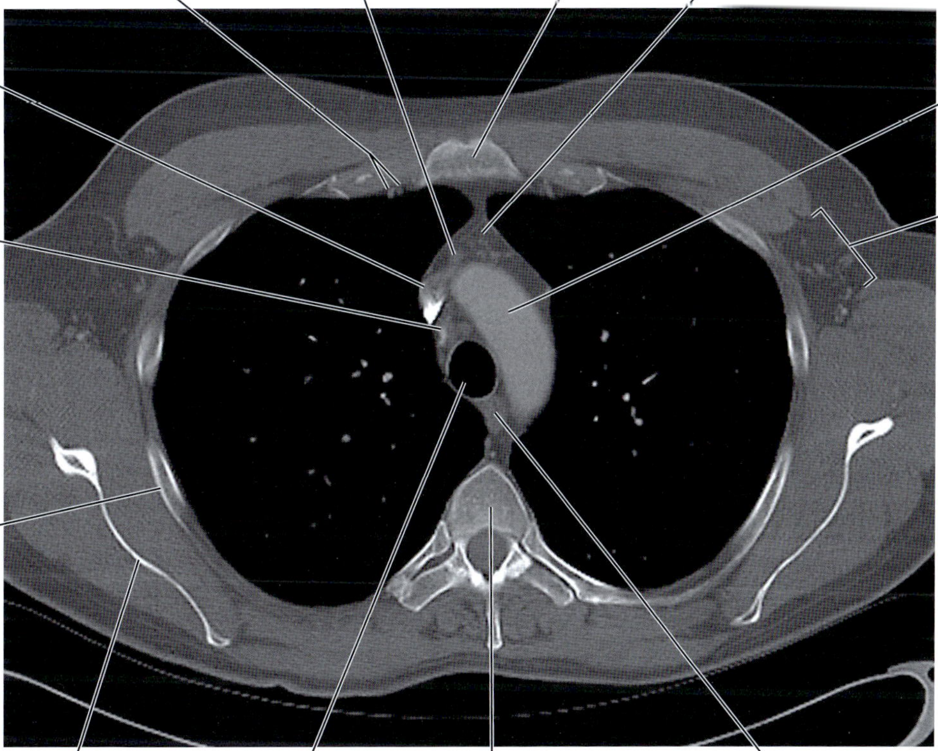
Right internal mammary a. & v.
Anterior mediastinal (para-aortic) lymph node (station 6)
Sternum (manubrium)
Anterior mediastinum
Superior vena cava
Aortic arch
Lower right paratracheal lymph node (station 4R)
Axilla
Rib
Scapula
Trachea
Vertebral body
Esophagus

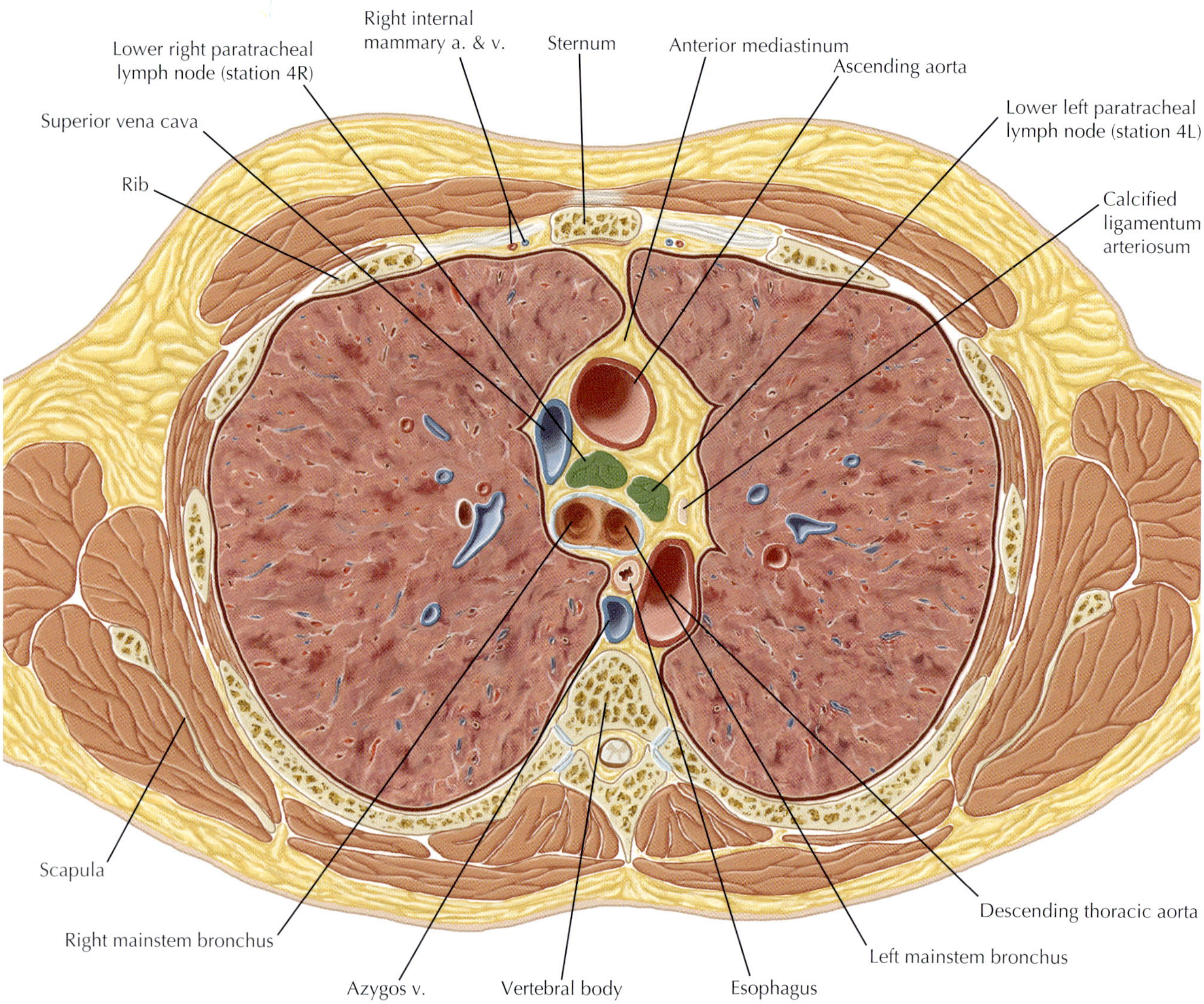

DIAGNOSTIC CONSIDERATION

High-attenuation foci are present in both lower paratracheal lymph nodes visible in this section, very faint within the right-sided lymph node. One lower paratracheal lymph node lies to the right of midline, whereas another lymph node lies to the left of midline—station 4R and 4L lymph nodes, respectively, in the AJCC lymph node classification system. Lower paratracheal (station 4) lymph nodes lie inferior to the cranial aspect of the aortic arch and cranial to the superior margin of the right upper lobe bronchus.

In this section, the calcified ligamentum arteriosum is visible. This is an important anatomical landmark because paratracheal lymph nodes lie medial to this structure and may be sampled with cervical mediastinoscopy, whereas prevascular, subaortic, and aortopulmonary window lymph nodes lie lateral to the ligamentum arteriosum and are not accessible with standard cervical mediastinoscopy.

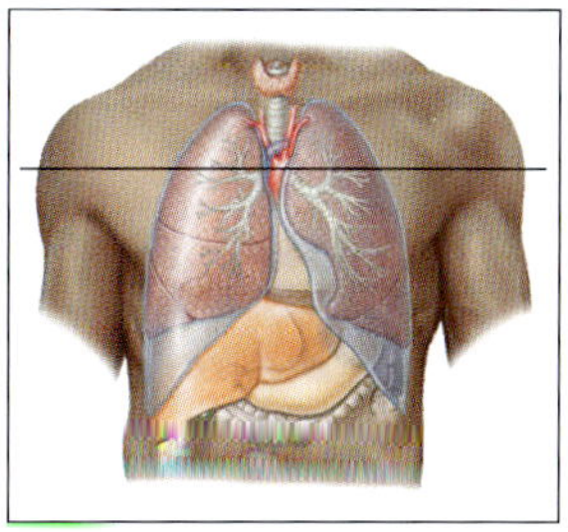

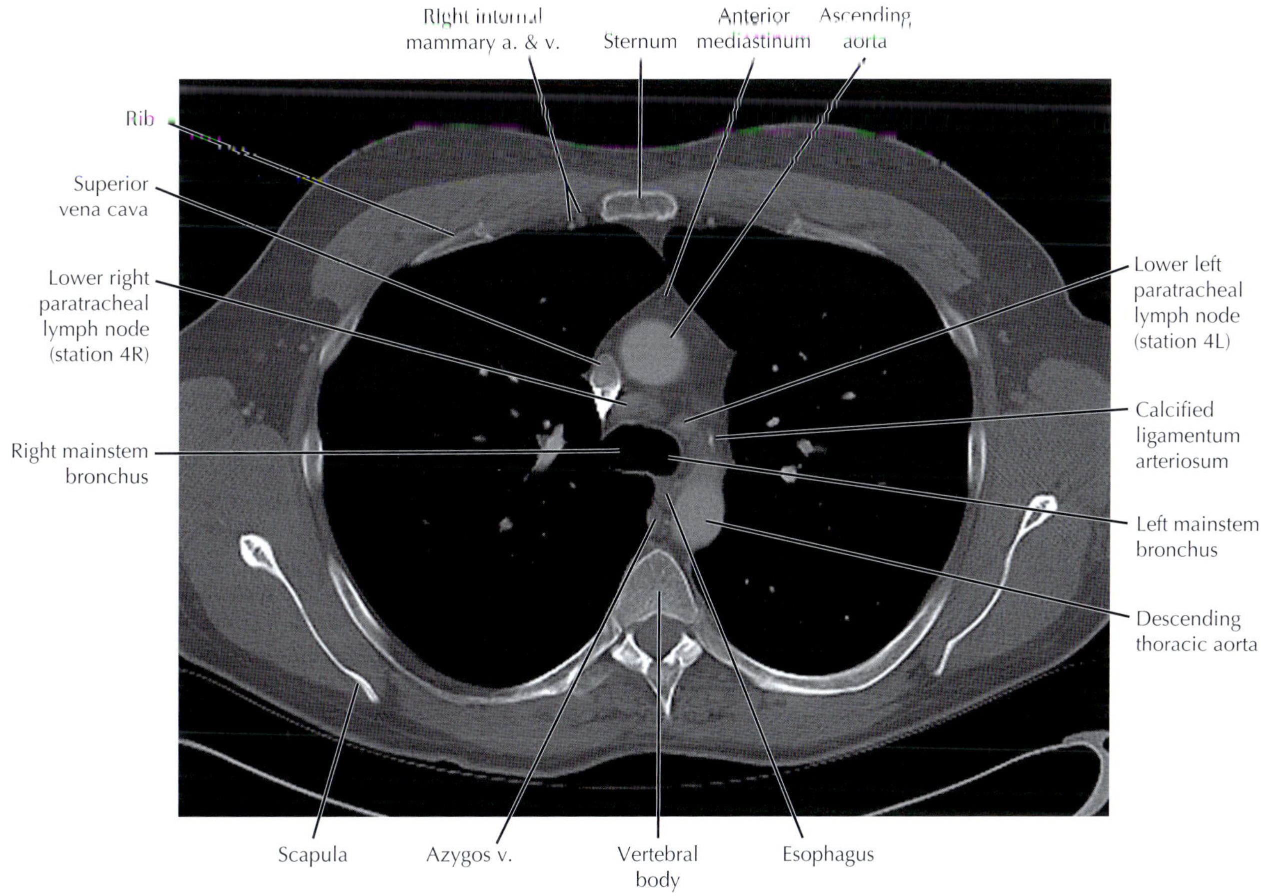
Right internal mammary a. & v.
Sternum
Anterior mediastinum
Ascending aorta
Rib
Superior vena cava
Lower right paratracheal lymph node (station 4R)
Right mainstem bronchus
Lower left paratracheal lymph node (station 4L)
Calcified ligamentum arteriosum
Left mainstem bronchus
Descending thoracic aorta
Scapula
Azygos v.
Vertebral body
Esophagus

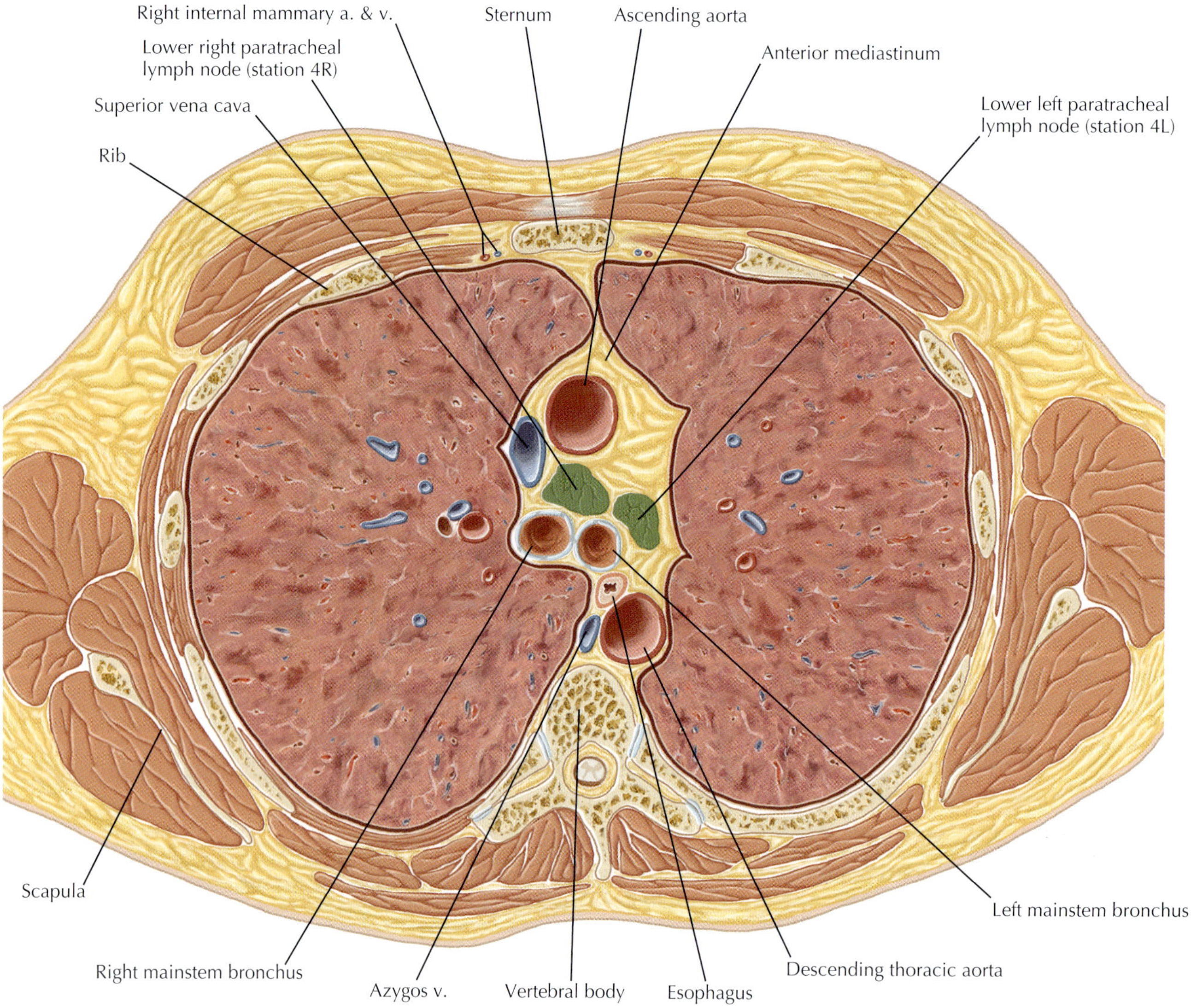

DIAGNOSTIC CONSIDERATION

High-attenuation foci, representing calcification, are readily visible within the right and left lower paratracheal lymph nodes. These nodes are accessible with cervical mediastinoscopy.

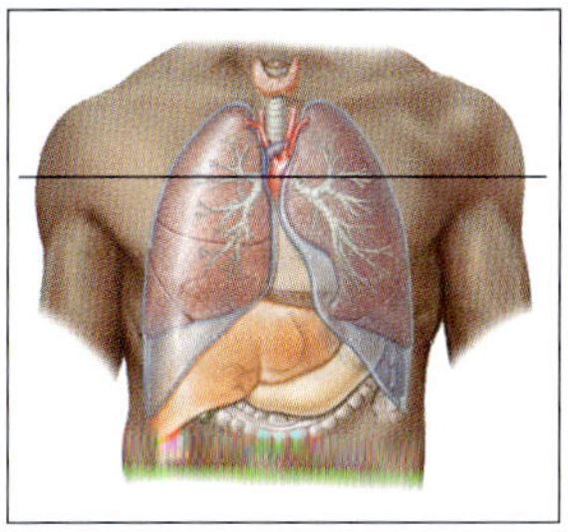

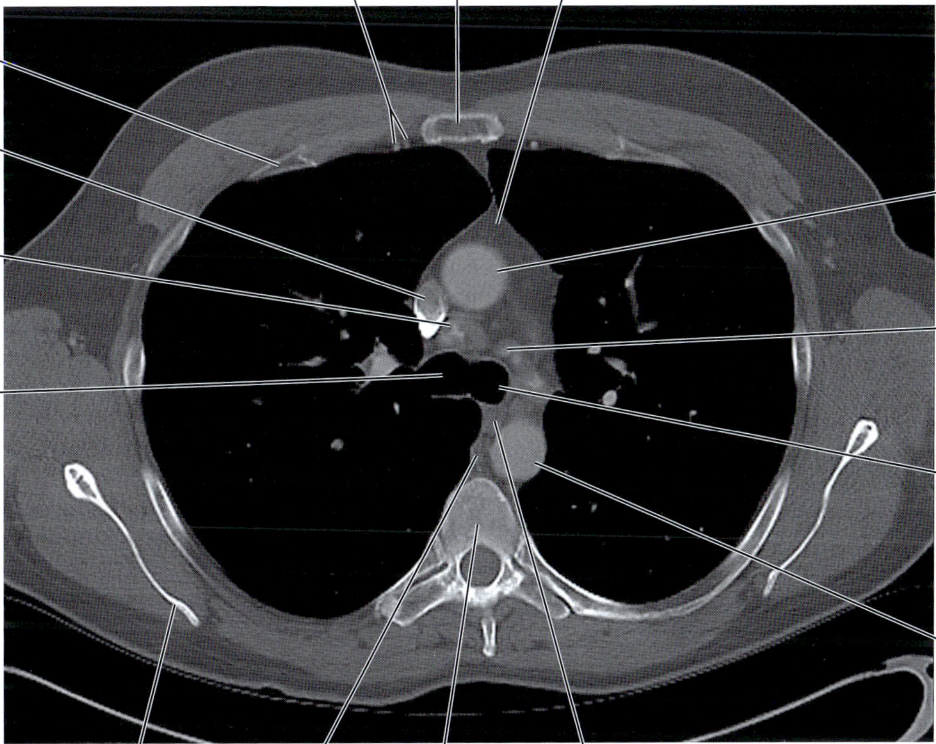
Right internal mammary a. & v.
Sternum
Anterior mediastinum
Rib
Superior vena cava
Lower right paratracheal lymph node (station 4R)
Right mainstem bronchus
Ascending aorta
Lower left paratracheal lymph node (station 4L)
Left mainstem bronchus
Descending thoracic aorta
Scapula
Azygos v.
Vertebral body
Esophagus

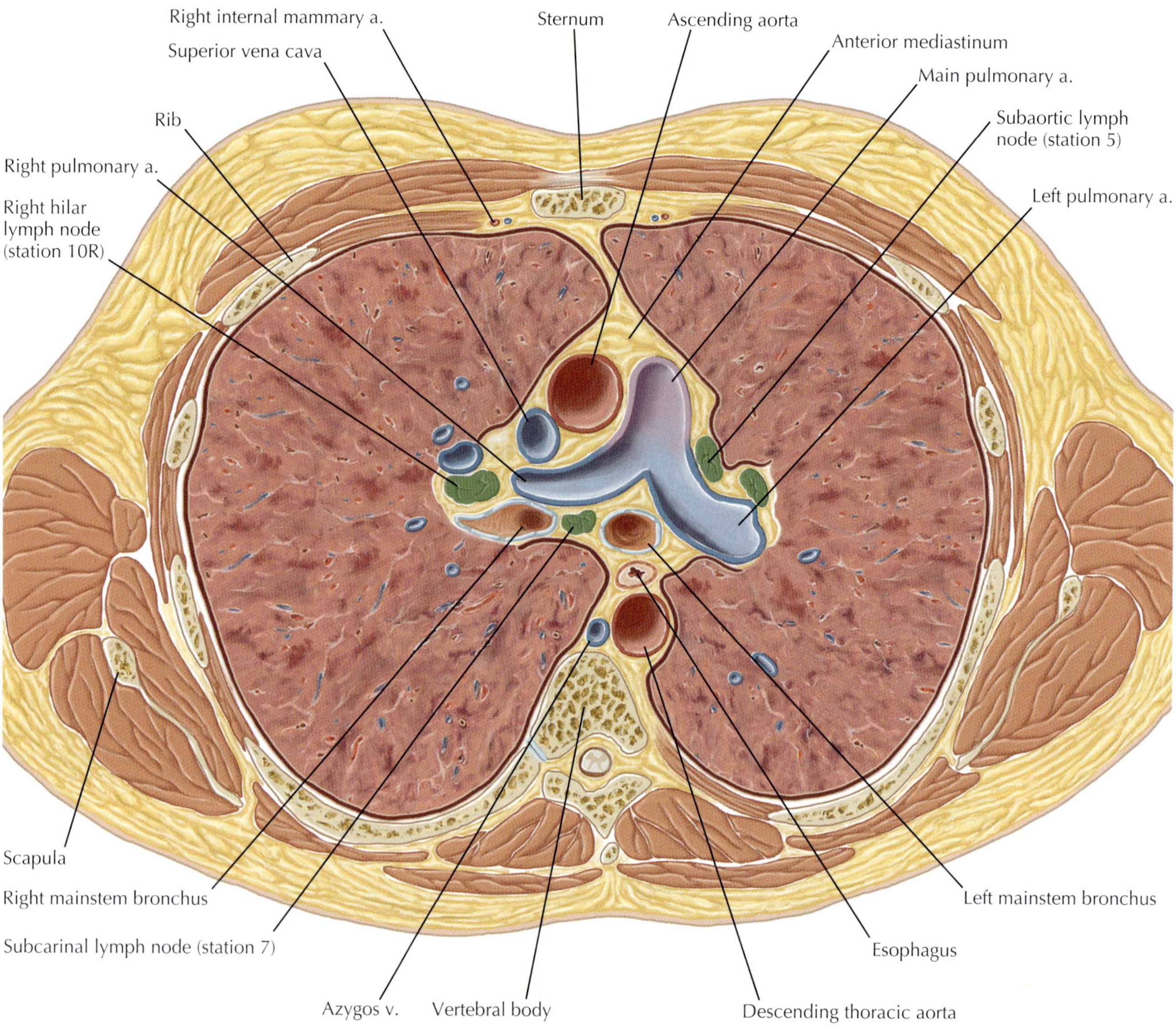

DIAGNOSTIC CONSIDERATION

Right hilar lymph nodes, station 10R in the AJCC lymph node classification system, are visible. Hilar lymph nodes are located caudal to the cranial portion of the right upper lobe bronchus and lie adjacent to the right mainstem bronchus and proximal bronchus intermedius. Hilar lymph nodes are located distal to the mediastinal pleural reflection. In other words, hilar lymph nodes, station 10 lymph nodes, as well as station 11-14 lymph nodes lie within the lung. In contrast, lymph nodes located in stations 1-9 in the AJCC lymph node classification system reside within the mediastinum. In patients with lung carcinoma, mediastinal lymph node involvement confers a worse prognosis compared with involved lymph nodes that reside within the lung.

In this image, a subaortic lymph node (station 5) is also visible. These lymph nodes lie lateral to the ligamentum arteriosum and medial to the origin of the first branch of the left pulmonary artery.

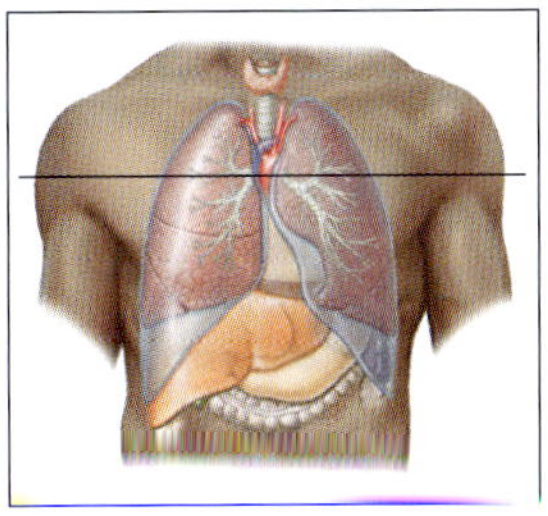

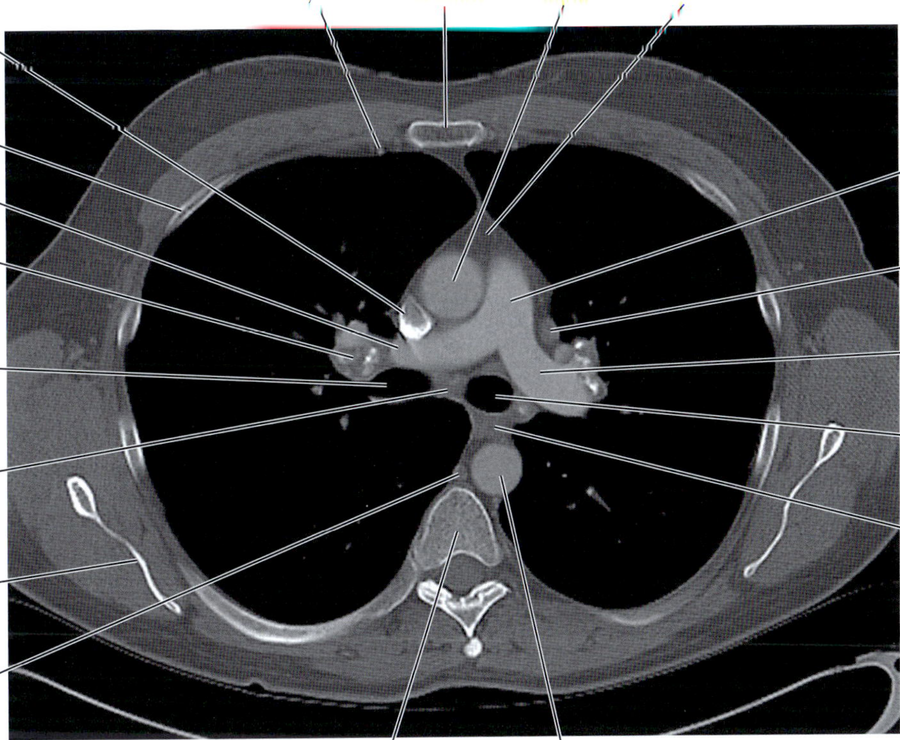
Right internal mammary a.
Sternum
Ascending aorta
Anterior mediastinum
Superior vena cava
Rib
Right pulmonary a.
Right hilar lymph node (station 10R)
Right mainstem bronchus
Subcarinal lymph node (station 7)
Scapula
Azygos v.
Vertebral body
Descending thoracic aorta
Main pulmonary a.
Subaortic lymph node (station 5)
Left pulmonary a.
Left mainstem bronchus
Esophagus

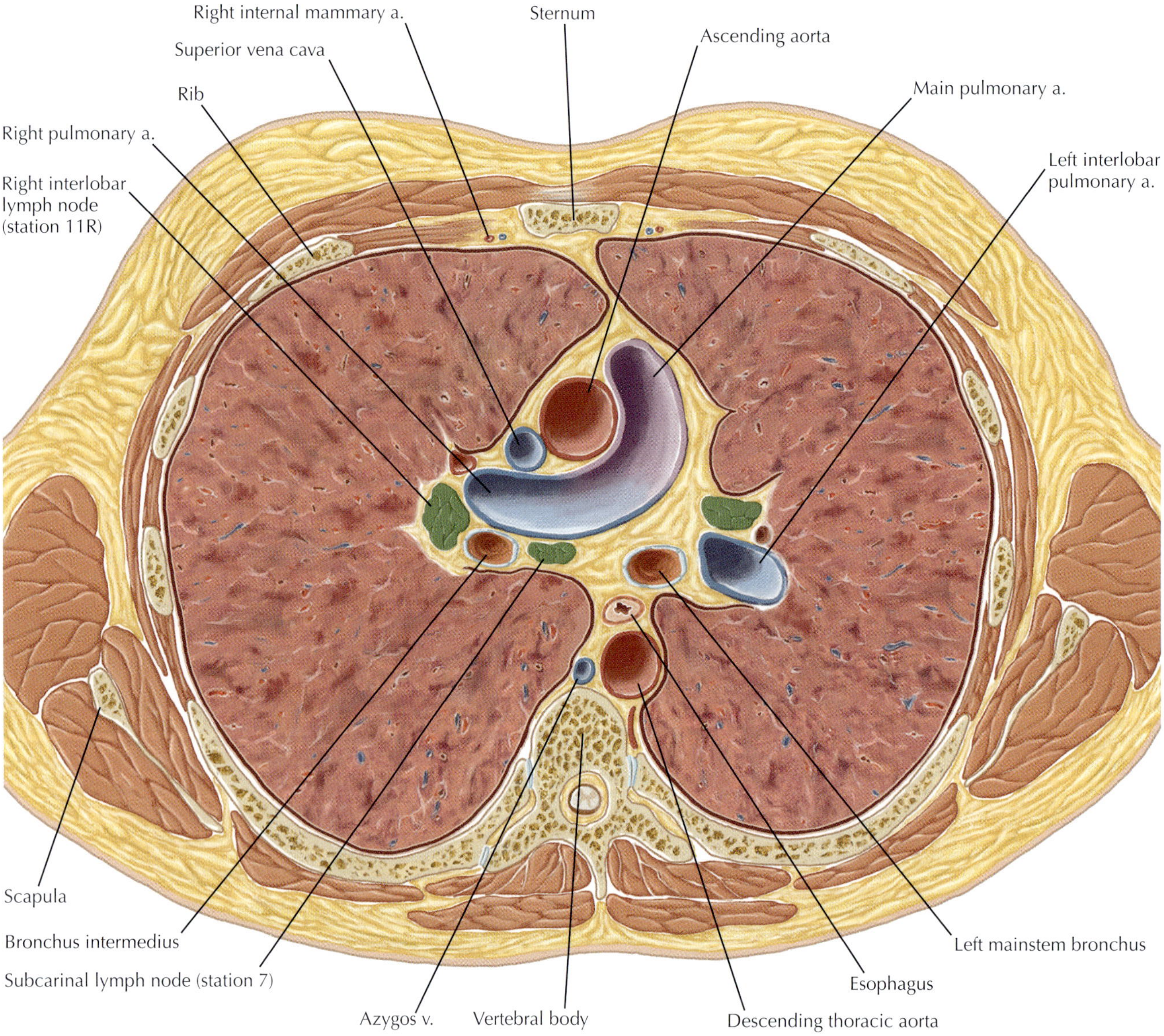

DIAGNOSTIC CONSIDERATION

With views progressively caudal to the pulmonary hilum, lymph nodes are consistently closely related to the pulmonary arteries. A calcified right interlobar lymph node (station 11R) is visible. The contour abnormality created by right hilar lymphadenopathy on chest radiographs is often caused by a combination of enlarged lymph nodes in the right hilar (station 10) and right interlobar (station 11) regions. Subcarinal lymph nodes (station 7), which reside within the mediastinum, are visible.

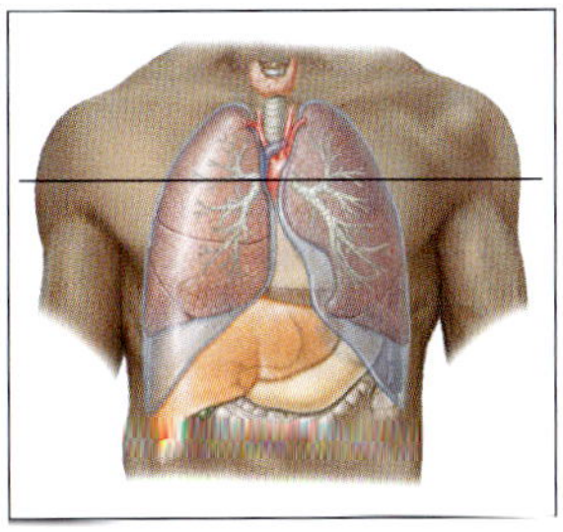

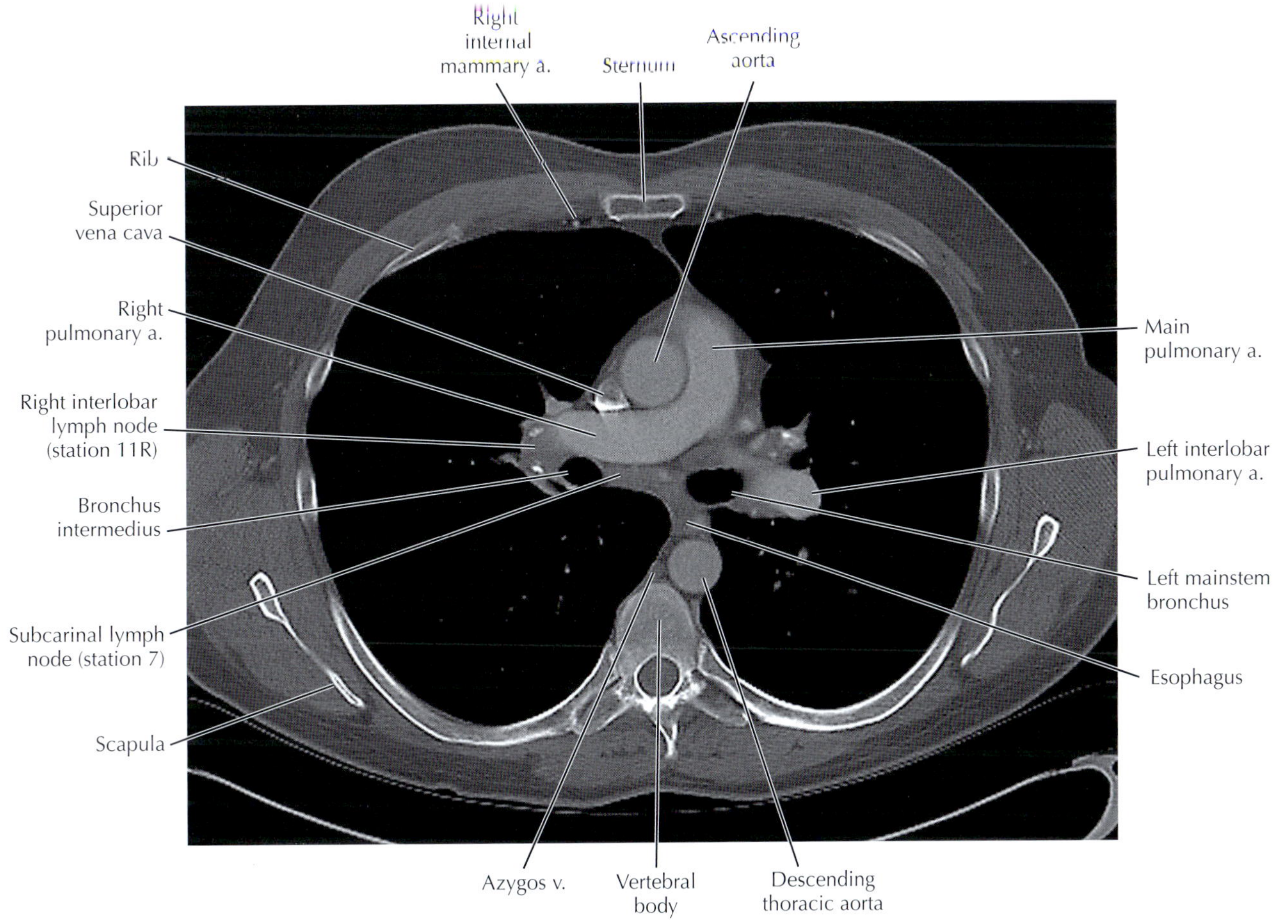
Right internal mammary a.
Sternum
Ascending aorta
Rib
Superior vena cava
Right pulmonary a.
Right interlobar lymph node (station 11R)
Bronchus intermedius
Subcarinal lymph node (station 7)
Scapula
Main pulmonary a.
Left interlobar pulmonary a.
Left mainstem bronchus
Esophagus
Azygos v.
Vertebral body
Descending thoracic aorta

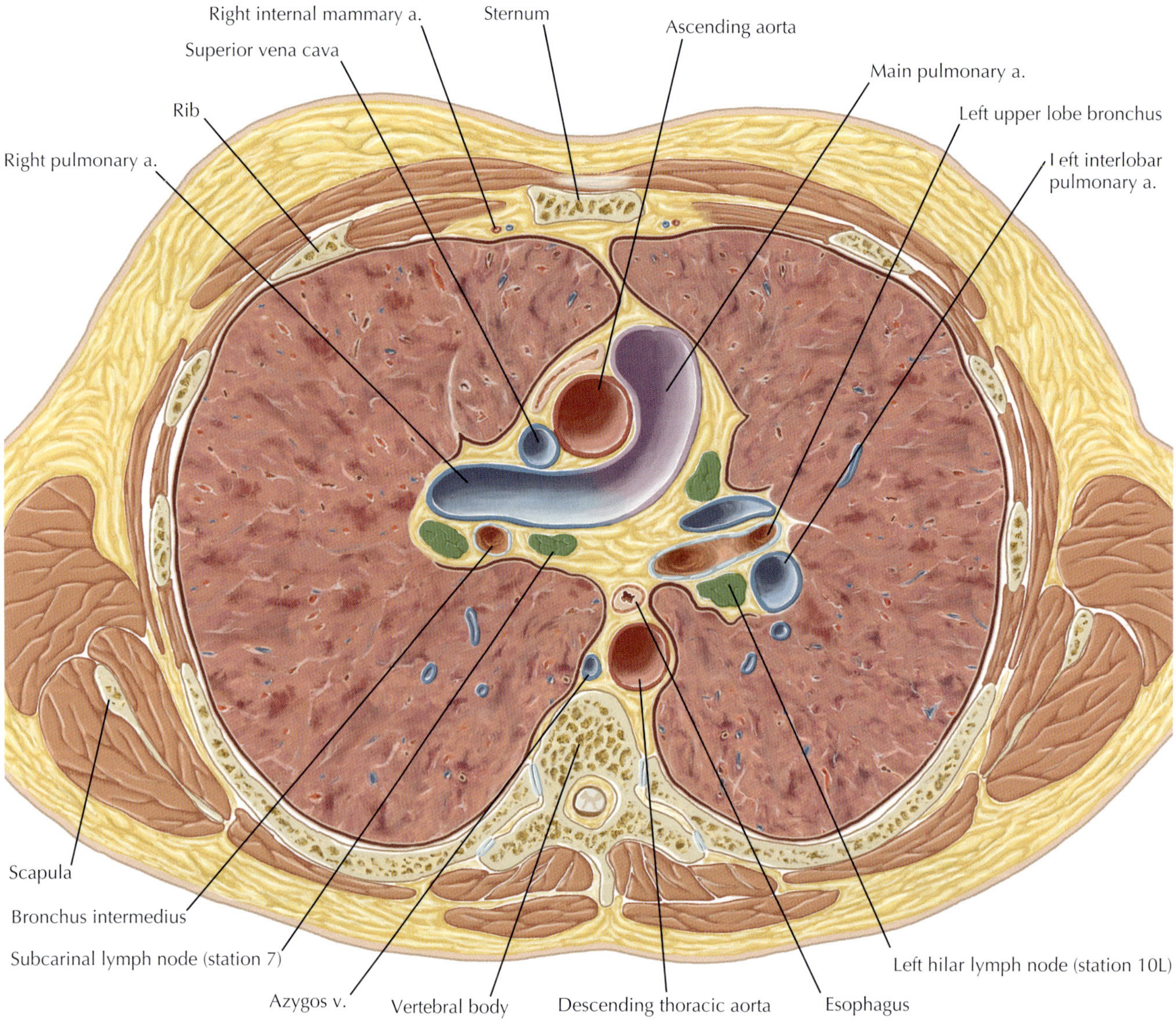

DIAGNOSTIC CONSIDERATION

This view is caudal to the foregoing images (Axial 1-6). Note how lymph nodes are closely associated with the pulmonary arteries. In the lower lobes, lymph nodes are often positioned medial to the adjacent pulmonary arteries and lateral to the bronchi.

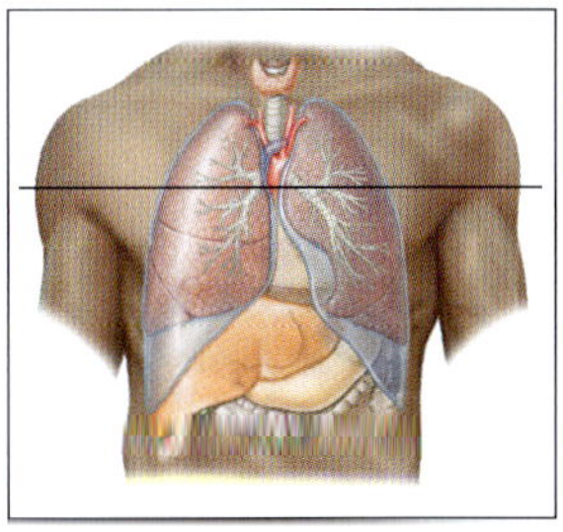

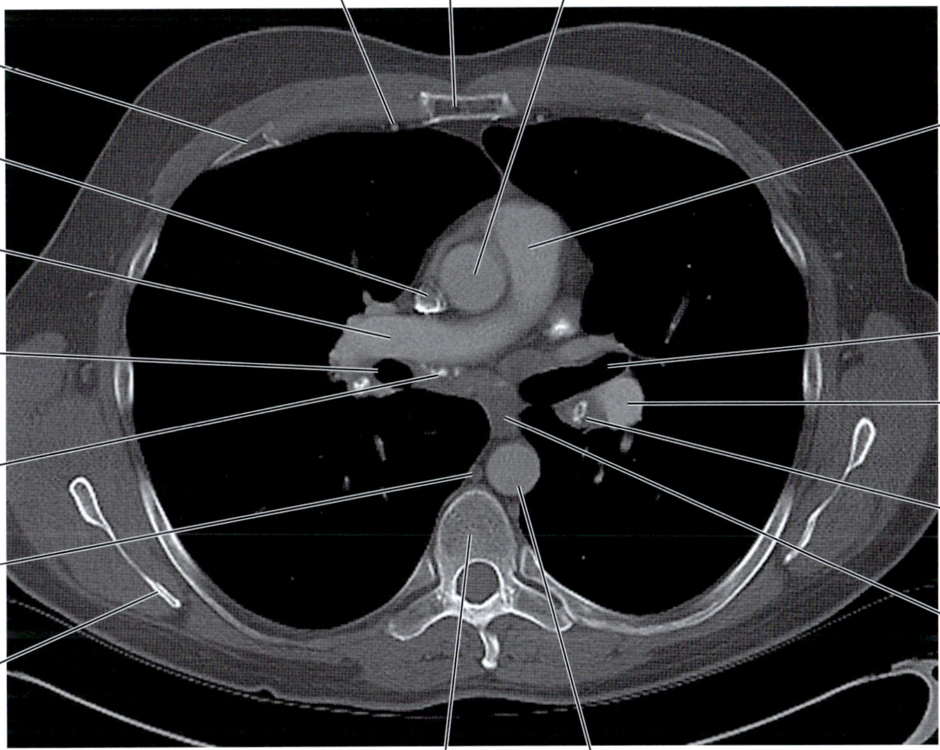
Right internal mammary a.
Sternum
Ascending aorta
Rib
Superior vena cava
Right pulmonary a.
Bronchus intermedius
Subcarinal lymph node (station 7)
Azygos v.
Scapula
Main pulmonary a.
Left upper lobe bronchus
Left interlobar pulmonary a.
Left hilar lymph node (station 10L)
Esophagus
Vertebral body
Descending thoracic aorta

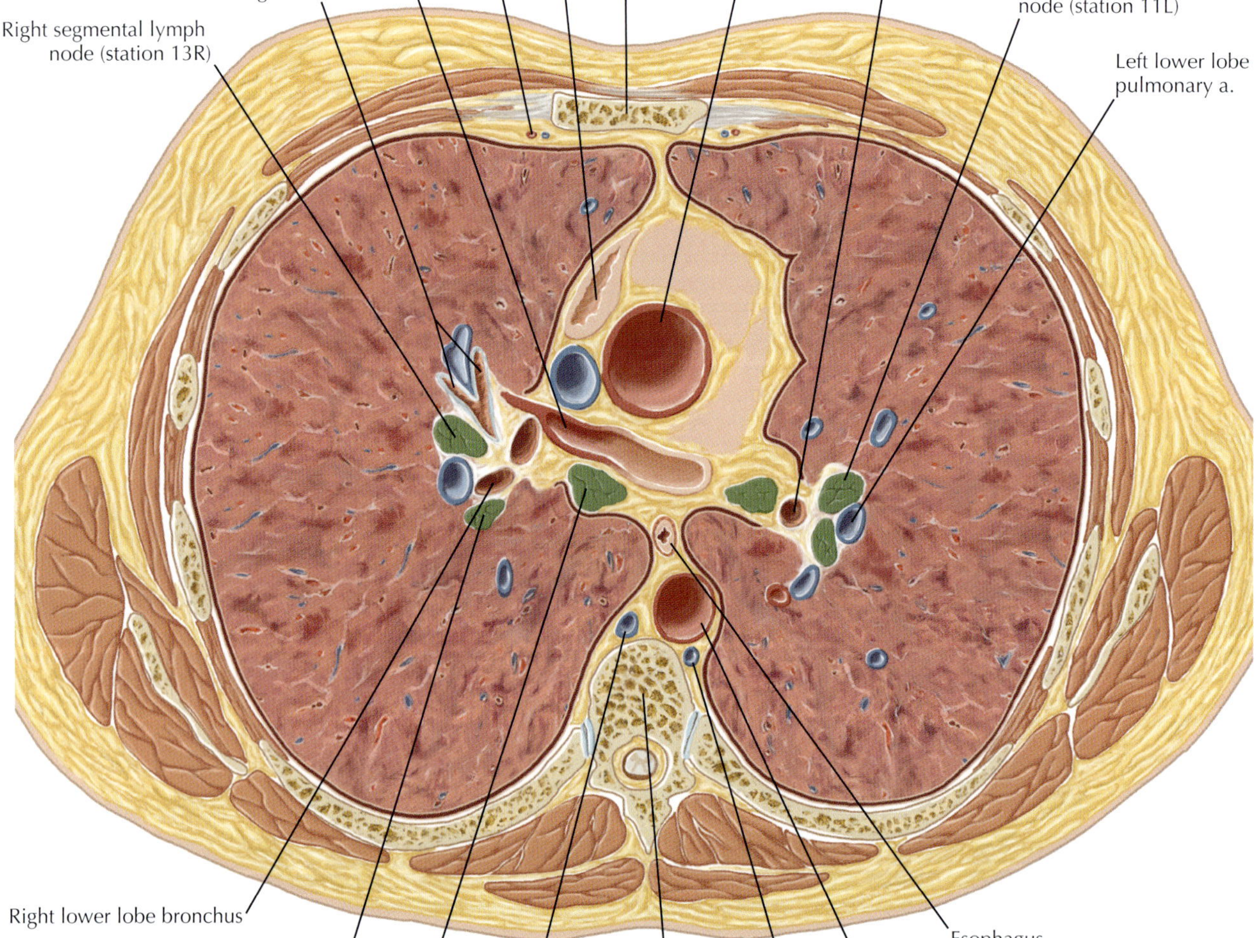

DIAGNOSTIC CONSIDERATION

At this level, segmental lymph nodes (station 13R) are seen just lateral to the lateral segmental right middle lobe bronchus, and lobar lymph nodes (station 12R) are seen adjacent to the right lower lobe bronchus. On the left, calcified interlobar lymph nodes (station 11L) are seen. Interlobar lymph nodes are typically found adjacent to and between proximal lobar bronchi. On the left, typically between the lingular and superior segmental bronchi.

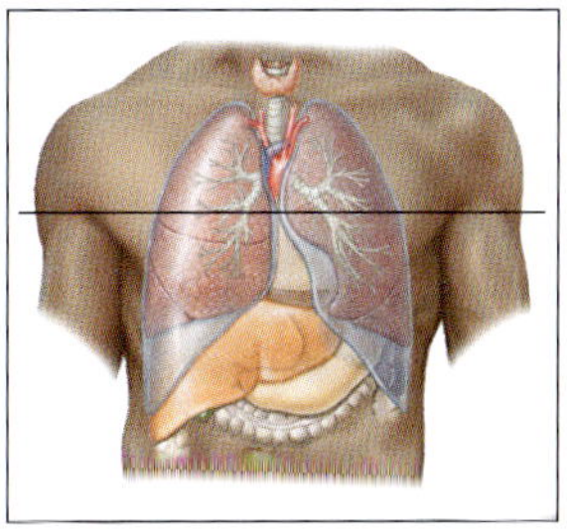

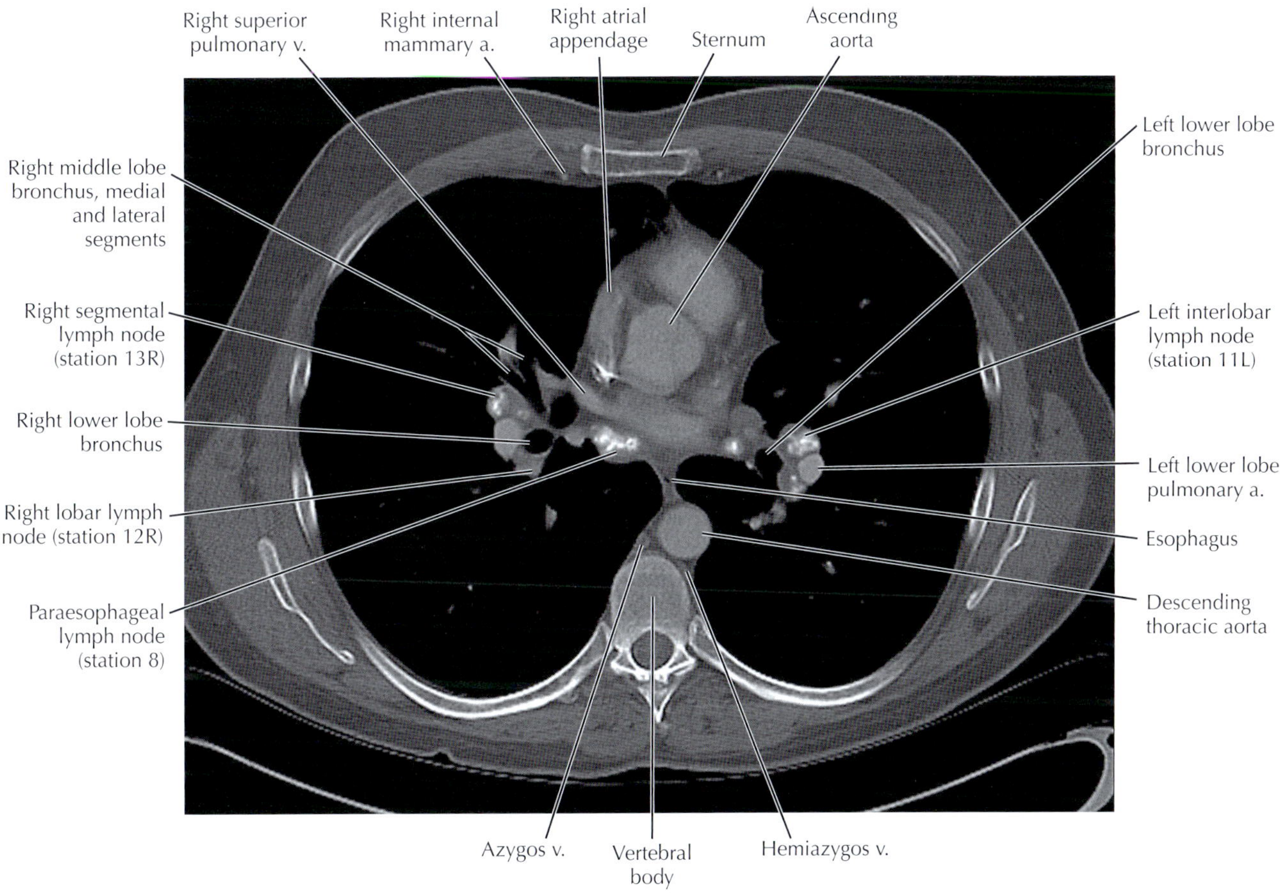

Right superior pulmonary v.
Right internal mammary a.
Right atrial appendage
Sternum
Ascending aorta
Left lower lobe bronchus
Right middle lobe bronchus, medial and lateral segments
Right segmental lymph node (station 13R)
Left interlobar lymph node (station 11L)
Right lower lobe bronchus
Left lower lobe pulmonary a.
Right lobar lymph node (station 12R)
Esophagus
Paraesophageal lymph node (station 8)
Descending thoracic aorta
Azygos v.
Vertebral body
Hemiazygos v.

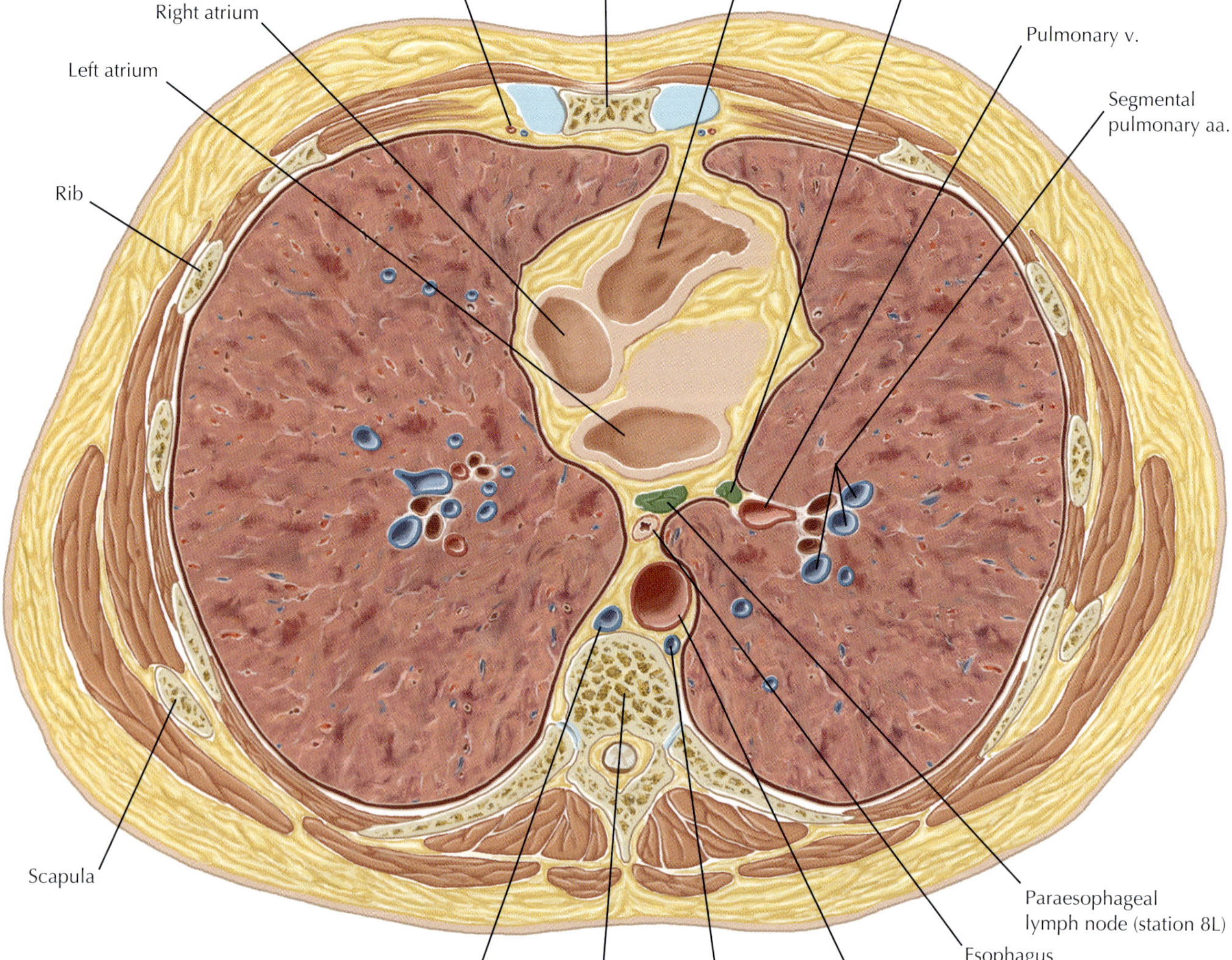

DIAGNOSTIC CONSIDERATION

Left inferior pulmonary ligament lymph nodes are visible. A small area of high attenuation, representing calcification, is visible within the lymph node. Inferior pulmonary ligament lymph nodes, also often referred to as pulmonary ligament lymph nodes, are usually found slightly medial and inferior to the inferior pulmonary veins.

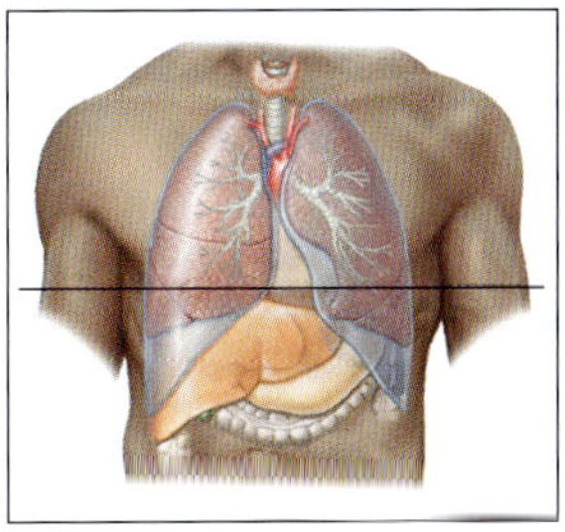

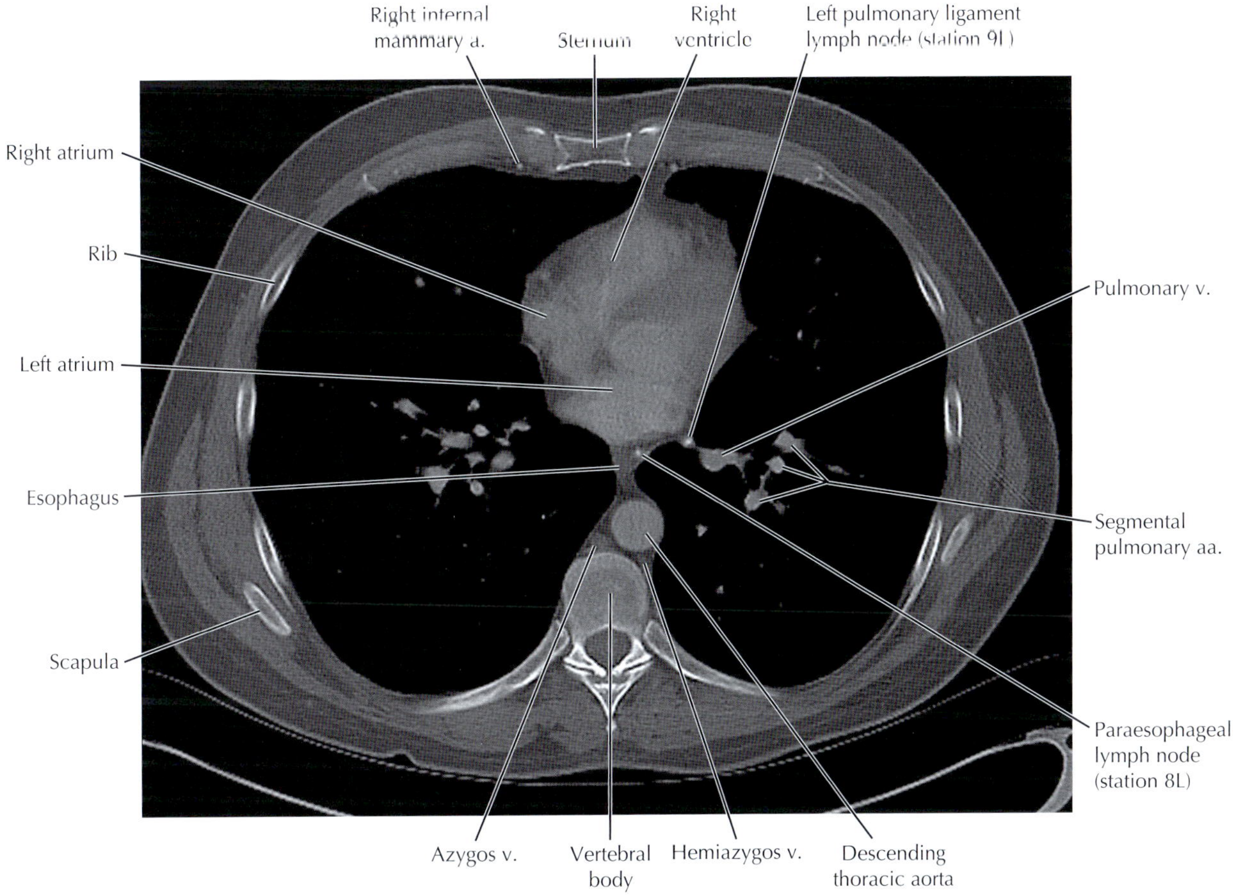
Right internal mammary a.
Sternum
Right ventricle
Left pulmonary ligament lymph node (station 9L)
Right atrium
Rib
Pulmonary v.
Left atrium
Esophagus
Segmental pulmonary aa.
Scapula
Paraesophageal lymph node (station 8L)
Azygos v.
Vertebral body
Hemiazygos v.
Descending thoracic aorta

Chapter 5 CISTERNA CHYLI AND THORACIC DUCT

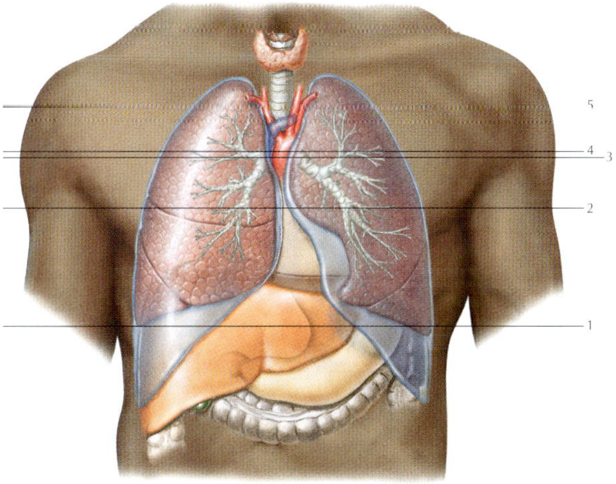

AXIAL 190

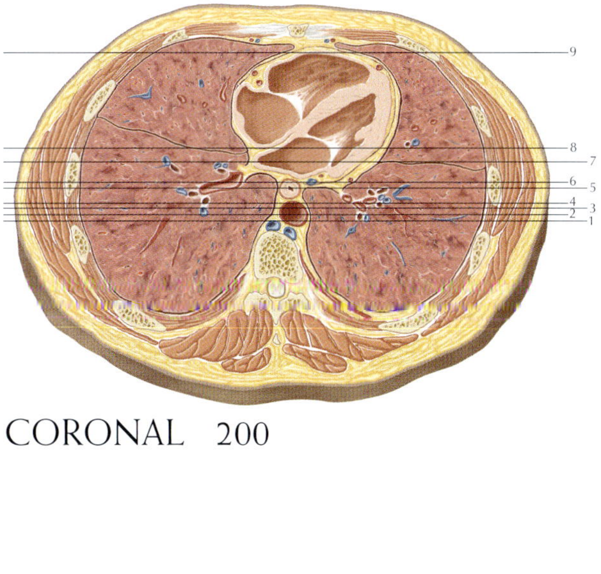

CORONAL 200

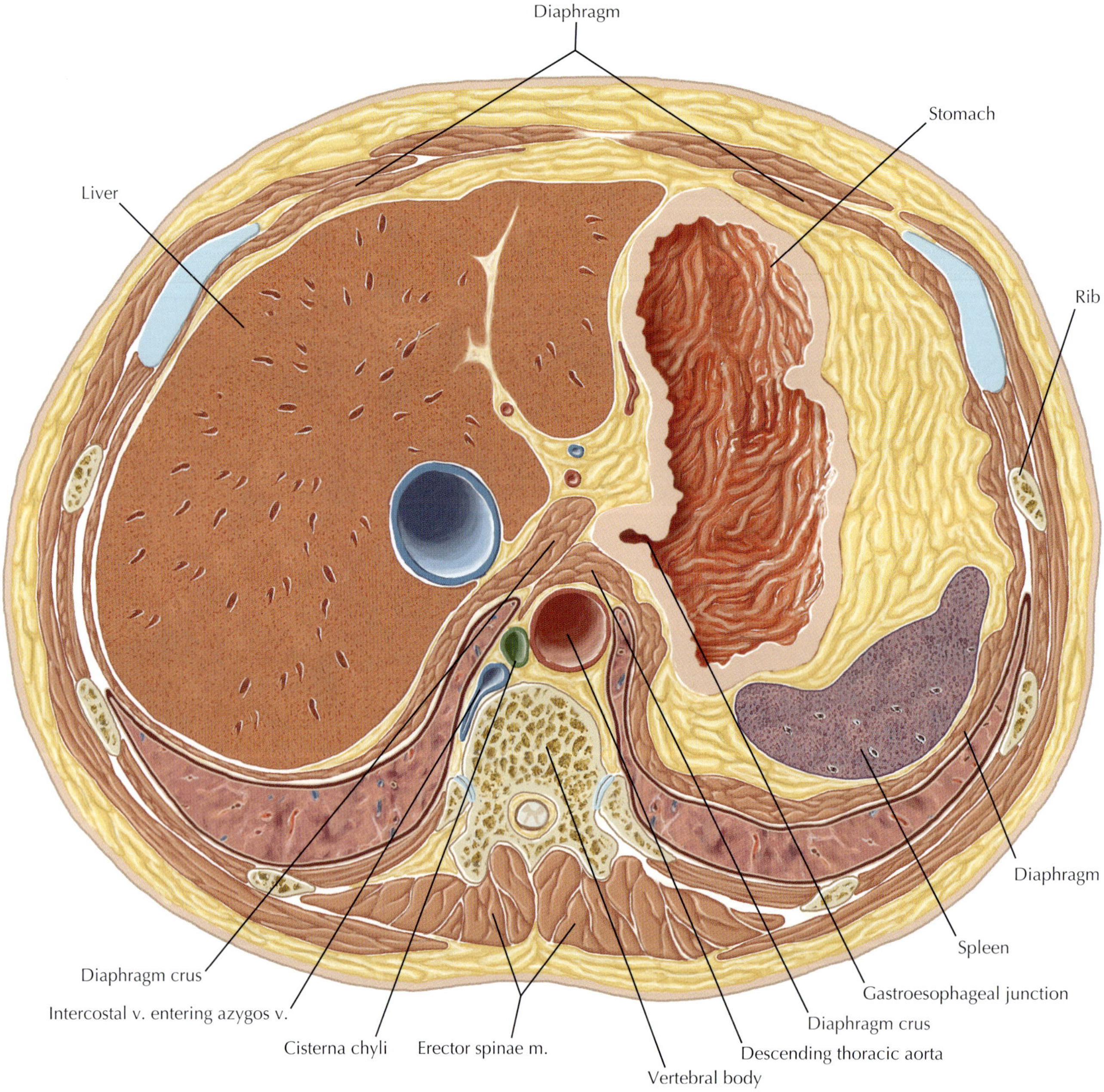

NORMAL ANATOMY

A normal structure is shown—the cisterna chyli—which is inconsistently seen on clinical thoracic CT scans. The cisterna chyli is typically located between the distal thoracic or upper abdominal aorta and azygos vein in the right posterior mediastinum or retrocrural space, posterior to the right diaphragmatic crus. The cisterna chyli receives lymph from the right and left lumbar lymphatic trunks, the intestinal lymphatic trunk, and the inferior intercostal lymph nodes. The cisterna chyli gives rise to the thoracic duct, whose course will be shown on subsequent images.

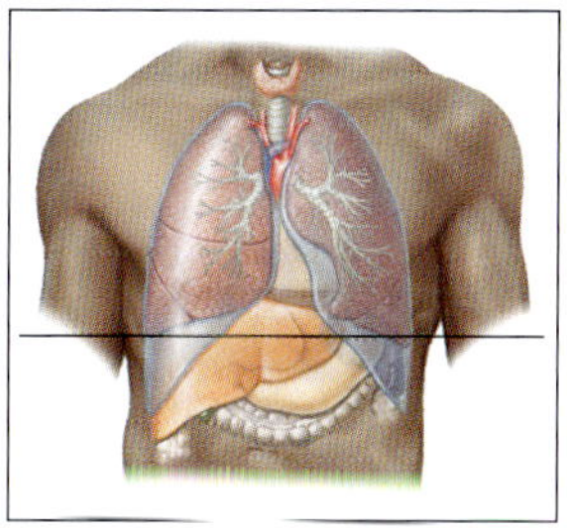

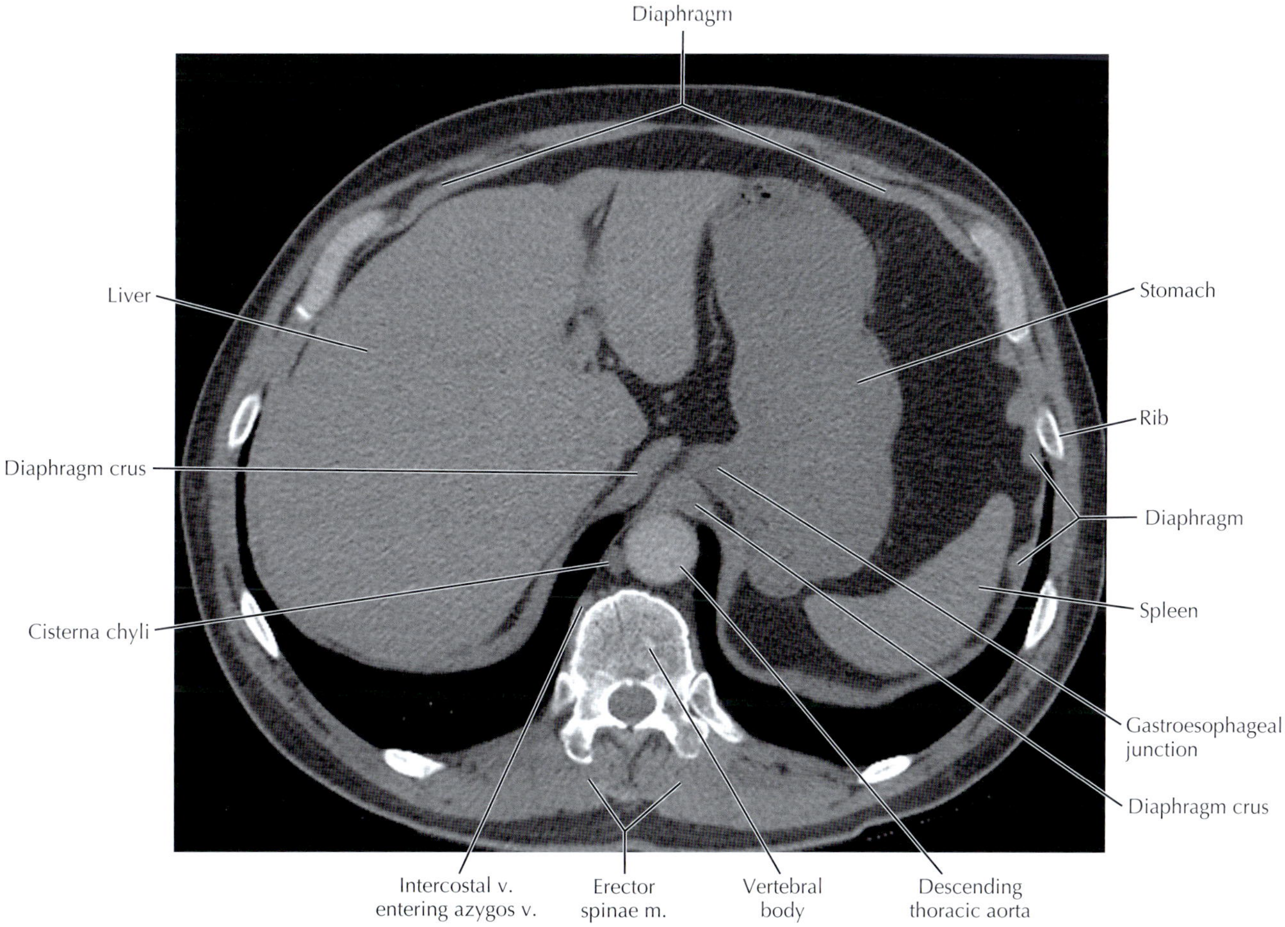
Diaphragm
Liver
Stomach
Rib
Diaphragm crus
Diaphragm
Spleen
Cisterna chyli
Gastroesophageal junction
Diaphragm crus
Intercostal v. entering azygos v.
Erector spinae m.
Vertebral body
Descending thoracic aorta

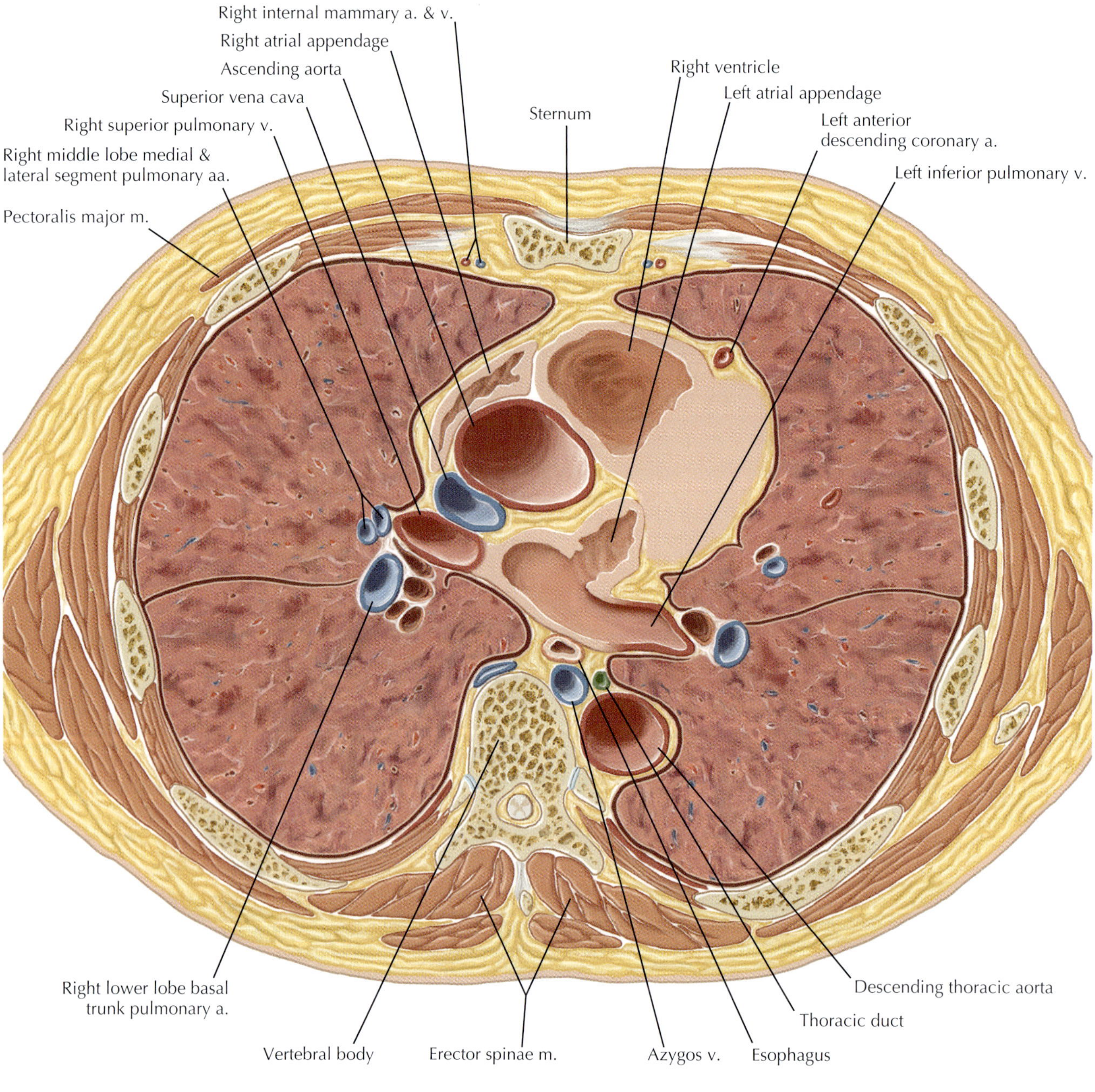

NORMAL ANATOMY

The thoracic duct is not always visible on thoracic CT scans, but is well seen in this patient. The thoracic duct originates from the cisterna chyli and ascends within the posterior mediastinum. The thoracic duct is well visualized adjacent to the azygos vein, posterior to the esophagus. Caudally, it usually ascends on the right side, often crossing to the left of midline at approximately the level of the 5th thoracic vertebral body. In this patient, the thoracic duct crossed midline at a more inferior level than is typically seen.

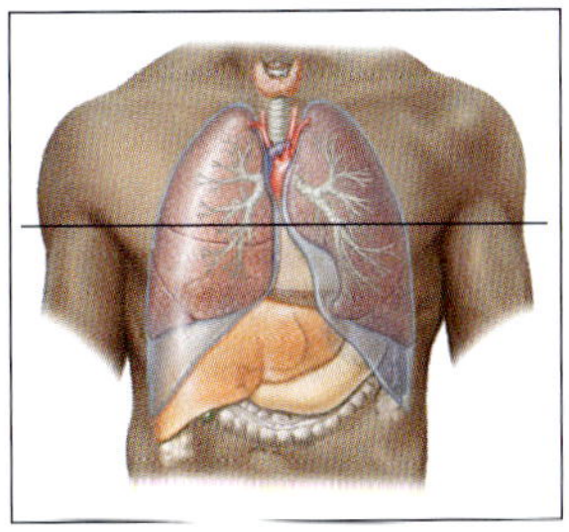

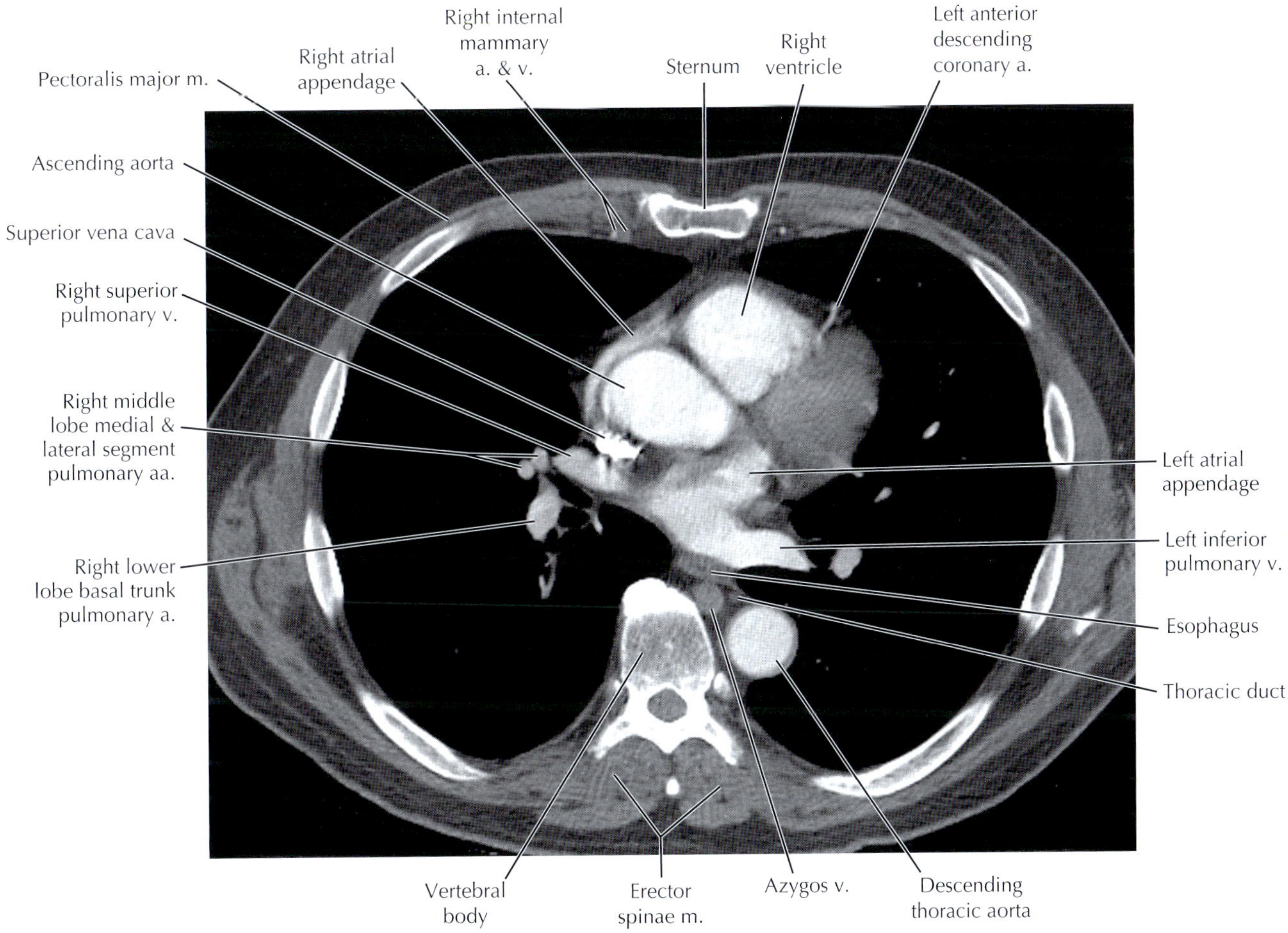
Pectoralis major m.
Right atrial appendage
Right internal mammary a. & v.
Sternum
Right ventricle
Left anterior descending coronary a.
Ascending aorta
Superior vena cava
Right superior pulmonary v.
Right middle lobe medial & lateral segment pulmonary aa.
Right lower lobe basal trunk pulmonary a.
Left atrial appendage
Left inferior pulmonary v.
Esophagus
Thoracic duct
Vertebral body
Erector spinae m.
Azygos v.
Descending thoracic aorta

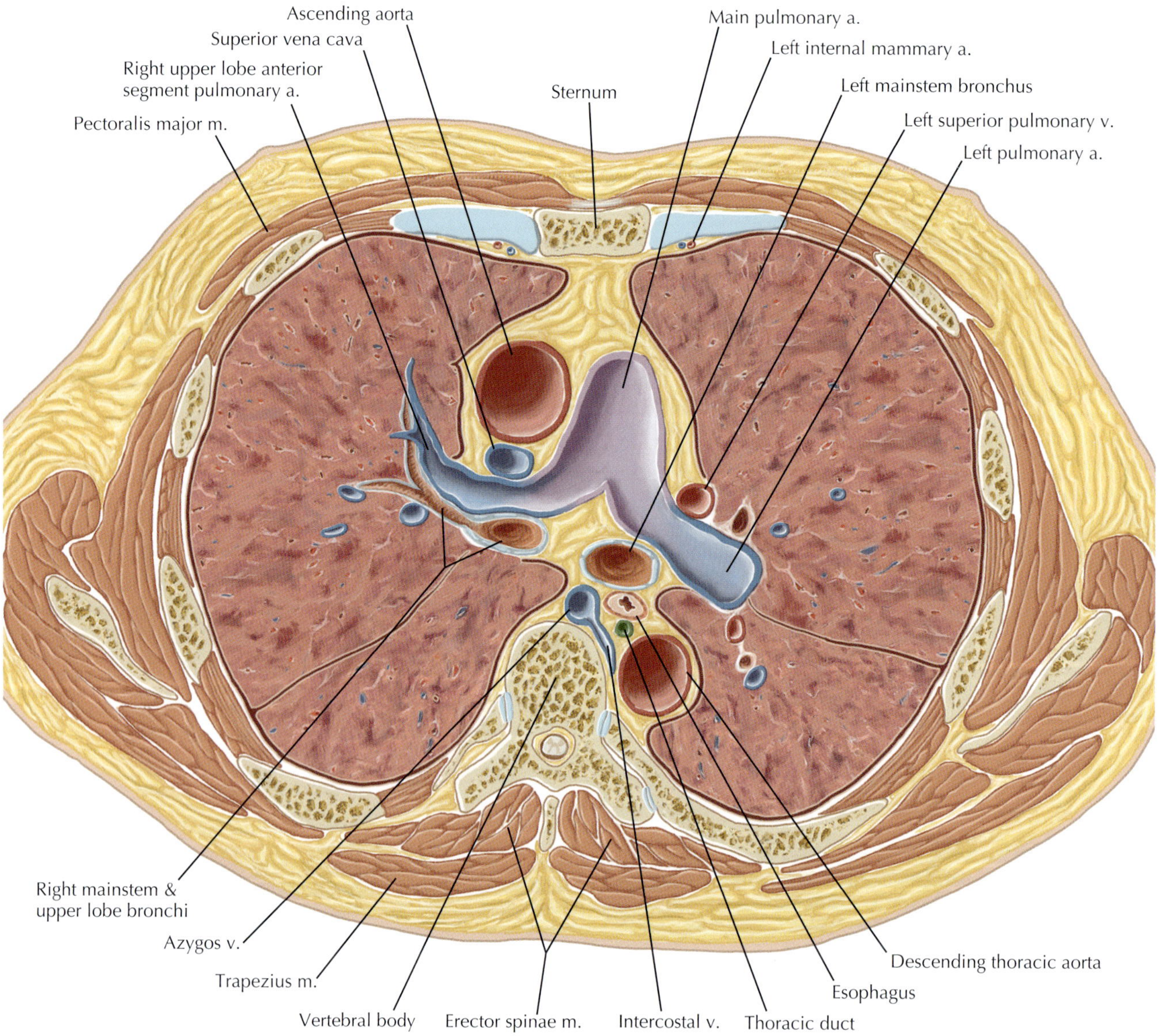

NORMAL ANATOMY

The thoracic duct is again seen coursing within the posterior mediastinum adjacent to the azygos vein and descending thoracic aorta and posterior to the esophagus.

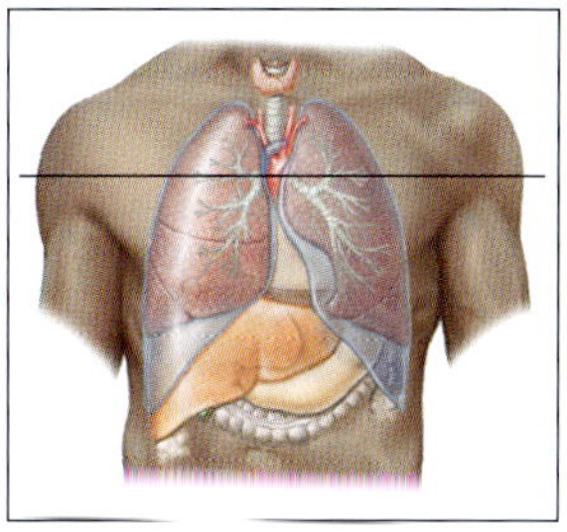

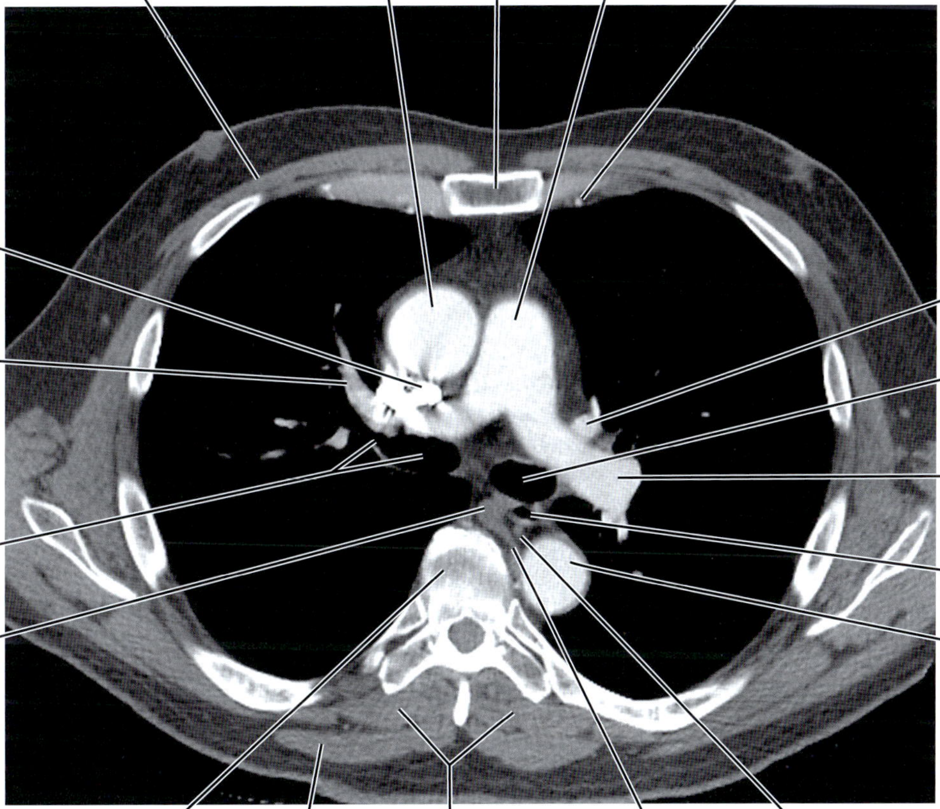
Pectoralis major m.
Ascending aorta
Sternum
Main pulmonary a.
Left internal mammary a.
Superior vena cava
Right upper lobe anterior segment pulmonary a.
Right mainstem & upper lobe bronchi
Azygos v.
Left superior pulmonary v.
Left mainstem bronchus
Left pulmonary a.
Esophagus
Descending thoracic aorta
Vertebral body
Trapezius m.
Erector spinae m.
Intercostal v.
Thoracic duct

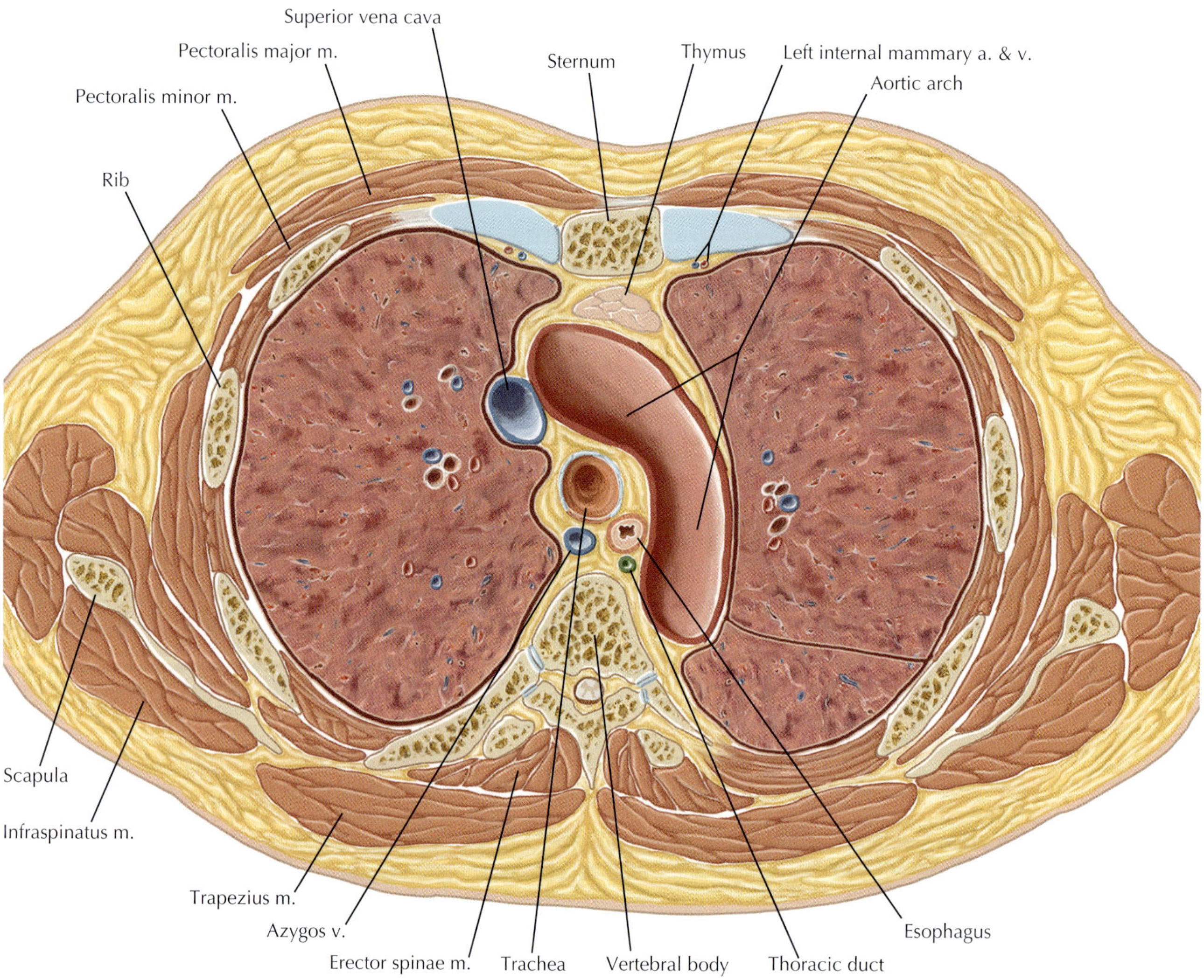

NORMAL ANATOMY

At the level of the aortic arch at the cranial aspect of the azygos vein, the thoracic duct is again seen to the left of midline, posterior to the esophagus.

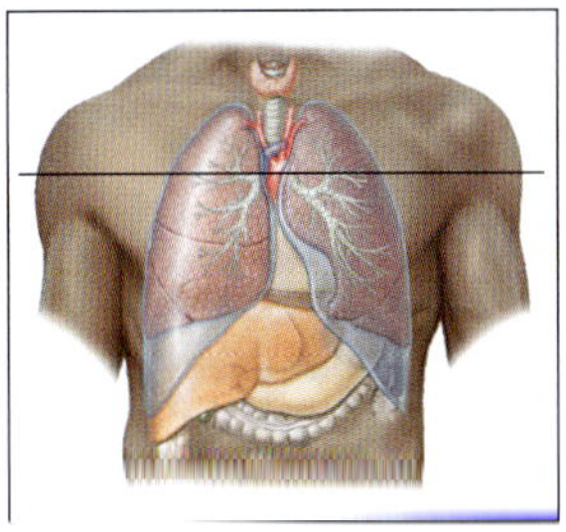

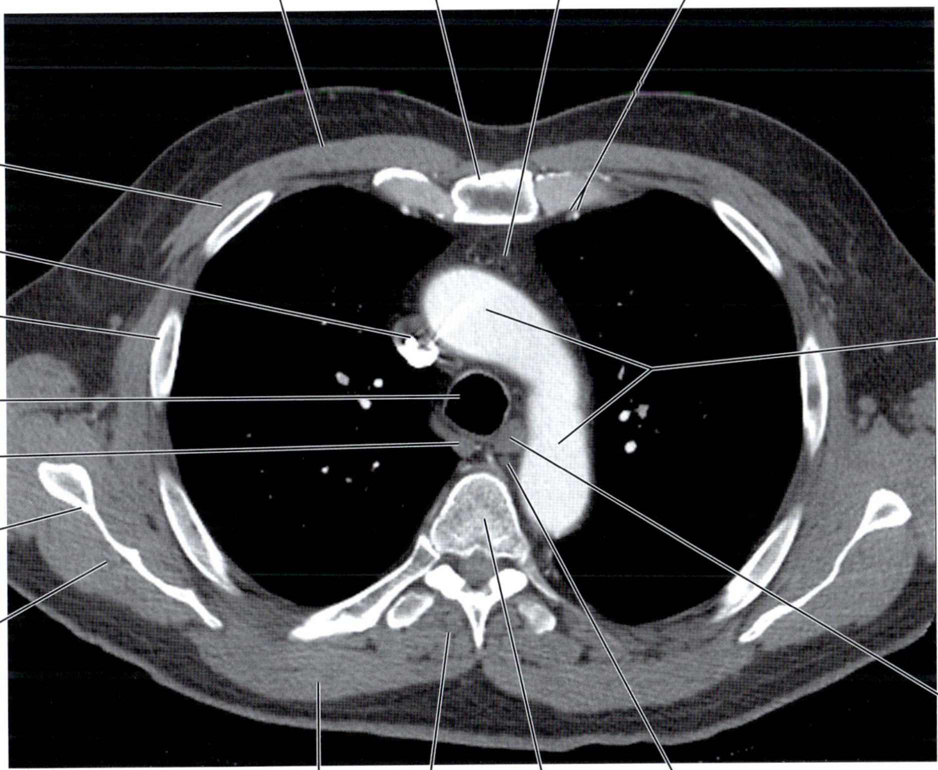
Pectoralis major m.
Sternum
Thymus
Left internal mammary a. & v.
Pectoralis minor m.
Superior vena cava
Rib
Trachea
Azygos v.
Scapula
Infraspinatus m.
Aortic arch
Esophagus
Trapezius m.
Erector spinae m.
Vertebral body
Thoracic duct

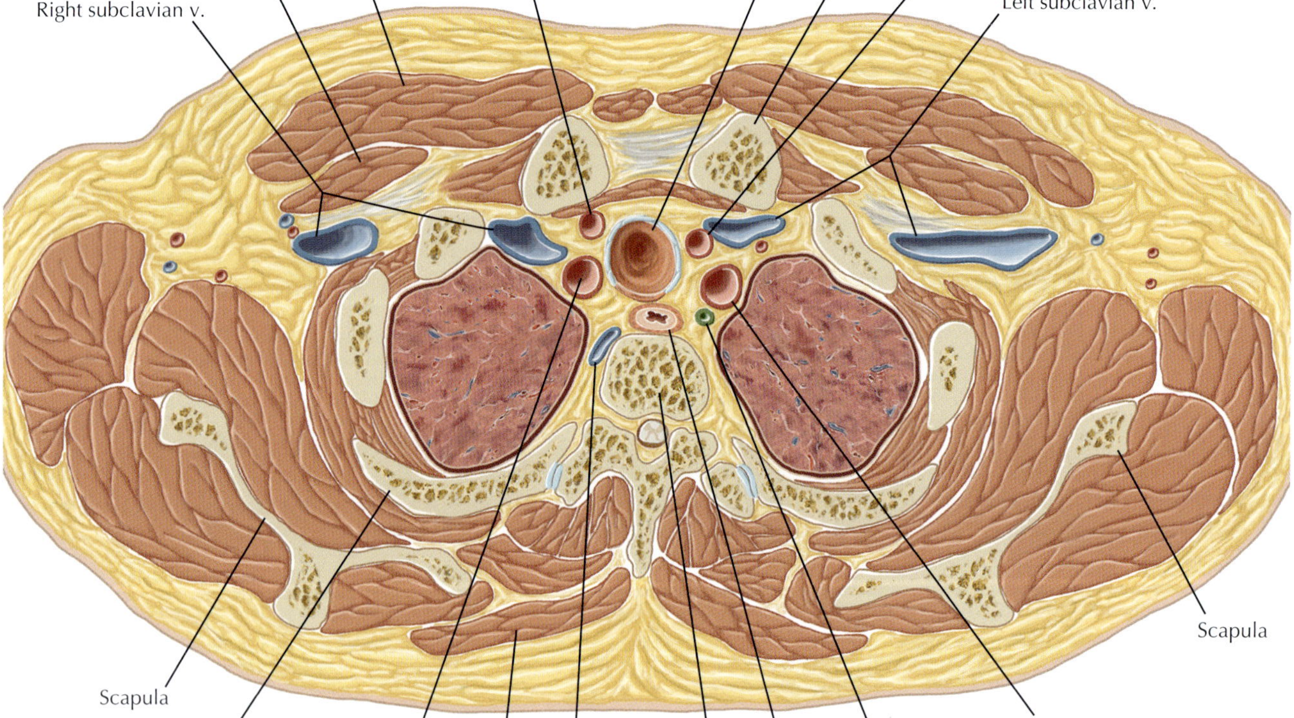

NORMAL ANATOMY

Within the superior mediastinum, the thoracic duct is visible to the left of midline. The thoracic duct courses cranially and eventually empties into the junction of the left subclavian and left internal jugular veins. The thoracic duct drains lymph from the entire body except for the right head and neck, right thorax, and right arm.

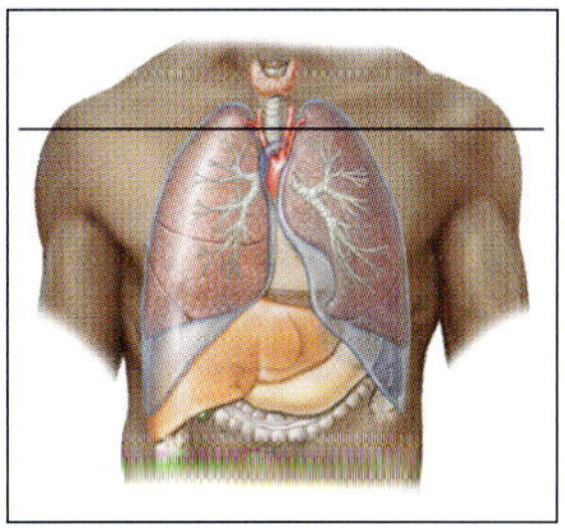

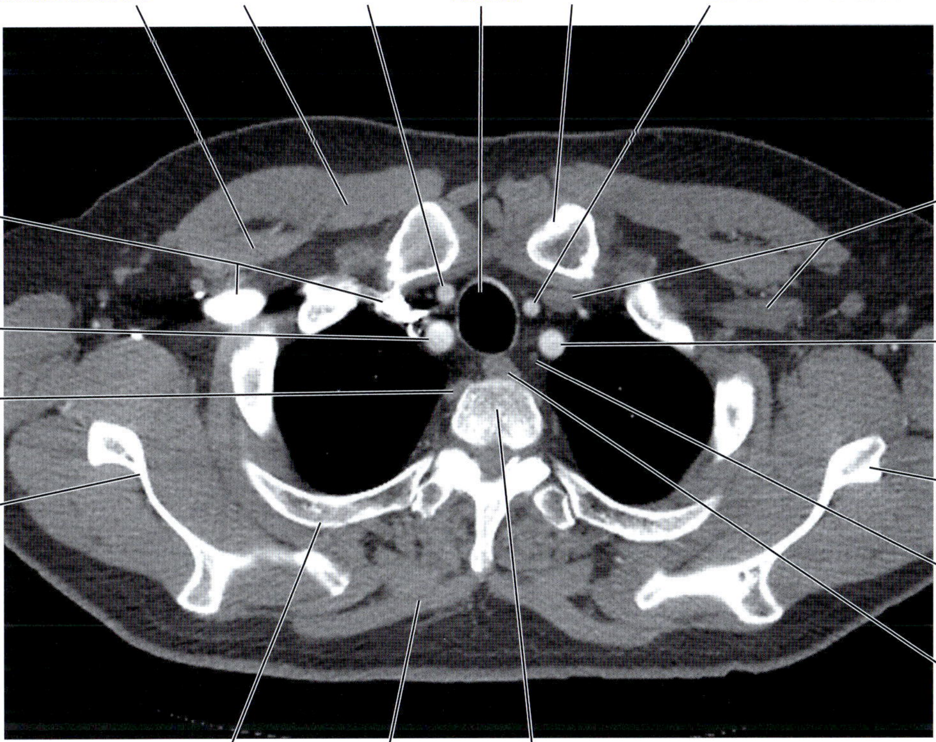
Pectoralis minor m.
Pectoralis major m.
Right common carotid a.
Trachea
Left clavicle
Left common carotid a.
Right subclavian v. (enhanced)
Right subclavian a.
Right superior intercostal v.
Scapula
Left subclavian v.
Left subclavian a.
Scapula
Thoracic duct
Esophagus
Rib
Trapezius m.
Vertebral body

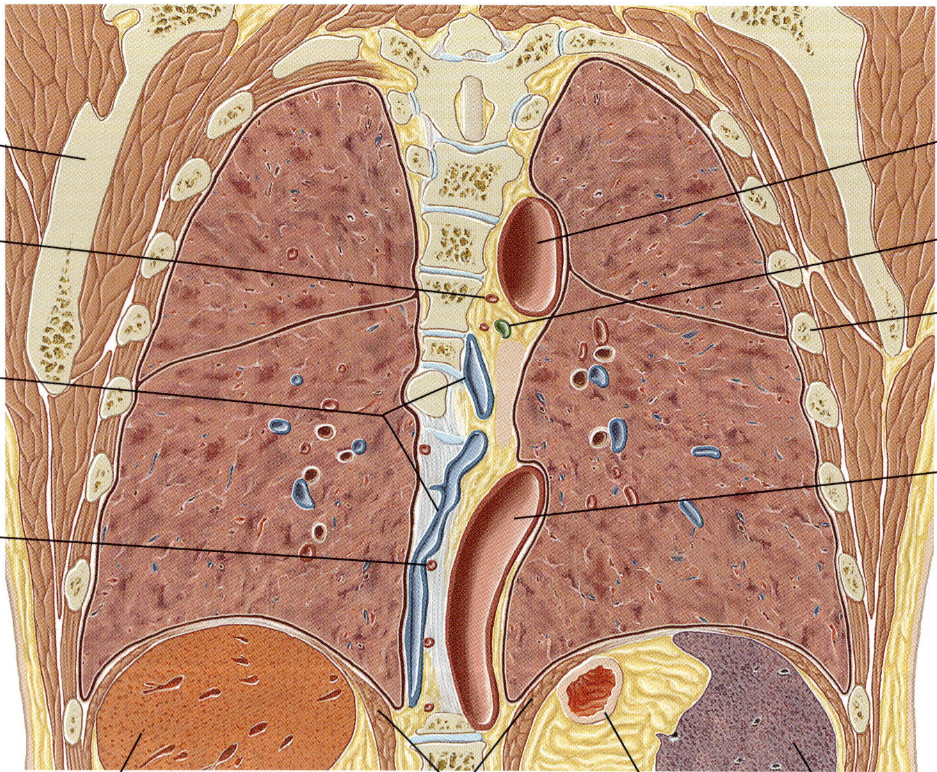

NORMAL ANATOMY

This coronal image, and those that follow, accompanies Cisterna Chyli/Thoracic Duct Axial 1-5 above and shows the position of the *cisterna chyli* and course of the *thoracic duct* in the coronal plane. The thoracic duct is not always visible on thoracic CT scans, but is well seen in this patient. The thoracic duct originates from the cisterna chyli and ascends within the posterior mediastinum. In this image, the thoracic duct is well visualized to the left of midline, in proximity to the azygos vein. The thoracic duct usually ascends on the right side, often crossing to the left of midline at approximately the level of the 5th thoracic vertebral body.

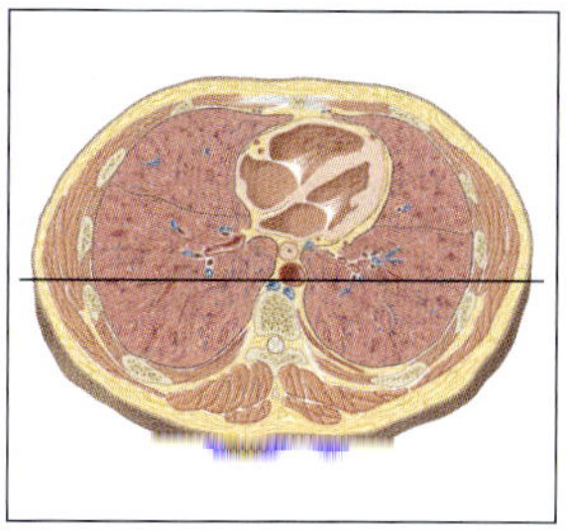

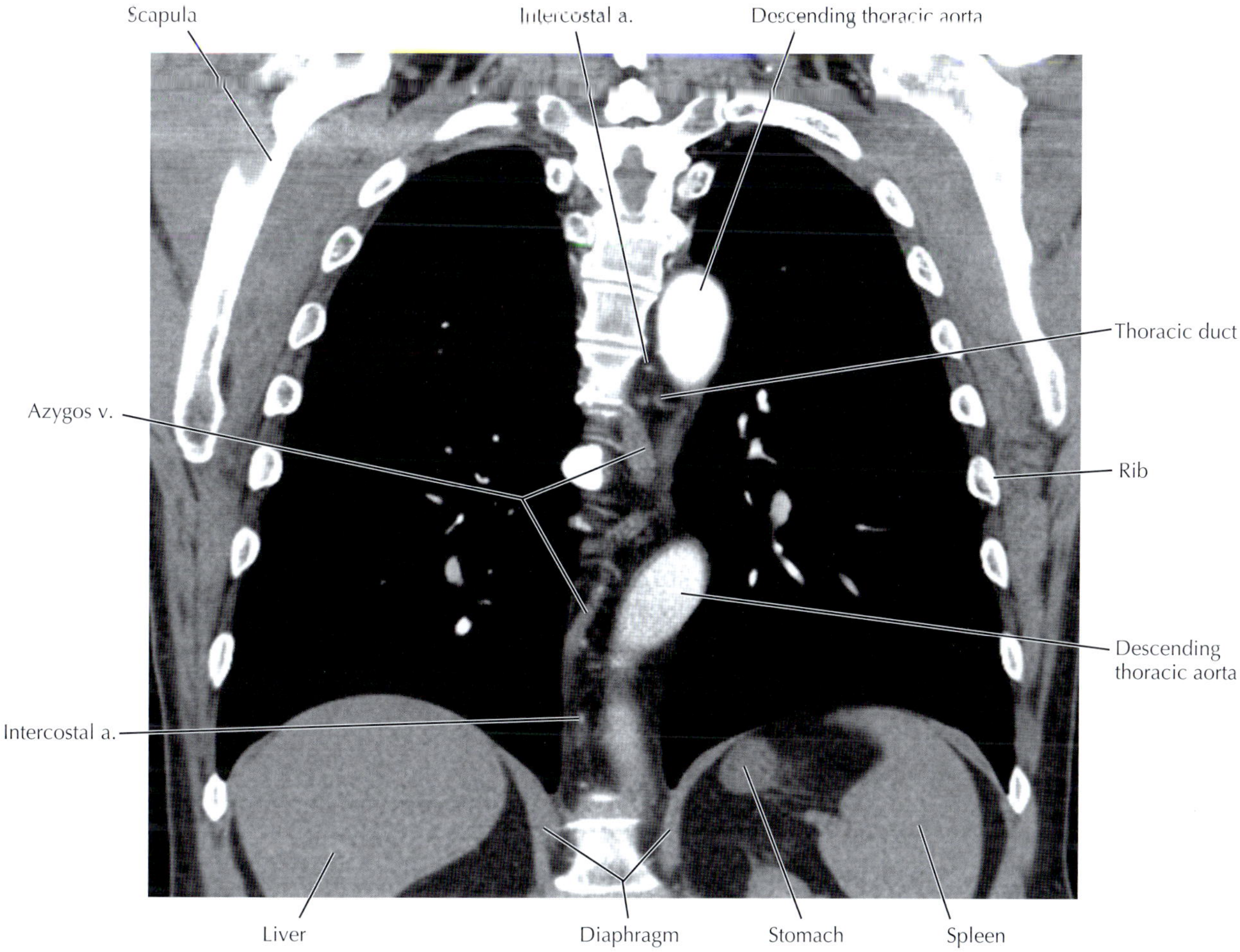
Scapula
Intercostal a.
Descending thoracic aorta
Thoracic duct
Azygos v.
Rib
Descending thoracic aorta
Intercostal a.
Liver
Diaphragm
Stomach
Spleen

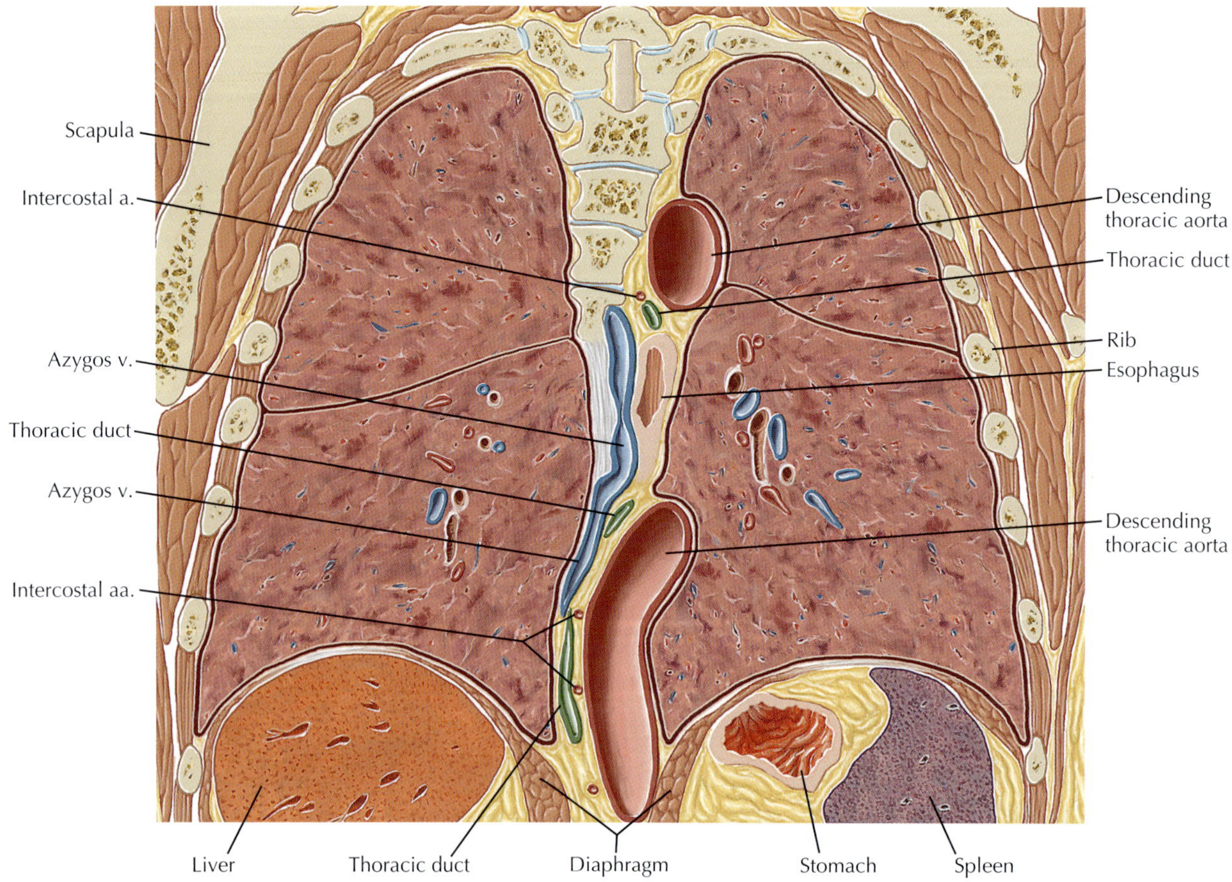

NORMAL ANATOMY

The thoracic duct is again seen coursing within the posterior mediastinum to the left of midline superiorly, in close proximity to the esophagus. Inferiorly, the thoracic duct is again visible medial to the azygos vein as it is crossing midline from right to left.

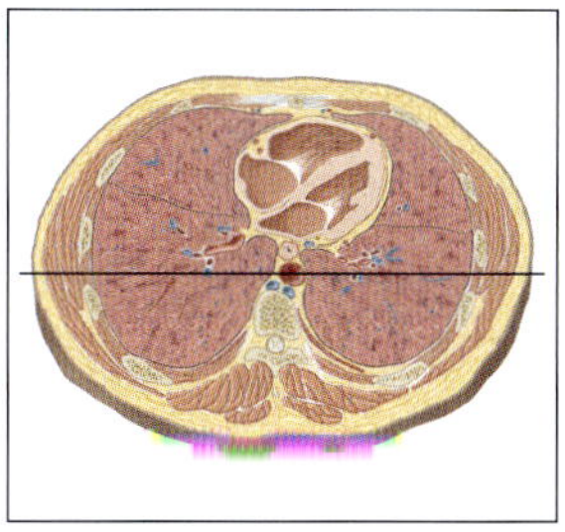

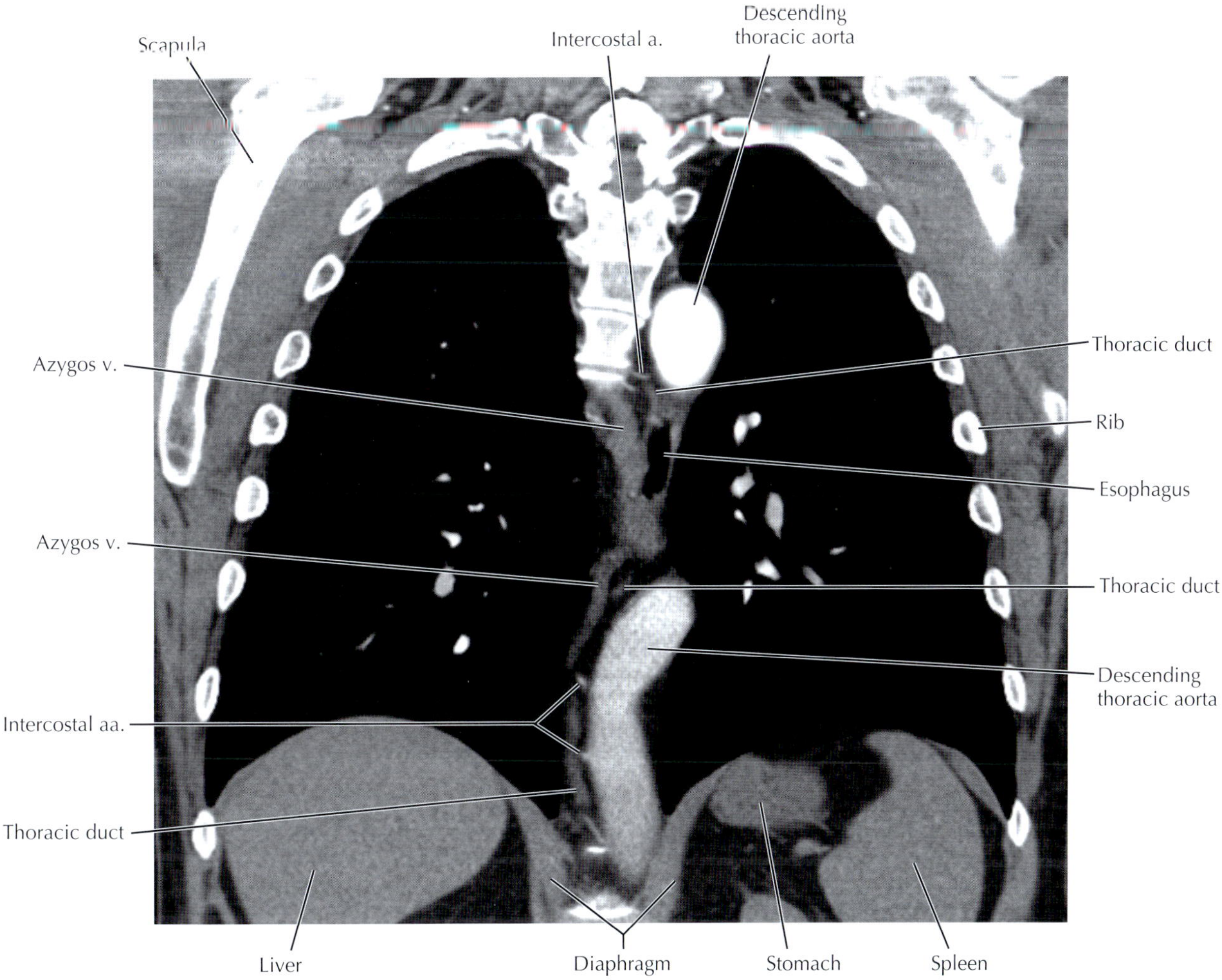
Scapula
Intercostal a.
Descending thoracic aorta
Thoracic duct
Azygos v.
Rib
Esophagus
Azygos v.
Thoracic duct
Descending thoracic aorta
Intercostal aa.
Thoracic duct
Liver
Diaphragm
Stomach
Spleen

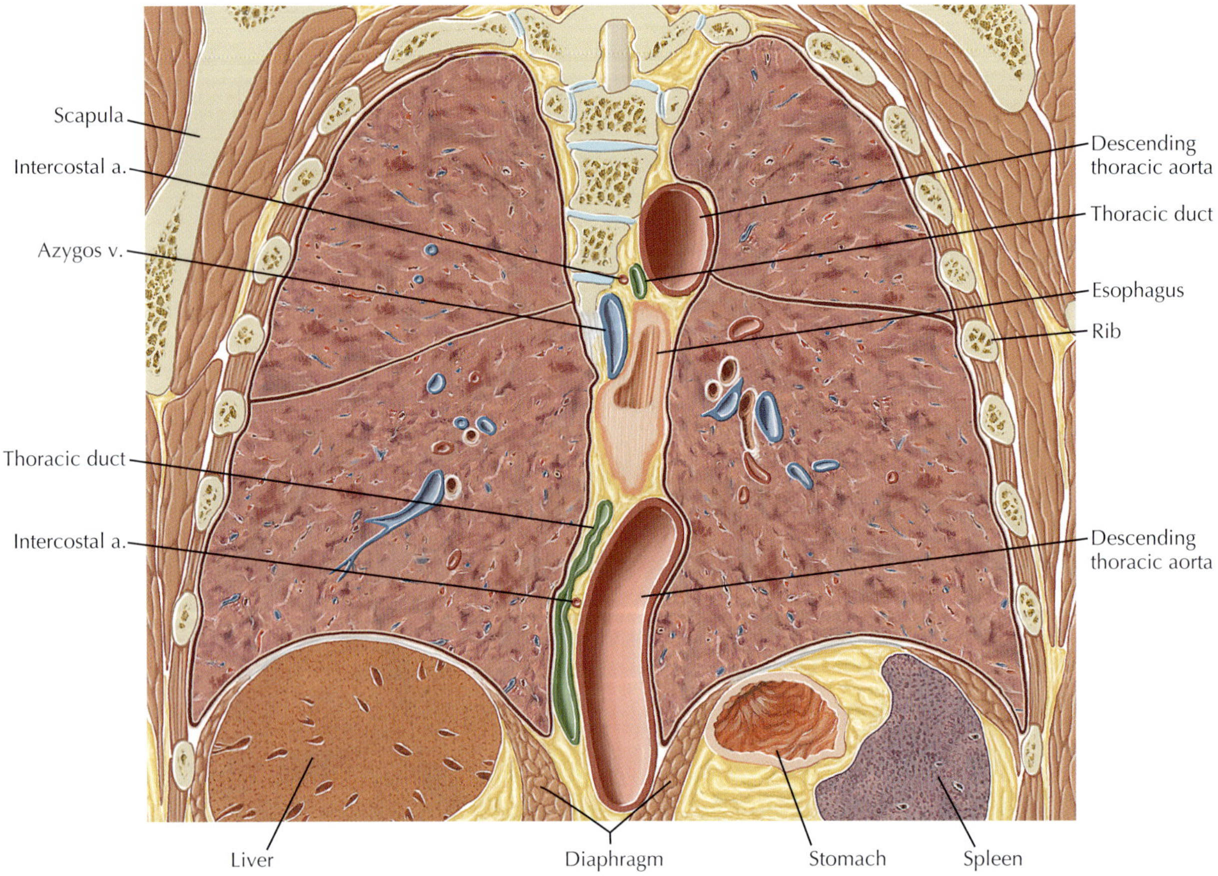

NORMAL ANATOMY

Slightly anterior to the two preceding views, the thoracic duct is shown on both sides of midline, to the right inferiorly and to the left superiorly.

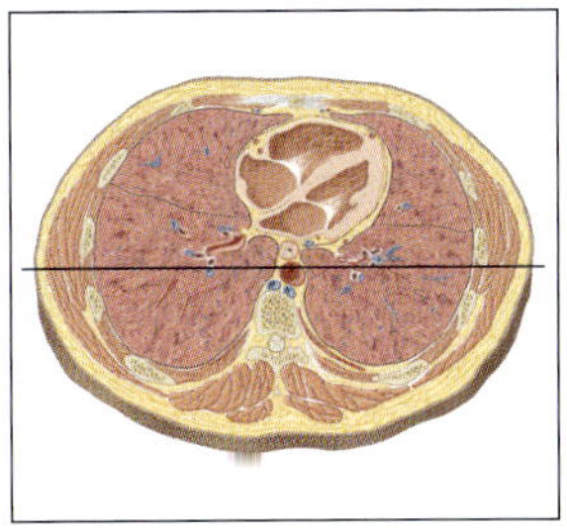

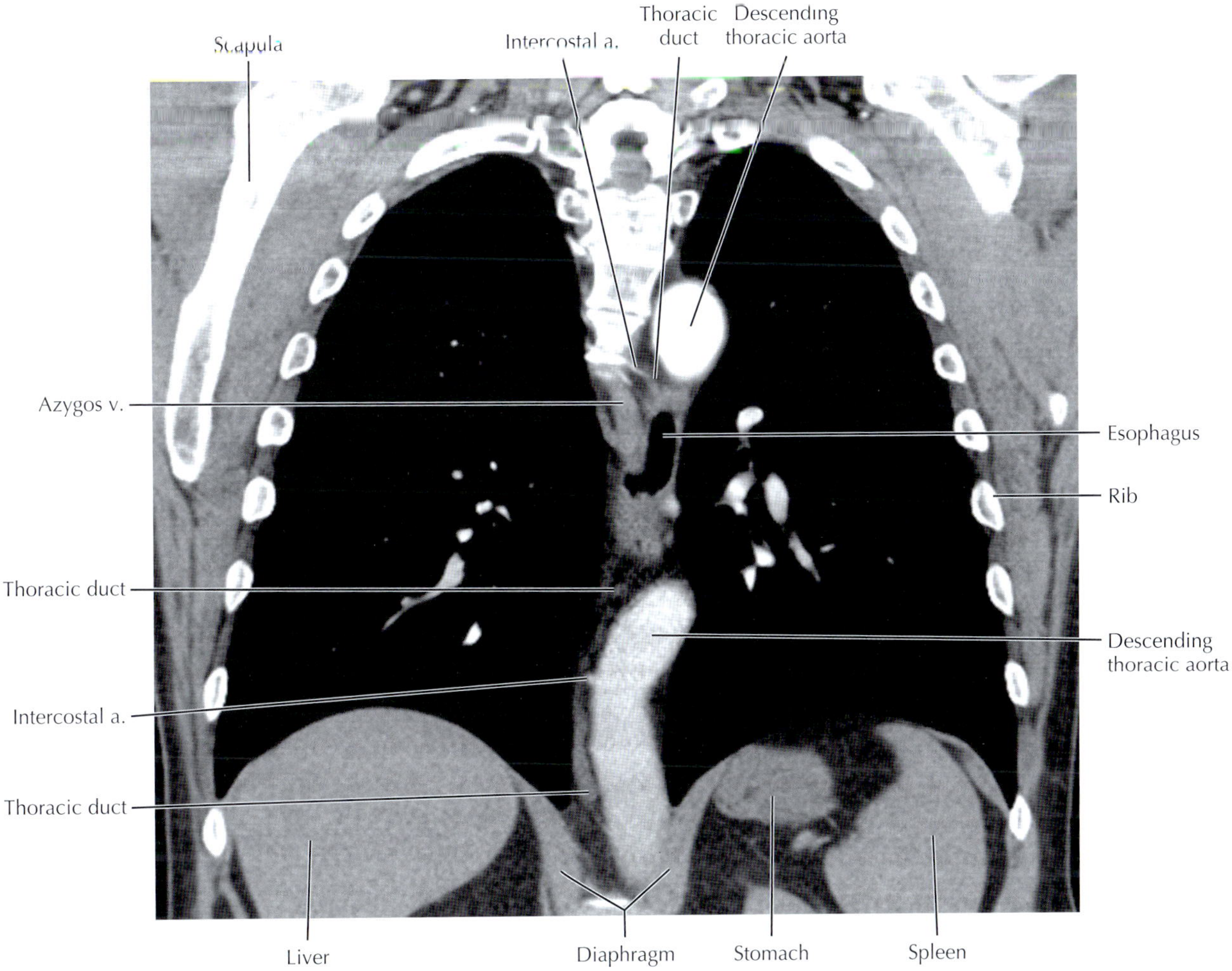
Scapula
Intercostal a.
Thoracic duct
Descending thoracic aorta
Azygos v.
Esophagus
Rib
Thoracic duct
Descending thoracic aorta
Intercostal a.
Thoracic duct
Liver
Diaphragm
Stomach
Spleen

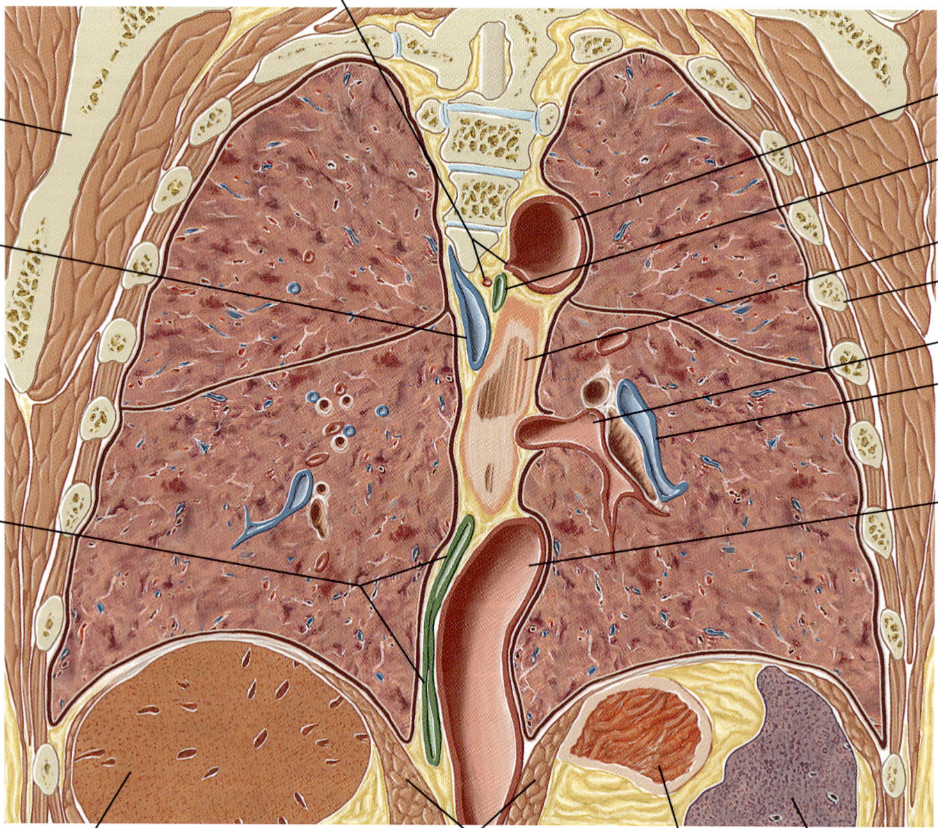

NORMAL ANATOMY

Still slightly more anteriorly located than preceding views, portions of the central pulmonary arteries and veins are shown. At this level, the thoracic duct is seen inferiorly, to the right of midline, adjacent to the descending thoracic aorta.

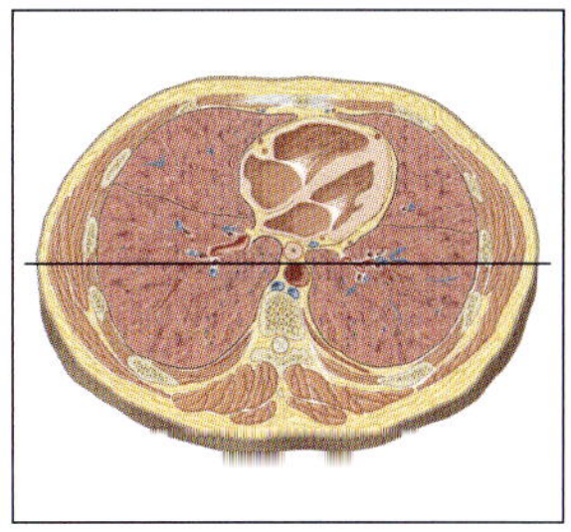

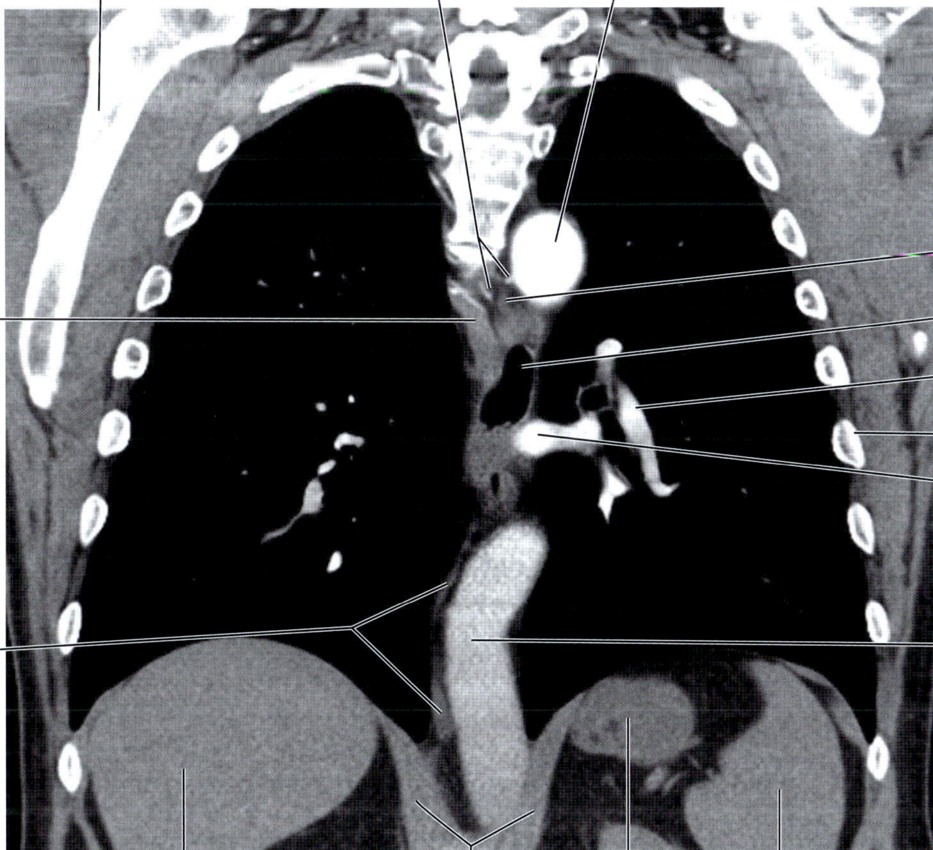
Scapula
Intercostal aa.
Descending thoracic aorta
Thoracic duct
Azygos v.
Esophagus
Pulmonary a.
Rib
Pulmonary v.
Thoracic duct
Descending thoracic aorta
Liver
Diaphragm
Stomach
Spleen

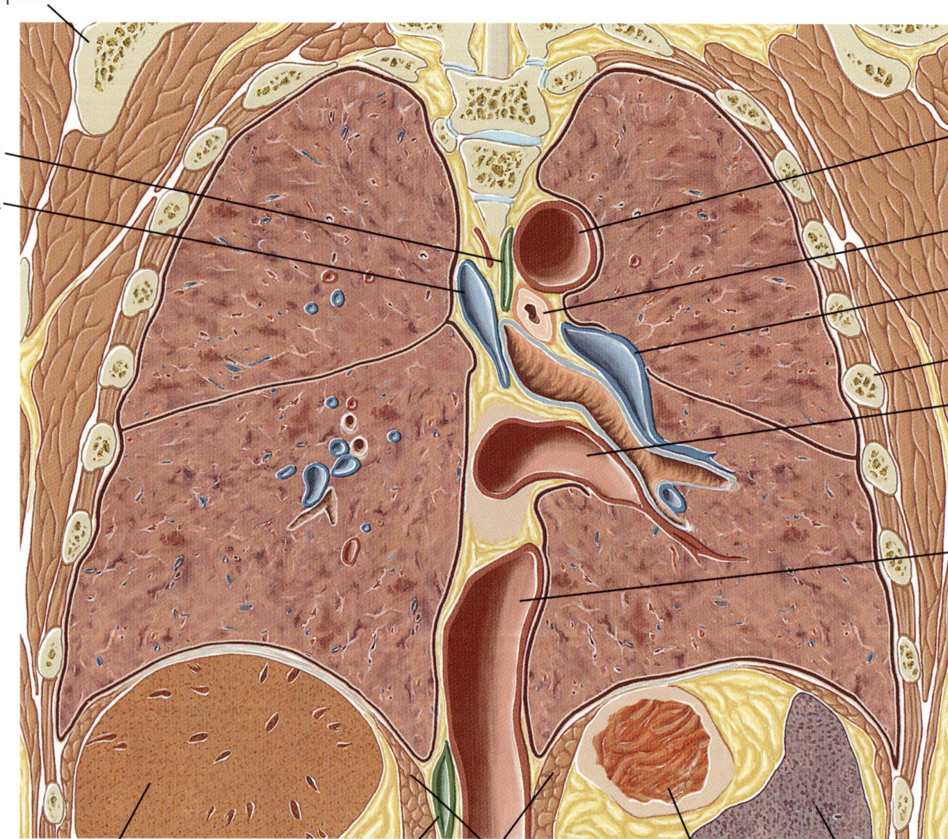

NORMAL ANATOMY

The left superior pulmonary vein is shown as it enters the left atrium. The cisterna chyli is now visible posteriorly on the right at the thoracoabdominal junction. The cranial portion of the thoracic duct is visible to the left of midline, adjacent to the esophagus and thoracic aorta.

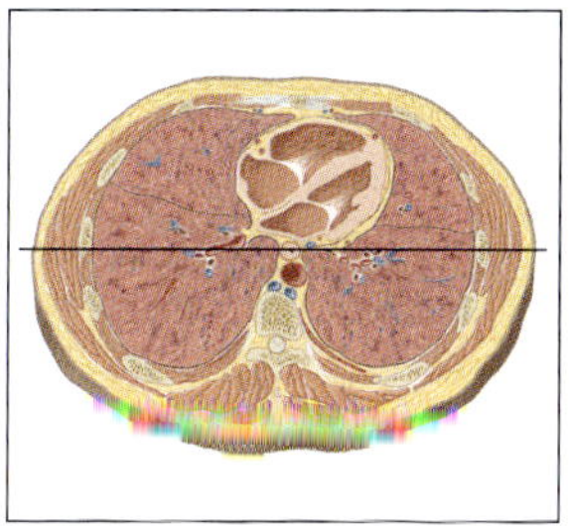

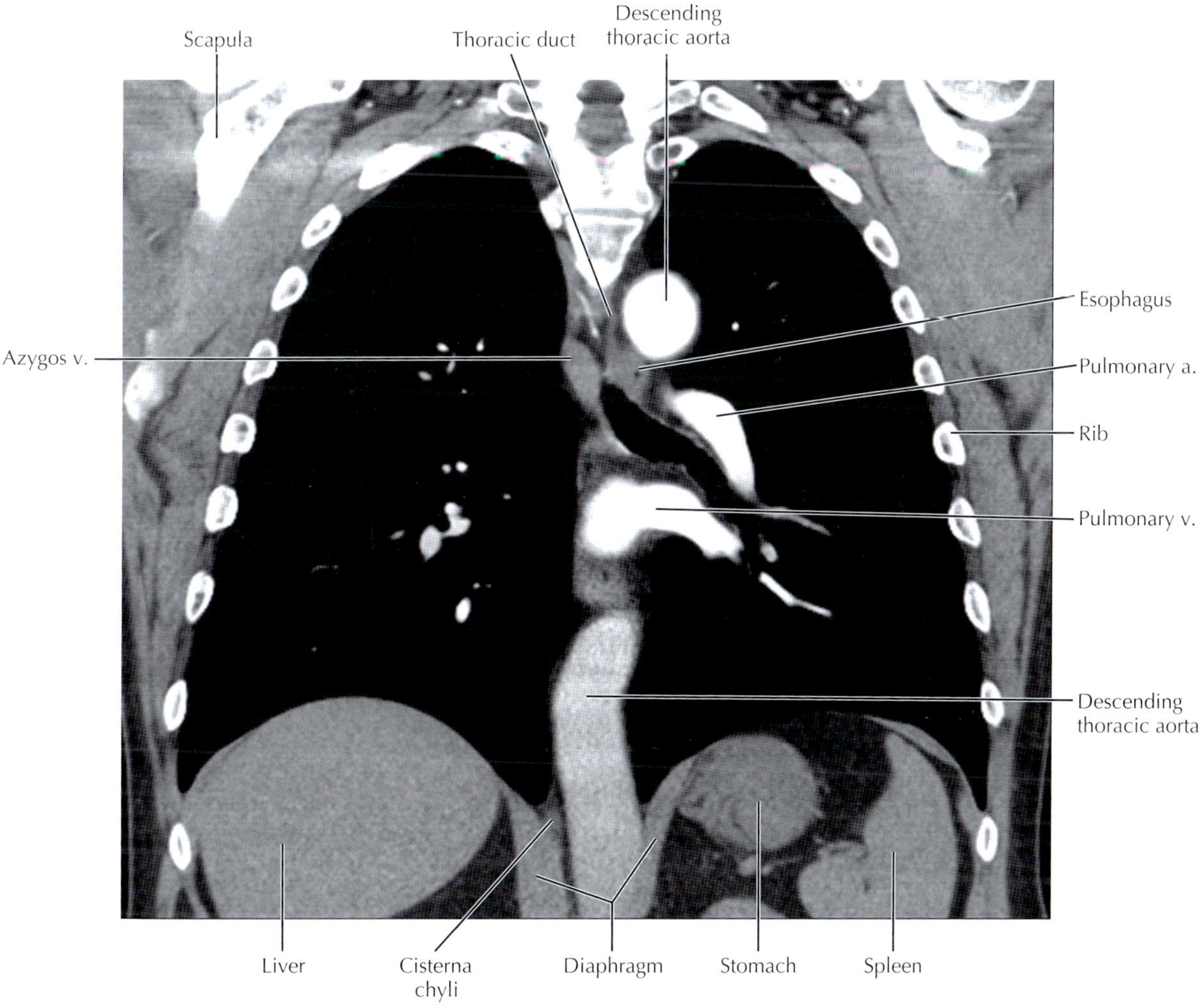
Scapula
Thoracic duct
Descending thoracic aorta
Esophagus
Azygos v.
Pulmonary a.
Rib
Pulmonary v.
Descending thoracic aorta
Liver
Cisterna chyli
Diaphragm
Stomach
Spleen

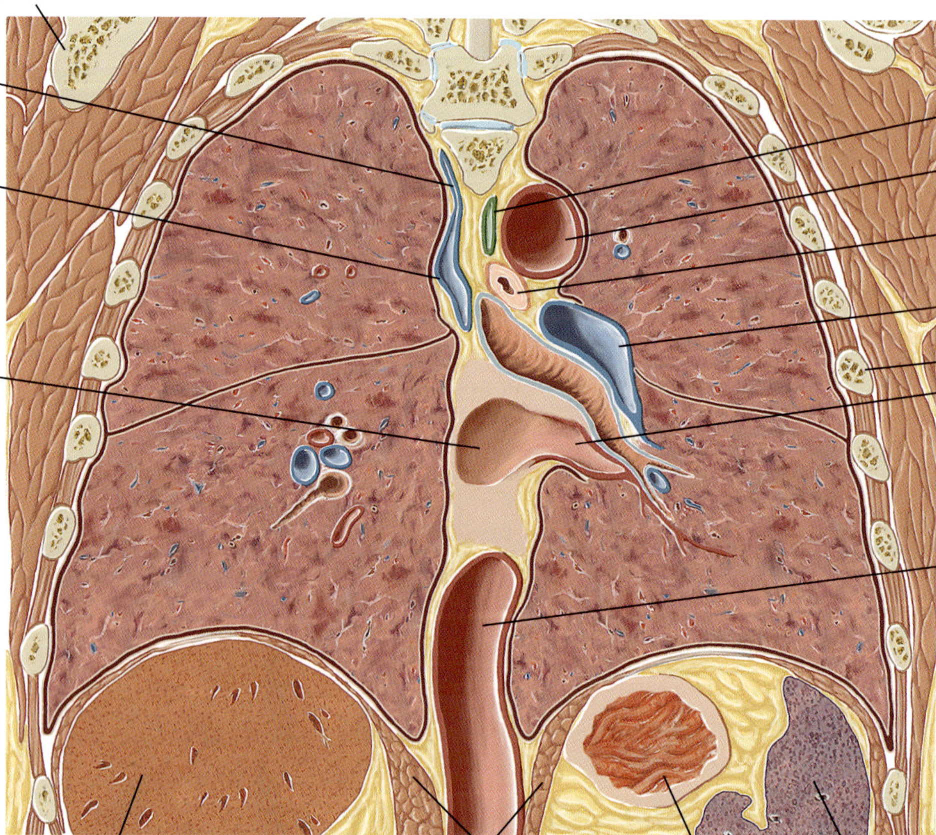

NORMAL ANATOMY

The cranial portion of the thoracic duct is shown in close proximity to the esophagus. The right superior intercostal vein, which drains the 2nd, 3rd, and 4th posterior intercostal veins, can be seen draining into the azygos vein.

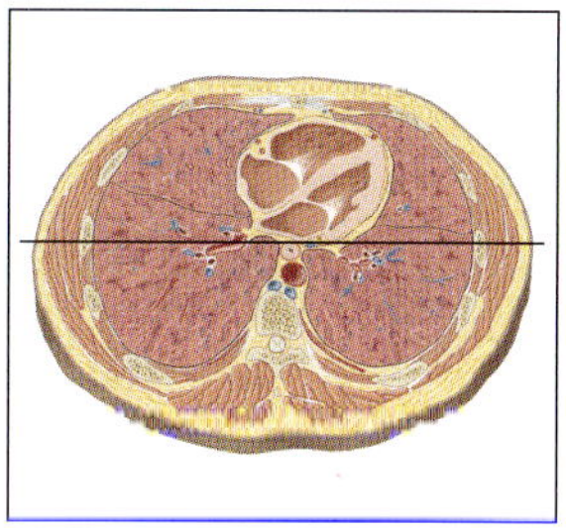

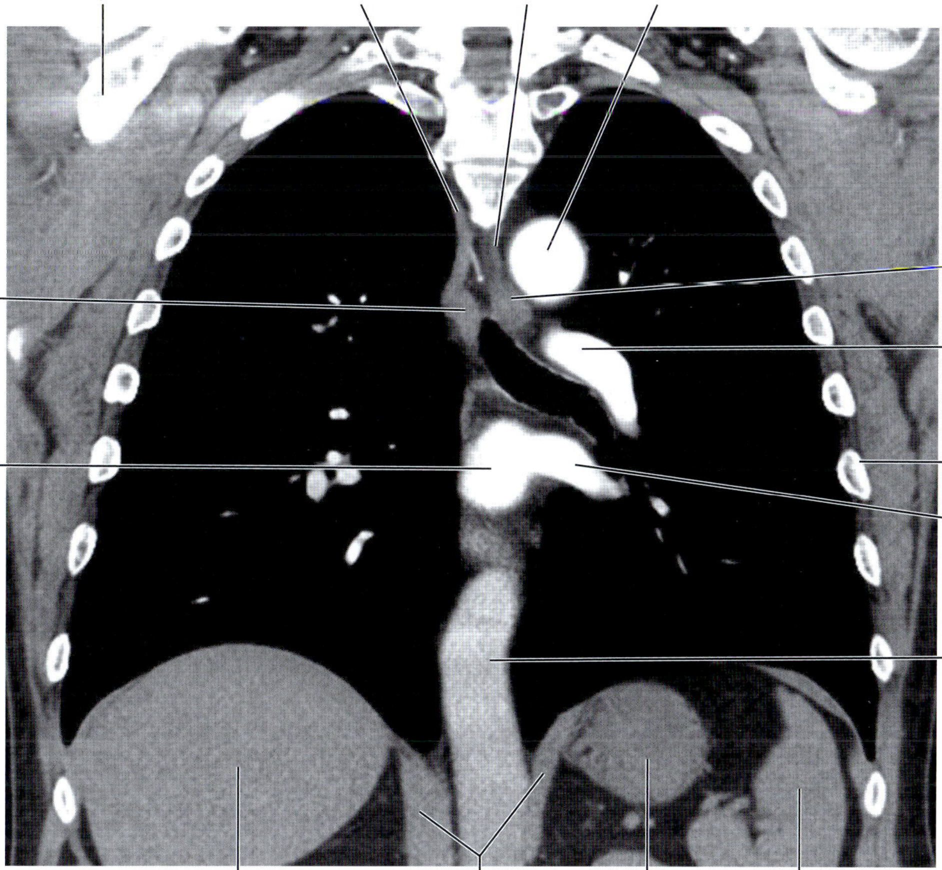
Scapula
Right superior intercostal v.
Thoracic duct
Descending thoracic aorta
Esophagus
Azygos v.
Pulmonary a.
Left atrium
Rib
Pulmonary v.
Descending thoracic aorta
Liver
Diaphragm
Stomach
Spleen

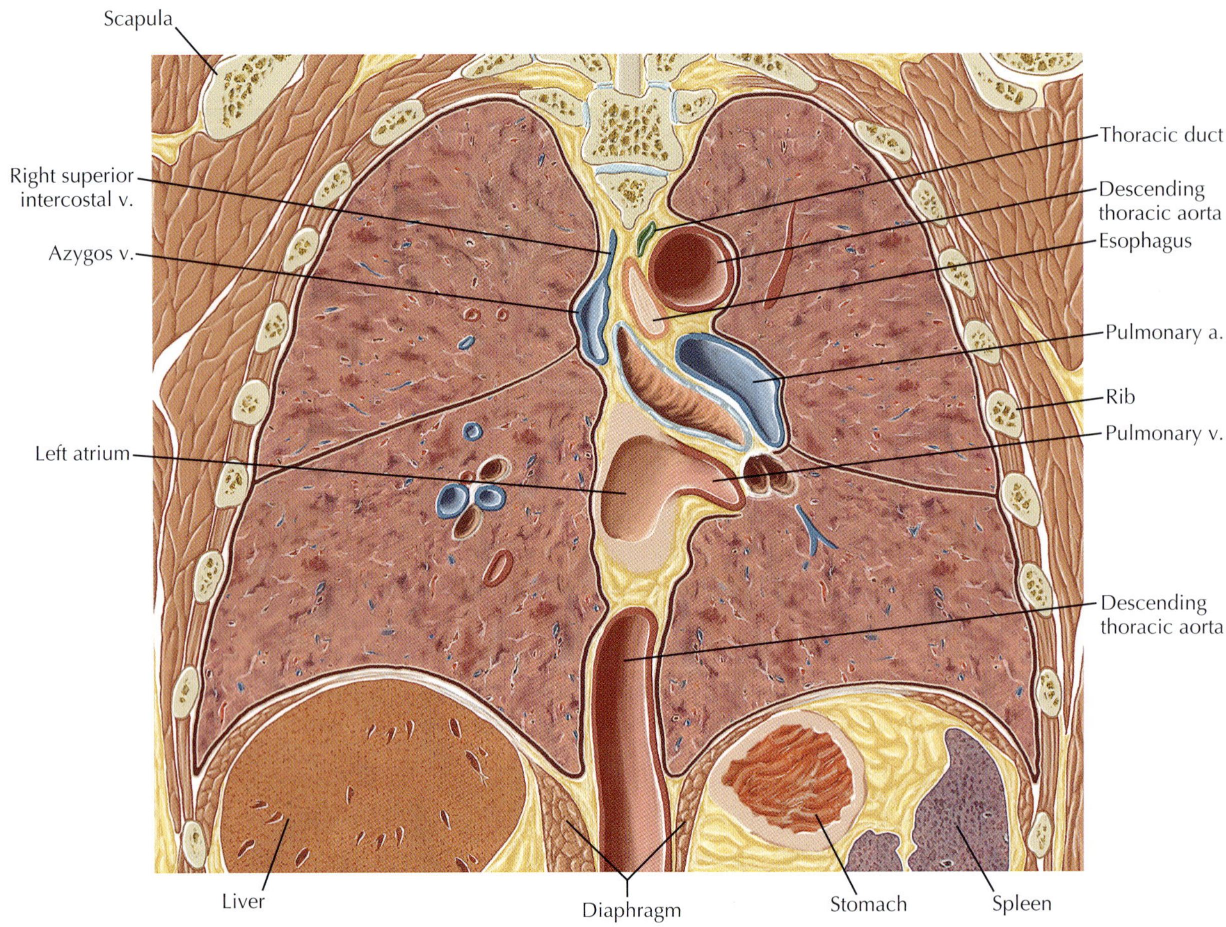

NORMAL ANATOMY

Again, the cranial portion of the thoracic duct is shown in close proximity to the esophagus, beginning to extend cranial to the thoracic aortic arch. The right superior intercostal vein is again seen draining into the azygos vein.

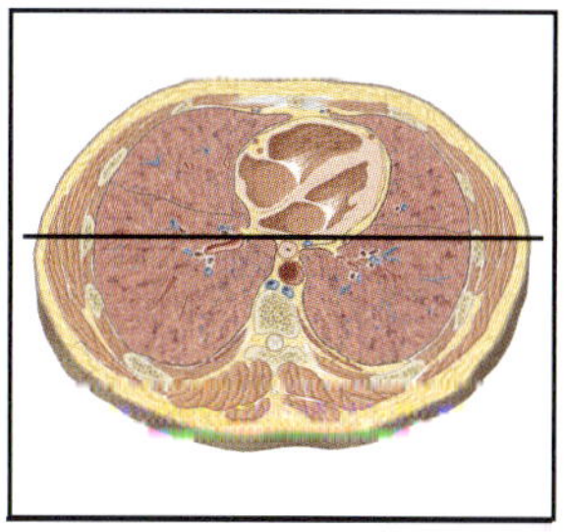

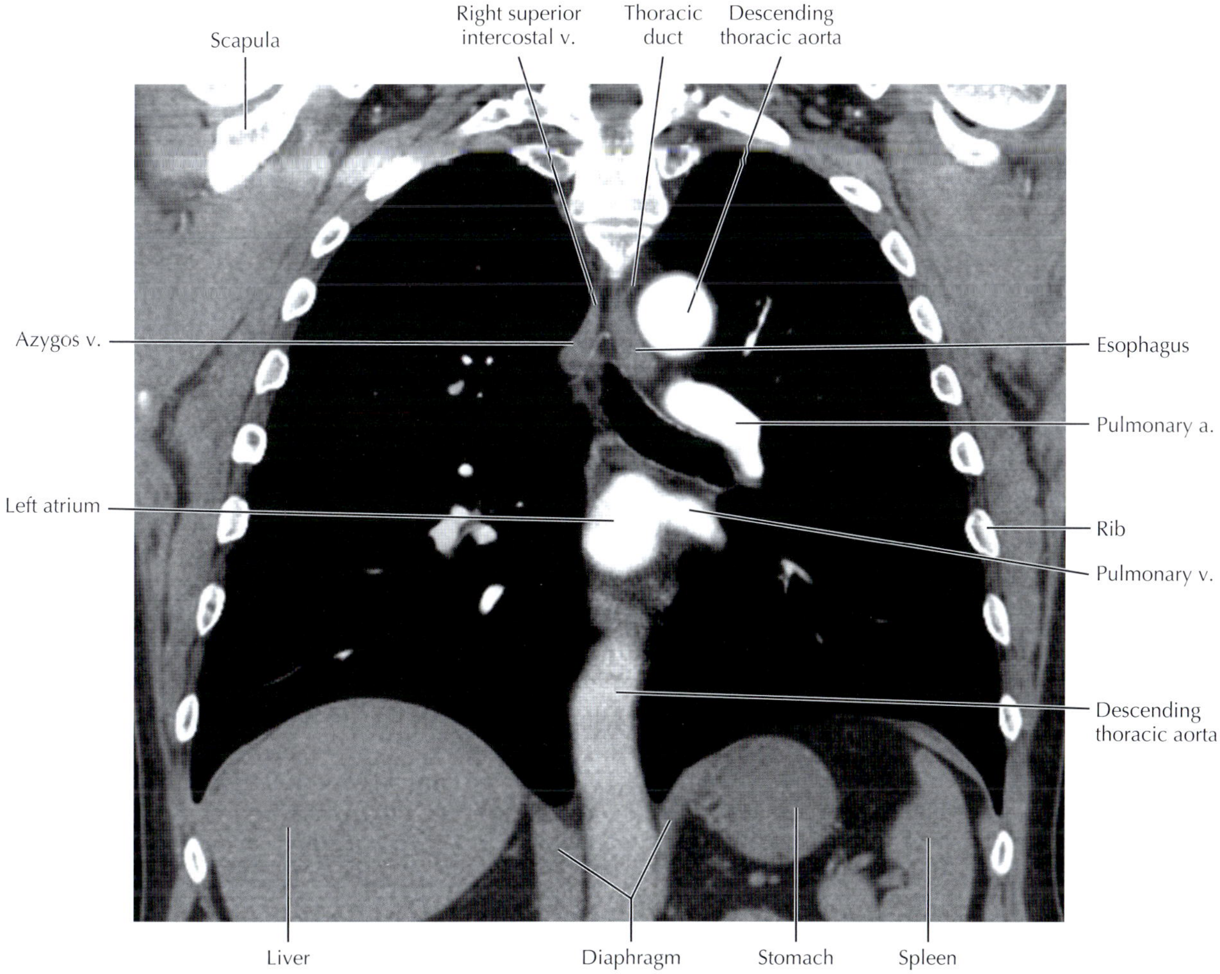
Scapula
Right superior intercostal v.
Thoracic duct
Descending thoracic aorta
Azygos v.
Esophagus
Pulmonary a.
Left atrium
Rib
Pulmonary v.
Descending thoracic aorta
Liver
Diaphragm
Stomach
Spleen

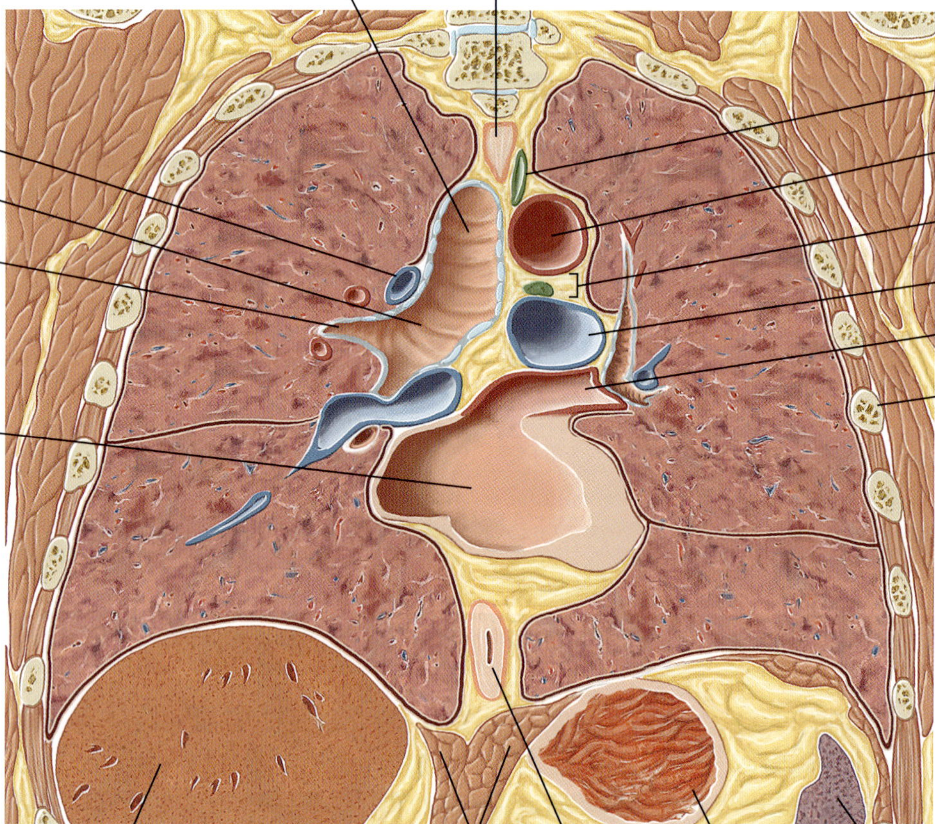

NORMAL ANATOMY

This view, anteriorly located relative to preceding views, shows the cranial portion of the thoracic duct adjacent to the esophagus, cranial to the thoracic aortic arch.

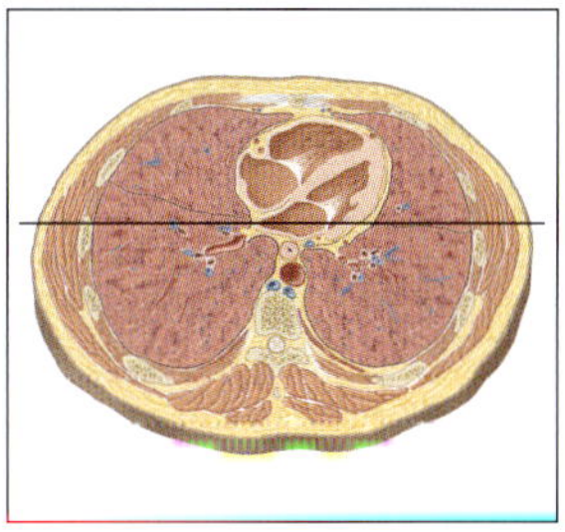

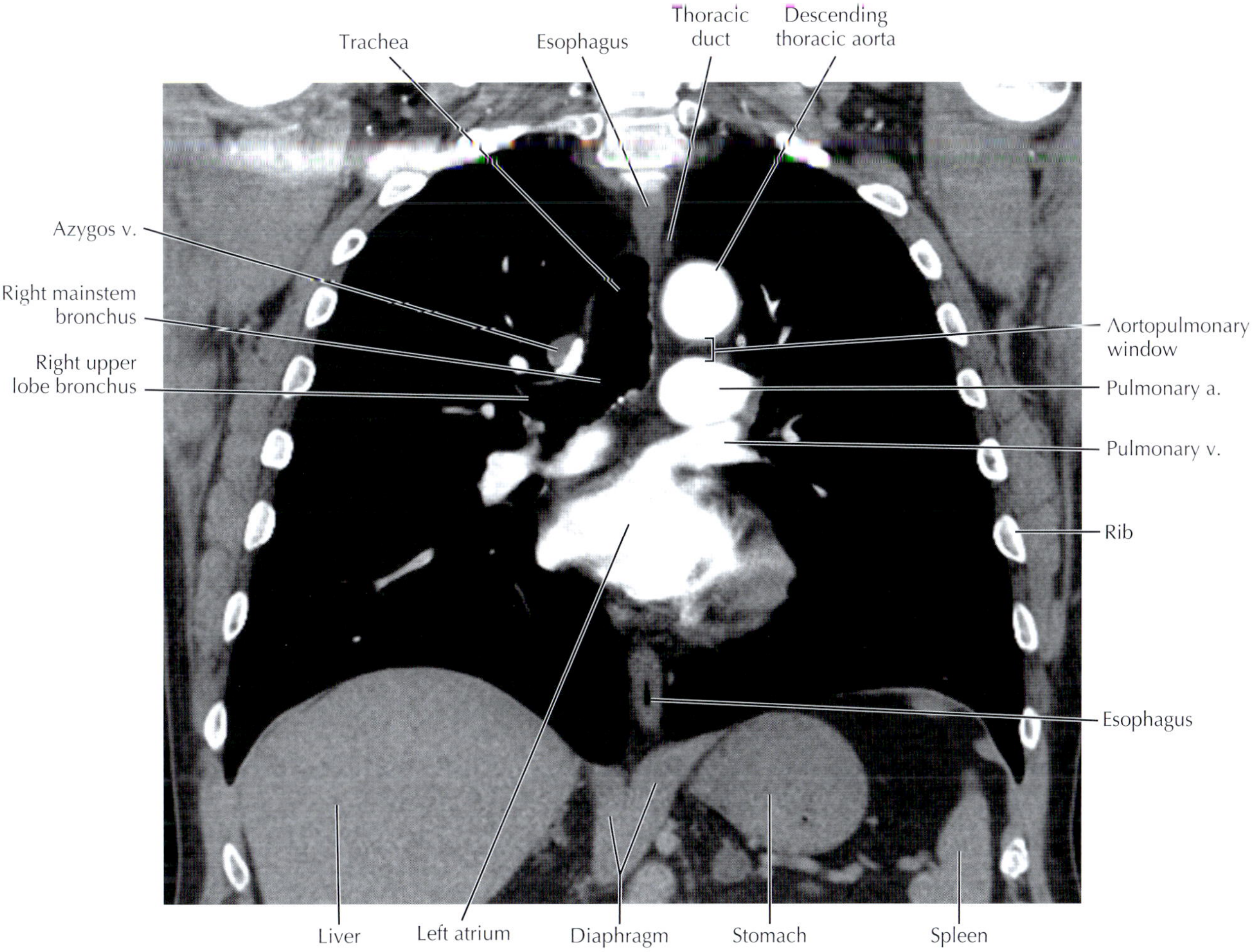
Trachea
Esophagus
Thoracic duct
Descending thoracic aorta
Azygos v.
Right mainstem bronchus
Right upper lobe bronchus
Aortopulmonary window
Pulmonary a.
Pulmonary v.
Rib
Esophagus
Liver
Left atrium
Diaphragm
Stomach
Spleen

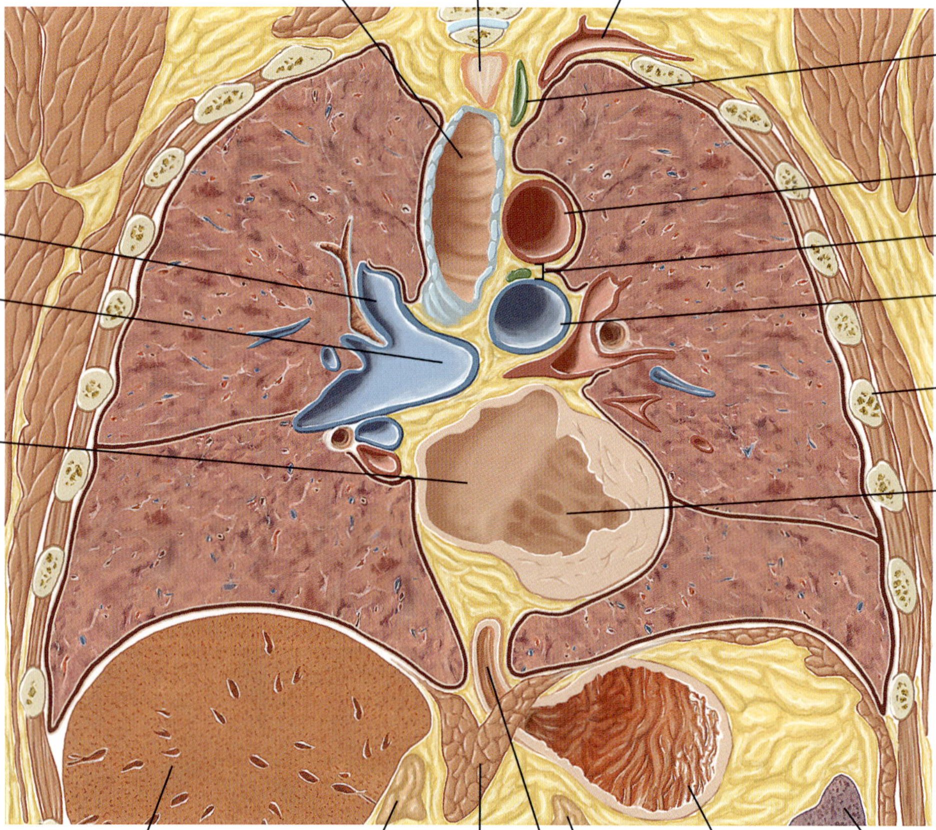

NORMAL ANATOMY

The most anteriorly positioned of the preceding views, detailing the course of the thoracic duct, shows the thoracic duct extending cranially toward the root of the neck, prior to entry into the junction of the left subclavian and internal jugular veins.

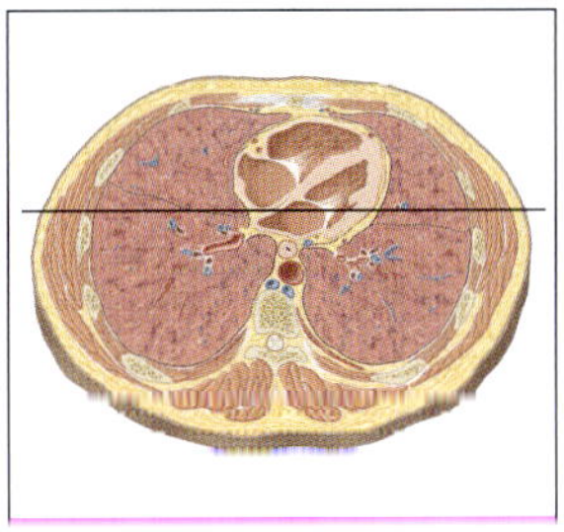

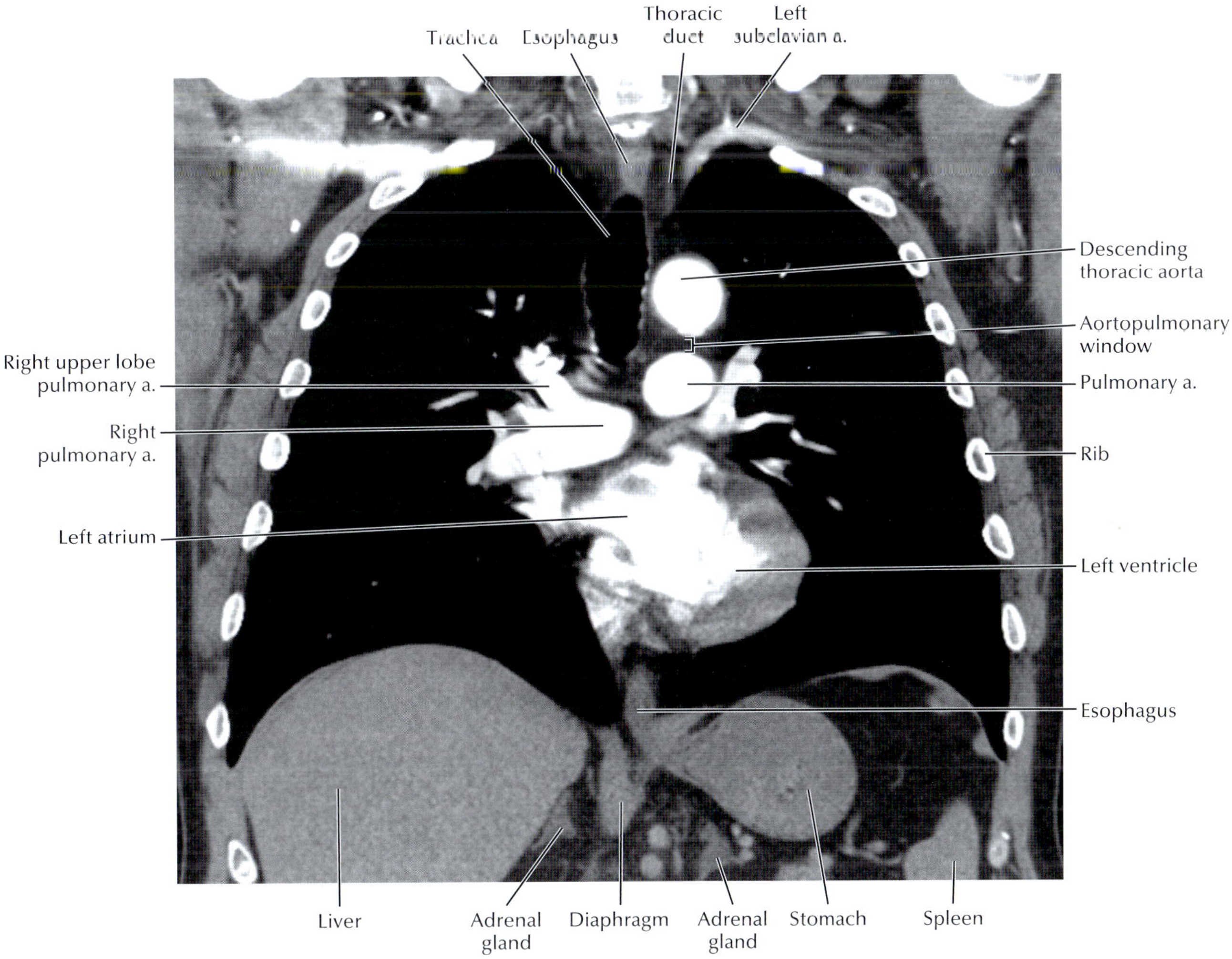
Trachea
Esophagus
Thoracic duct
Left subclavian a.
Descending thoracic aorta
Aortopulmonary window
Right upper lobe pulmonary a.
Pulmonary a.
Right pulmonary a.
Rib
Left atrium
Left ventricle
Esophagus
Liver
Adrenal gland
Diaphragm
Adrenal gland
Stomach
Spleen

Chapter 6 VENOUS ANATOMY AND VARIANTS

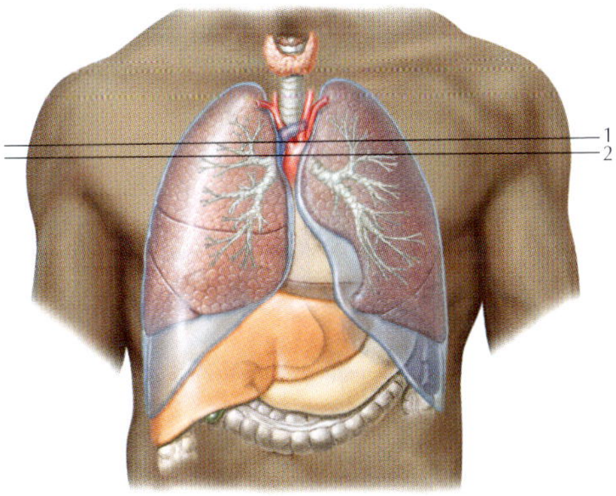

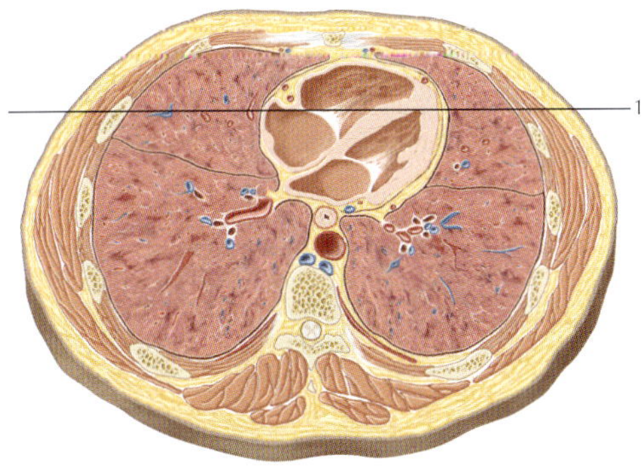

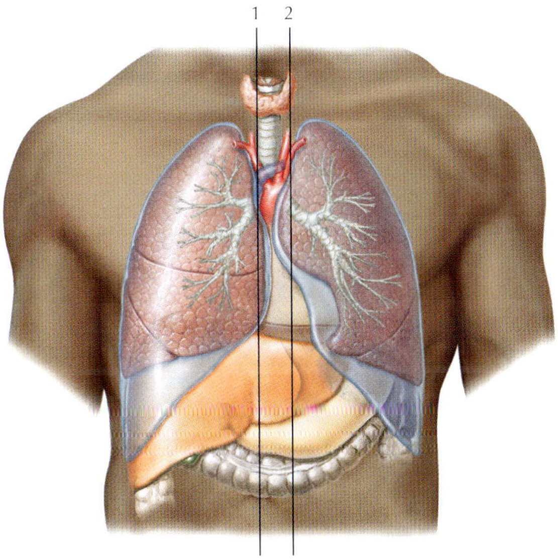

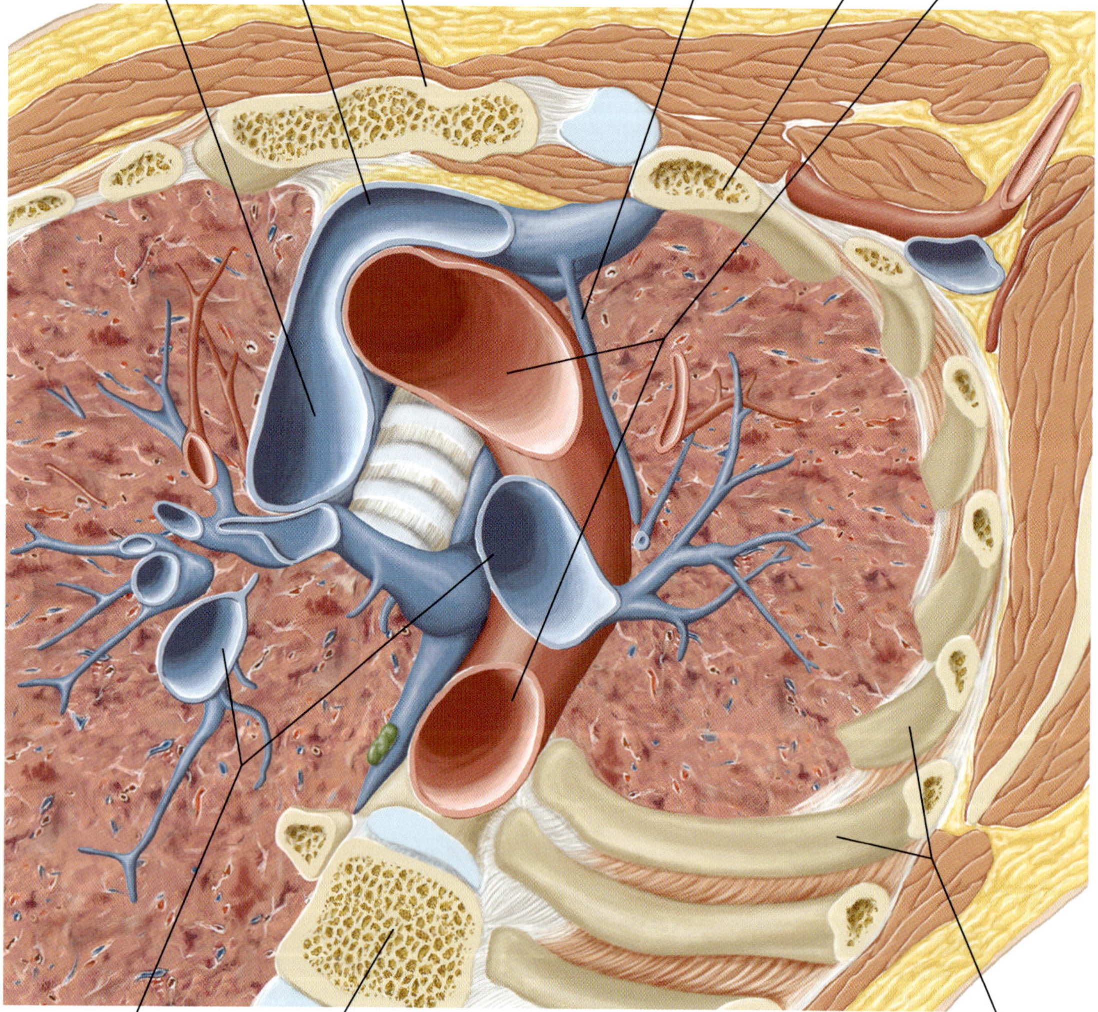

NORMAL VARIANT

An axial volume rendered image of the thorax showing the normal *left superior intercostal vein* coursing along the lateral aspect of the aortic arch, emptying into the left brachiocephalic vein. The left superior intercostal vein typically drains the 2nd, 3rd, and 4th intercostal veins on the left, and connects the left brachiocephalic and accessory hemiazygos veins. The left superior intercostal vein provides a collateral pathway for blood flow from the upper extremities and trunk to the heart in the setting of venous stenosis or obstruction.

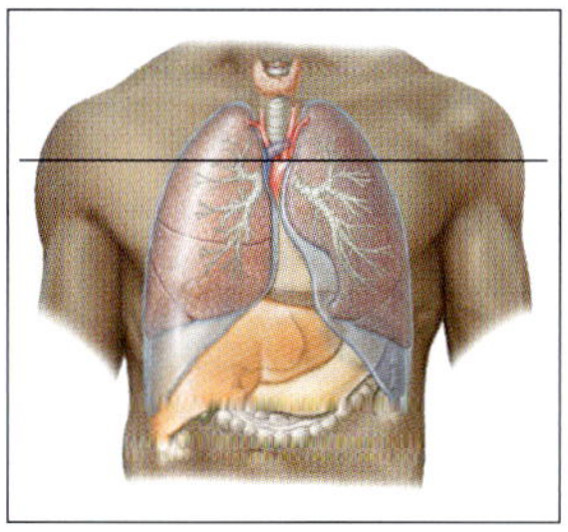

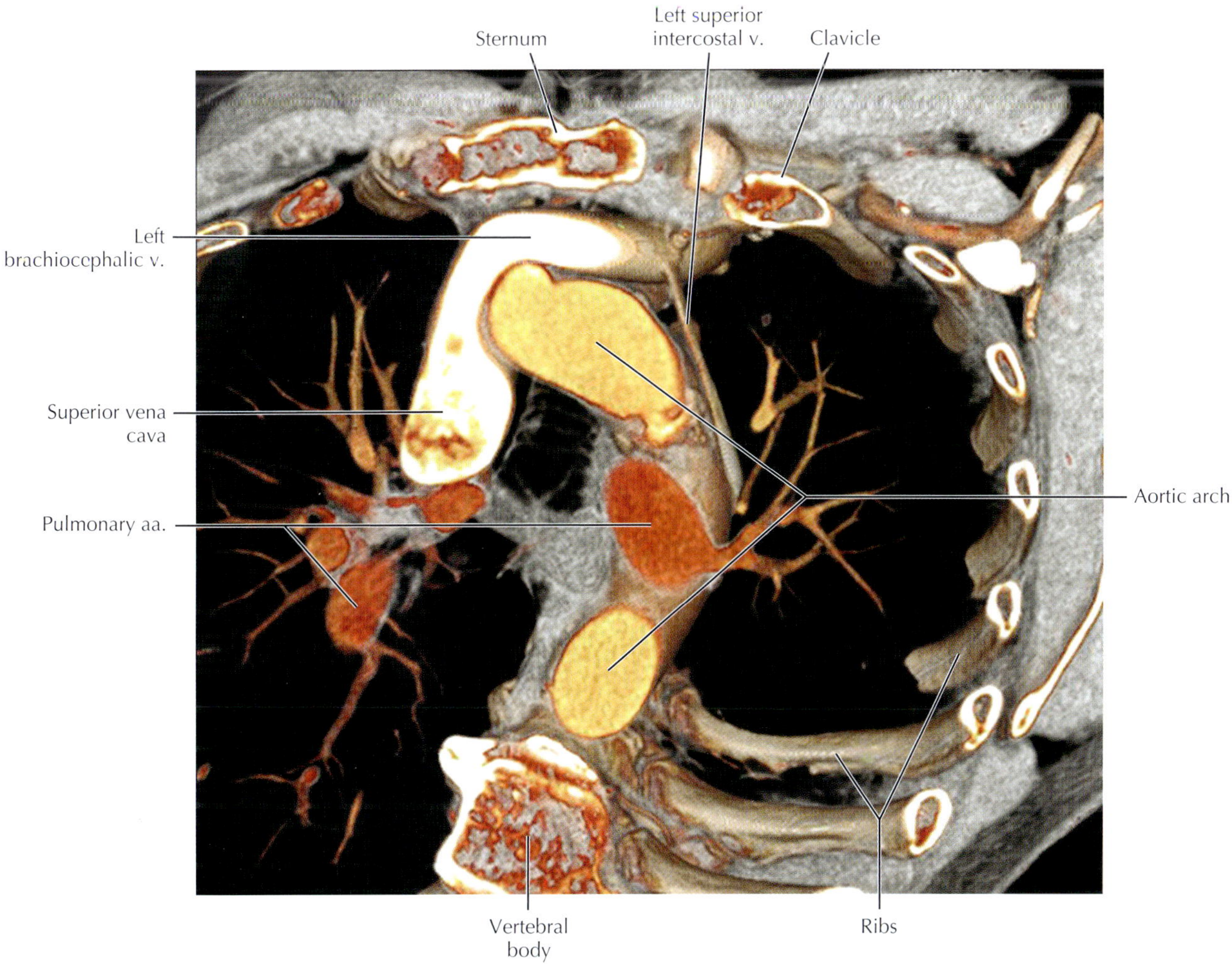
Sternum
Left superior intercostal v.
Clavicle
Left brachiocephalic v.
Superior vena cava
Pulmonary aa.
Aortic arch
Vertebral body
Ribs

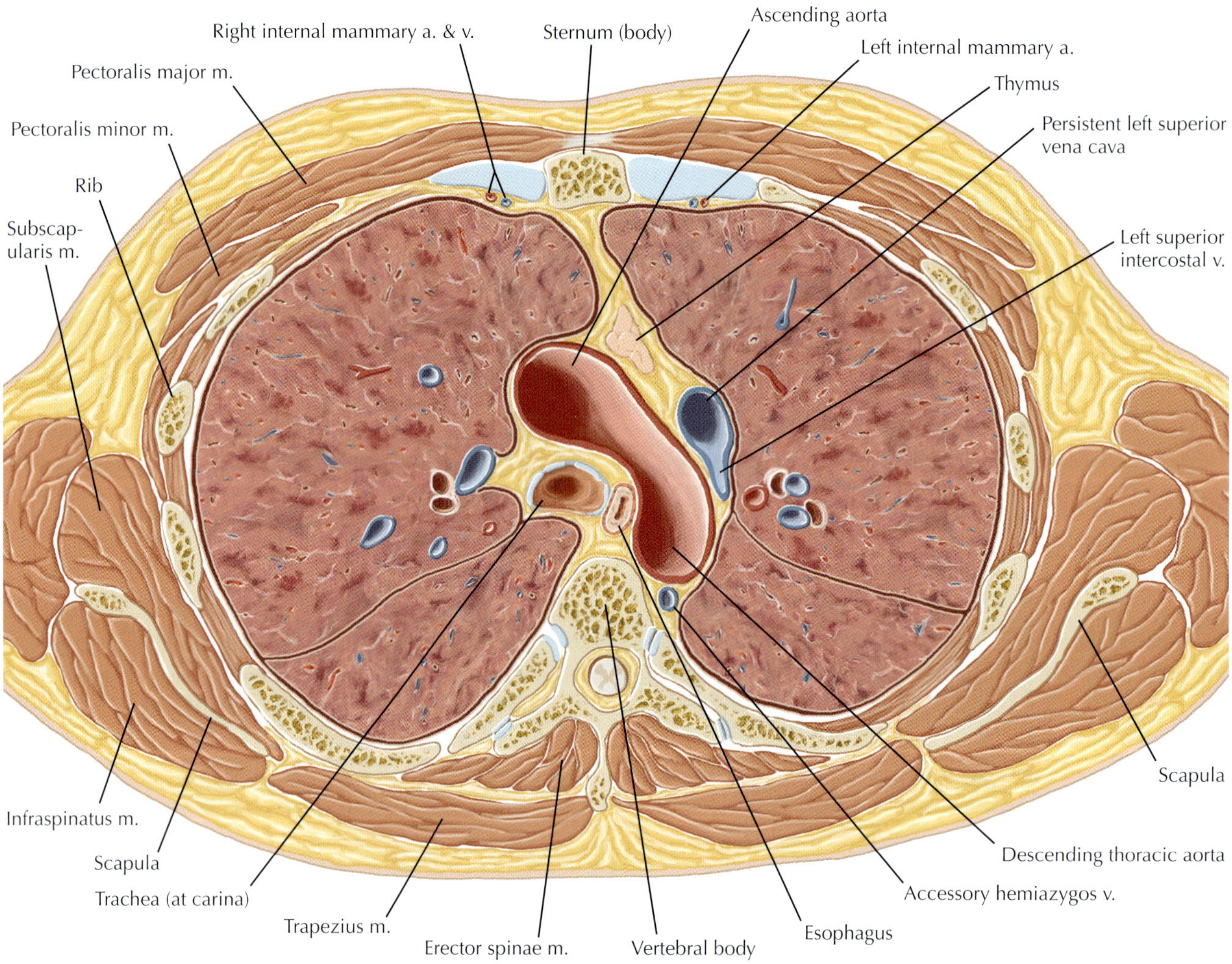

NORMAL VARIANT

This scan, performed at the caudal surface of the aortic arch, shows a common venous anomaly affecting the thorax—the *persistent left superior vena cava*. The prevalence of this anomaly is estimated at nearly 0.3% of the general population, and it may occasionally be associated with other congenital cardiovascular anomalies. In its most common form, the persistent left superior vena cava forms at the confluence of the left internal jugular and subclavian veins and descends along the left aspect of the aortic arch and mediastinum, passing anterior to the left hilum, crossing the posterior wall of the left atrium, eventually emptying into the coronary sinus. Rarely, the persistent left superior vena cava empties into the left atrium, creating a right-to-left shunt. The enhanced persistent left superior vena cava is shown as it passes lateral to the aortic arch.

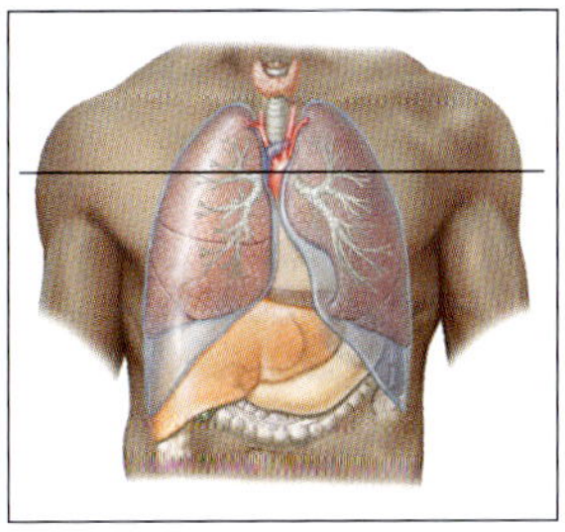

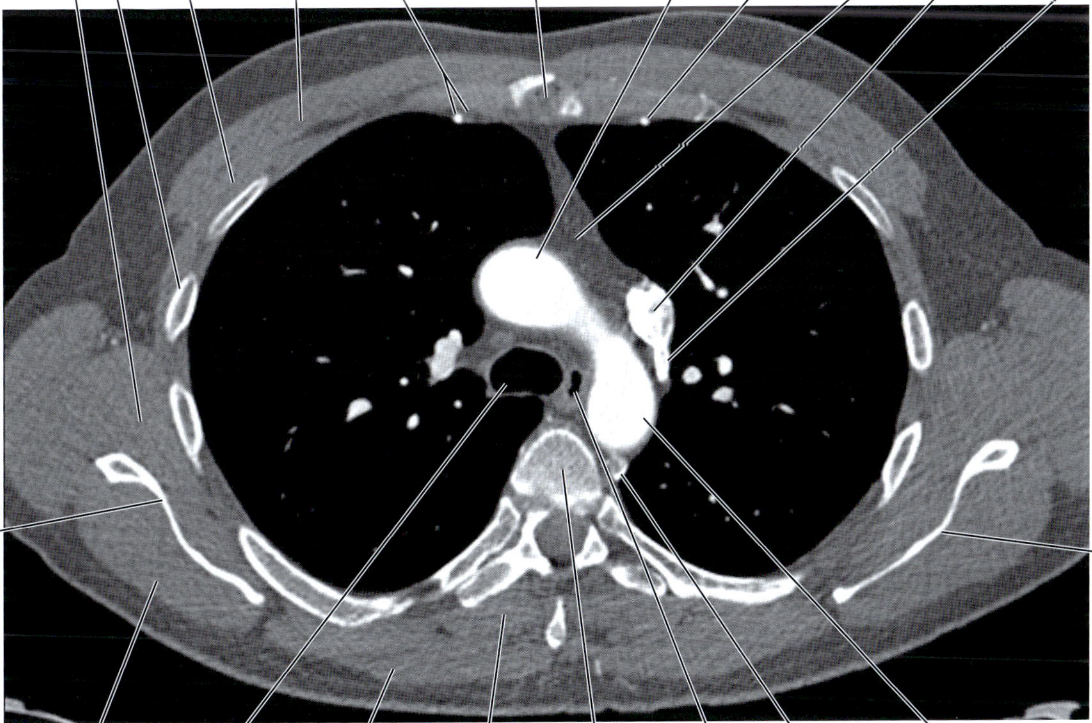
Subscapularis m.
Rib
Pectoralis minor m.
Pectoralis major m.
Right internal mammary a. & v.
Sternomanubrial junction
Ascending aorta
Left internal mammary a.
Thymus
Persistent left superior vena cava
Left superior intercostal v.
Scapula
Scapula
Infraspinatus m.
Trachea (at carina)
Trapezius m.
Erector spinae m.
Vertebral body
Esophagus
Accessory hemiazygos v.
Descending thoracic aorta

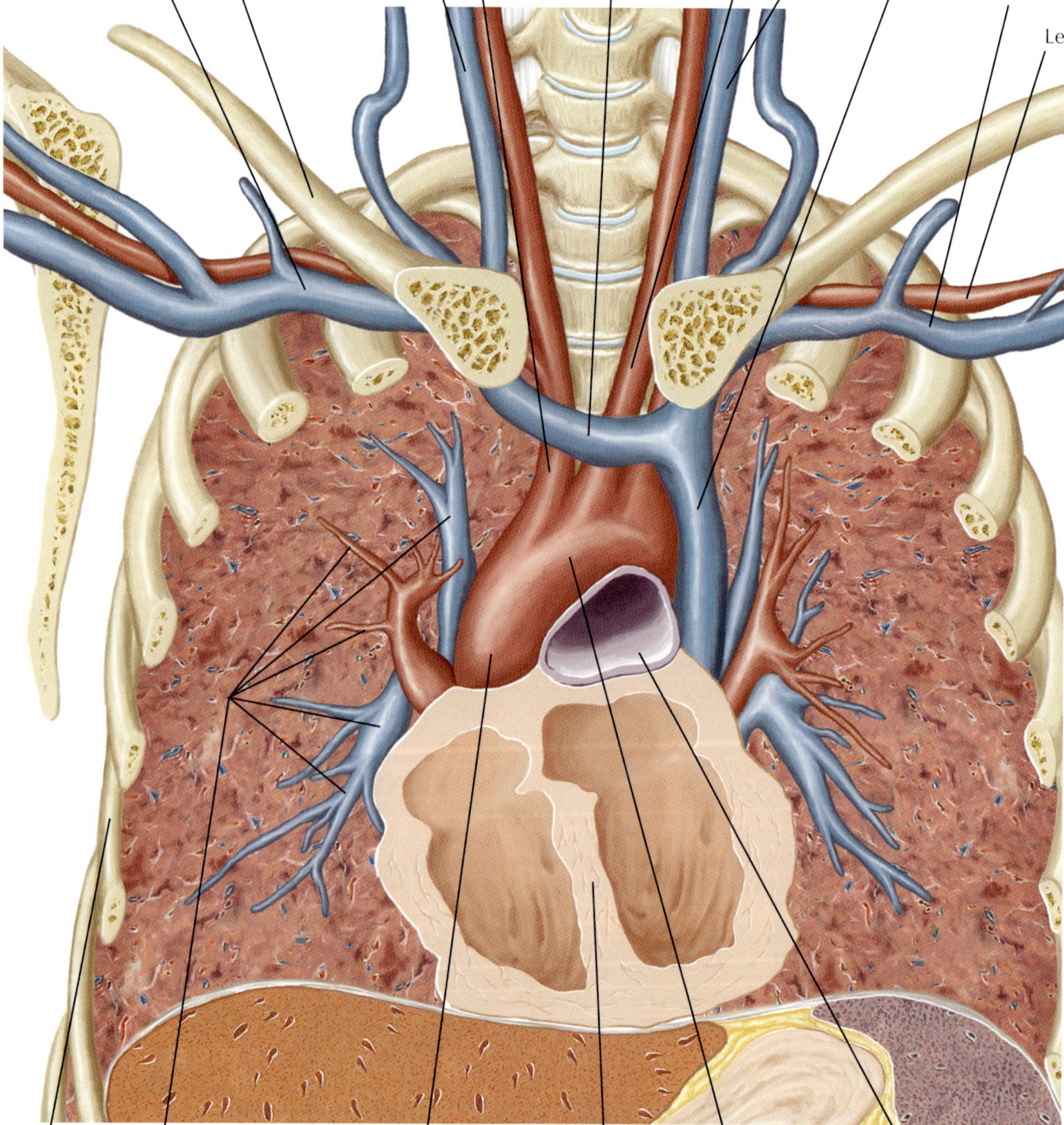

NORMAL VARIANT

A coronal volume rendered image of the thorax, providing a different perspective of the *persistent left superior vena cava* that was shown above. The origin of persistent left superior vena cava at the confluence of the left subclavian and internal jugular veins is clearly shown, as well as the course of this venous anomaly as it descends along the left aspect of the aortic arch and mediastinum, eventually emptying into the coronary sinus.

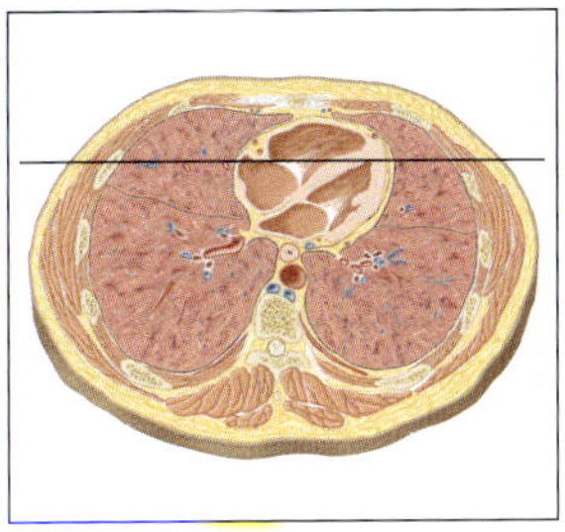

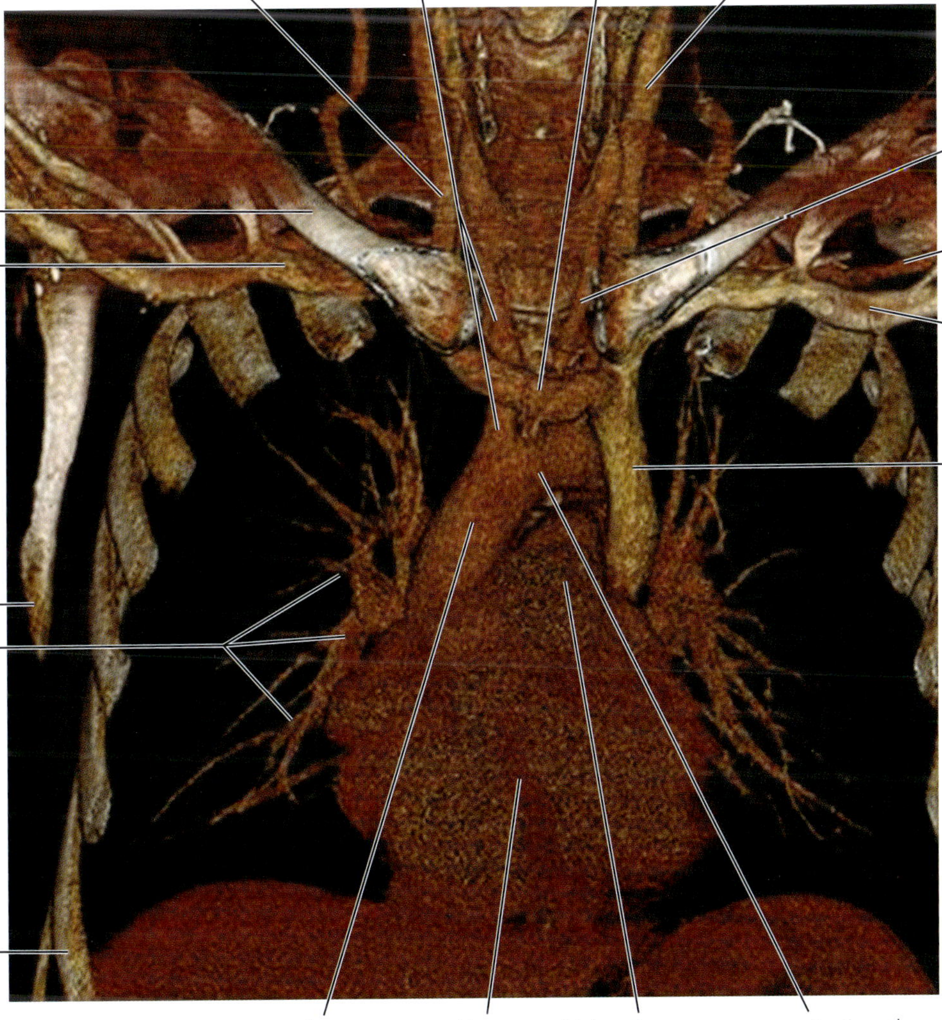
Right internal jugular v.
Right brachiocephalic a.
Left brachiocephalic v.
Left internal jugular v.
Left common carotid a.
Clavicle
Right subclavian v.
Left subclavian a.
Left subclavian v.
Persistent left superior vena cava
Scapula
Pulmonary aa. & vv.
Rib
Ascending aorta
Heart
Main pulmonary a.
Aortic arch

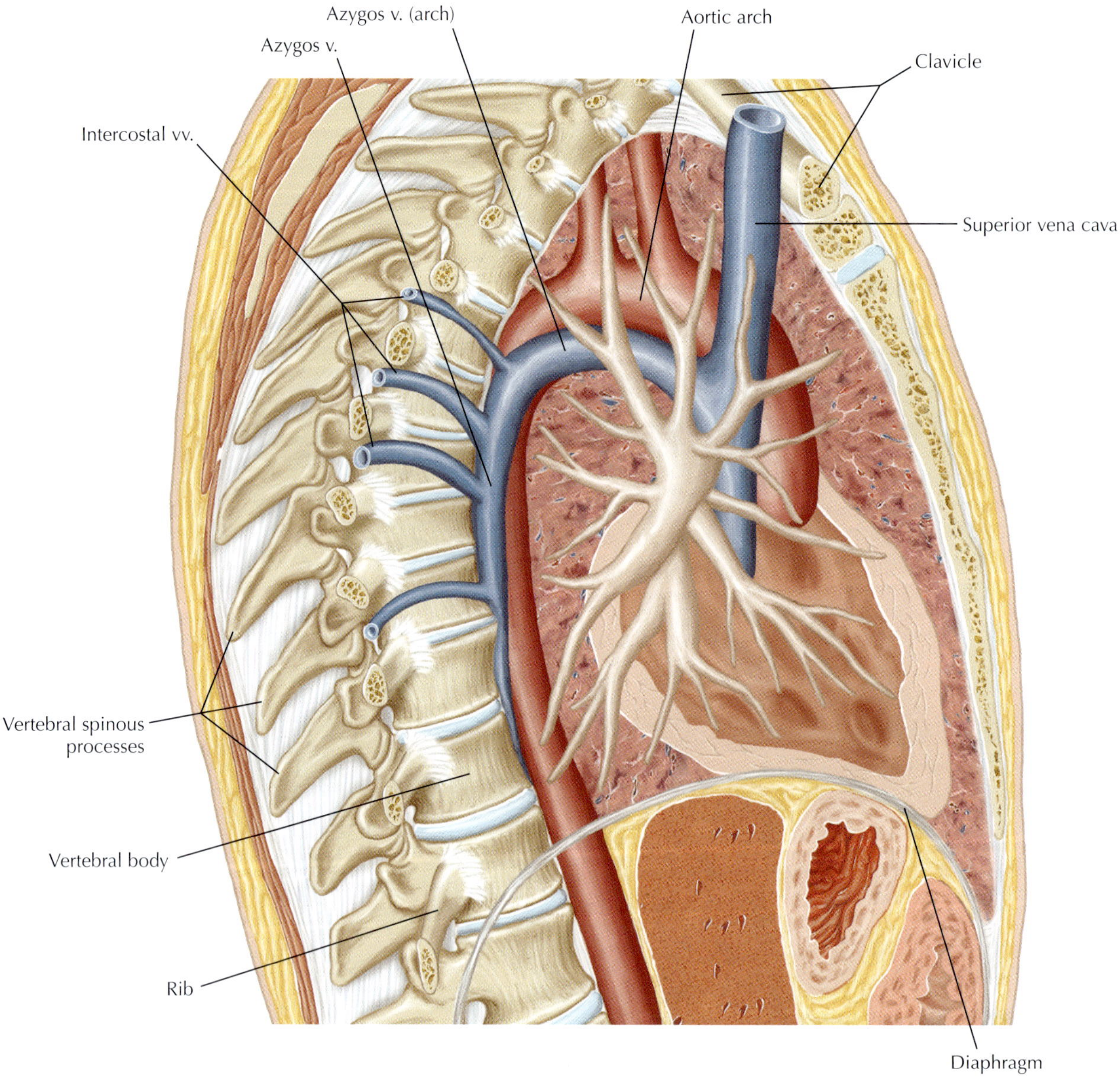

PATHOLOGIC PROCESS

An oblique, sagittal volume rendered image performed in a patient with a right subclavian venous stenosis. This condition causes blood from the right upper extremity and chest wall to route through various chest wall and thoracic veins as the body attempts to bypass the obstructed subclavian vein. When the right upper extremity venous system is injected with intravenous contrast for thoracic CT, this situation creates a unique opportunity to demonstrate the intercostal and azygos venous systems of the thorax. The arch of the azygos vein is well visualized. The azygos vein normally courses within the posterior mediastinum on the right, adjacent to the lower eight thoracic vertebral bodies, eventually extending anteriorly, superior to the root of the right lung, to empty into the superior vena cava. The azygos vein typically receives blood flow from intercostal veins, mediastinal veins, bronchial veins, esophageal veins, and the paravertebral venous plexus. When thoracic veins become obstructed, the azygos system assumes the role of a major collateral pathway for blood flow from the upper extremities and thorax to reach the heart.

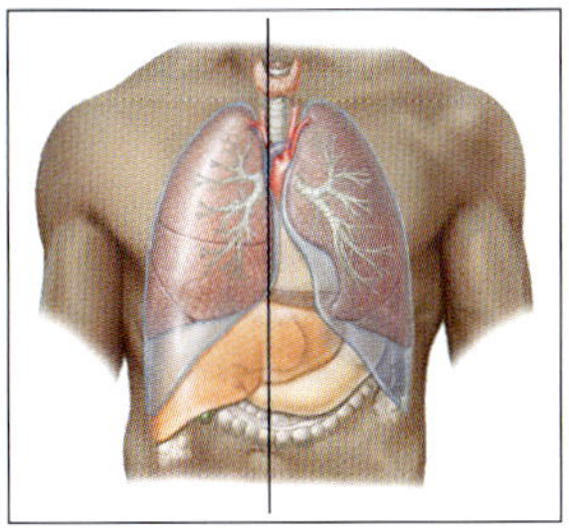

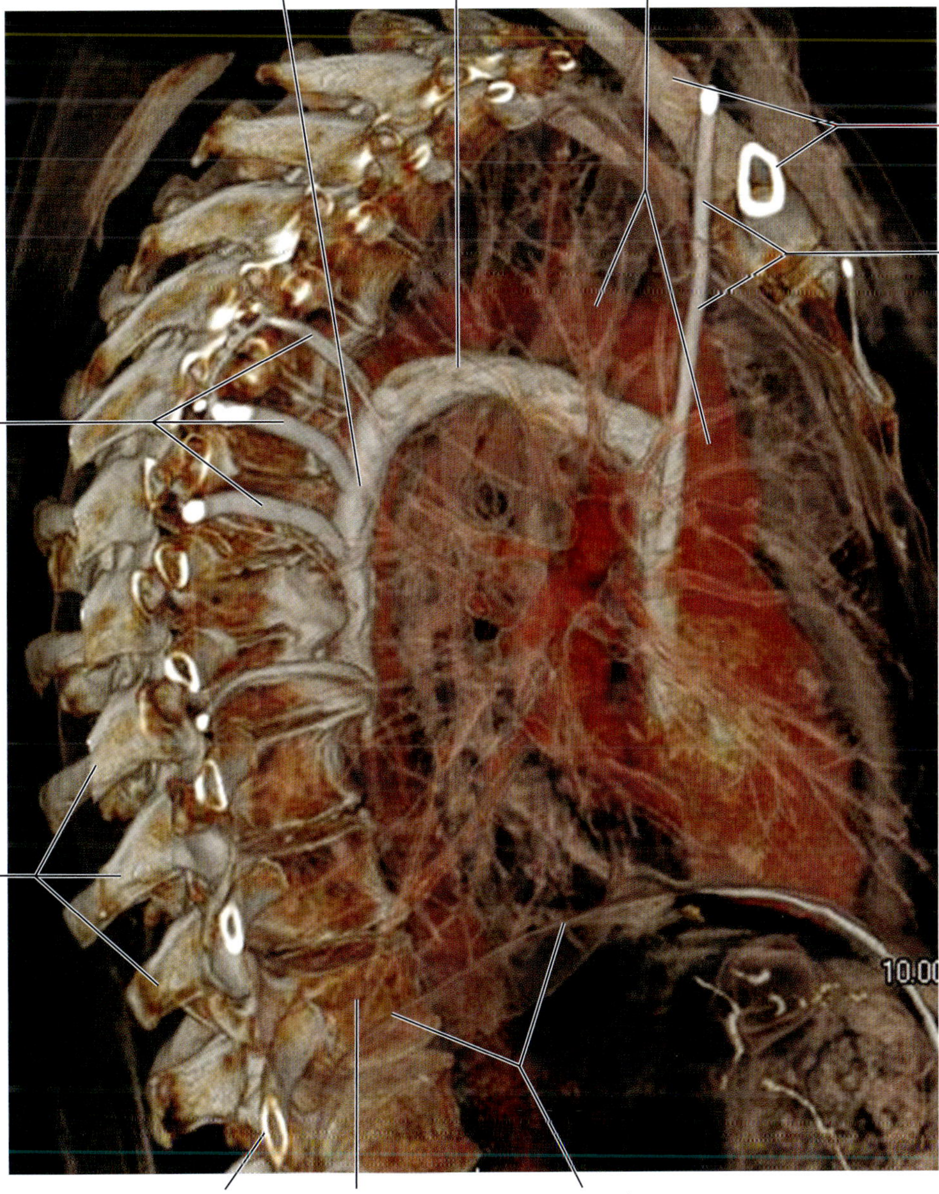
Azygos v.
Azygos v. (arch)
Aortic arch
Clavicle
Superior vena cava
Intercostal vv.
Vertebral spinous processes
Rib
Vertebral body
Diaphragm
10.00

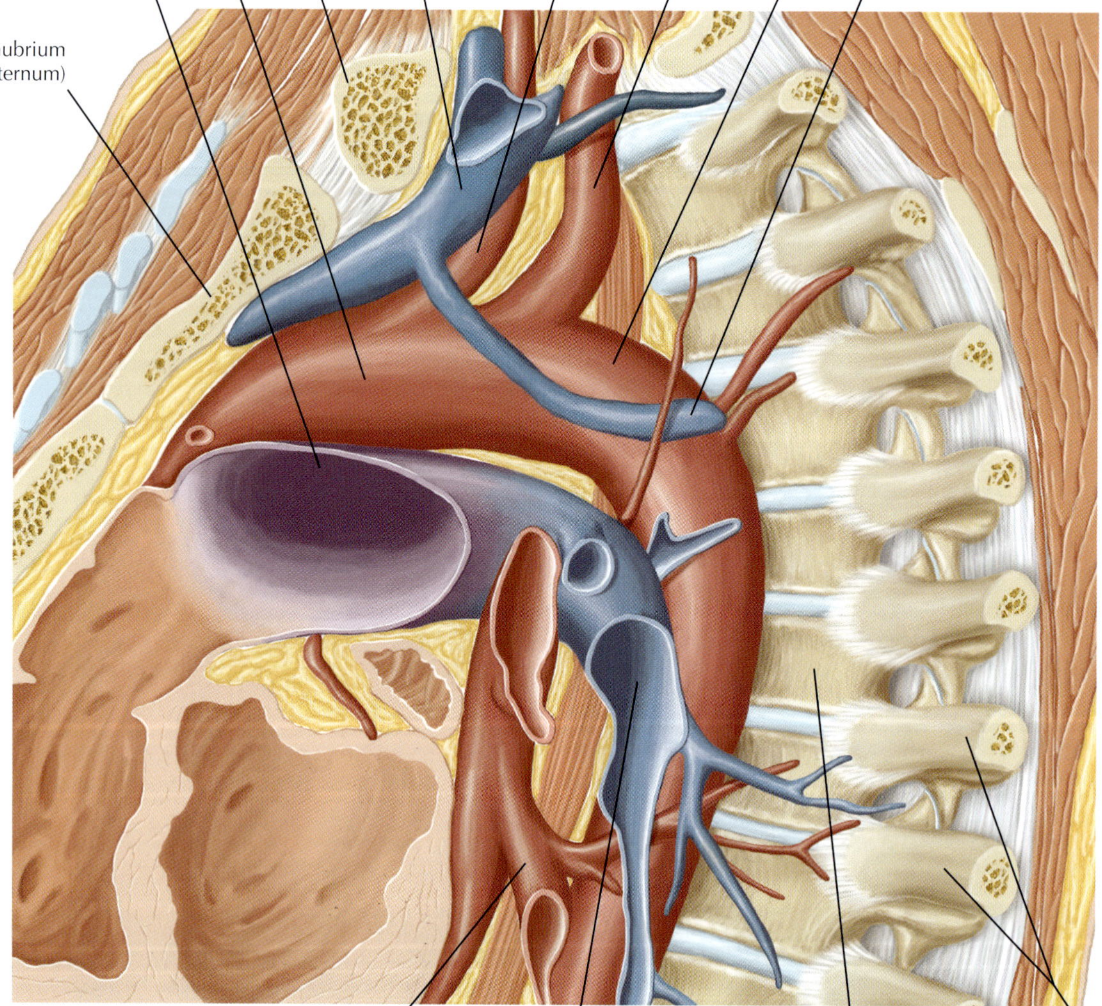

NORMAL VARIANT

An oblique sagittal volume rendered image of the thorax that represents a different perspective of the *left superior intercostal vein* as it courses from posterior to anterior, adjacent to the aortic arch, emptying into the left brachiocephalic vein. The left superior intercostal vein typically drains the 2nd, 3rd, and 4th intercostal veins on the left, and connects the left brachiocephalic and accessory hemiazygos veins. The left superior intercostal vein provides a collateral pathway for blood flow from the upper extremities and trunk to the heart in the setting of venous stenosis or obstruction.

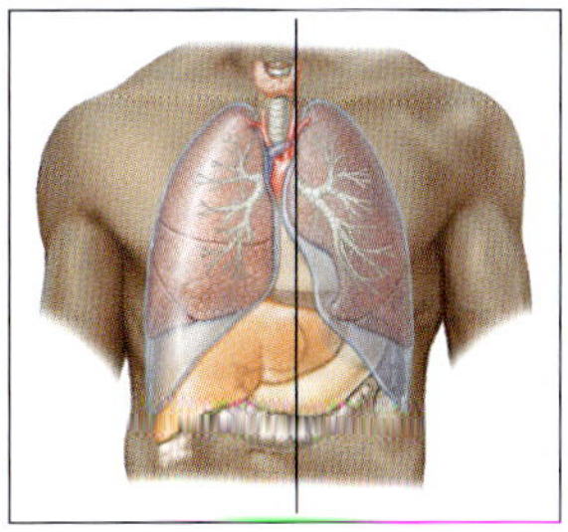

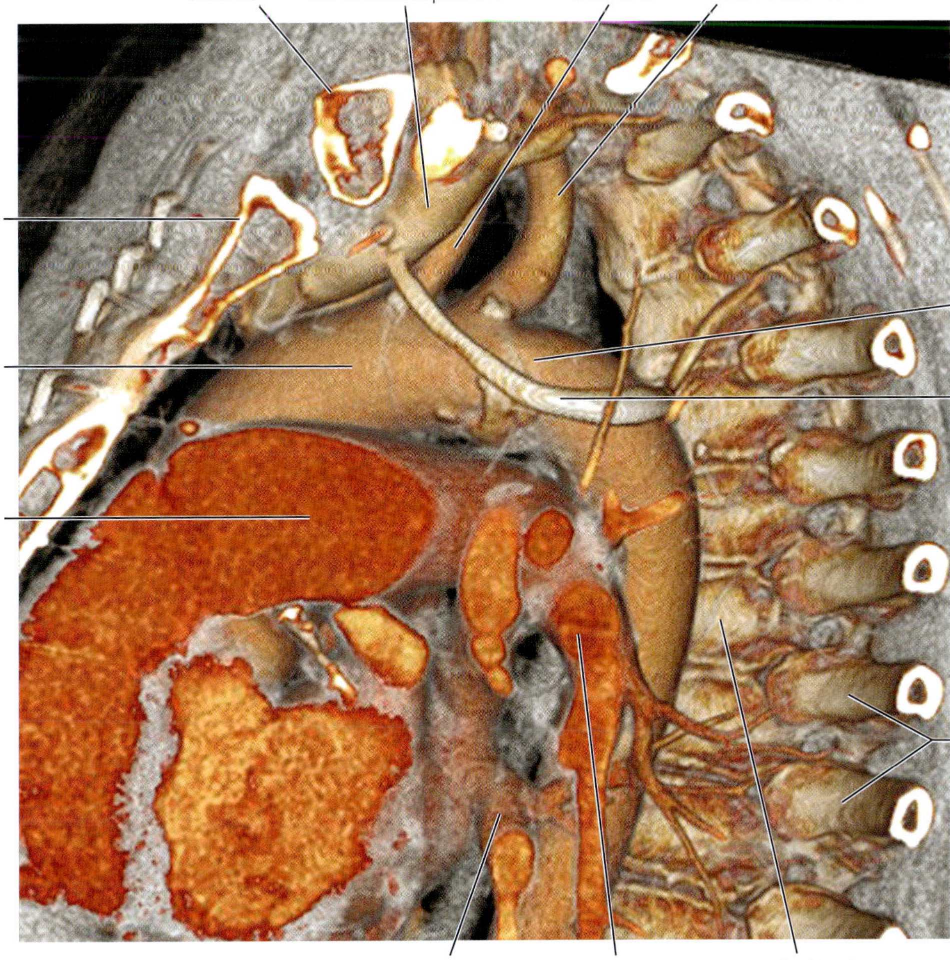
Clavicle
Left brachiocephalic v.
Left common carotid a.
Left subclavian a.
Manubrium (sternum)
Descending thoracic aorta
Aortic arch
Left superior intercostal v.
Main pulmonary a.
Ribs
Pulmonary v.
Left pulmonary a.
Vertebral body

PART 2 CARDIAC ANATOMY

Chapter 7 OVERVIEW OF CARDIAC ANATOMY

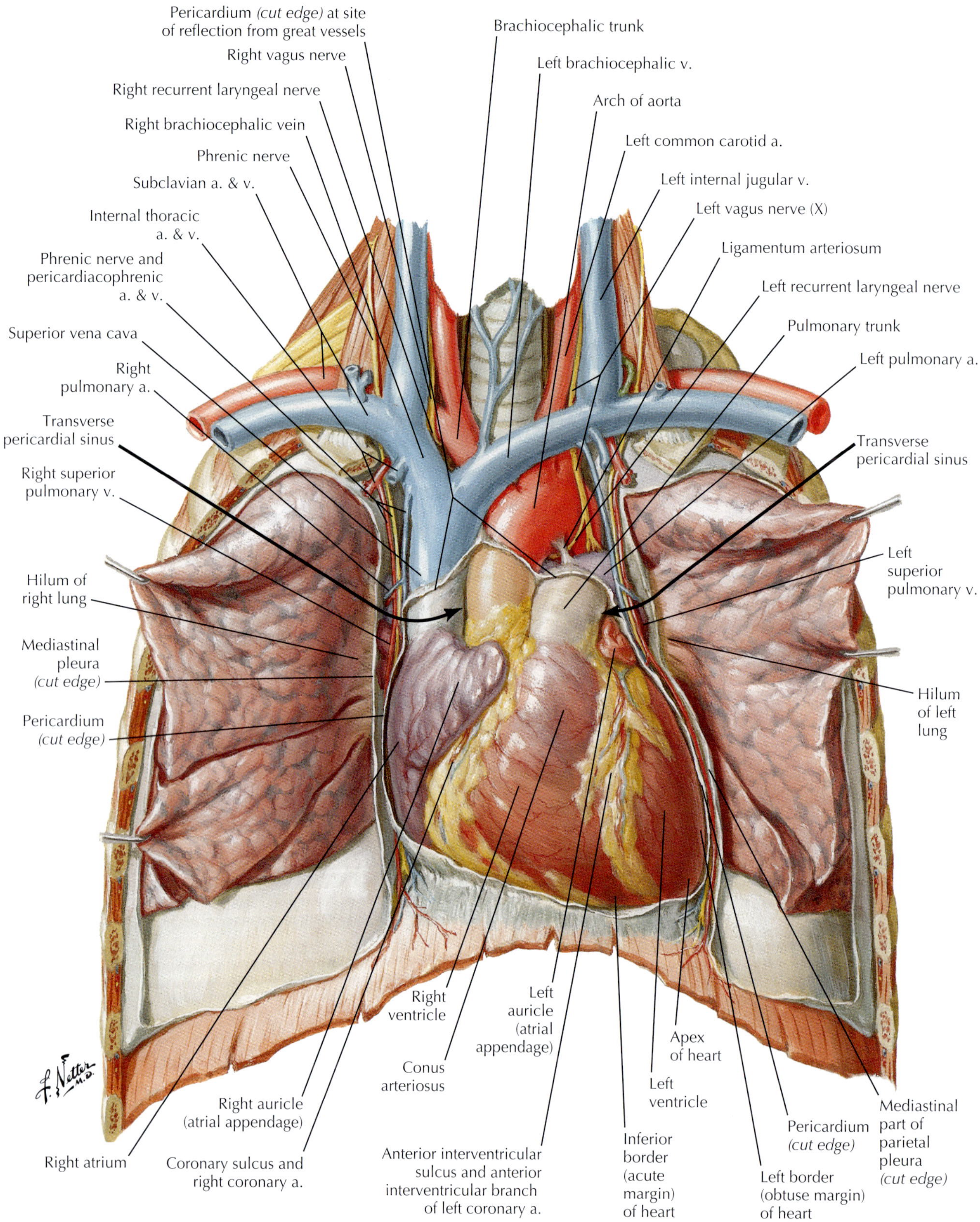
Pericardium (cut edge) at site of reflection from great vessels
Right vagus nerve
Right recurrent laryngeal nerve
Right brachiocephalic vein
Phrenic nerve
Subclavian a. & v.
Internal thoracic a. & v.
Phrenic nerve and pericardiacophrenic a. & v.
Superior vena cava
Right pulmonary a.
Transverse pericardial sinus
Right superior pulmonary v.
Hilum of right lung
Mediastinal pleura (cut edge)
Pericardium (cut edge)
Brachiocephalic trunk
Left brachiocephalic v.
Arch of aorta
Left common carotid a.
Left internal jugular v.
Left vagus nerve (X)
Ligamentum arteriosum
Left recurrent laryngeal nerve
Pulmonary trunk
Left pulmonary a.
Transverse pericardial sinus
Left superior pulmonary v.
Hilum of left lung
Right atrium
Right auricle (atrial appendage)
Coronary sulcus and right coronary a.
Right ventricle
Conus arteriosus
Left auricle (atrial appendage)
Anterior interventricular sulcus and anterior interventricular branch of left coronary a.
Inferior border (acute margin) of heart
Apex of heart
Left ventricle
Left border (obtuse margin) of heart
Pericardium (cut edge)
Mediastinal part of parietal pleura (cut edge)

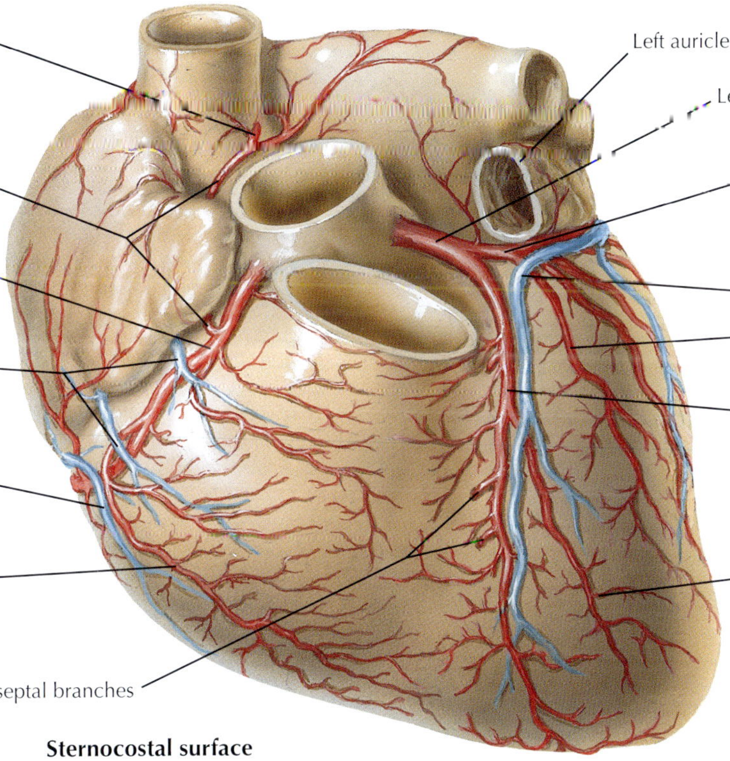

Sternocostal surface

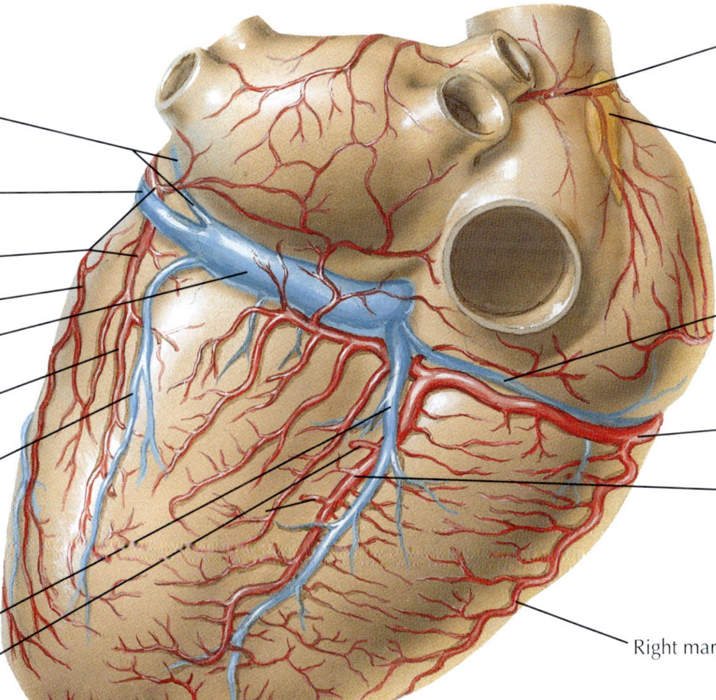

Diaphragmatic surface

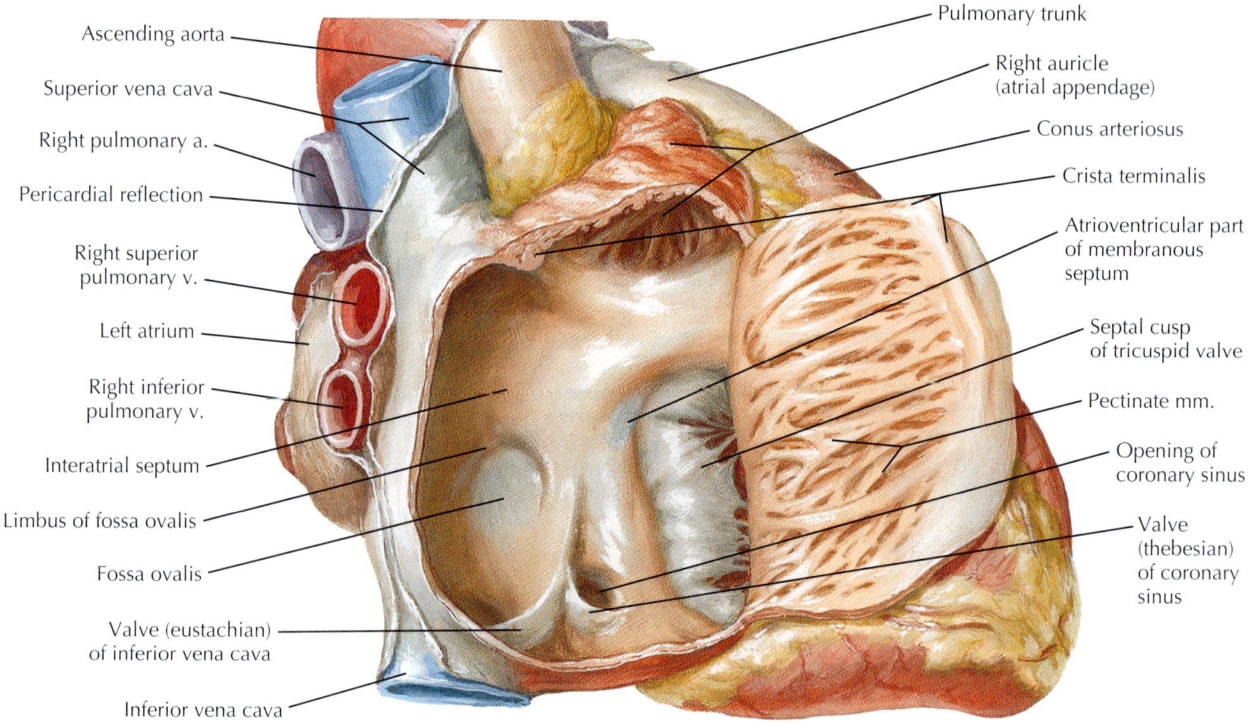

Opened right atrium: right lateral view

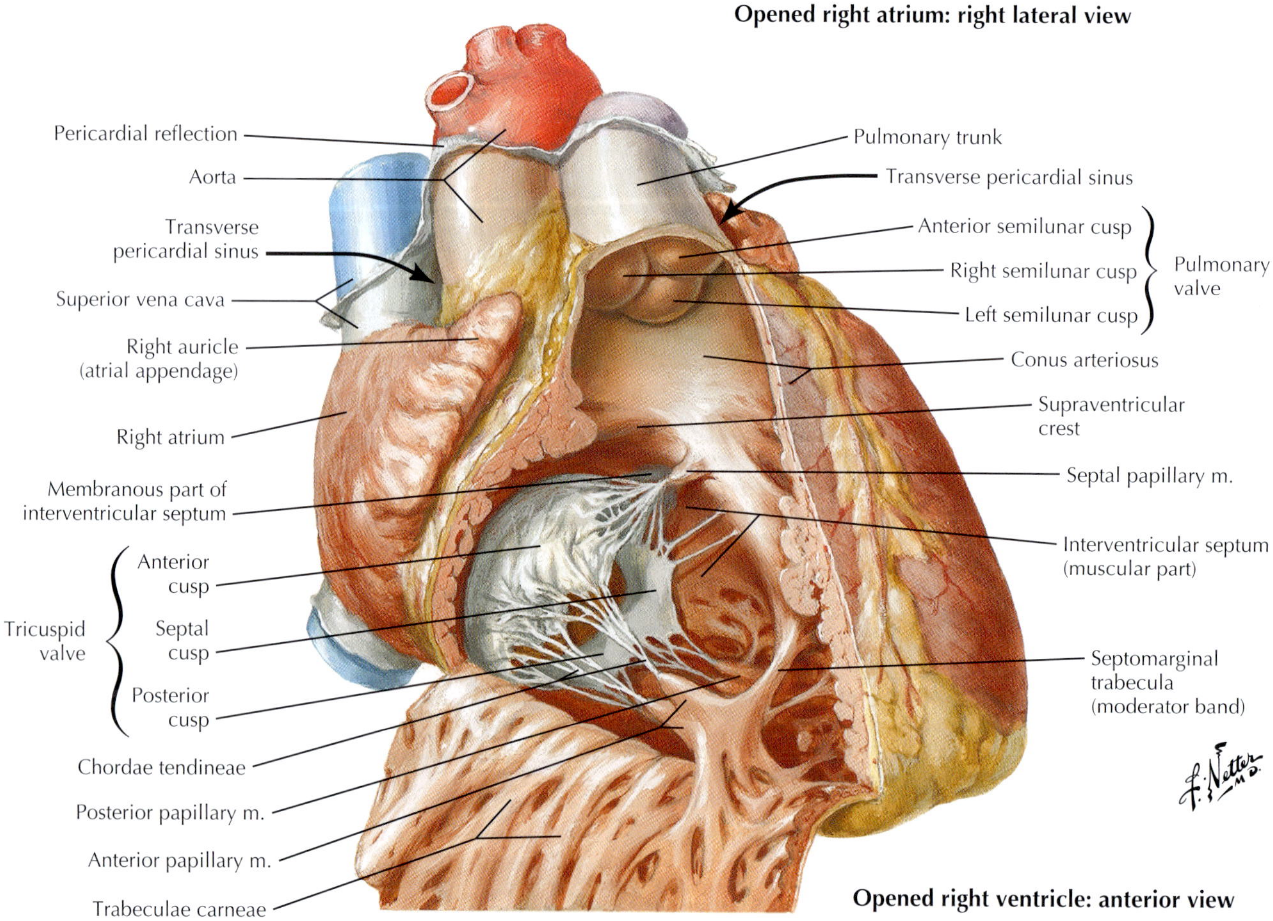

Opened right ventricle: anterior view

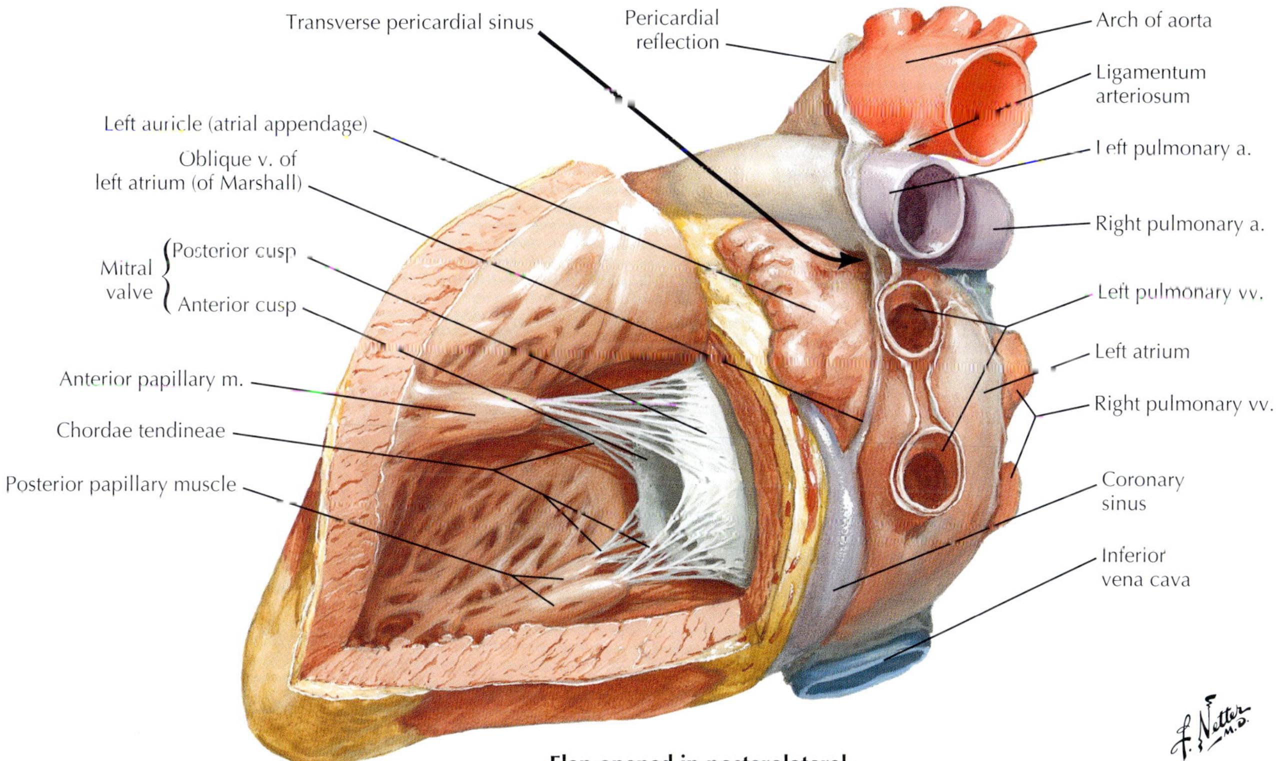

Flap opened in posterolateral wall of left ventricle

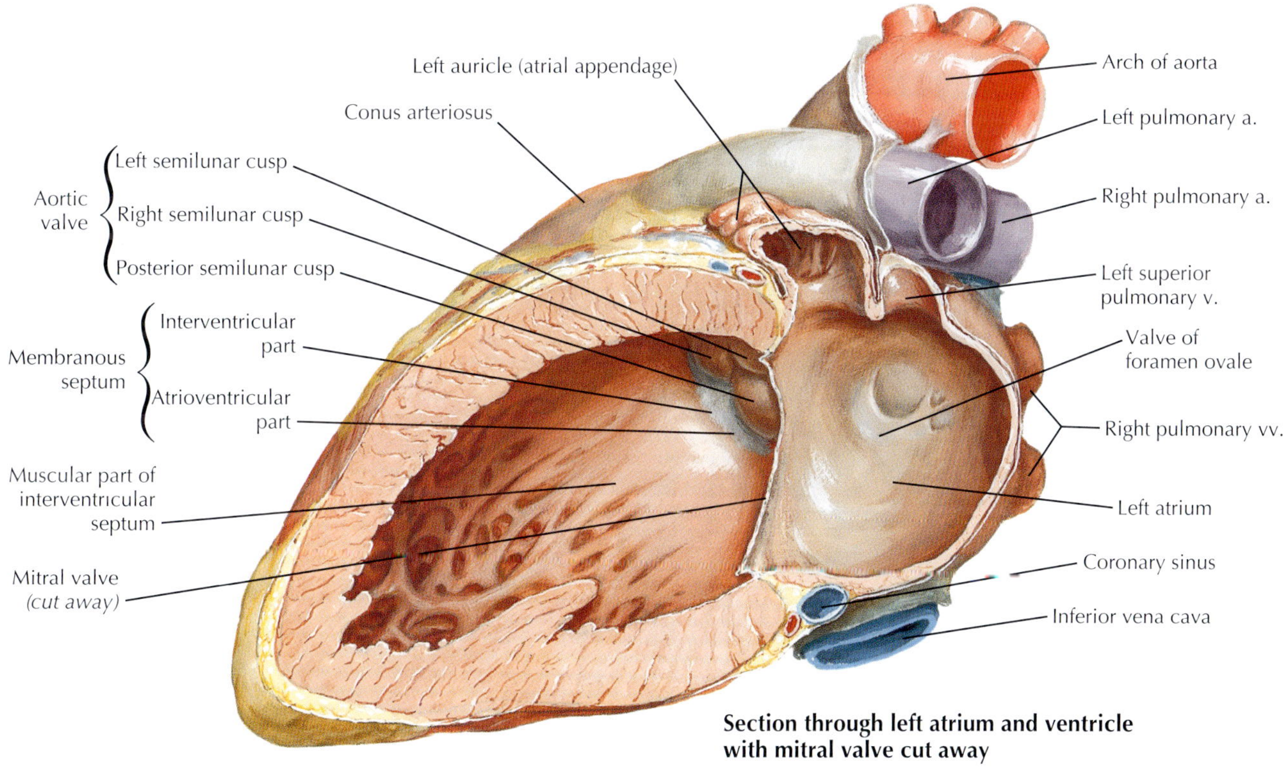

Section through left atrium and ventricle with mitral valve cut away

Atria, Ventricles, and Interventricular Septum

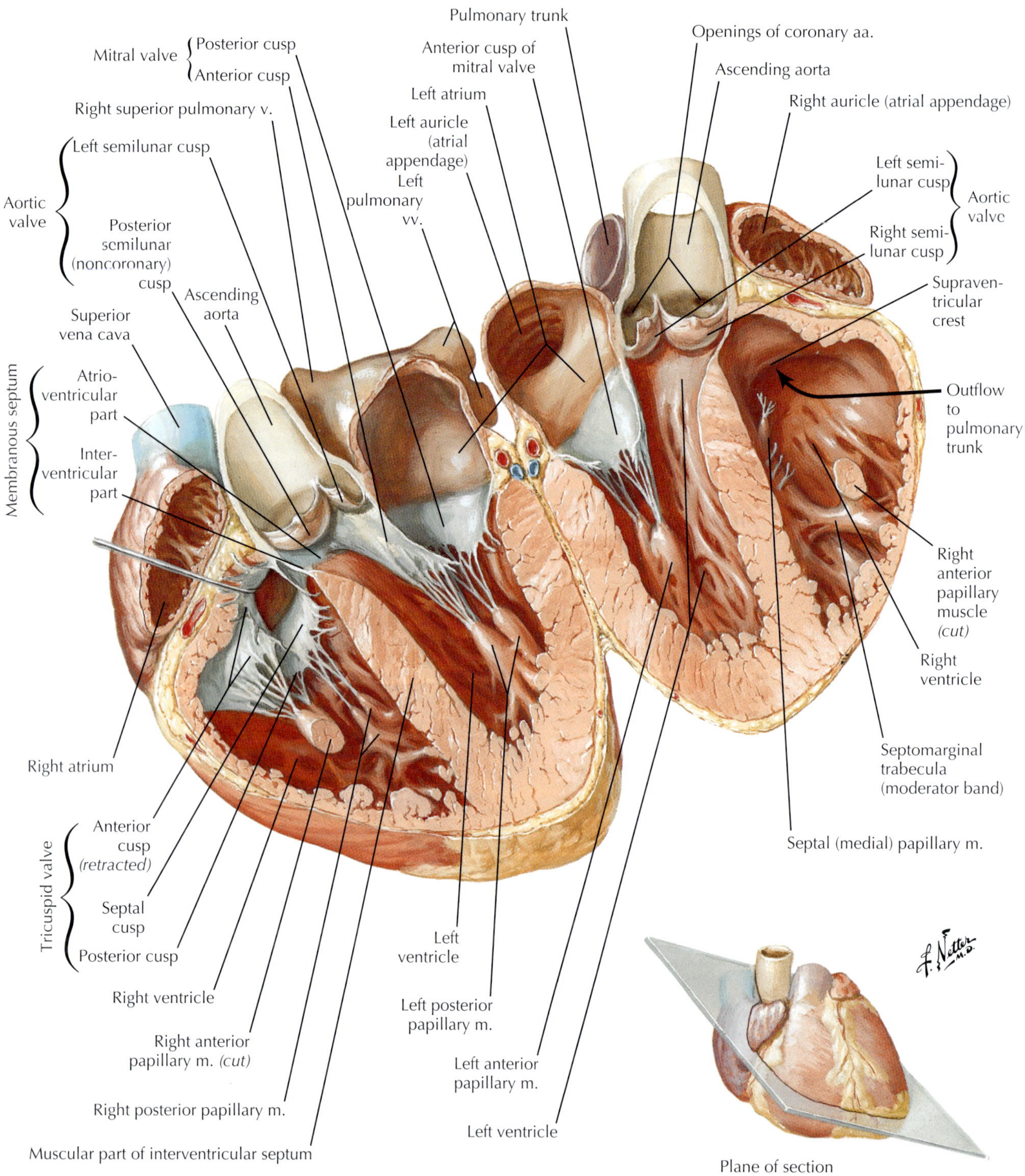

Chapter 8

CARDIAC ANATOMY USING CT

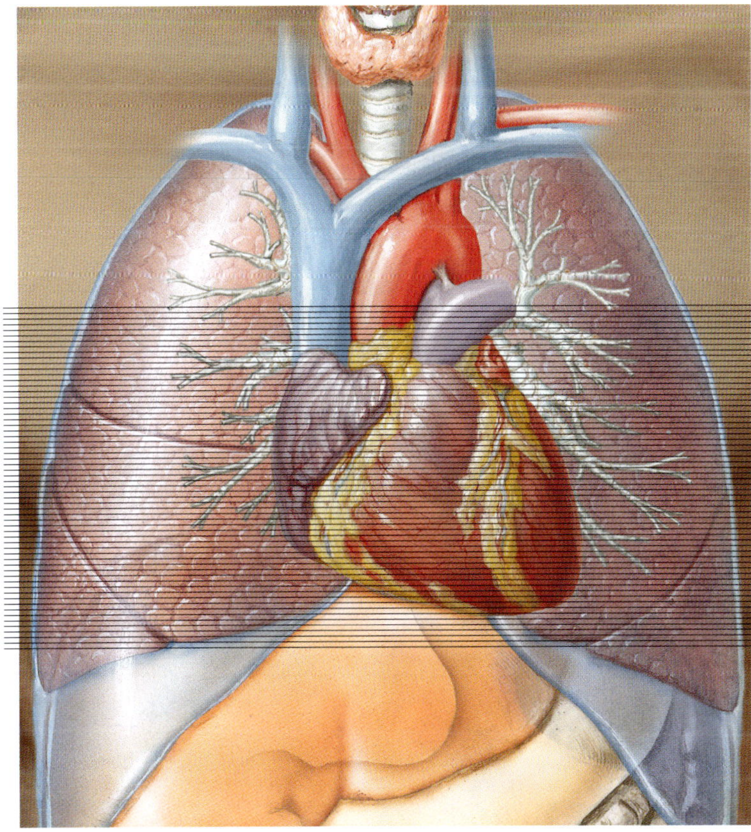

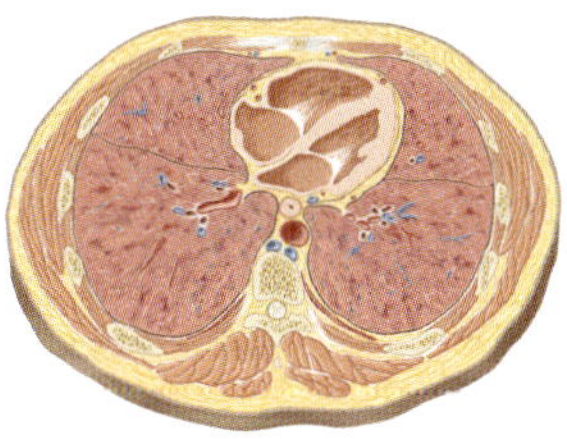

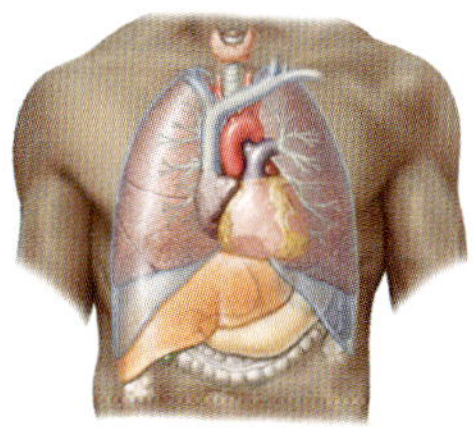

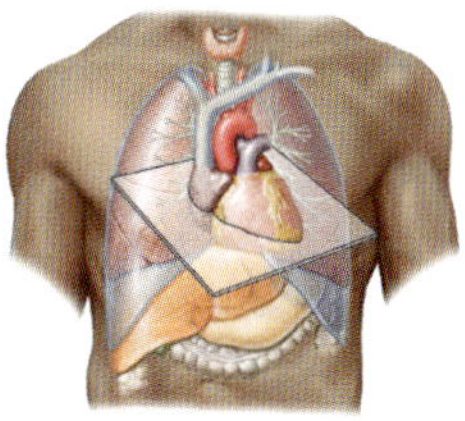

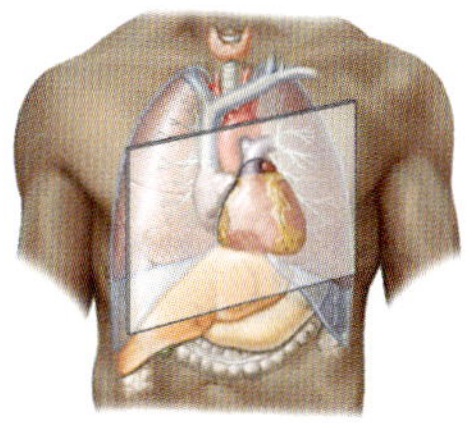

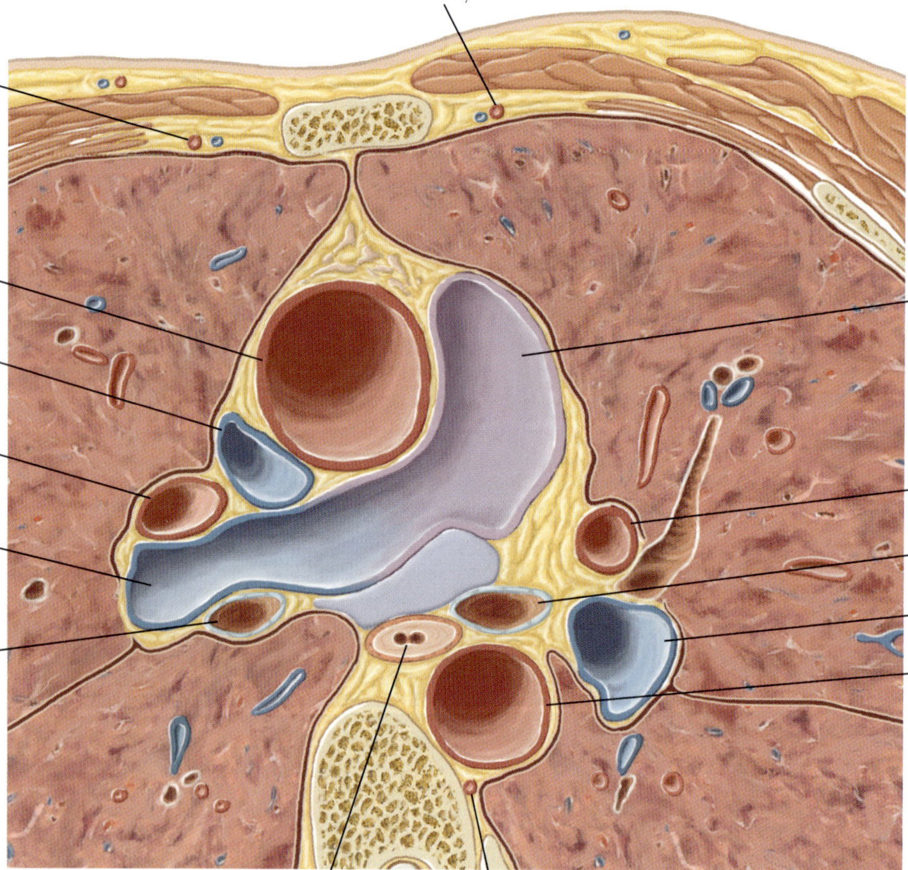

TECHNICAL CONSIDERATION

Typically, cardiac CT axial examinations are specifically tailored to image the heart, and therefore the imaging volume is restricted to only a portion of the thorax. Often the examination begins just below the carina, as this first plate shows. Note how the contrast bolus shows bright enhancement of the left-sided cardiovascular structures—the aorta and pulmonary veins—whereas right-sided structures (pulmonary arteries) are poorly enhanced. This is purposely accomplished by following the intravenous contrast bolus with a saline injection to "wash out" dense intravenous contrast from the right heart and thereby improve visualization of the right coronary artery.

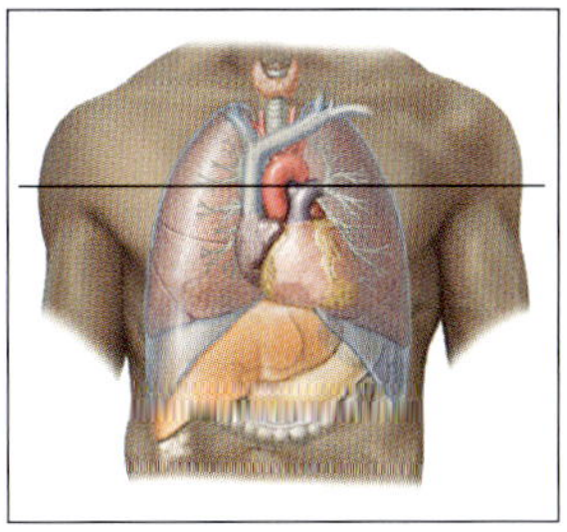

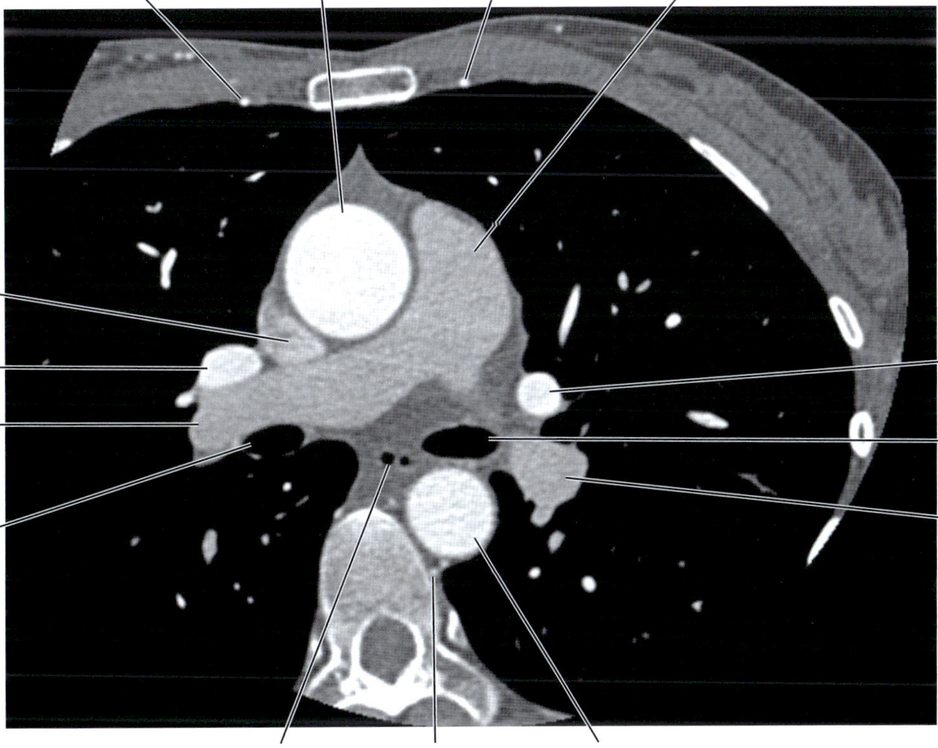
Right internal mammary a.
Ascending aorta
Left internal mammary a.
Main pulmonary a.
Superior vena cava
Pulmonary v.
Right interlobar pulmonary a.
Bronchus intermedius
Pulmonary v.
Left mainstem bronchus
Left interlobar pulmonary a.
Esophagus
Intercostal a.
Descending thoracic aorta

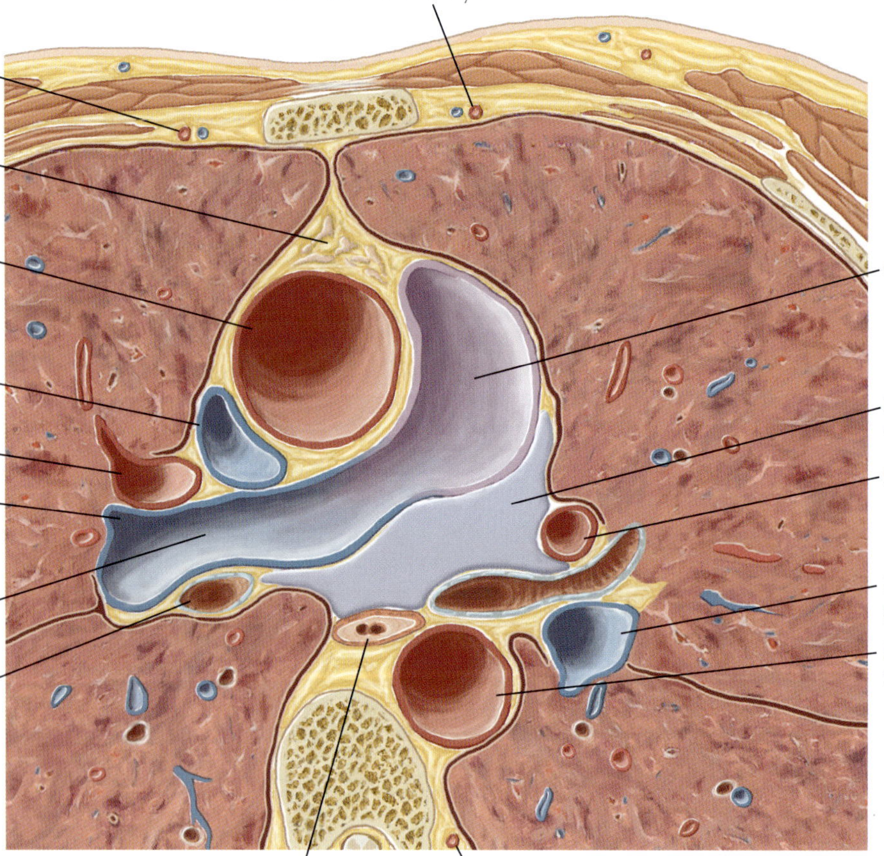

NORMAL ANATOMY

Several millimeters inferior to Axial 1 again shows intense enhancement of left-sided cardiovascular structures—the ascending and descending thoracic aorta and pulmonary veins. A small amount of normal pericardial fluid is seen within the left pulmonic recess of the transverse sinus of the pericardium. The origin of the right middle lobe pulmonary artery is visible, marking the distal aspect of the right interlobar pulmonary artery and the beginning of the right lower lobe pulmonary artery.

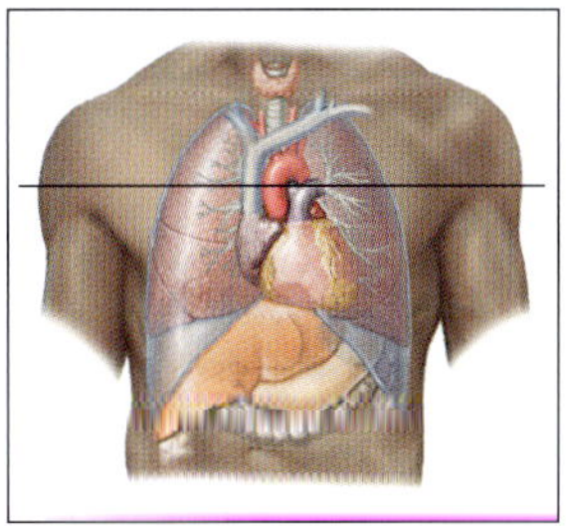

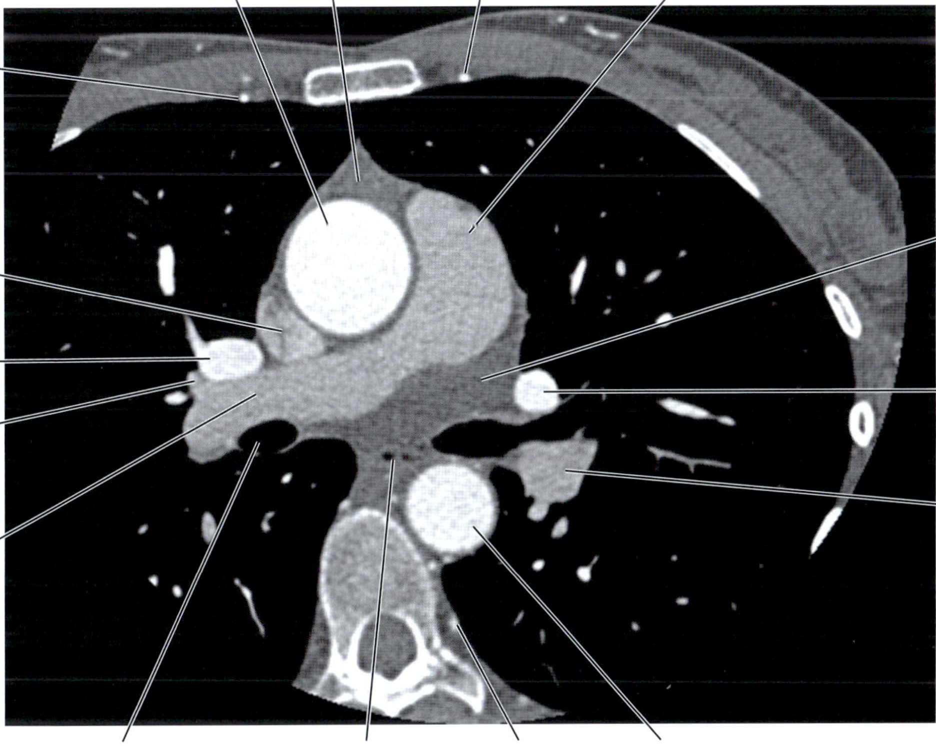
Ascending aorta
Anterior mediastinum
Left internal mammary a.
Main pulmonary a.
Right internal mammary a.
Superior vena cava
Pulmonary v.
Right middle lobe medial segment pulmonary a.
Right interlobar pulmonary a.
Pericardial fluid (left pulmonic recess)
Pulmonary v.
Left interlobar pulmonary a.
Bronchus intermedius
Esophagus
Intercostal a.
Descending thoracic aorta

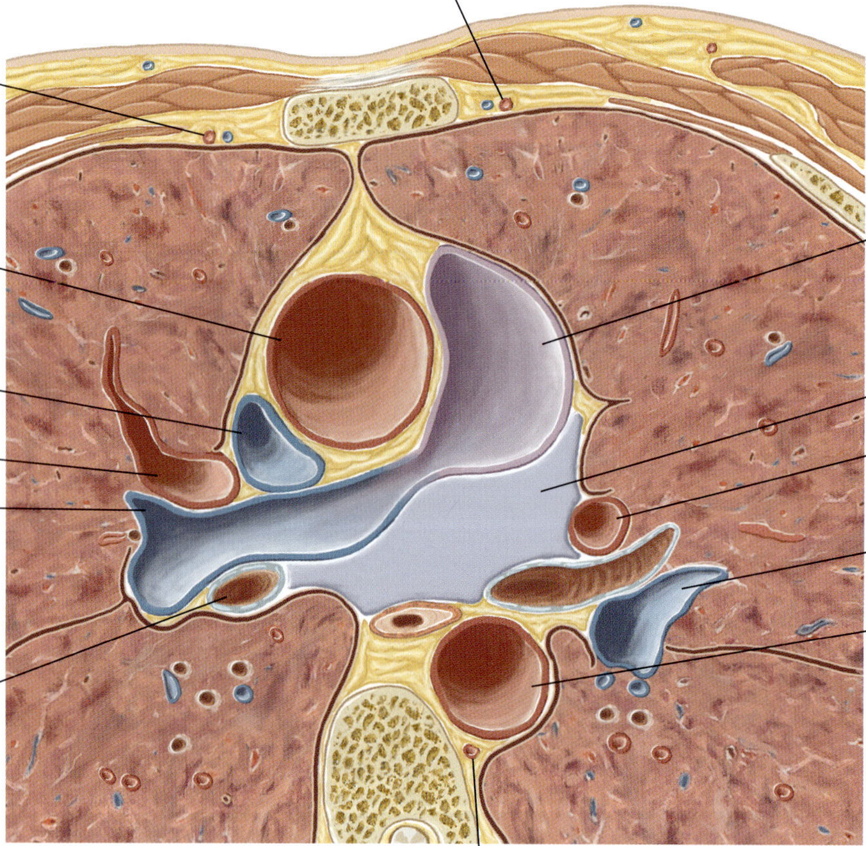

NORMAL VARIANT

The medial segment of the right middle lobe and lingular arteries are visible at this level. Usually the right middle lobe pulmonary artery arises from the distal right interlobar pulmonary artery and branches into medial and lateral segments. However, in this patient, the medial and lateral segments of the right middle lobe pulmonary artery arise directly from the right interlobar pulmonary artery.

NORMAL ANATOMY

The pericardial space is divided into the **pericardium proper,** consisting of a postcaval recess and right and left pulmonary vein recesses, and the **transverse** and **oblique** sinuses. The transverse sinus lies posterior to the ascending aorta and main pulmonary artery and cranial to the left atrium. The transverse sinus is further subdivided into superior and inferior aortic recesses and right and left pulmonic recesses. The oblique sinus also contains the posterior pericardial recess. Small amounts of fluid are commonly seen within some of these compartments in normal patients during thoracic and cardiovascular CT examinations.

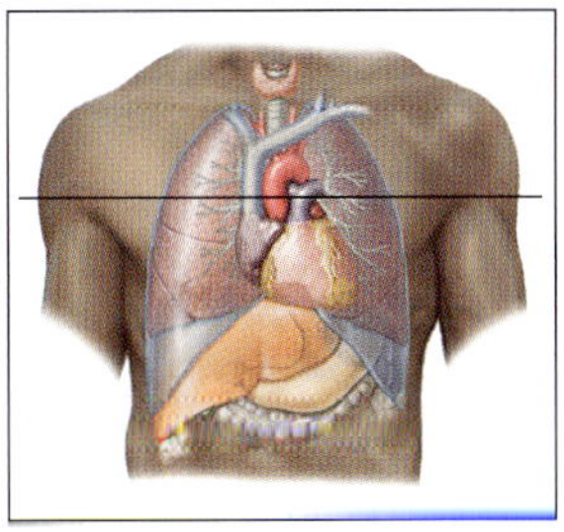

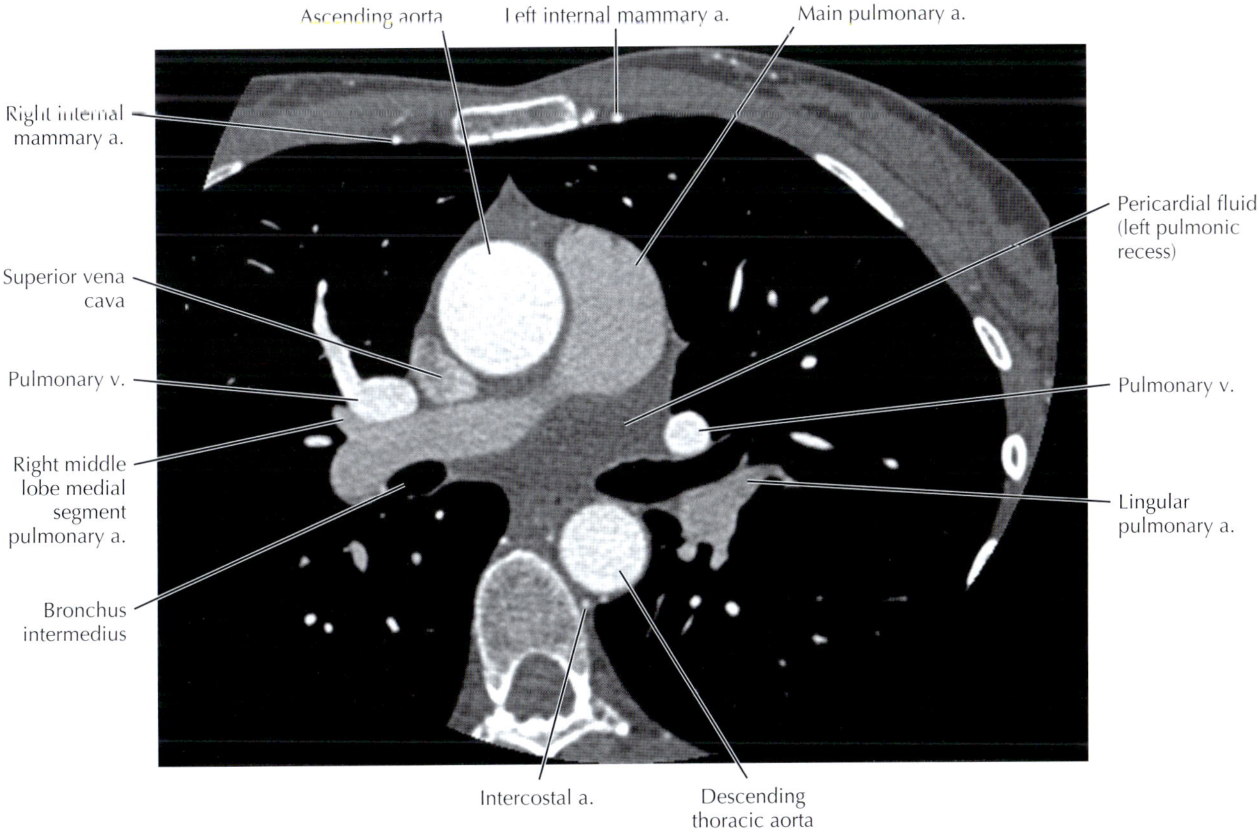

Ascending aorta
Left internal mammary a.
Main pulmonary a.
Right internal mammary a.
Pericardial fluid (left pulmonic recess)
Superior vena cava
Pulmonary v.
Pulmonary v.
Right middle lobe medial segment pulmonary a.
Lingular pulmonary a.
Bronchus intermedius
Intercostal a.
Descending thoracic aorta

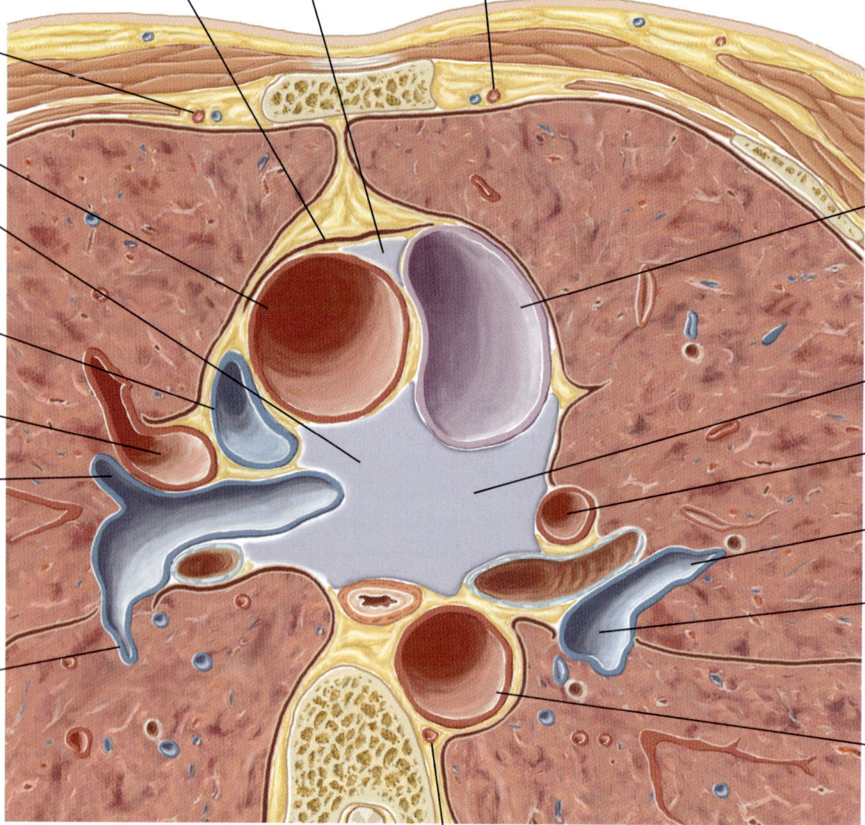

NORMAL ANATOMY

Along the anterior aspect of the ascending aorta and main pulmonary artery, the normal pericardium is visible. A small amount of fluid immediately subjacent to the pericardium in this region, interposed between the ascending aorta and main pulmonary artery (*), is within the anterior portion of the superior recess of the transverse sinus.

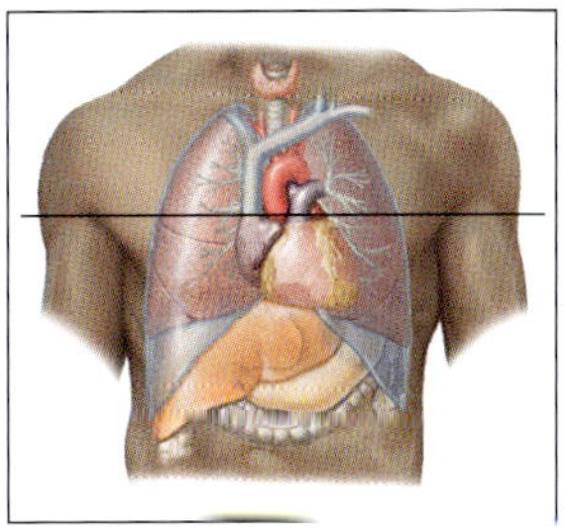

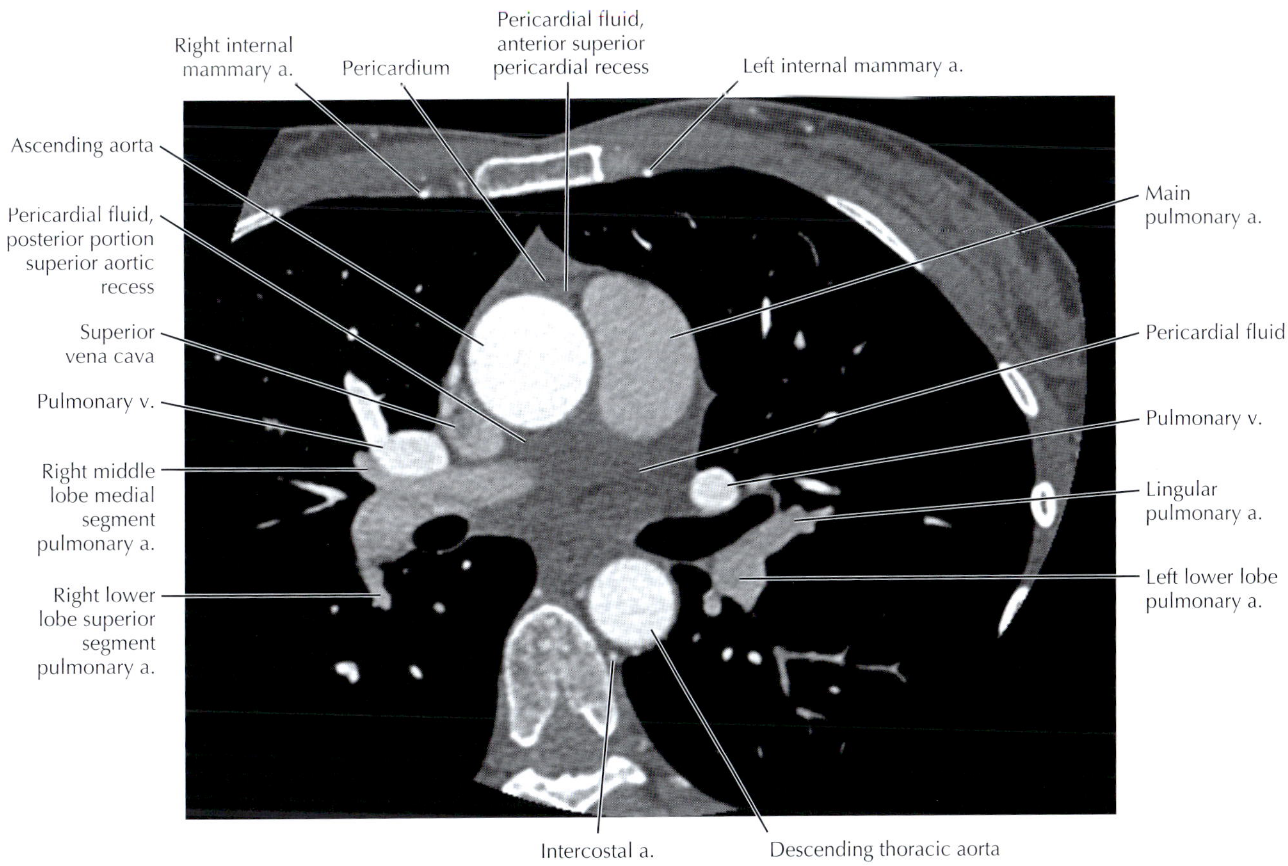
Right internal mammary a.
Pericardium
Pericardial fluid, anterior superior pericardial recess
Left internal mammary a.
Ascending aorta
Pericardial fluid, posterior portion superior aortic recess
Superior vena cava
Pulmonary v.
Right middle lobe medial segment pulmonary a.
Right lower lobe superior segment pulmonary a.
Main pulmonary a.
Pericardial fluid
Pulmonary v.
Lingular pulmonary a.
Left lower lobe pulmonary a.
Intercostal a.
Descending thoracic aorta

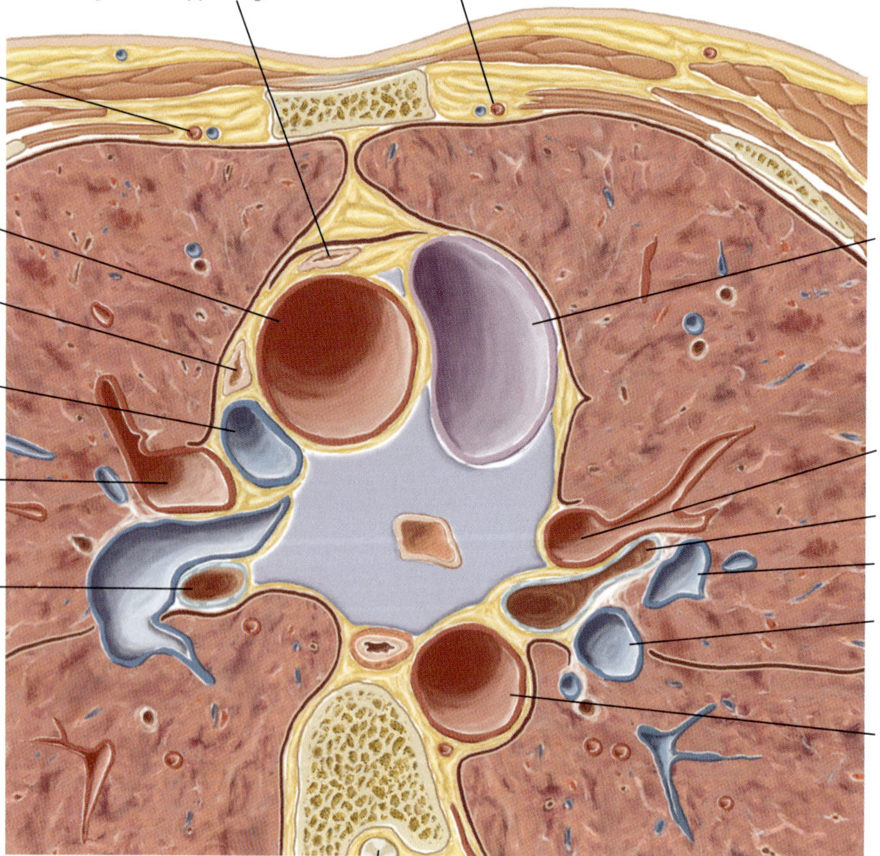
Left internal mammary a.
Right atrial appendage
Right internal mammary a.
Ascending aorta
Right atrial appendage
Superior vena cava
Pulmonary v.
Bronchus intermedius
Main pulmonary a.
Pulmonary v.
Lingular bronchus
Lingular pulmonary a.
Left lower lobe pulmonary a.
Descending thoracic aorta
Spinal cord

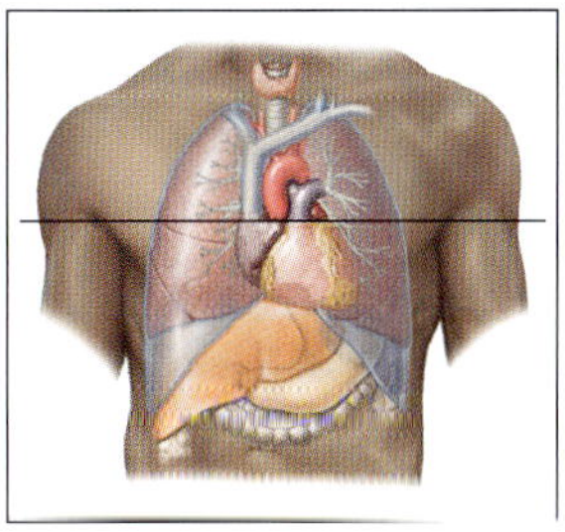

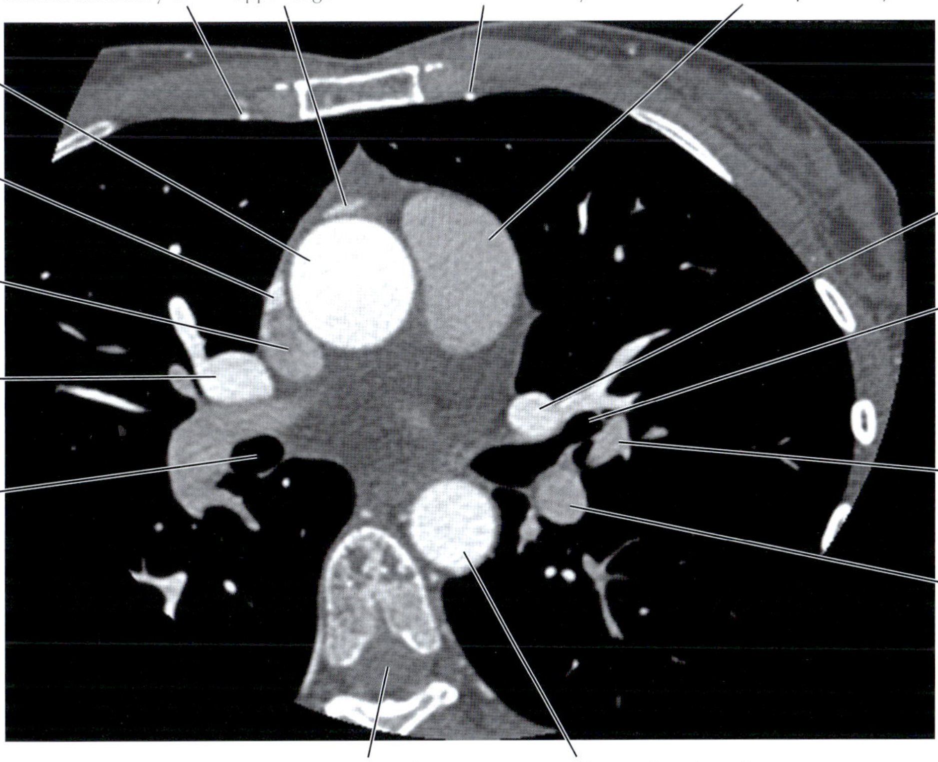
Right internal mammary a.
Right atrial appendage
Left internal mammary a.
Main pulmonary a.
Ascending aorta
Right atrial appendage
Superior vena cava
Pulmonary v.
Bronchus intermedius
Pulmonary v.
Lingular bronchus
Lingular pulmonary a.
Left lower lobe pulmonary a.
Spinal cord
Descending thoracic aorta

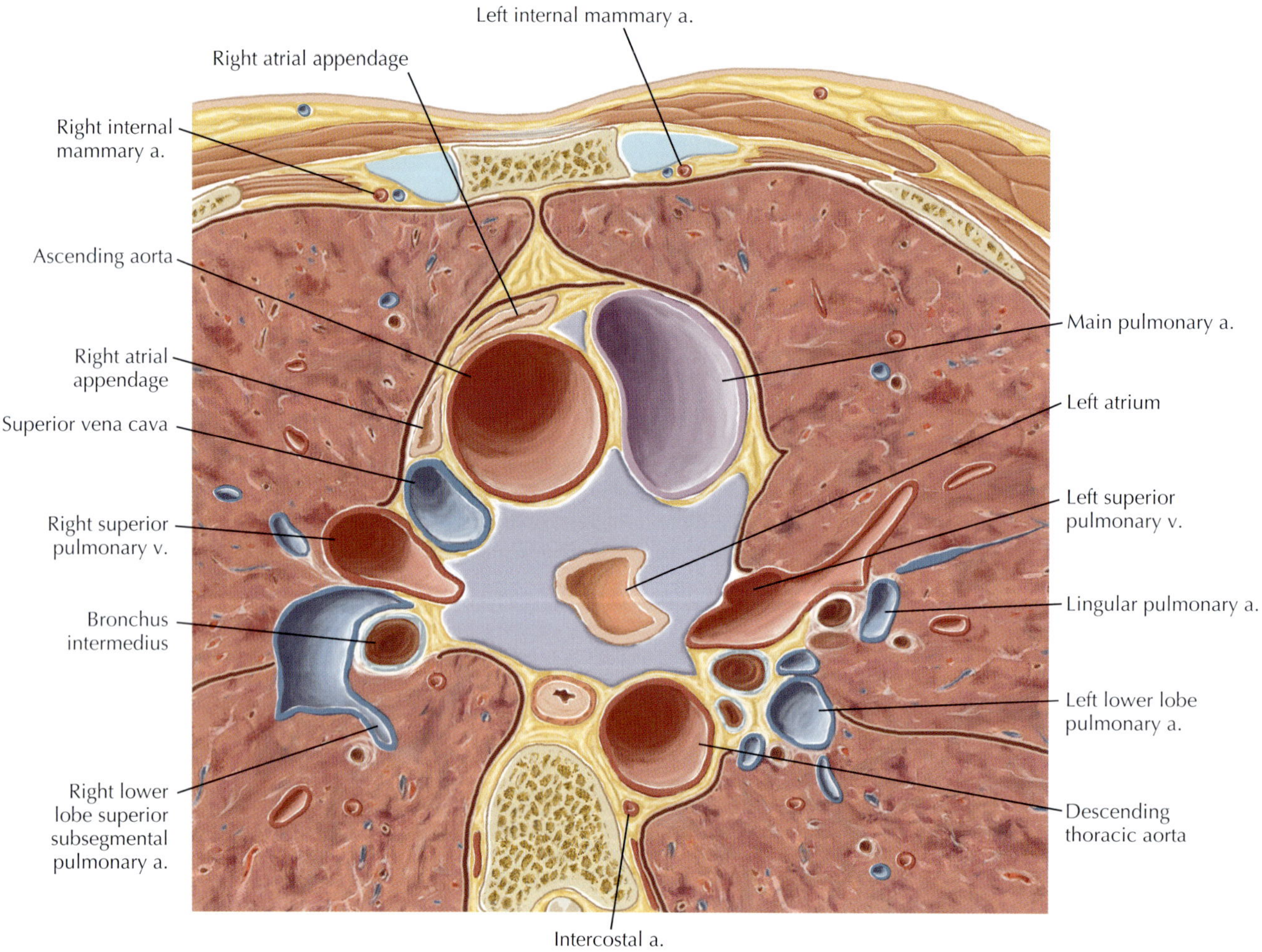
Left internal mammary a.
Right atrial appendage
Right internal mammary a.
Ascending aorta
Right atrial appendage
Superior vena cava
Right superior pulmonary v.
Bronchus intermedius
Right lower lobe superior subsegmental pulmonary a.
Main pulmonary a.
Left atrium
Left superior pulmonary v.
Lingular pulmonary a.
Left lower lobe pulmonary a.
Descending thoracic aorta
Intercostal a.

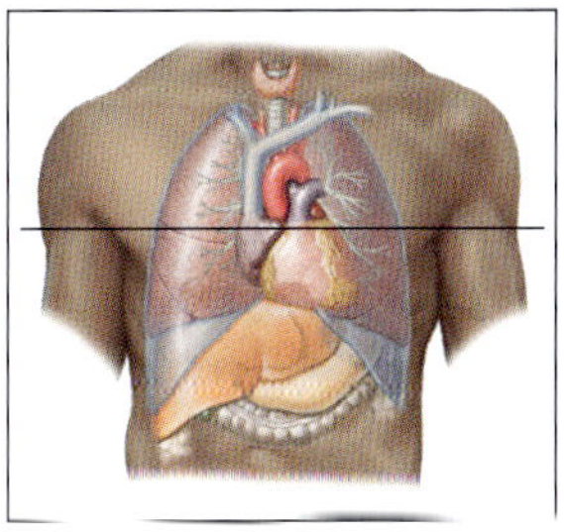

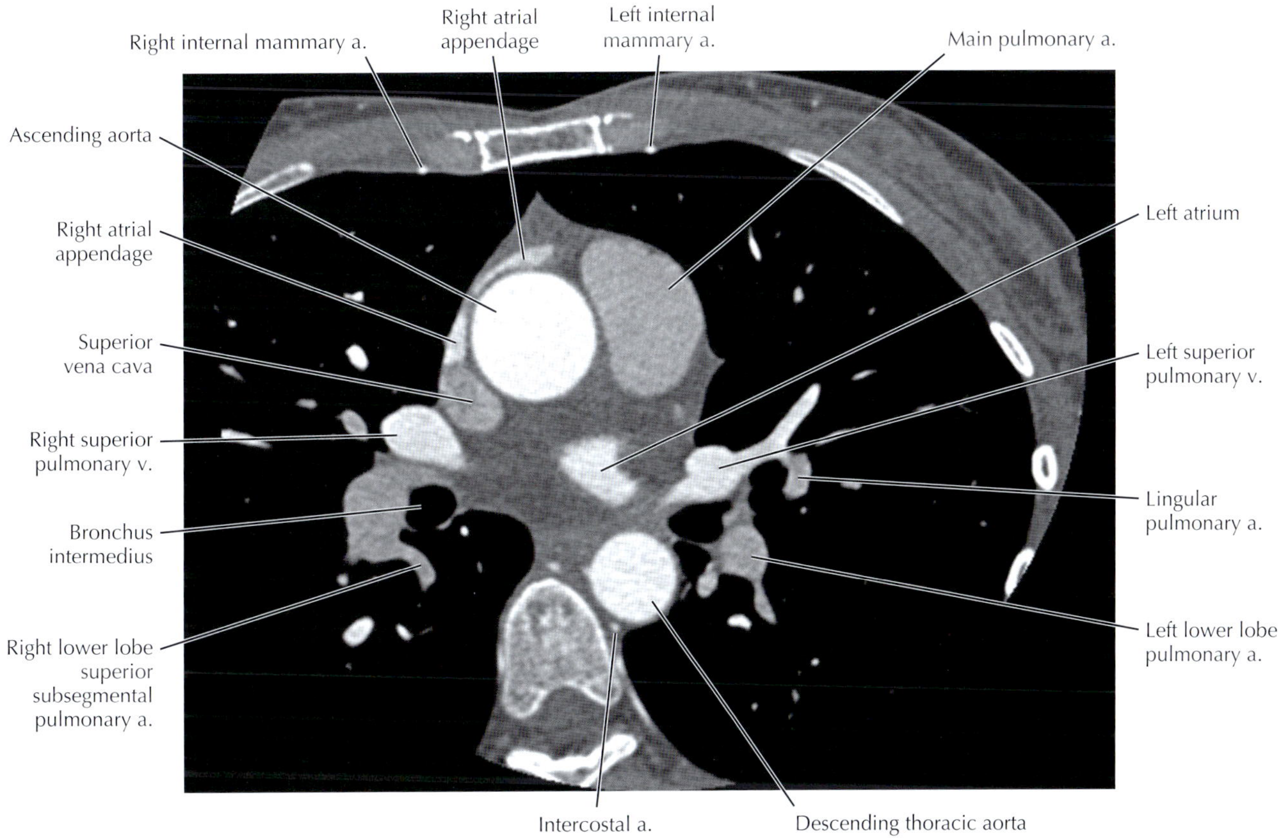
Right internal mammary a.
Right atrial appendage
Left internal mammary a.
Main pulmonary a.
Ascending aorta
Right atrial appendage
Superior vena cava
Right superior pulmonary v.
Bronchus intermedius
Right lower lobe superior subsegmental pulmonary a.
Left atrium
Left superior pulmonary v.
Lingular pulmonary a.
Left lower lobe pulmonary a.
Intercostal a.
Descending thoracic aorta

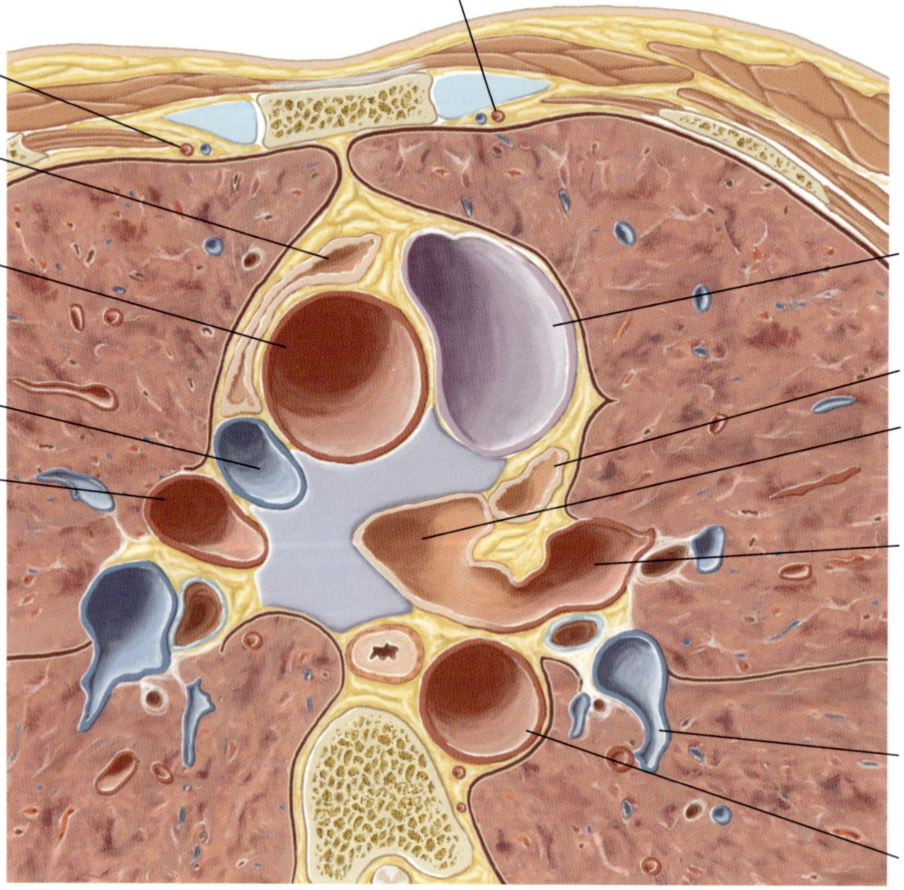
Left internal mammary a.
Right internal mammary a.
Right atrial appendage
Ascending aorta
Superior vena cava
Right superior pulmonary v.
Main pulmonary a.
Left atrial appendage
Left atrium
Left superior pulmonary v.
Left lower lobe superior segment pulmonary a.
Descending thoracic aorta

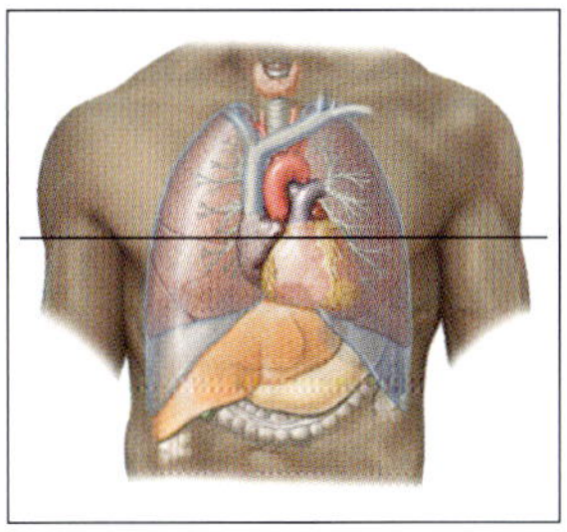

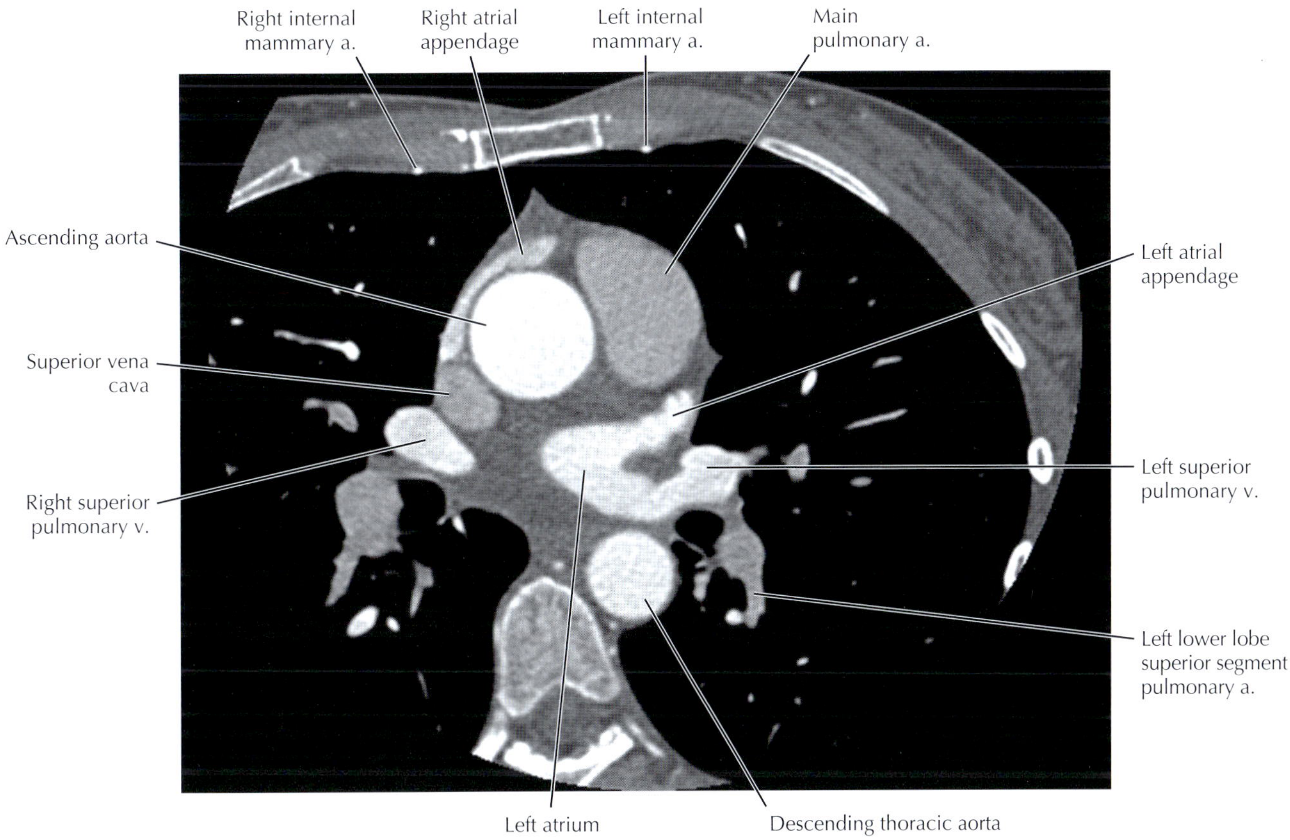
Right internal mammary a.
Right atrial appendage
Left internal mammary a.
Main pulmonary a.
Ascending aorta
Superior vena cava
Right superior pulmonary v.
Left atrial appendage
Left superior pulmonary v.
Left lower lobe superior segment pulmonary a.
Left atrium
Descending thoracic aorta

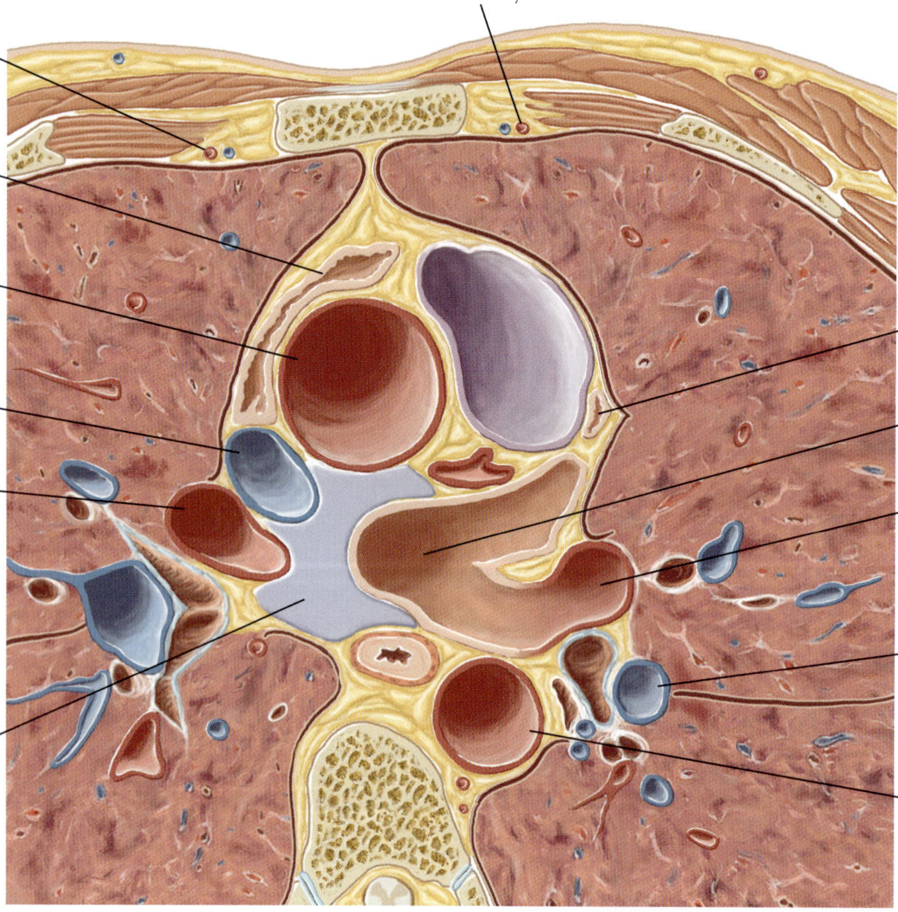
Left internal mammary a.
Right internal mammary a.
Right atrial appendage
Ascending aorta
Superior vena cava
Right superior pulmonary v.
Oblique sinus of pericardium
Left atrial appendage
Left atrium
Left superior pulmonary v.
Left lower lobe basal trunk pulmonary a.
Descending thoracic aorta

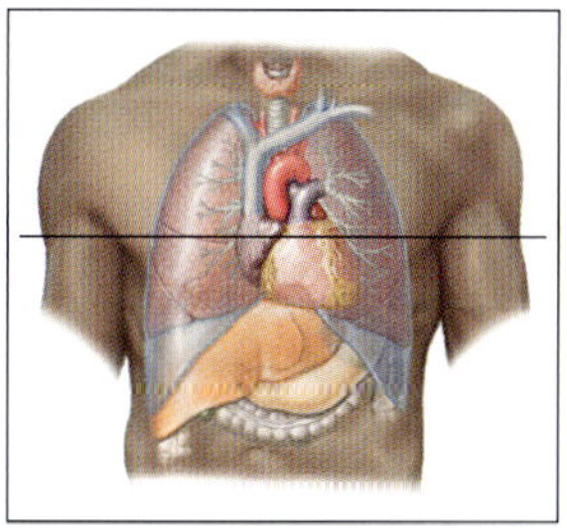

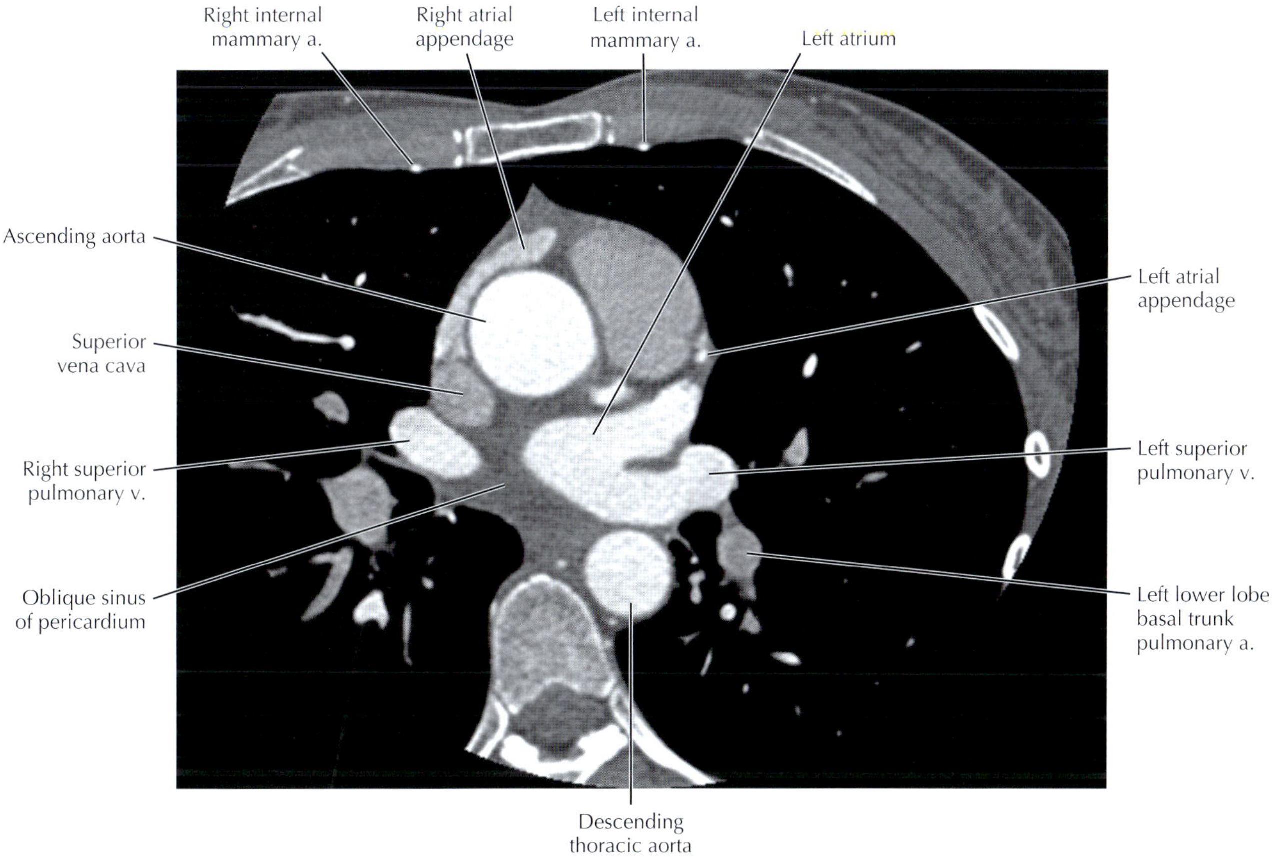
Right internal mammary a.
Right atrial appendage
Left internal mammary a.
Left atrium
Ascending aorta
Superior vena cava
Right superior pulmonary v.
Oblique sinus of pericardium
Left atrial appendage
Left superior pulmonary v.
Left lower lobe basal trunk pulmonary a.
Descending thoracic aorta

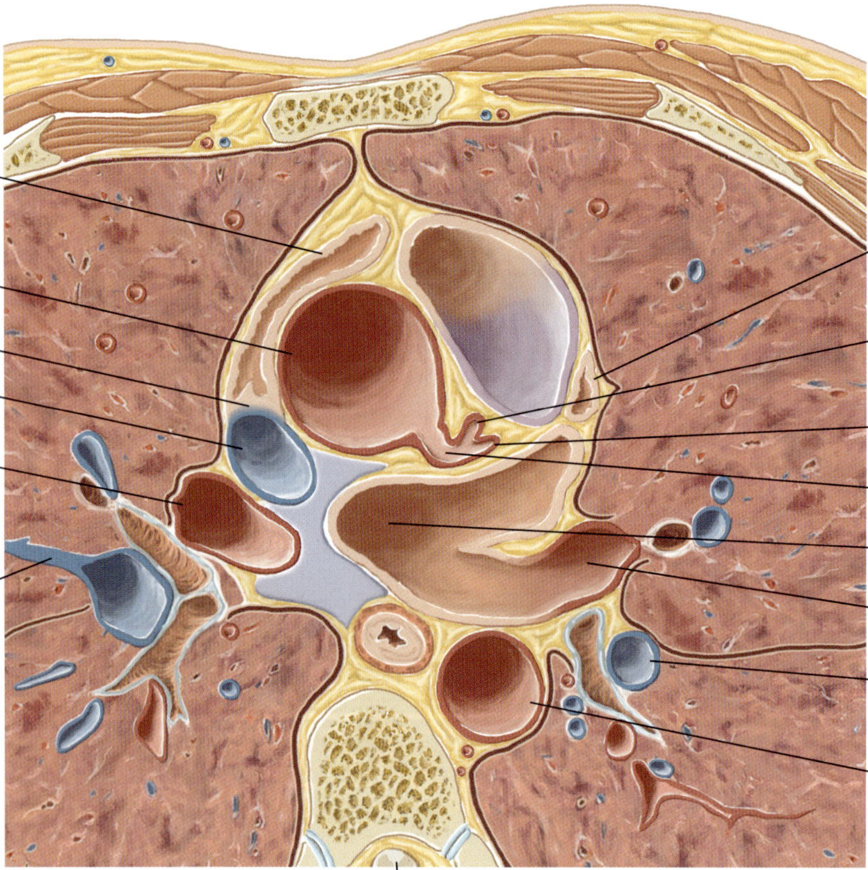

NORMAL ANATOMY

The crista terminalis is now just visible and will be readily visualized on views that follow. The crista terminalis is a vertical fibromuscular ridge that separates the smooth portion of the right atrium, which receives the superior and inferior vena cavae and coronary sinus, from the right atrial appendage and the remainder of the right atrium containing pectinate muscles. The crista terminalis extends superiorly from the anterior margin of the superior vena cava along the lateral wall of the right atrium inferiorly toward the inferior vena cava. A prominent crista terminalis can occasionally be mistaken for a right atrial mass on imaging studies.

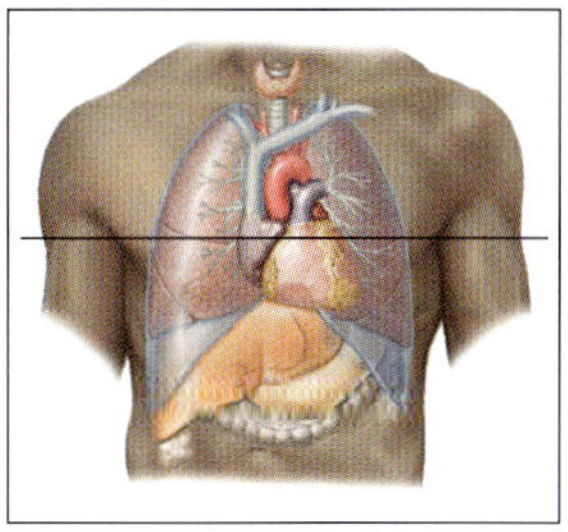

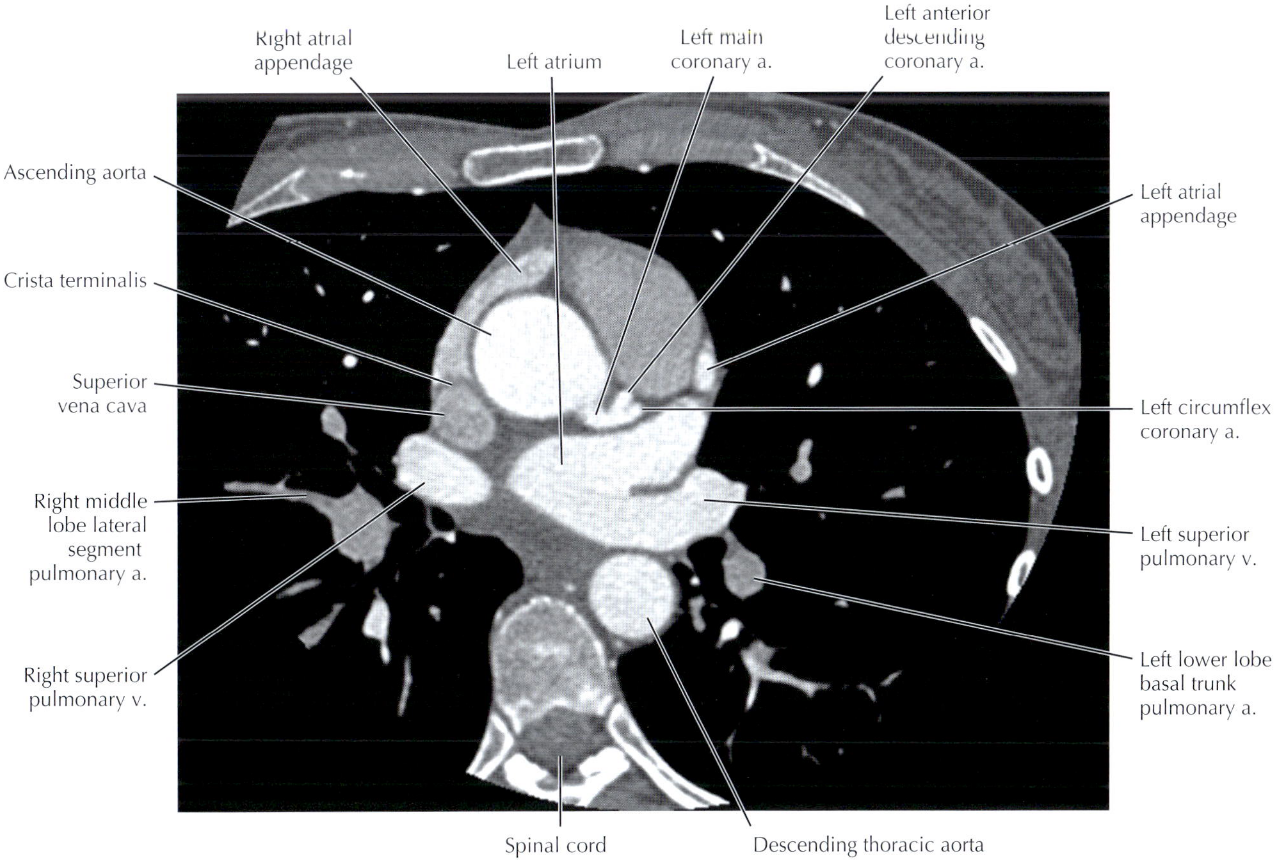
Right atrial appendage
Left atrium
Left main coronary a.
Left anterior descending coronary a.
Ascending aorta
Left atrial appendage
Crista terminalis
Superior vena cava
Left circumflex coronary a.
Right middle lobe lateral segment pulmonary a.
Left superior pulmonary v.
Right superior pulmonary v.
Left lower lobe basal trunk pulmonary a.
Spinal cord
Descending thoracic aorta

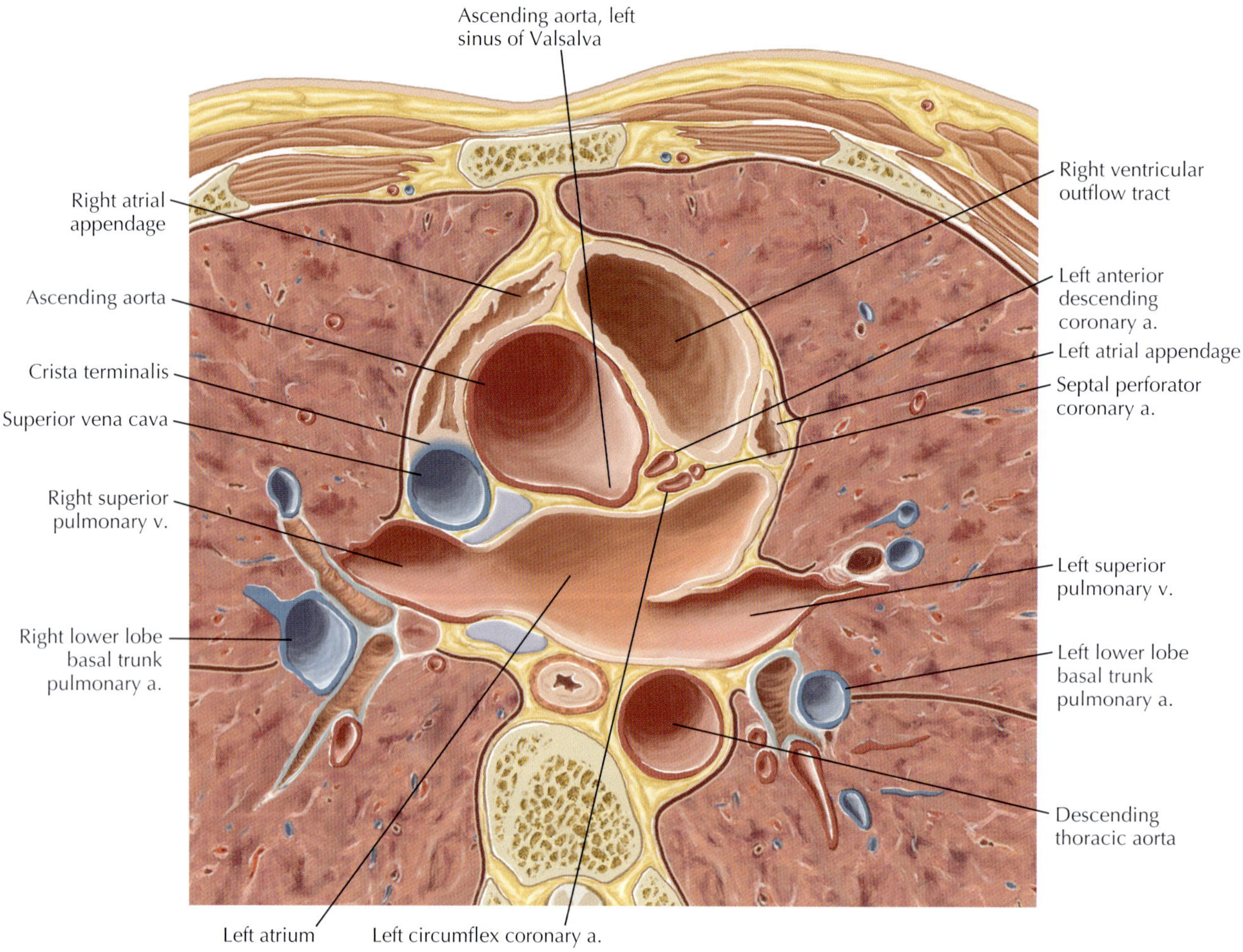
Ascending aorta, left sinus of Valsalva
Right atrial appendage
Ascending aorta
Crista terminalis
Superior vena cava
Right superior pulmonary v.
Right lower lobe basal trunk pulmonary a.
Right ventricular outflow tract
Left anterior descending coronary a.
Left atrial appendage
Septal perforator coronary a.
Left superior pulmonary v.
Left lower lobe basal trunk pulmonary a.
Descending thoracic aorta
Left atrium
Left circumflex coronary a.

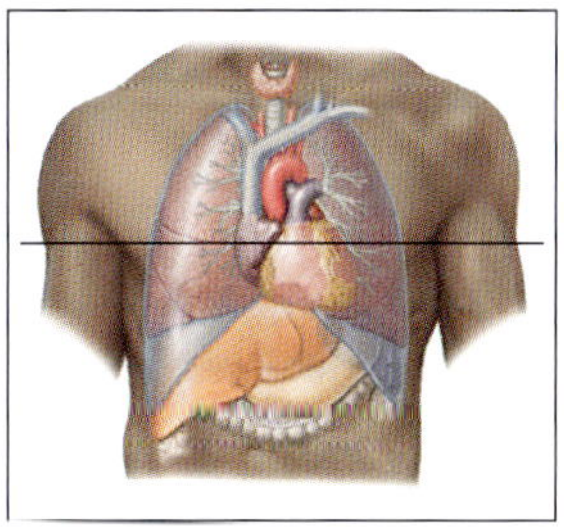

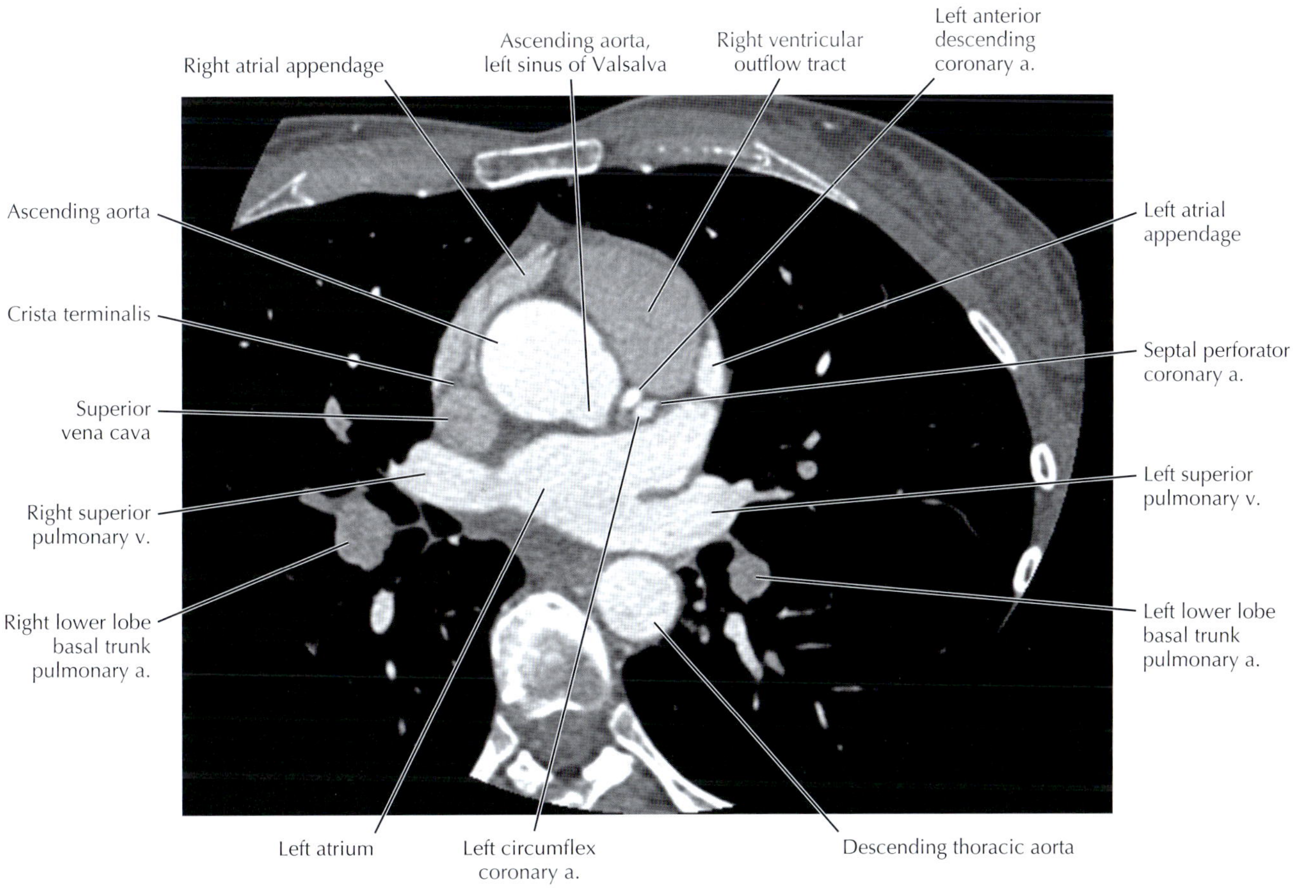
Right atrial appendage
Ascending aorta, left sinus of Valsalva
Right ventricular outflow tract
Left anterior descending coronary a.
Ascending aorta
Crista terminalis
Superior vena cava
Right superior pulmonary v.
Right lower lobe basal trunk pulmonary a.
Left atrial appendage
Septal perforator coronary a.
Left superior pulmonary v.
Left lower lobe basal trunk pulmonary a.
Left atrium
Left circumflex coronary a.
Descending thoracic aorta

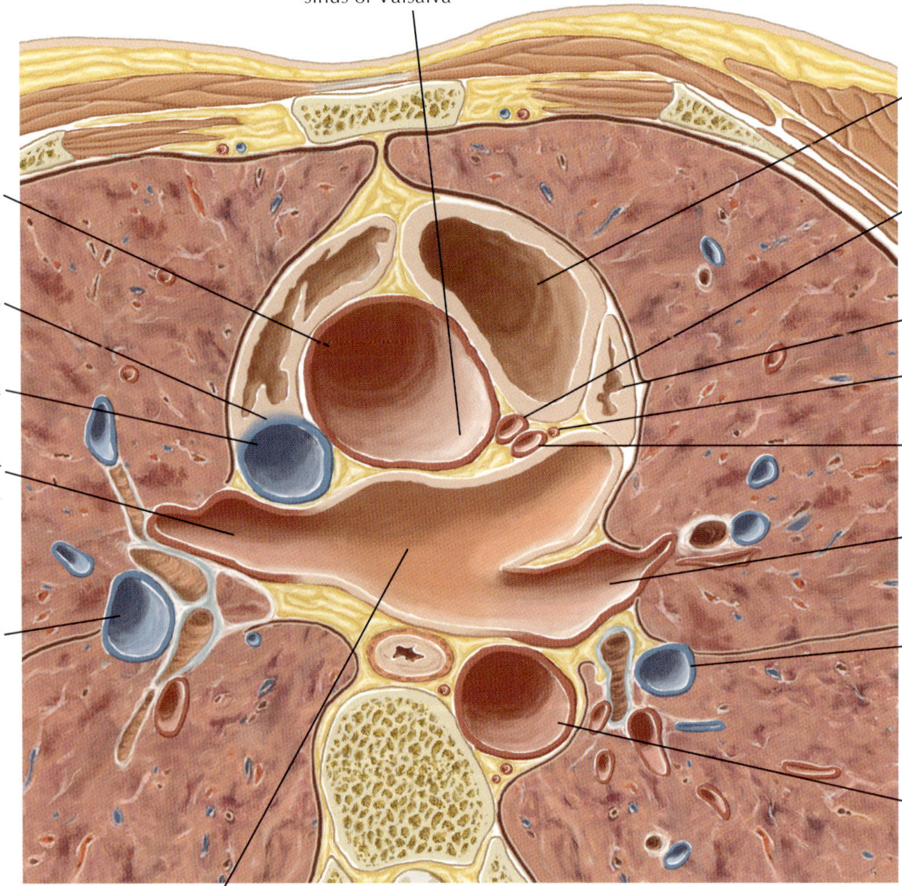

NORMAL ANATOMY

This image shows the origin of the first septal perforator branch of the proximal left anterior descending coronary artery (also known as the anterior interventricular branch of the left coronary artery). The first septal perforator coronary artery provides blood flow to the interventricular septum and conduction system of the heart. Disruption of blood flow within the proximal segment of the left anterior descending artery and first septal perforator vessel, as may occur with significant atherosclerosis in the left main or proximal left anterior descending coronary arteries, may result in cardiac dysrhythmias and a large myocardial infarction, leading to sudden cardiac death.

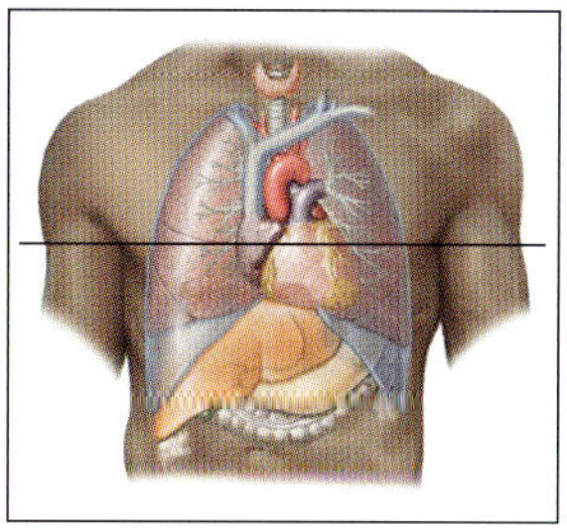

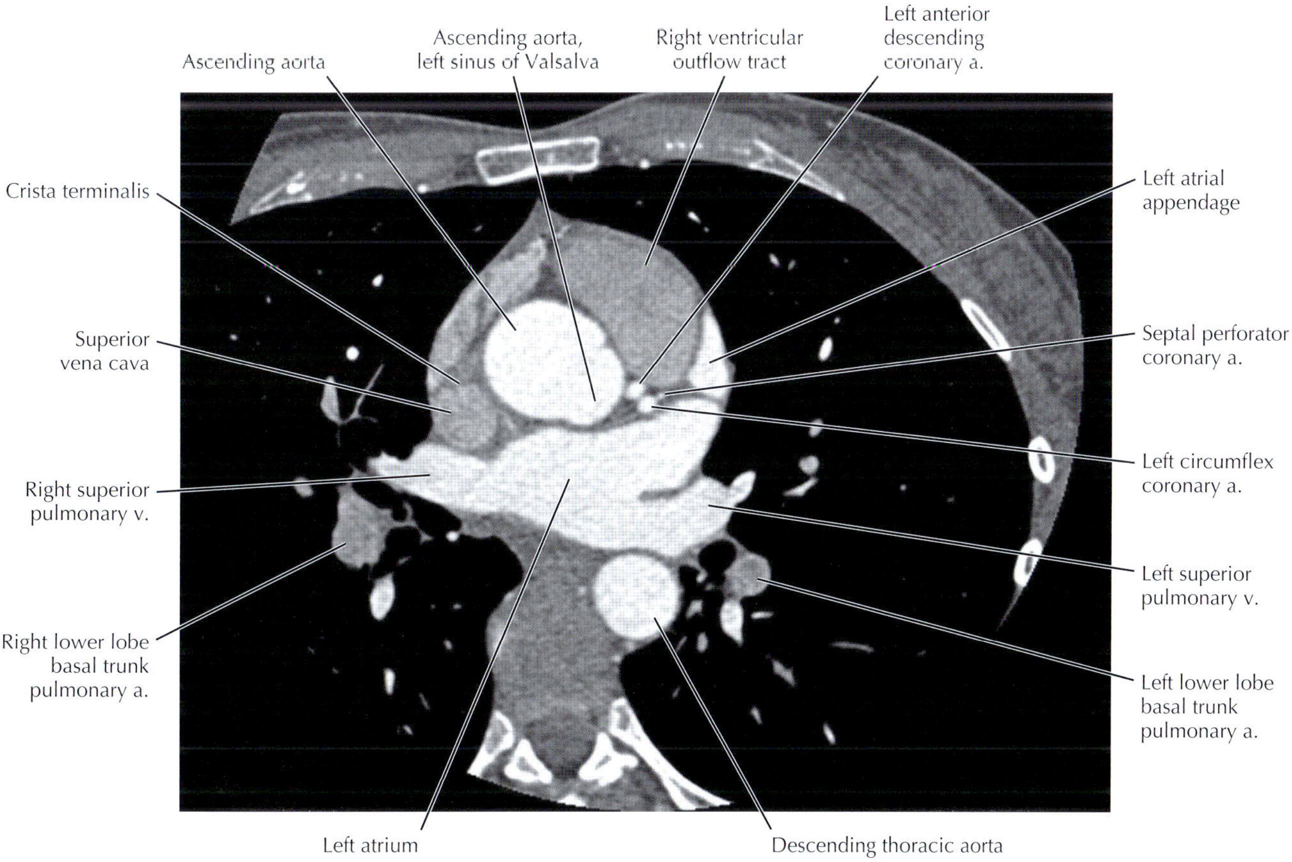
Ascending aorta
Ascending aorta, left sinus of Valsalva
Right ventricular outflow tract
Left anterior descending coronary a.
Crista terminalis
Left atrial appendage
Superior vena cava
Septal perforator coronary a.
Left circumflex coronary a.
Right superior pulmonary v.
Left superior pulmonary v.
Right lower lobe basal trunk pulmonary a.
Left lower lobe basal trunk pulmonary a.
Left atrium
Descending thoracic aorta

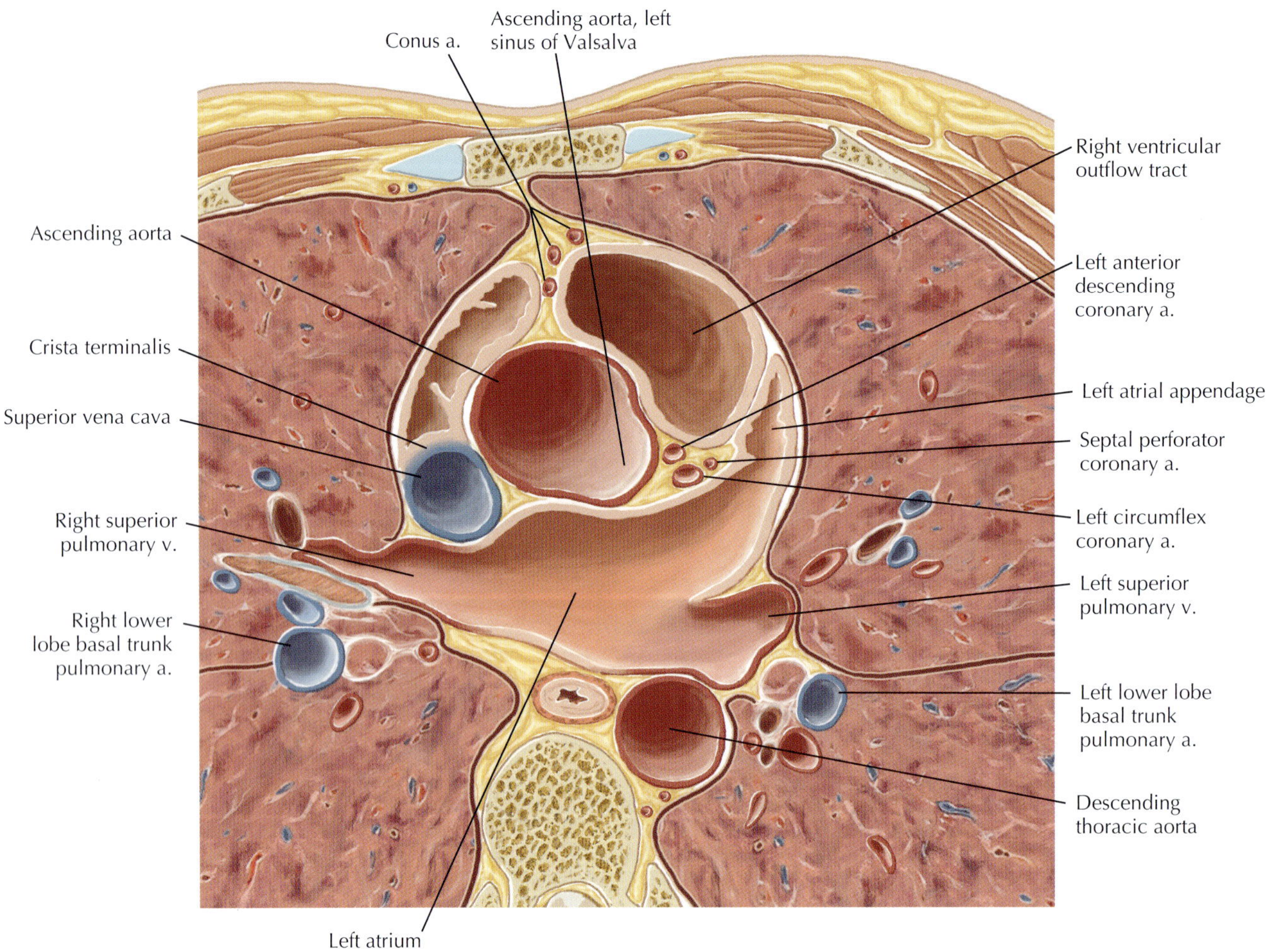
Conus a.
Ascending aorta, left sinus of Valsalva
Right ventricular outflow tract
Ascending aorta
Left anterior descending coronary a.
Crista terminalis
Left atrial appendage
Superior vena cava
Septal perforator coronary a.
Left circumflex coronary a.
Right superior pulmonary v.
Left superior pulmonary v.
Right lower lobe basal trunk pulmonary a.
Left lower lobe basal trunk pulmonary a.
Descending thoracic aorta
Left atrium

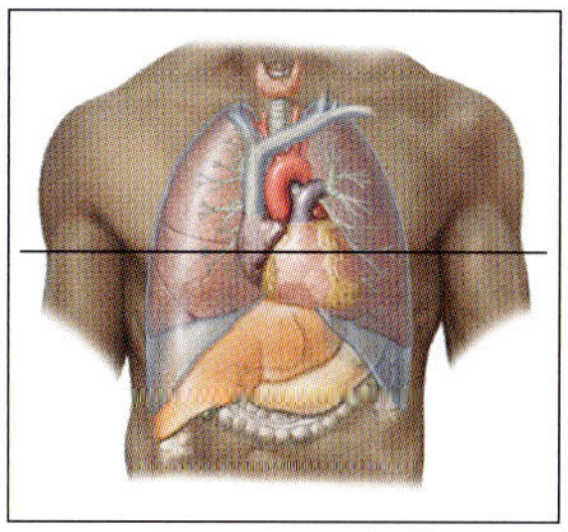

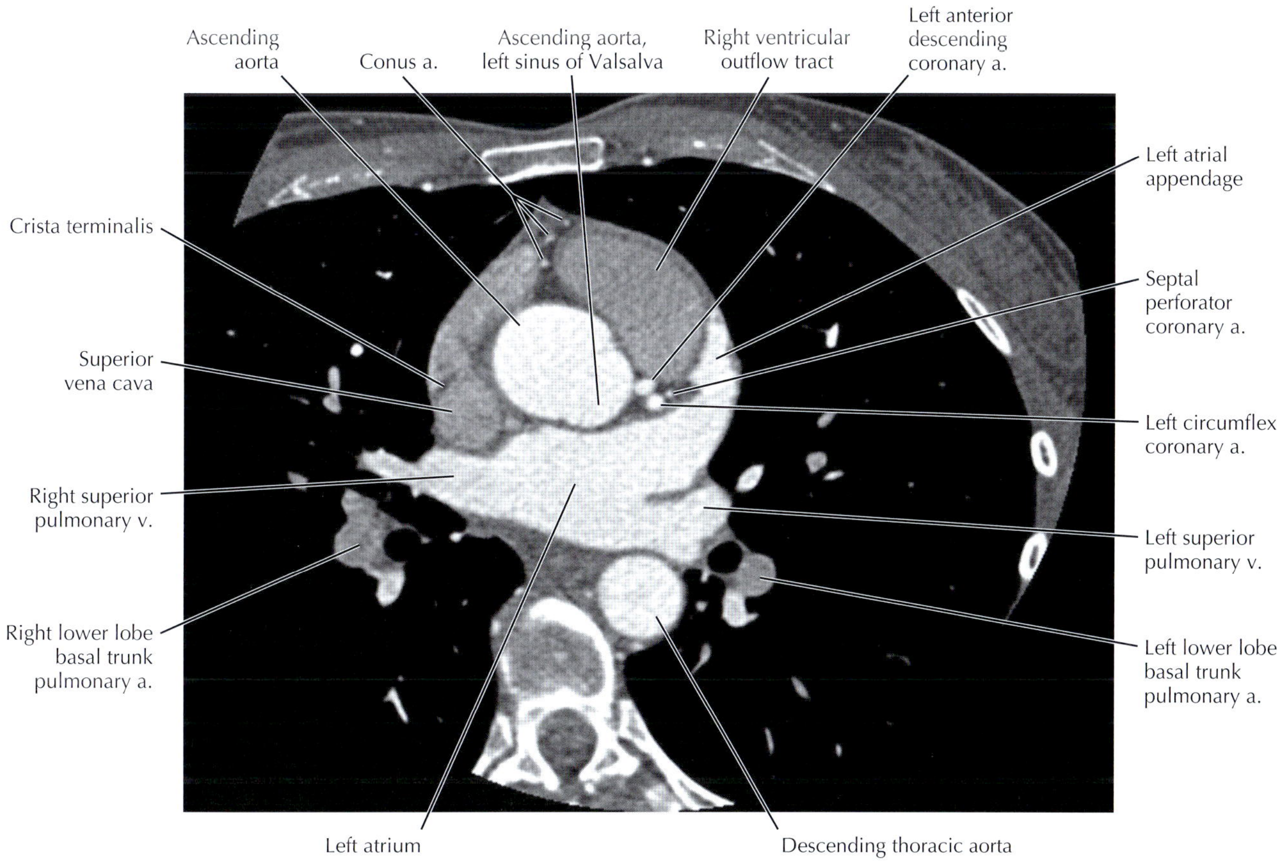
Ascending aorta
Conus a.
Ascending aorta, left sinus of Valsalva
Right ventricular outflow tract
Left anterior descending coronary a.
Left atrial appendage
Crista terminalis
Septal perforator coronary a.
Superior vena cava
Left circumflex coronary a.
Right superior pulmonary v.
Left superior pulmonary v.
Right lower lobe basal trunk pulmonary a.
Left lower lobe basal trunk pulmonary a.
Left atrium
Descending thoracic aorta

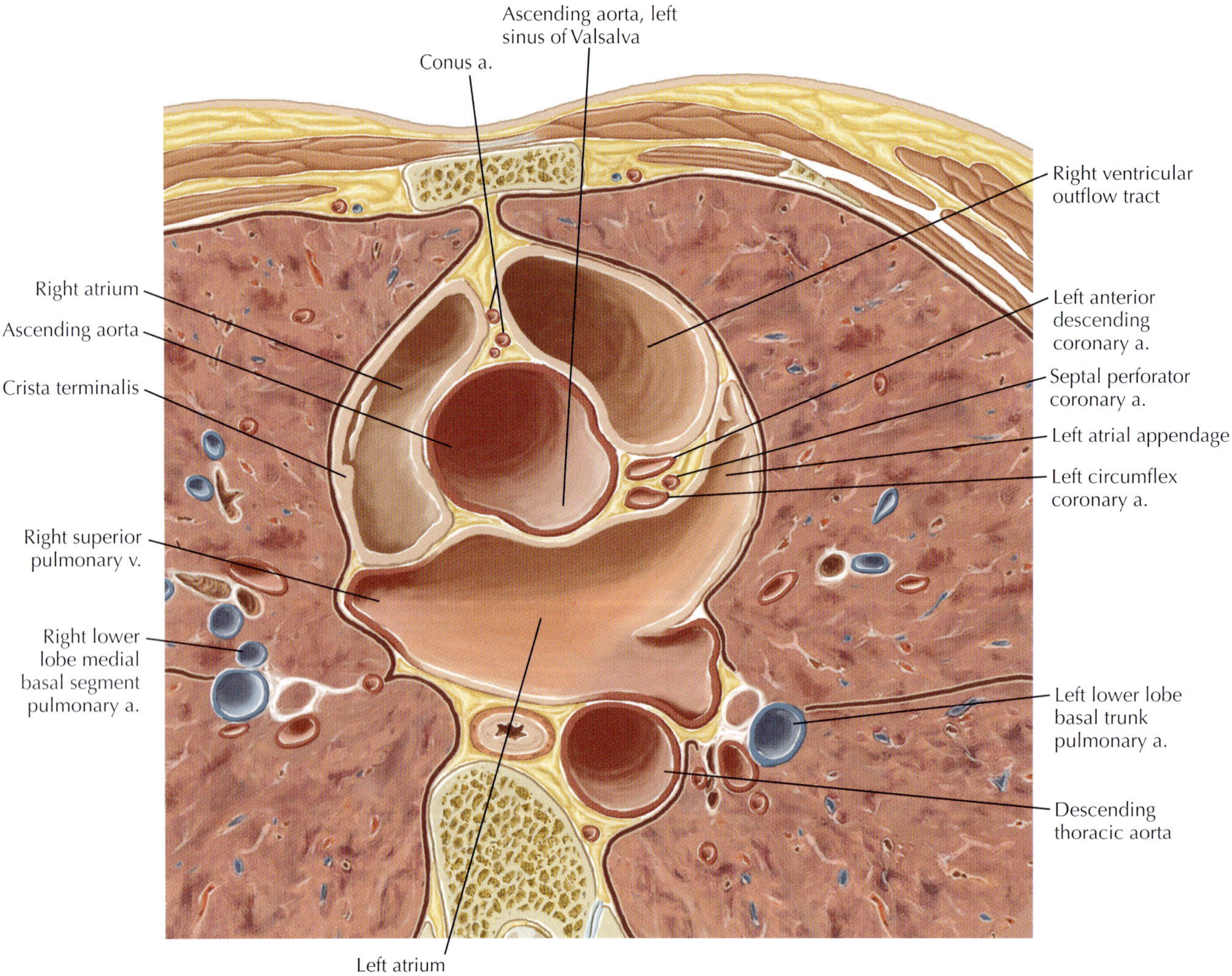
Ascending aorta, left sinus of Valsalva
Conus a.
Right ventricular outflow tract
Right atrium
Ascending aorta
Crista terminalis
Left anterior descending coronary a.
Septal perforator coronary a.
Left atrial appendage
Left circumflex coronary a.
Right superior pulmonary v.
Right lower lobe medial basal segment pulmonary a.
Left lower lobe basal trunk pulmonary a.
Descending thoracic aorta
Left atrium

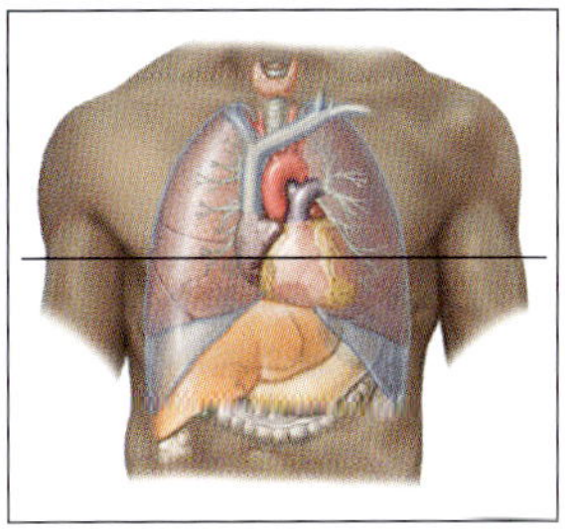

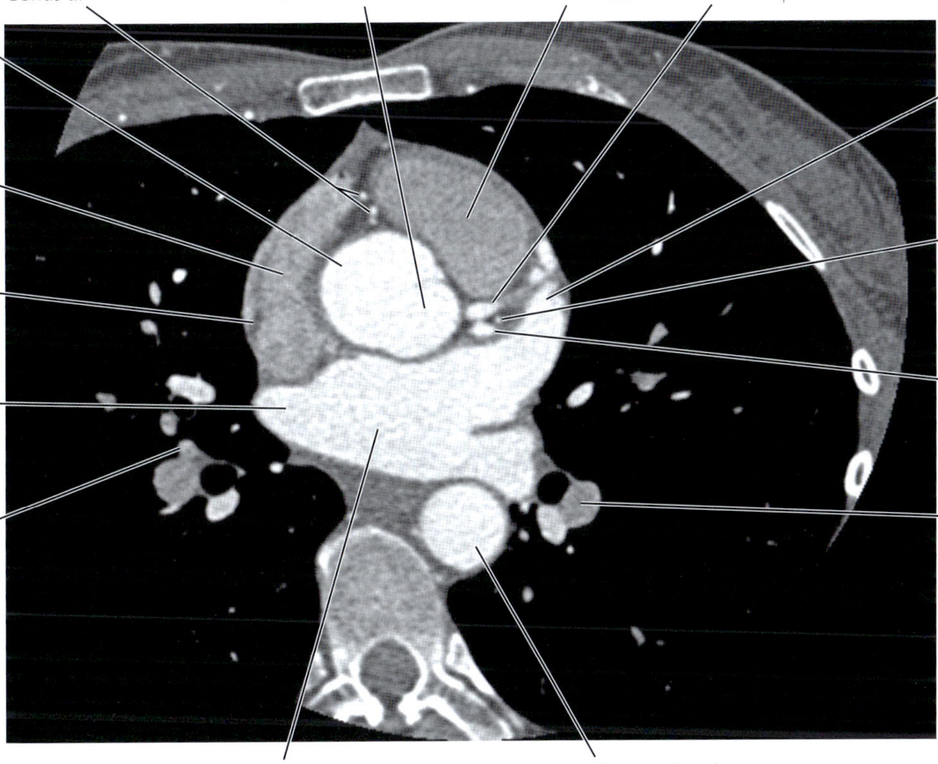
Conus a.
Ascending aorta, left sinus of Valsalva
Right ventricular outflow tract
Left anterior descending coronary a.
Ascending aorta
Left atrial appendage
Right atrium
Septal perforator coronary a.
Crista terminalis
Left circumflex coronary a.
Right superior pulmonary v.
Right lower lobe medial basal segment pulmonary a.
Left lower lobe basal trunk pulmonary a.
Left atrium
Descending thoracic aorta

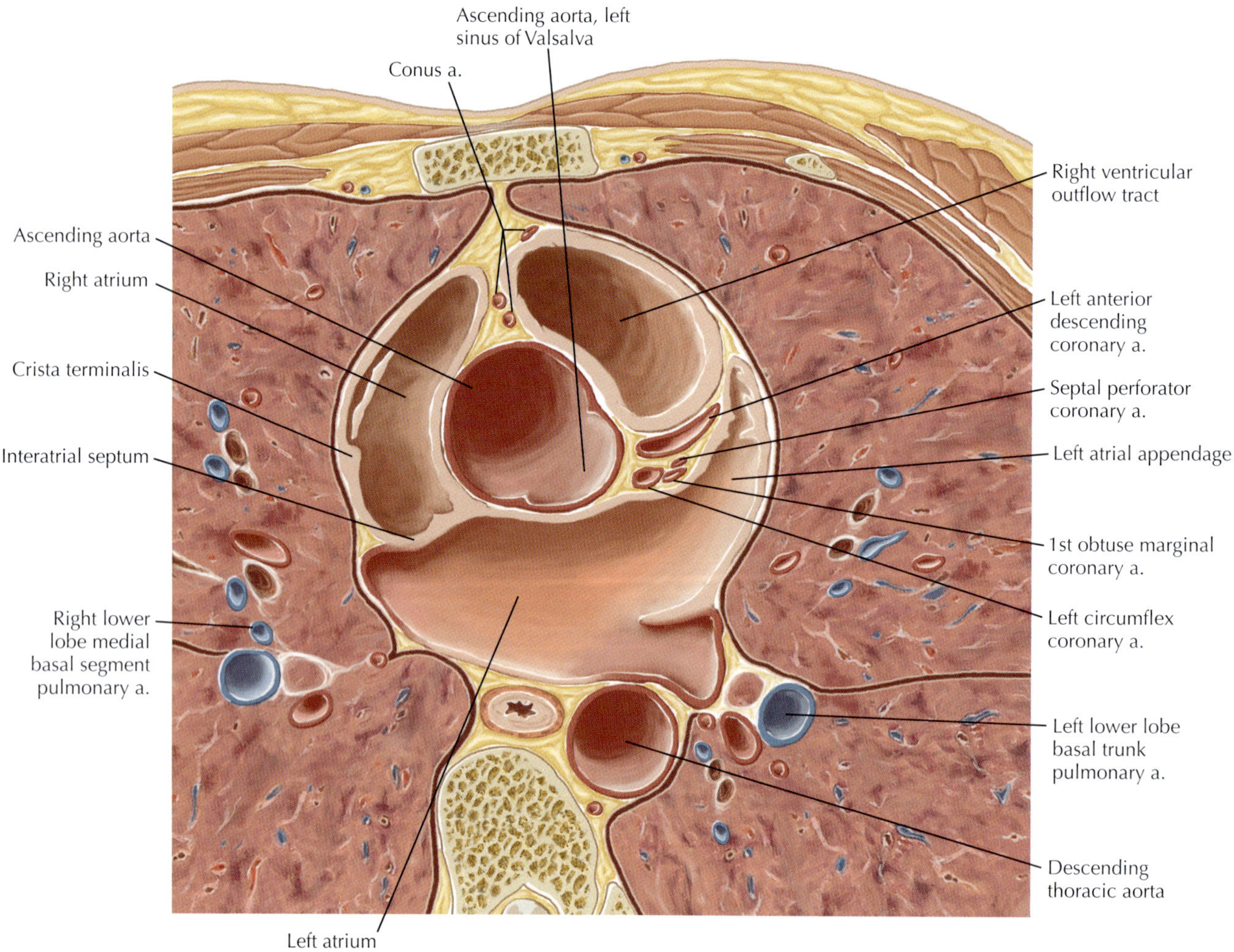
Ascending aorta, left sinus of Valsalva
Conus a.
Ascending aorta
Right atrium
Crista terminalis
Interatrial septum
Right lower lobe medial basal segment pulmonary a.
Left atrium
Right ventricular outflow tract
Left anterior descending coronary a.
Septal perforator coronary a.
Left atrial appendage
1st obtuse marginal coronary a.
Left circumflex coronary a.
Left lower lobe basal trunk pulmonary a.
Descending thoracic aorta

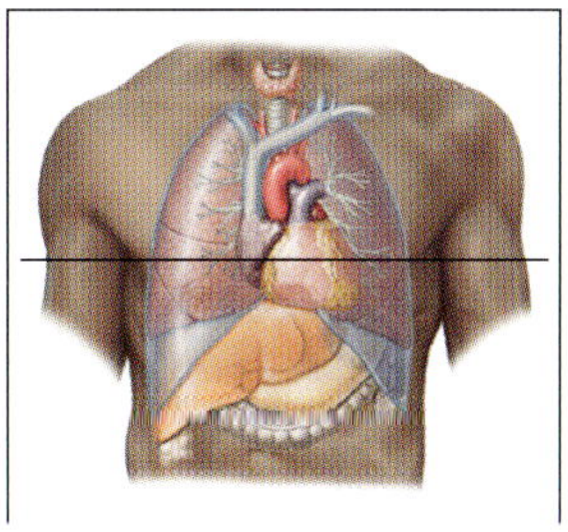

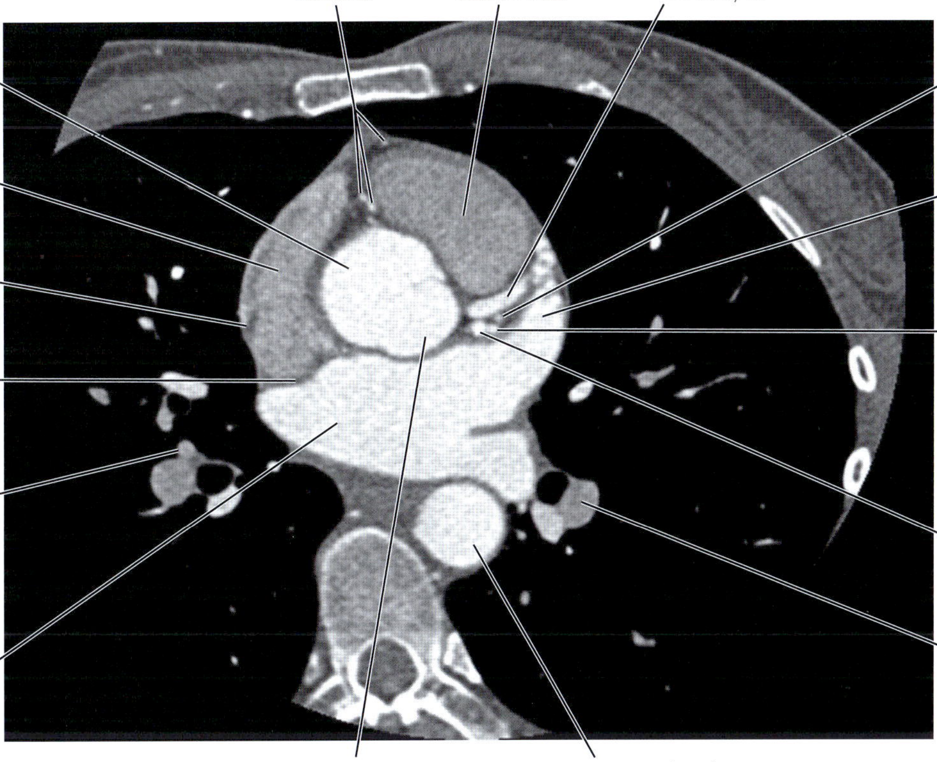
Conus a.
Right ventricular outflow tract
Left anterior descending coronary a.
Ascending aorta
Right atrium
Crista terminalis
Interatrial septum
Right lower lobe medial basal segment pulmonary a.
Left atrium
Septal perforator coronary a.
Left atrial appendage
1st obtuse marginal coronary a.
Left circumflex coronary a.
Left lower lobe basal trunk pulmonary a.
Ascending aorta, left sinus of Valsalva
Descending thoracic aorta

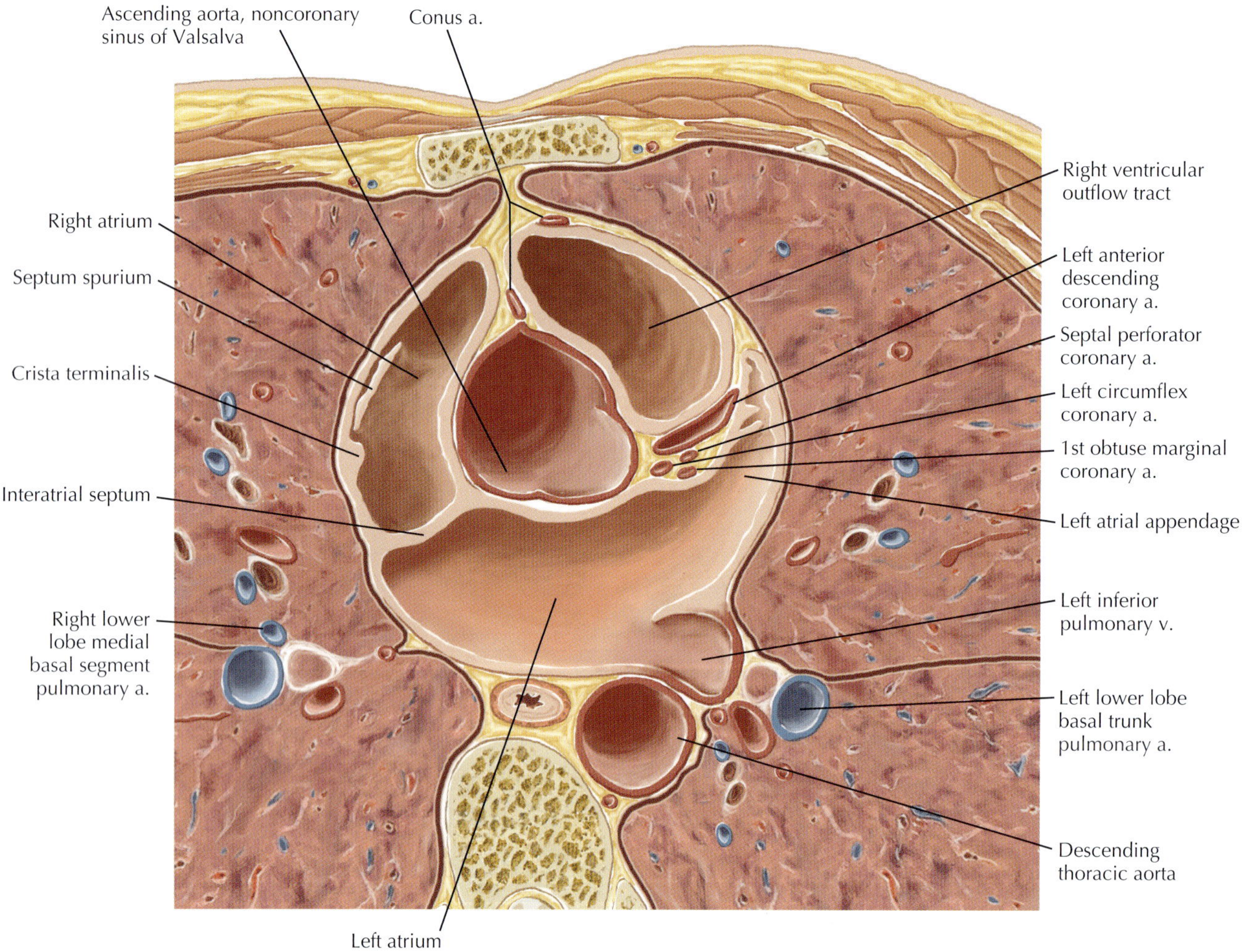

NORMAL ANATOMY

A linear low-attenuation structure extending anteriorly from the crista terminalis is visible; this structure represents the septum spurium. The septum spurium is the most prominent of the anterior pectinate muscles arising from the crista terminalis.

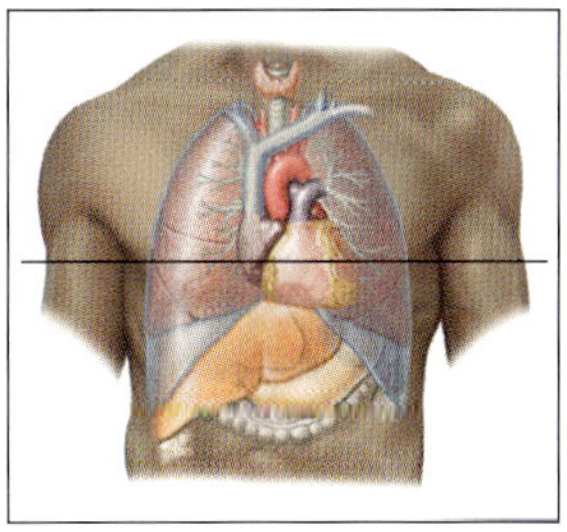

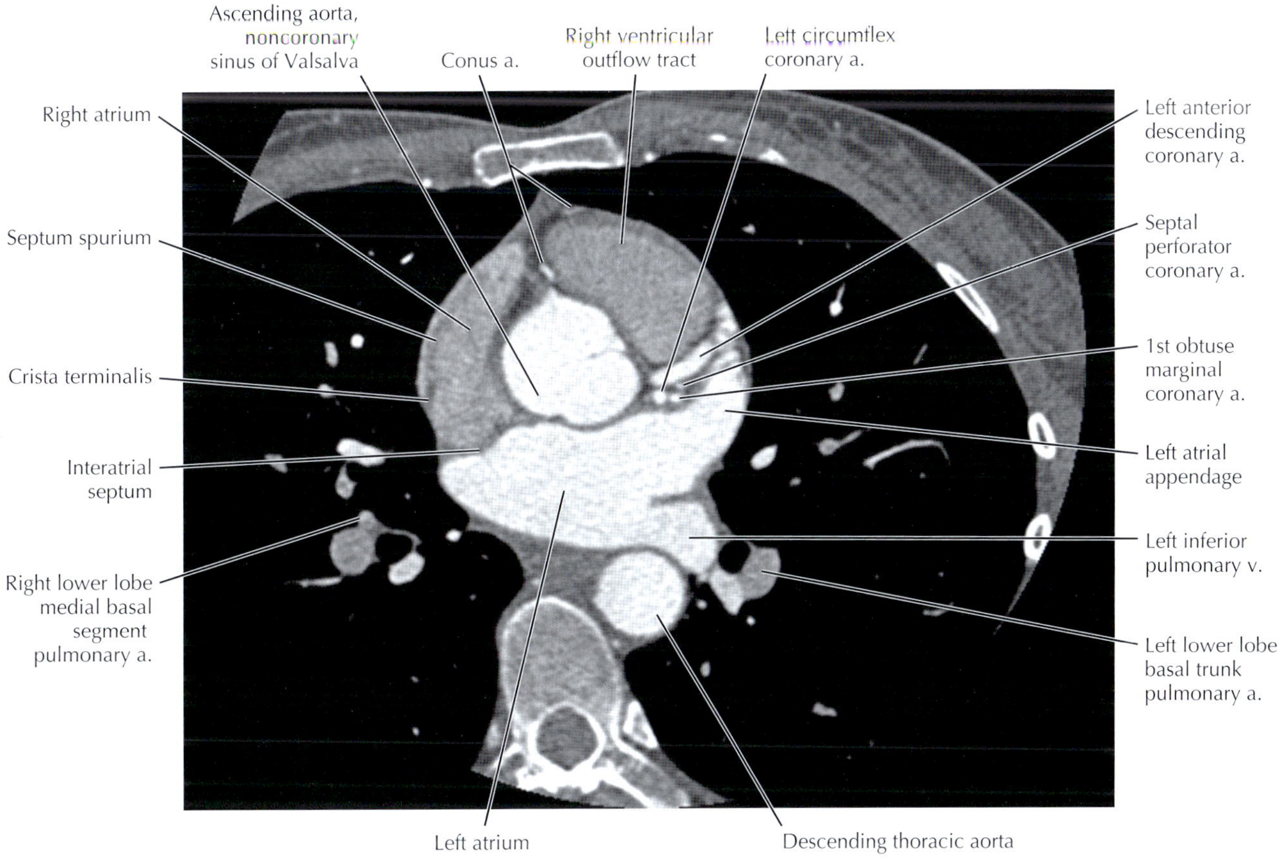
Ascending aorta, noncoronary sinus of Valsalva
Conus a.
Right ventricular outflow tract
Left circumflex coronary a.
Right atrium
Left anterior descending coronary a.
Septum spurium
Septal perforator coronary a.
Crista terminalis
1st obtuse marginal coronary a.
Interatrial septum
Left atrial appendage
Left inferior pulmonary v.
Right lower lobe medial basal segment pulmonary a.
Left lower lobe basal trunk pulmonary a.
Left atrium
Descending thoracic aorta

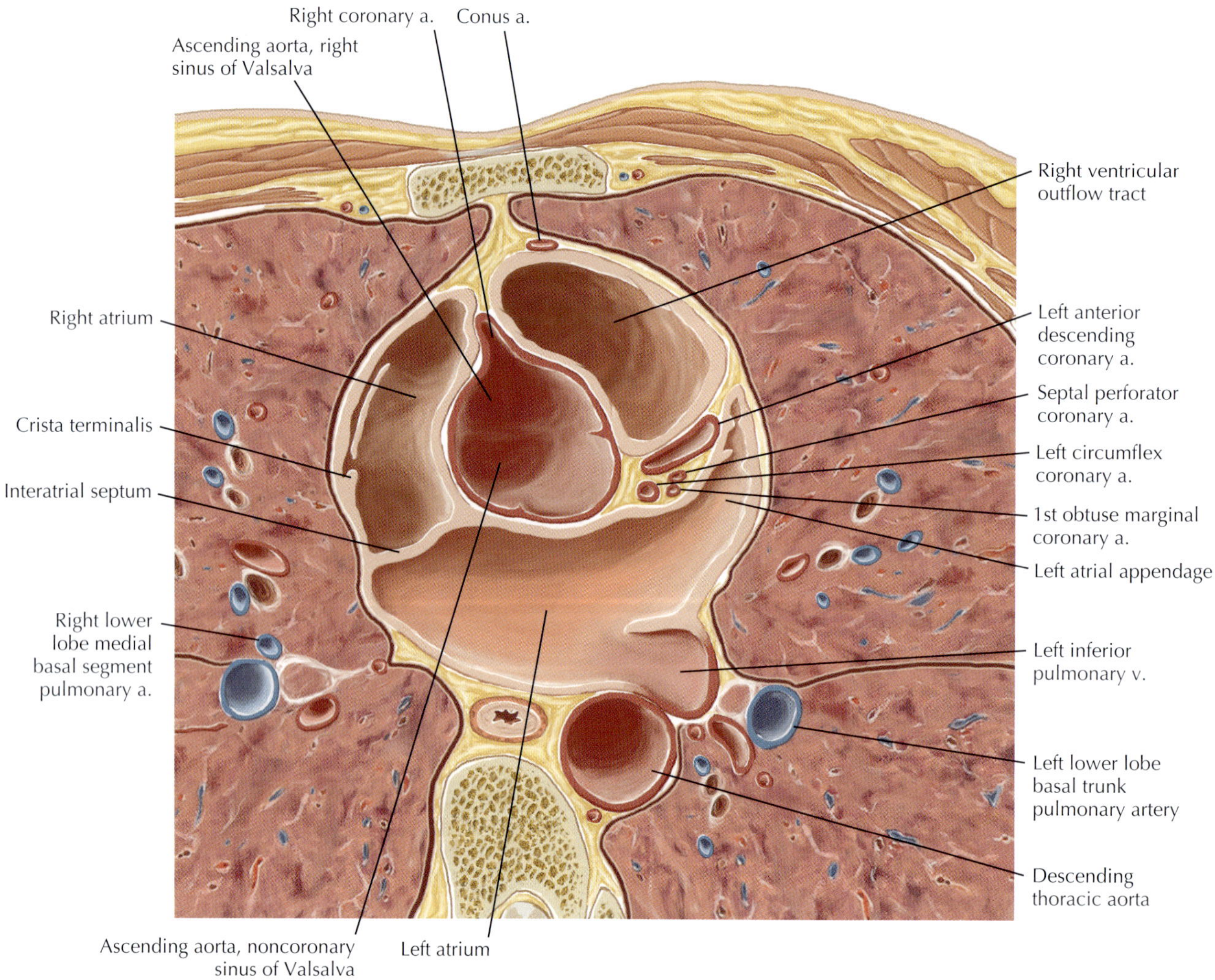
Right coronary a.
Conus a.
Ascending aorta, right sinus of Valsalva
Right ventricular outflow tract
Right atrium
Left anterior descending coronary a.
Septal perforator coronary a.
Crista terminalis
Left circumflex coronary a.
Interatrial septum
1st obtuse marginal coronary a.
Left atrial appendage
Right lower lobe medial basal segment pulmonary a.
Left inferior pulmonary v.
Left lower lobe basal trunk pulmonary artery
Descending thoracic aorta
Ascending aorta, noncoronary sinus of Valsalva
Left atrium

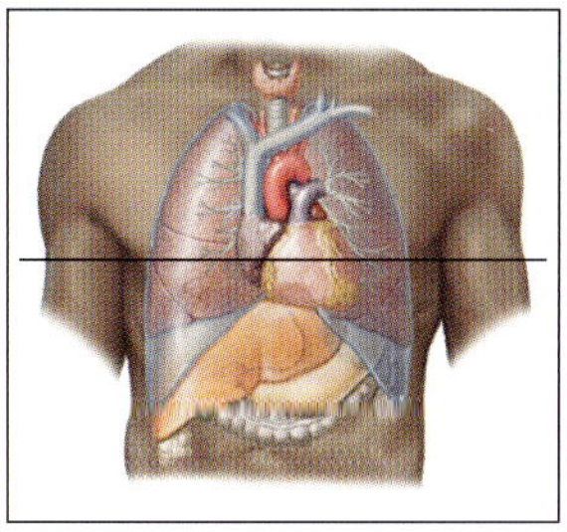

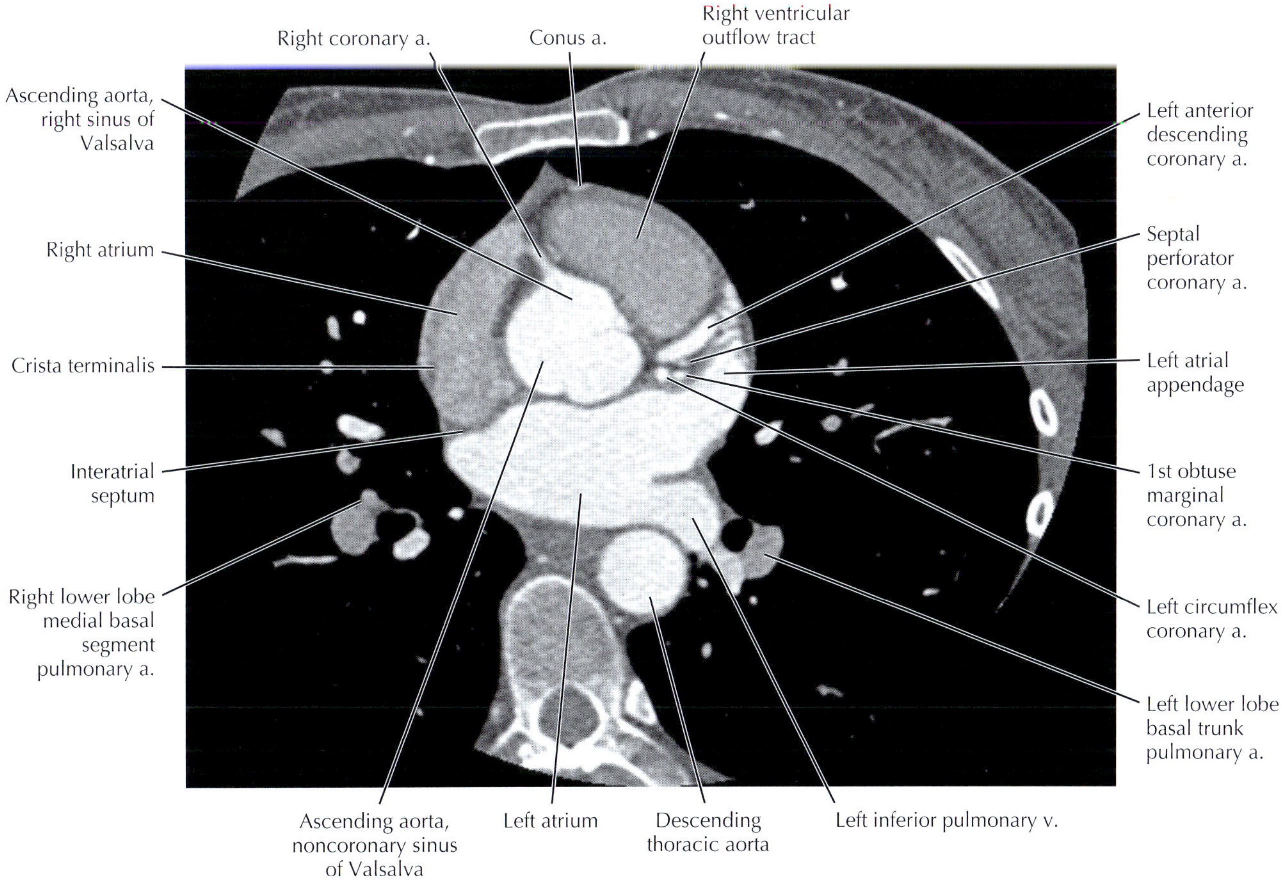
Right coronary a.
Conus a.
Right ventricular outflow tract
Ascending aorta, right sinus of Valsalva
Right atrium
Crista terminalis
Interatrial septum
Right lower lobe medial basal segment pulmonary a.
Left anterior descending coronary a.
Septal perforator coronary a.
Left atrial appendage
1st obtuse marginal coronary a.
Left circumflex coronary a.
Left lower lobe basal trunk pulmonary a.
Ascending aorta, noncoronary sinus of Valsalva
Left atrium
Descending thoracic aorta
Left inferior pulmonary v.

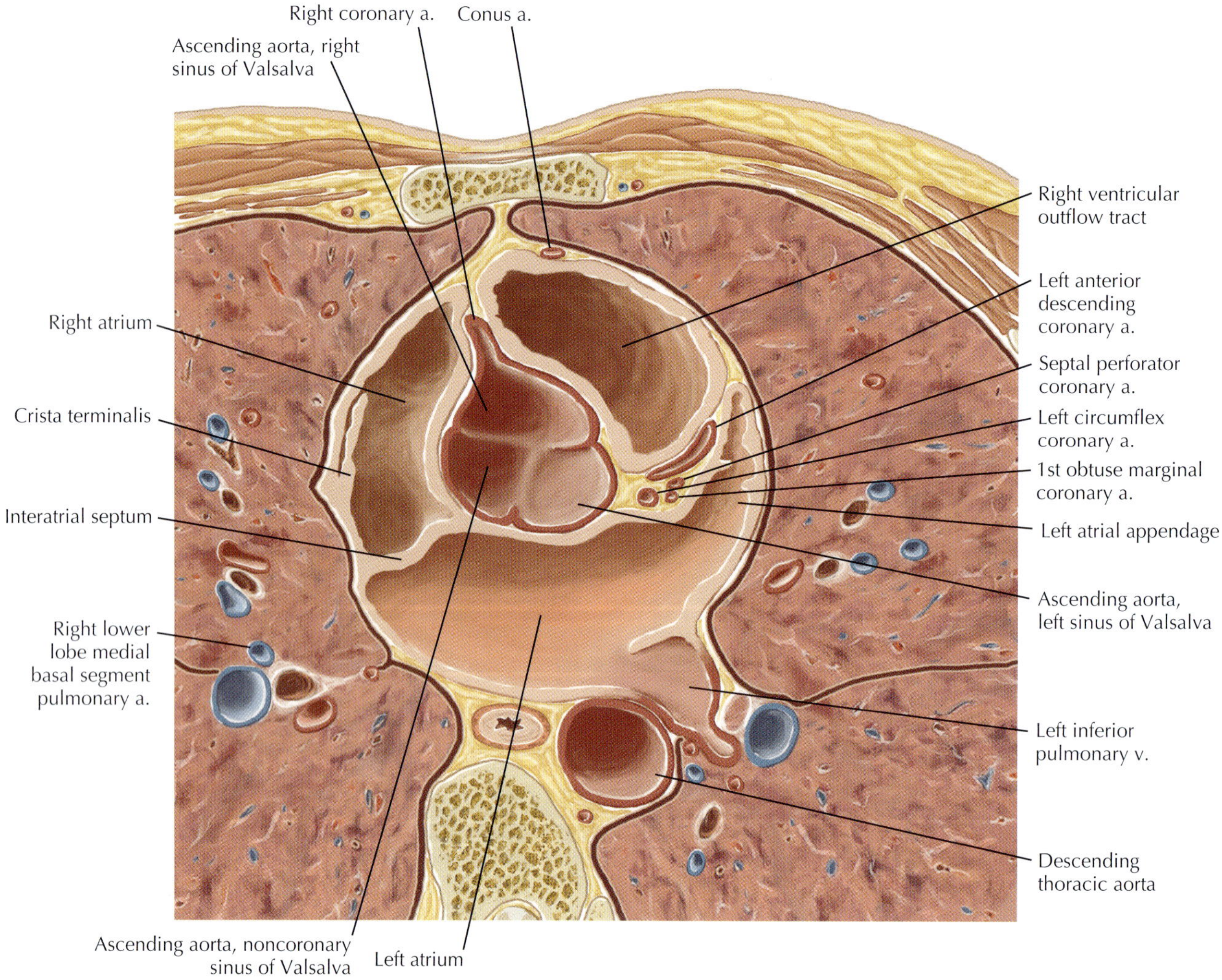
Right coronary a.
Conus a.
Ascending aorta, right sinus of Valsalva
Right ventricular outflow tract
Left anterior descending coronary a.
Right atrium
Septal perforator coronary a.
Crista terminalis
Left circumflex coronary a.
1st obtuse marginal coronary a.
Interatrial septum
Left atrial appendage
Ascending aorta, left sinus of Valsalva
Right lower lobe medial basal segment pulmonary a.
Left inferior pulmonary v.
Descending thoracic aorta
Ascending aorta, noncoronary sinus of Valsalva
Left atrium

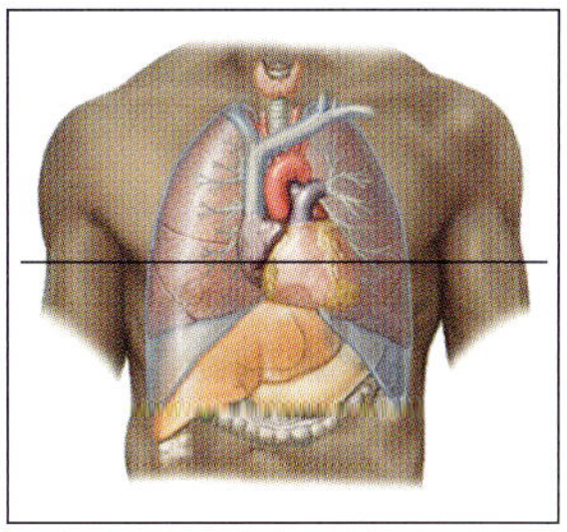

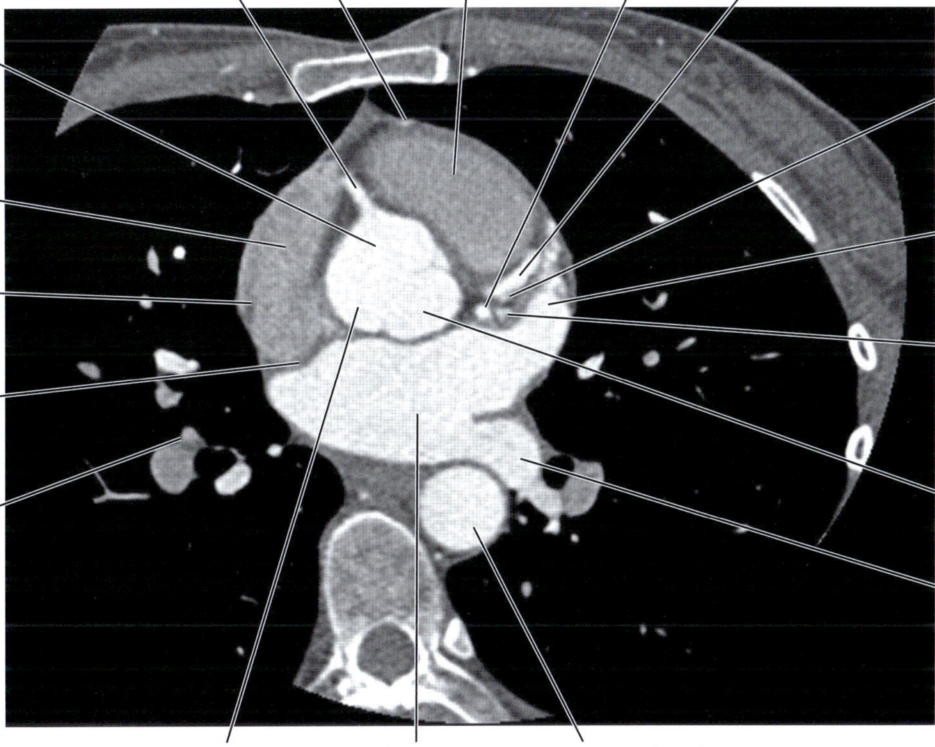
Right coronary a.
Conus a.
Right ventricular outflow tract
Left circumflex coronary a.
Left anterior descending coronary a.
Ascending aorta, right sinus of Valsalva
Septal perforator coronary a.
Right atrium
Left atrial appendage
Crista terminalis
1st obtuse marginal coronary a.
Interatrial septum
Right lower lobe medial basal segment pulmonary a.
Ascending aorta, left sinus of Valsalva
Left inferior pulmonary v.
Ascending aorta, noncoronary sinus of Valsalva
Left atrium
Descending thoracic aorta

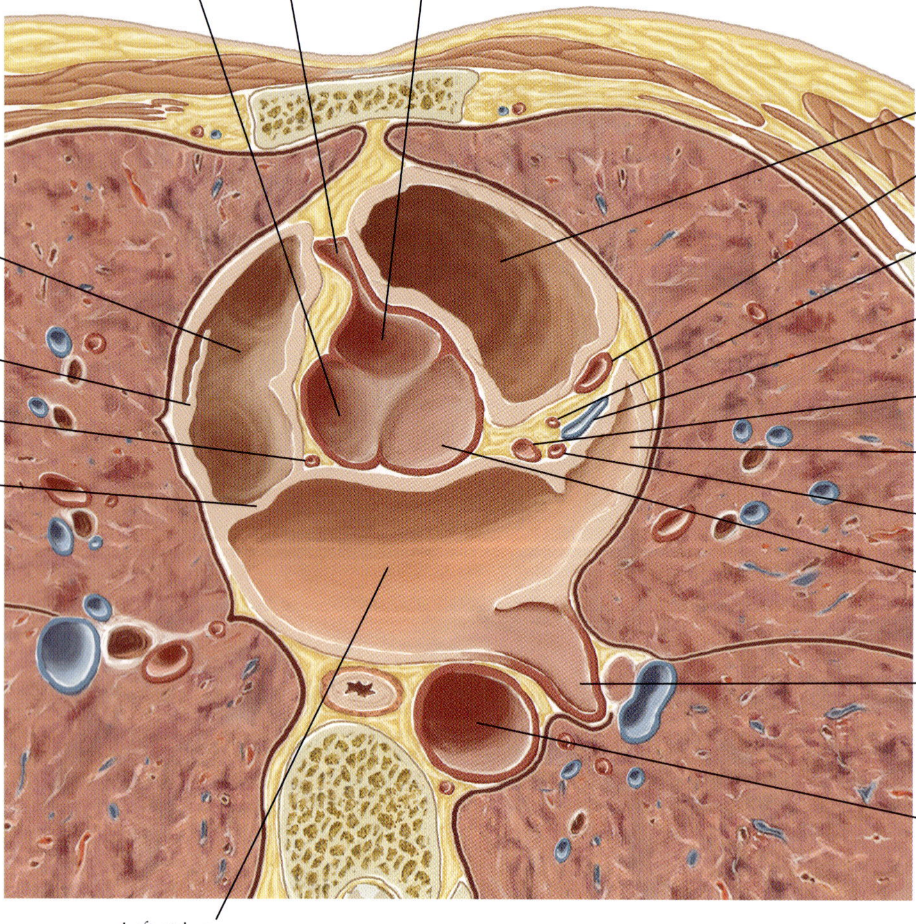

Right coronary a.
Ascending aorta, right sinus of Valsalva
Ascending aorta, noncoronary sinus of Valsalva
Right atrium
Crista terminalis
Sinoatrial node a.
Interatrial septum
Left atrium
Right ventricular outflow tract
Left anterior descending coronary a.
Septal perforator coronary a.
Anterior interventricular coronary v.
Left circumflex coronary a.
Left atrial appendage
1st obtuse marginal coronary a.
Ascending aorta, left sinus of Valsalva
Left inferior pulmonary v.
Descending thoracic aorta

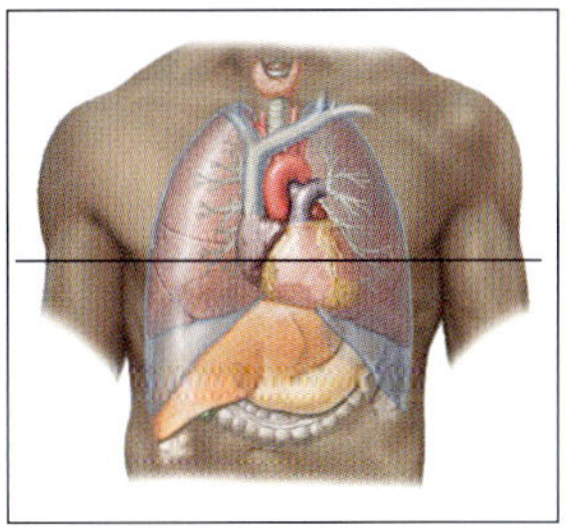

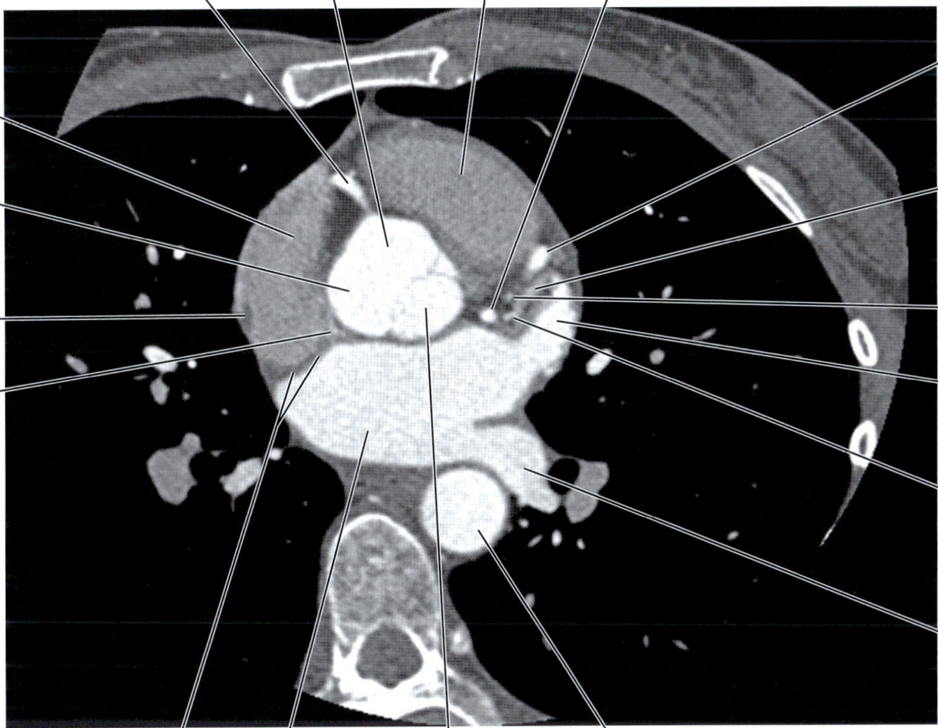
Right coronary a.
Ascending aorta, right sinus of Valsalva
Right ventricular outflow tract
Left circumflex coronary a.
Left anterior descending coronary a.
Right atrium
Ascending aorta, noncoronary sinus of Valsalva
Anterior interventricular coronary v.
Crista terminalis
Septal perforator coronary a.
Sinoatrial node a.
Left atrial appendage
1st obtuse marginal coronary a.
Left inferior pulmonary v.
Interatrial septum
Left atrium
Ascending aorta, left sinus of Valsalva
Descending thoracic aorta

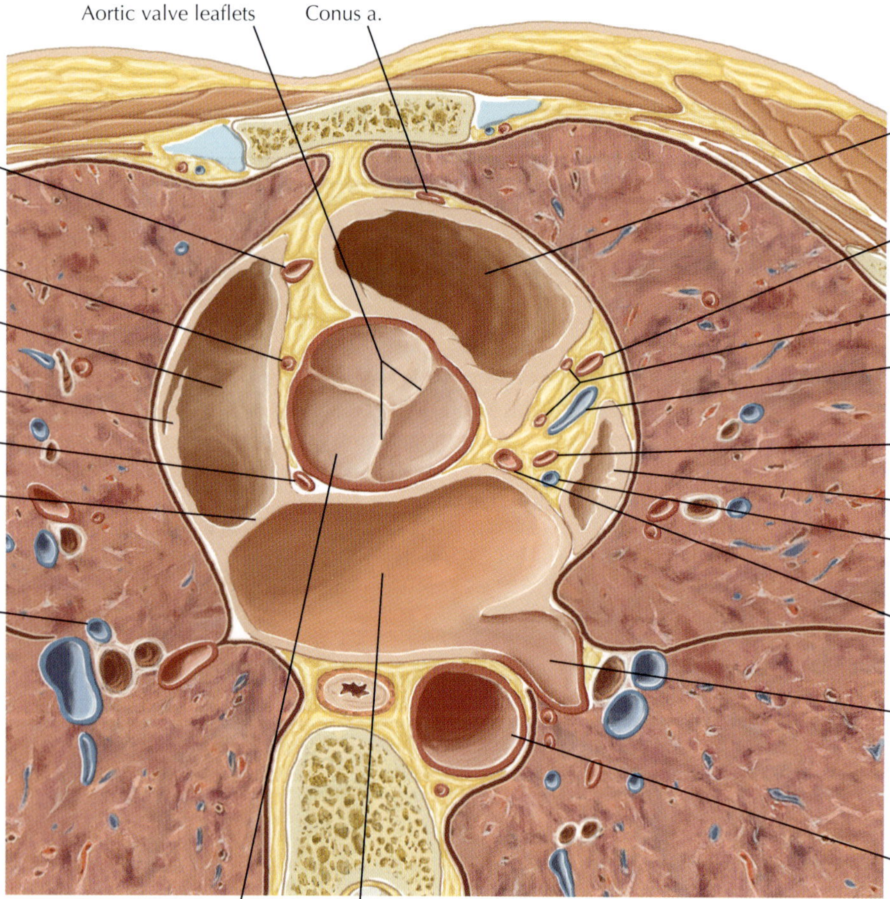

NORMAL ANATOMY

The sinoatrial nodal coronary artery is visible. The sinoatrial node is the source of the cardiac impulse and is typically located at the junction of the superior vena cava and right atrium, in the superior end of the crista terminalis. The sinoatrial nodal artery usually arises as a single branch from the right coronary artery, as in this patient (see Axials 20 to 25), or, less commonly, the sinoatrial nodal artery may arise from the left circumflex coronary artery. The sinoatrial nodal artery may be followed superiorly toward the location of the sinoatrial node.

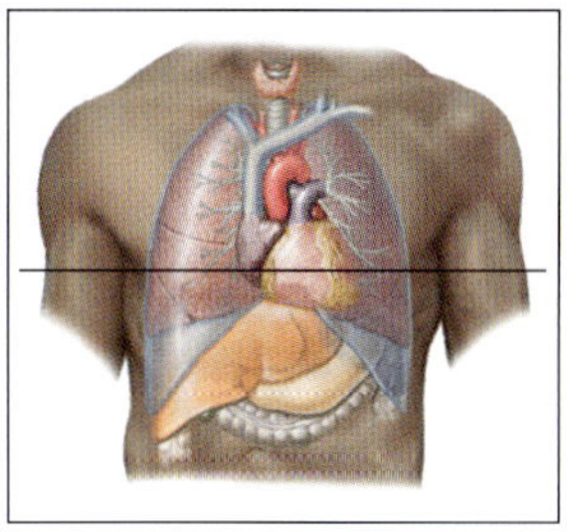

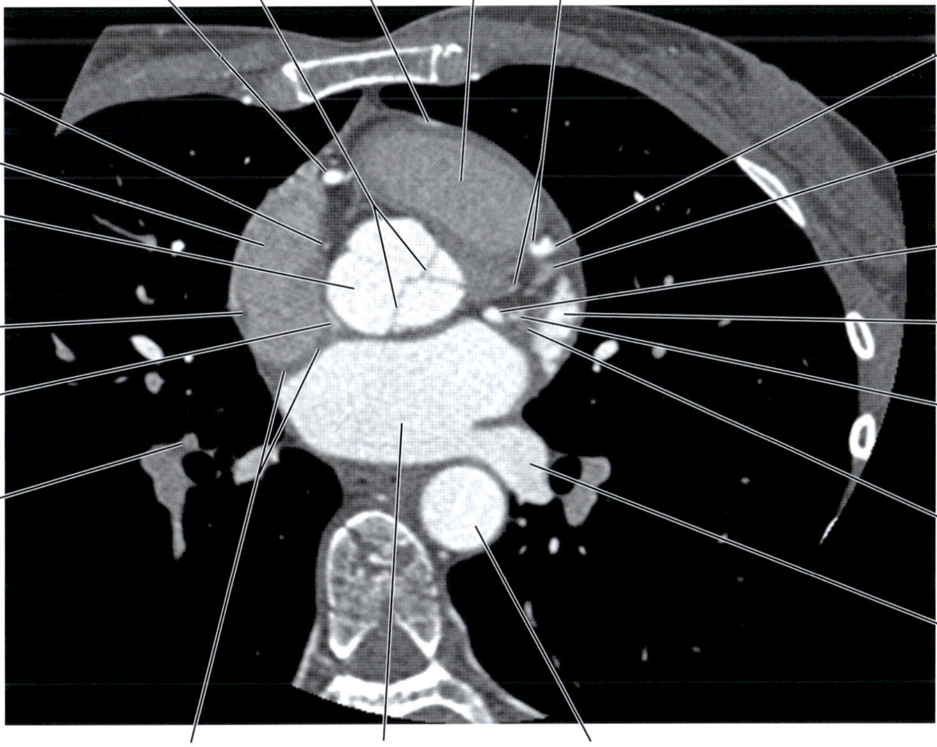
Right coronary a.
Aortic valve leaflets
Conus a.
Right ventricular outflow tract
Septal perforator coronary aa.
Sinoatrial node a.
Right atrium
Ascending aorta, noncoronary sinus of Valsalva
Crista terminalis
Sinoatrial node a.
Right lower lobe medial basal segment pulmonary a.
Left anterior descending coronary a.
Anterior interventricular coronary v.
Left circumflex coronary a.
Left atrial appendage
1st obtuse marginal coronary a.
Great cardiac v.
Left inferior pulmonary v.
Interatrial septum
Left atrium
Descending thoracic aorta

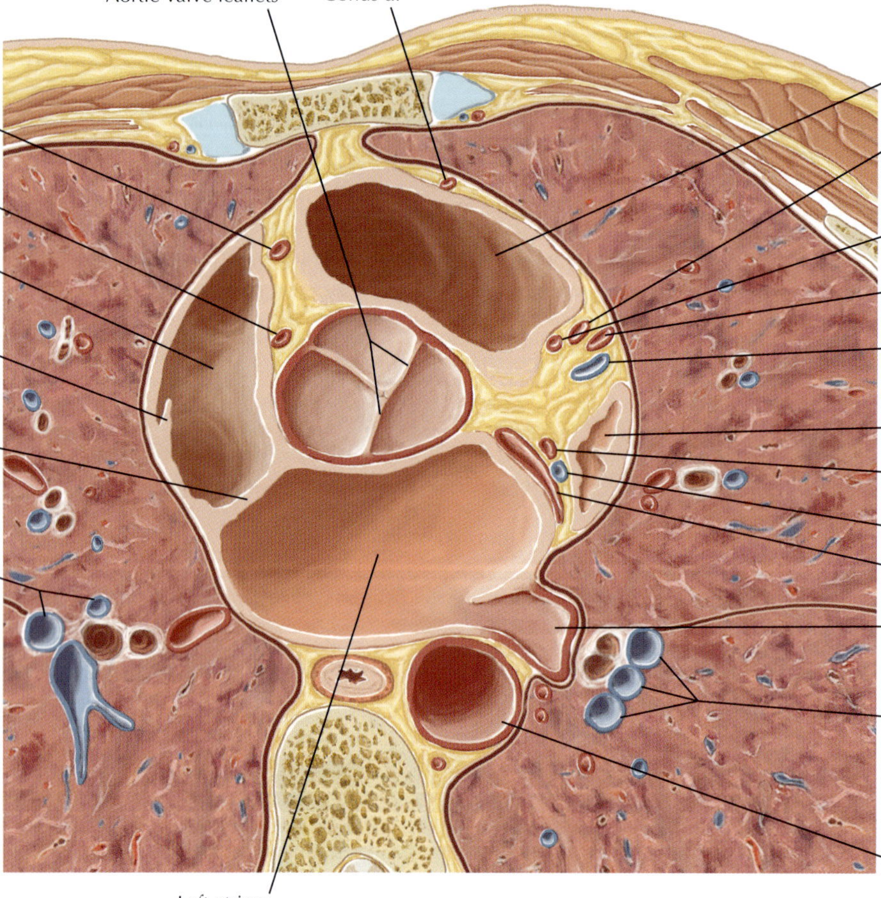
Aortic valve leaflets
Conus a.
Right coronary a.
Sinoatrial node a.
Right atrium
Crista terminalis
Interatrial septum
Right lower lobe anterior & medial basal segment pulmonary aa.
Left atrium
Right ventricular outflow tract
Left anterior descending coronary a.
Septal perforator coronary a.
1st diagonal coronary a.
Anterior interventricular coronary v.
Left atrial appendage
1st obtuse marginal coronary a.
Great cardiac v.
Left circumflex coronary a.
Left inferior pulmonary v.
Left lower lobe anterior-medial, lateral, & posterior basal segment pulmonary aa.
Descending thoracic aorta

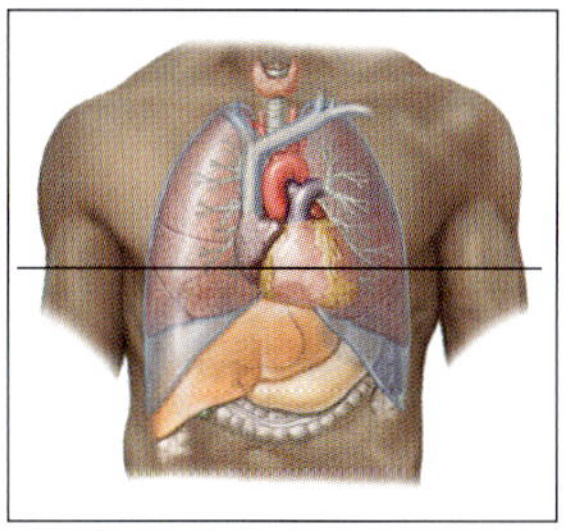

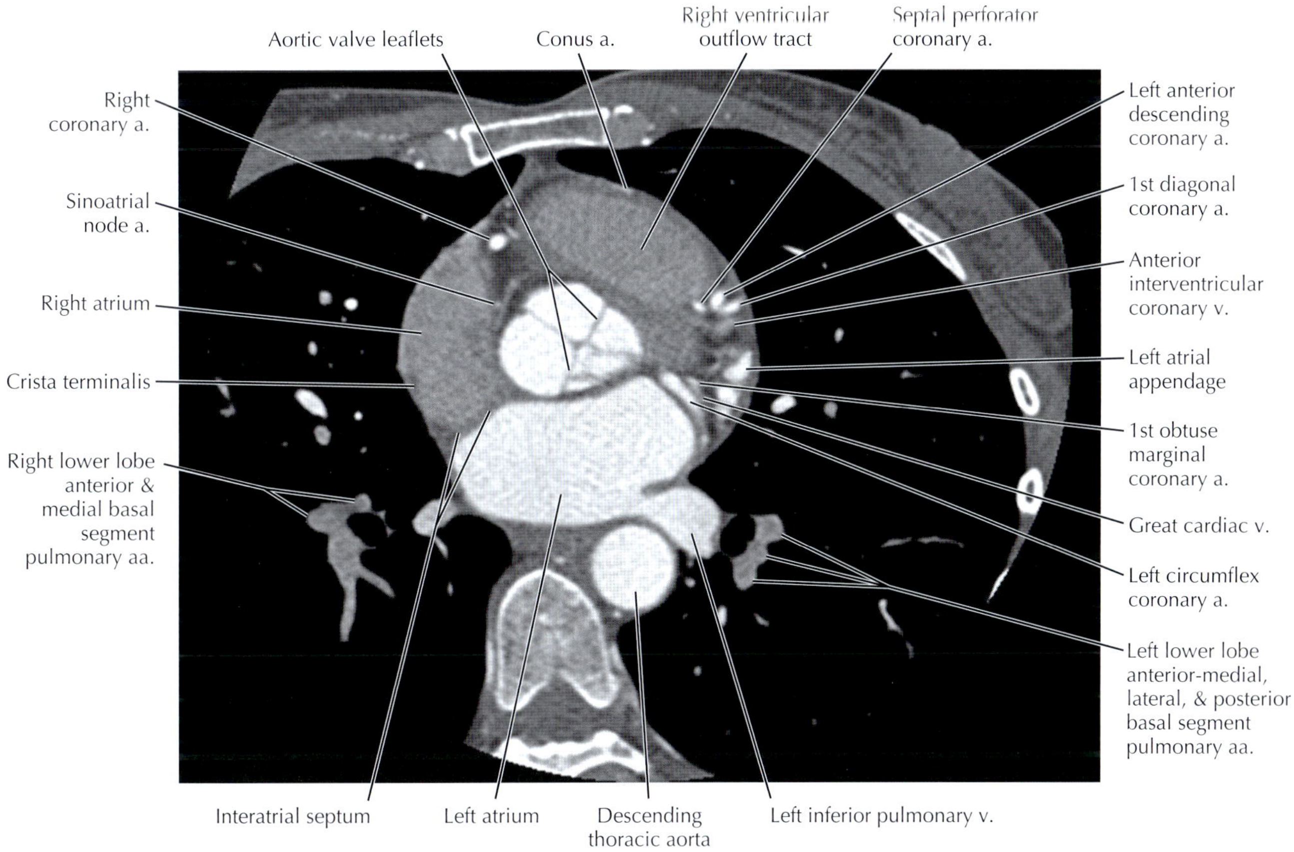
Aortic valve leaflets
Conus a.
Right ventricular outflow tract
Septal perforator coronary a.
Right coronary a.
Sinoatrial node a.
Right atrium
Crista terminalis
Right lower lobe anterior & medial basal segment pulmonary aa.
Left anterior descending coronary a.
1st diagonal coronary a.
Anterior interventricular coronary v.
Left atrial appendage
1st obtuse marginal coronary a.
Great cardiac v.
Left circumflex coronary a.
Left lower lobe anterior-medial, lateral, & posterior basal segment pulmonary aa.
Interatrial septum
Left atrium
Descending thoracic aorta
Left inferior pulmonary v.

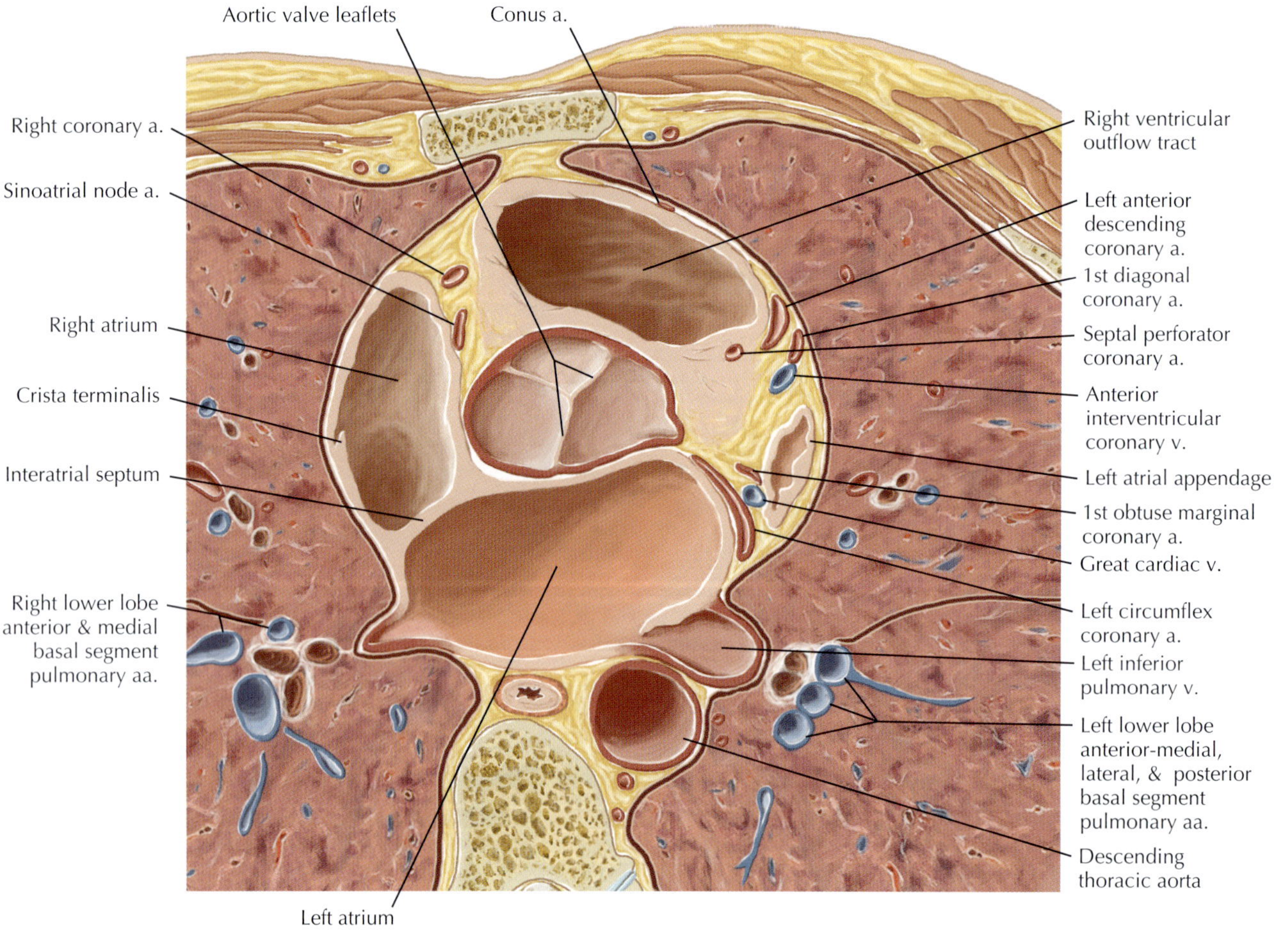
Aortic valve leaflets
Conus a.
Right coronary a.
Sinoatrial node a.
Right atrium
Crista terminalis
Interatrial septum
Right lower lobe anterior & medial basal segment pulmonary aa.
Left atrium
Right ventricular outflow tract
Left anterior descending coronary a.
1st diagonal coronary a.
Septal perforator coronary a.
Anterior interventricular coronary v.
Left atrial appendage
1st obtuse marginal coronary a.
Great cardiac v.
Left circumflex coronary a.
Left inferior pulmonary v.
Left lower lobe anterior-medial, lateral, & posterior basal segment pulmonary aa.
Descending thoracic aorta

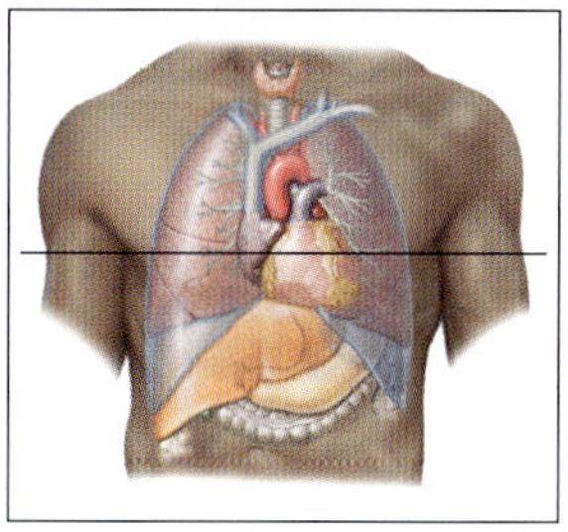

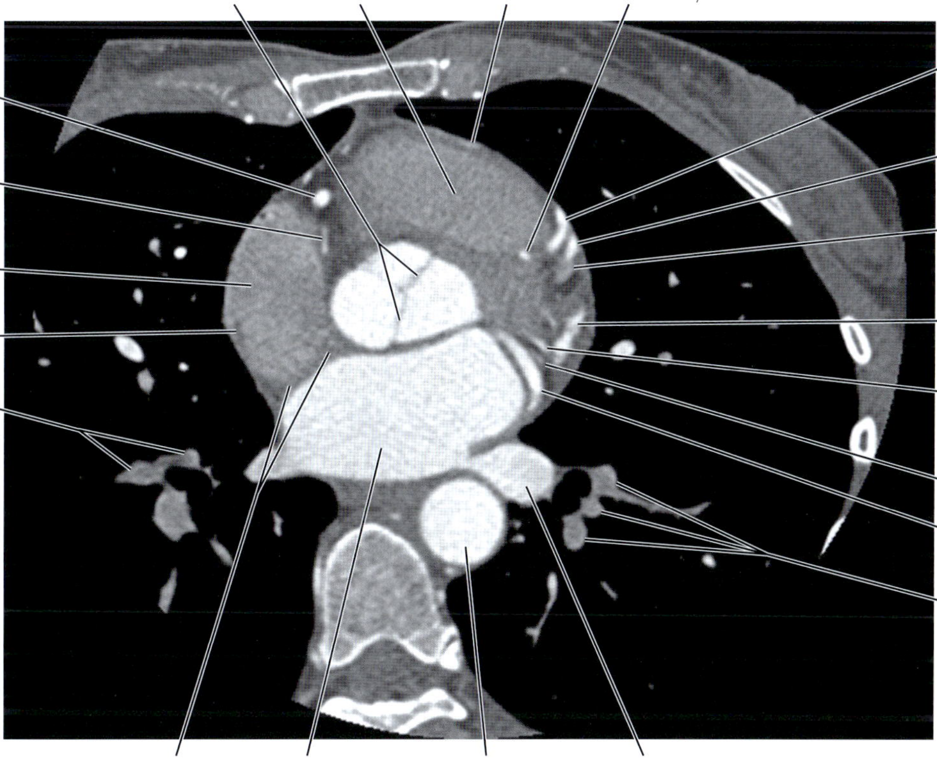
Aortic valve leaflets
Right ventricular outflow tract
Conus a.
Septal perforator coronary a.
Right coronary a.
Sinoatrial node a.
Right atrium
Crista terminalis
Right lower lobe anterior & medial basal segment pulmonary aa.
Left anterior descending coronary a.
1st diagonal coronary a.
Anterior interventricular coronary v.
Left atrial appendage
1st obtuse marginal coronary a.
Great cardiac v.
Left circumflex coronary a.
Left lower lobe anterior-medial, lateral, & posterior basal segment pulmonary aa.
Interatrial septum
Left atrium
Descending thoracic aorta
Left inferior pulmonary v.

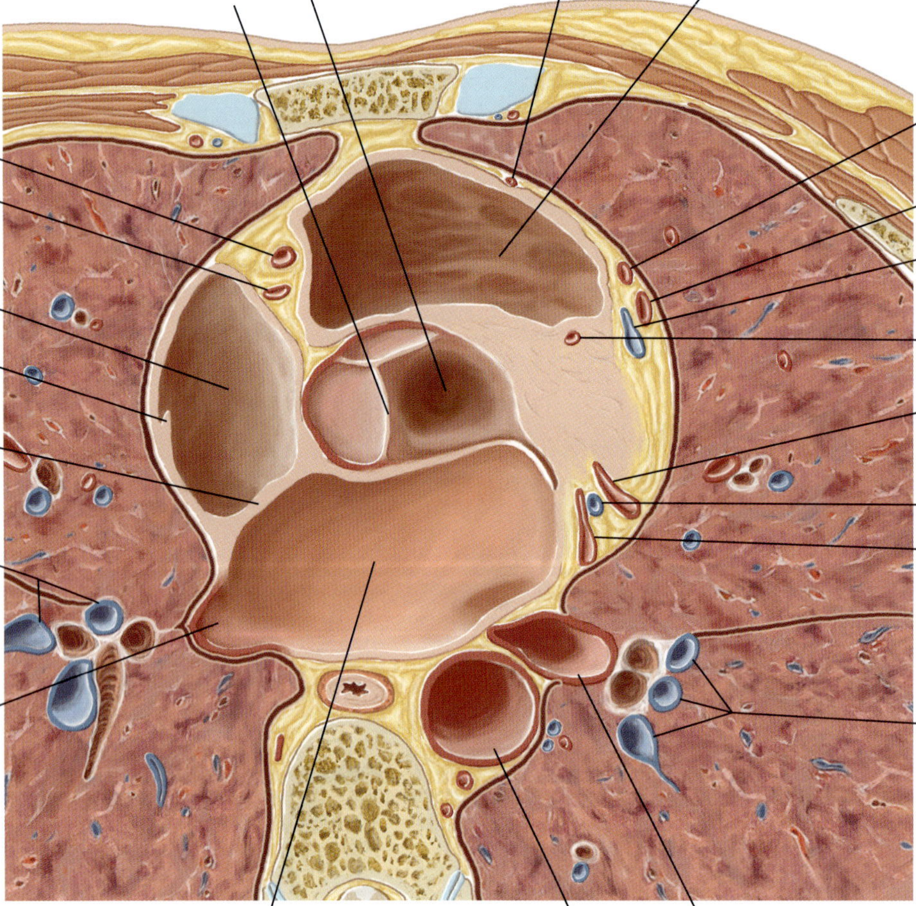
Left ventricular outflow tract
Aortic valve leaflet
Conus a.
Right ventricle
Right coronary a.
Sinoatrial node a.
Right atrium
Crista terminalis
Interatrial septum
Right lower lobe anterior & medial basal segment pulmonary aa.
Right inferior pulmonary v.
Left anterior descending coronary a.
1st diagonal coronary a.
Anterior interventricular coronary v.
Septal perforator coronary a.
1st obtuse marginal coronary a.
Great cardiac v.
Left circumflex coronary a.
Left lower lobe anterior-medial, lateral, & posterior basal segment pulmonary aa.
Left atrium
Left inferior pulmonary v.
Descending thoracic aorta

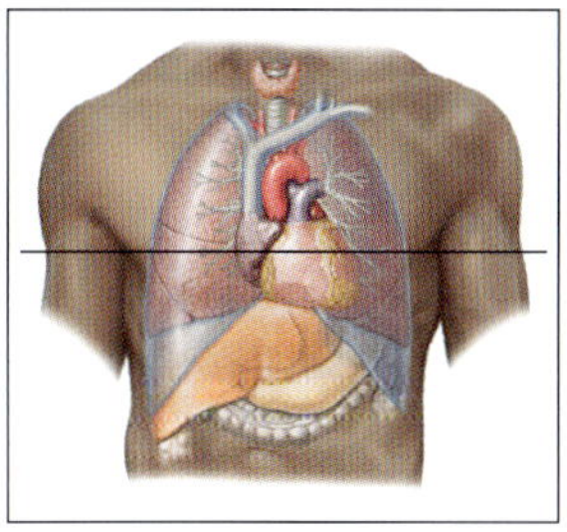

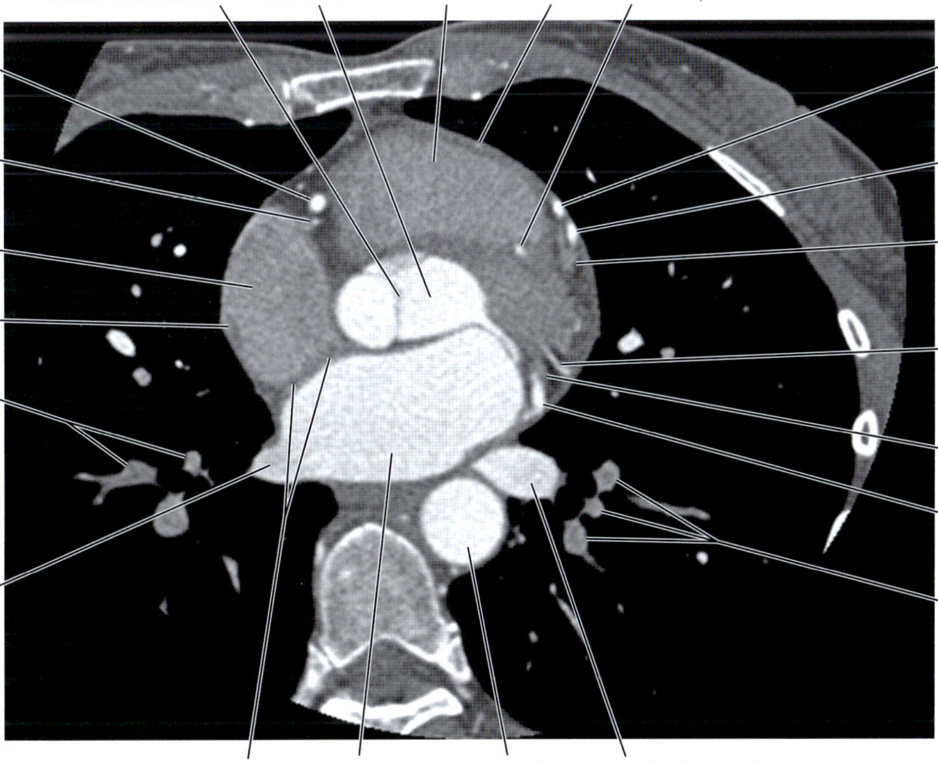
Aortic valve leaflet
Left ventricular outflow tract
Right ventricle
Conus a.
Septal perforator coronary a.
Right coronary a.
Sinoatrial node a.
Right atrium
Crista terminalis
Right lower lobe anterior & medial basal segment pulmonary aa.
Right inferior pulmonary v.
Left anterior descending coronary a.
1st diagonal coronary a.
Anterior interventricular coronary v.
1st obtuse marginal coronary a.
Great cardiac v.
Left circumflex coronary a.
Left lower lobe anterior-medial, lateral, & posterior basal segment pulmonary aa.
Interatrial septum
Left atrium
Descending thoracic aorta
Left inferior pulmonary v.

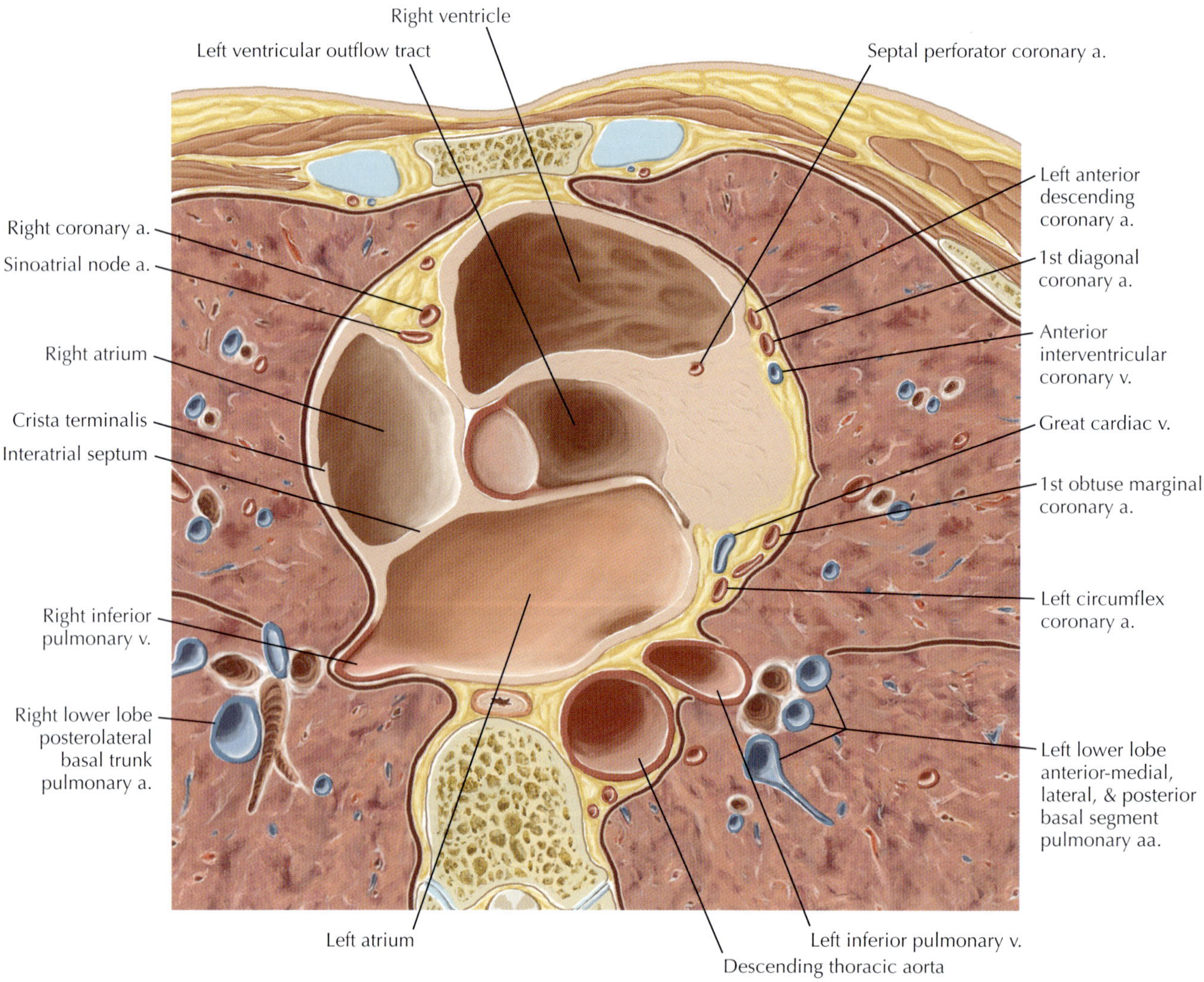
Right ventricle
Left ventricular outflow tract
Septal perforator coronary a.
Left anterior descending coronary a.
1st diagonal coronary a.
Anterior interventricular coronary v.
Great cardiac v.
1st obtuse marginal coronary a.
Left circumflex coronary a.
Left lower lobe anterior-medial, lateral, & posterior basal segment pulmonary aa.
Right coronary a.
Sinoatrial node a.
Right atrium
Crista terminalis
Interatrial septum
Right inferior pulmonary v.
Right lower lobe posterolateral basal trunk pulmonary a.
Left atrium
Left inferior pulmonary v.
Descending thoracic aorta

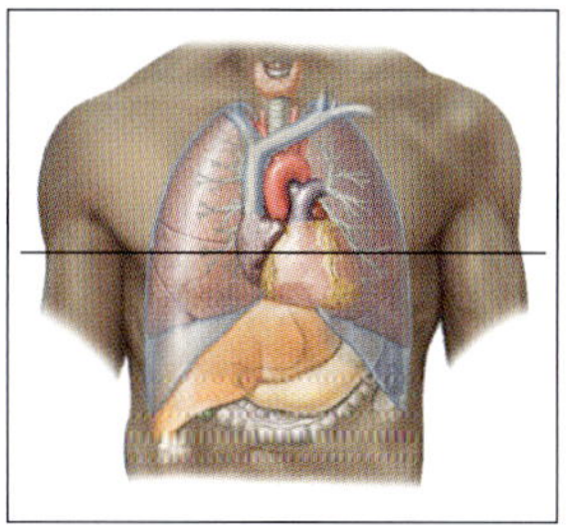

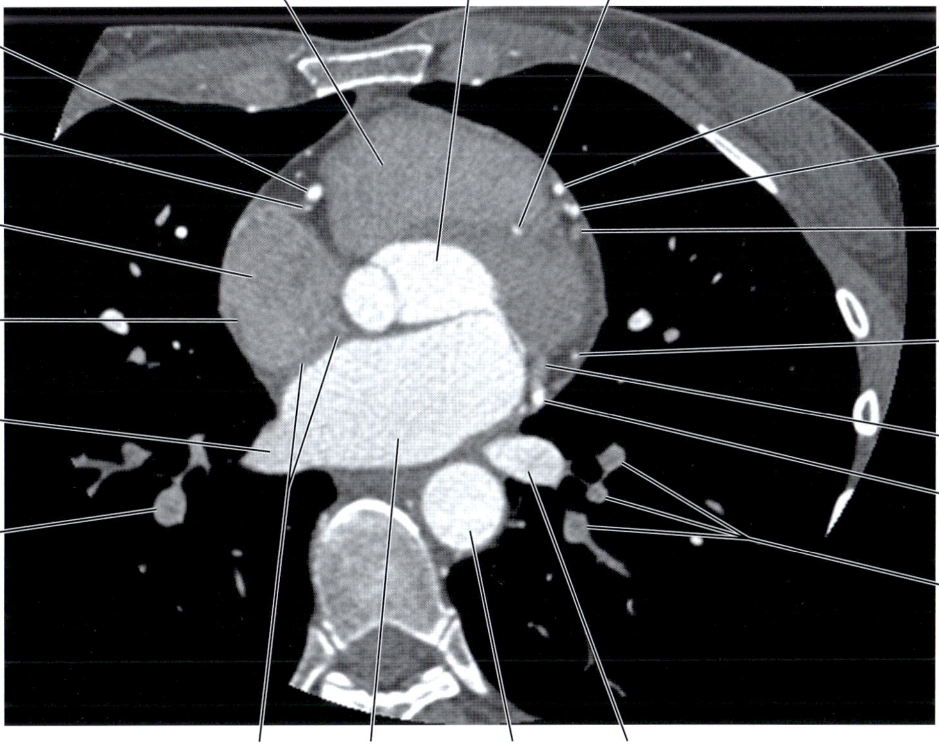
Right ventricle
Left ventricular outflow tract
Septal perforator coronary a.
Right coronary a.
Sinoatrial node a.
Right atrium
Crista terminalis
Right inferior pulmonary v.
Right lower lobe posterolateral basal trunk pulmonary a.
Left anterior descending coronary a.
1st diagonal coronary a.
Anterior interventricular coronary v.
1st obtuse marginal coronary a.
Great cardiac v.
Left circumflex coronary a.
Left lower lobe anterior-medial, lateral, & posterior basal segment pulmonary aa.
Interatrial septum
Left atrium
Descending thoracic aorta
Left inferior pulmonary v.

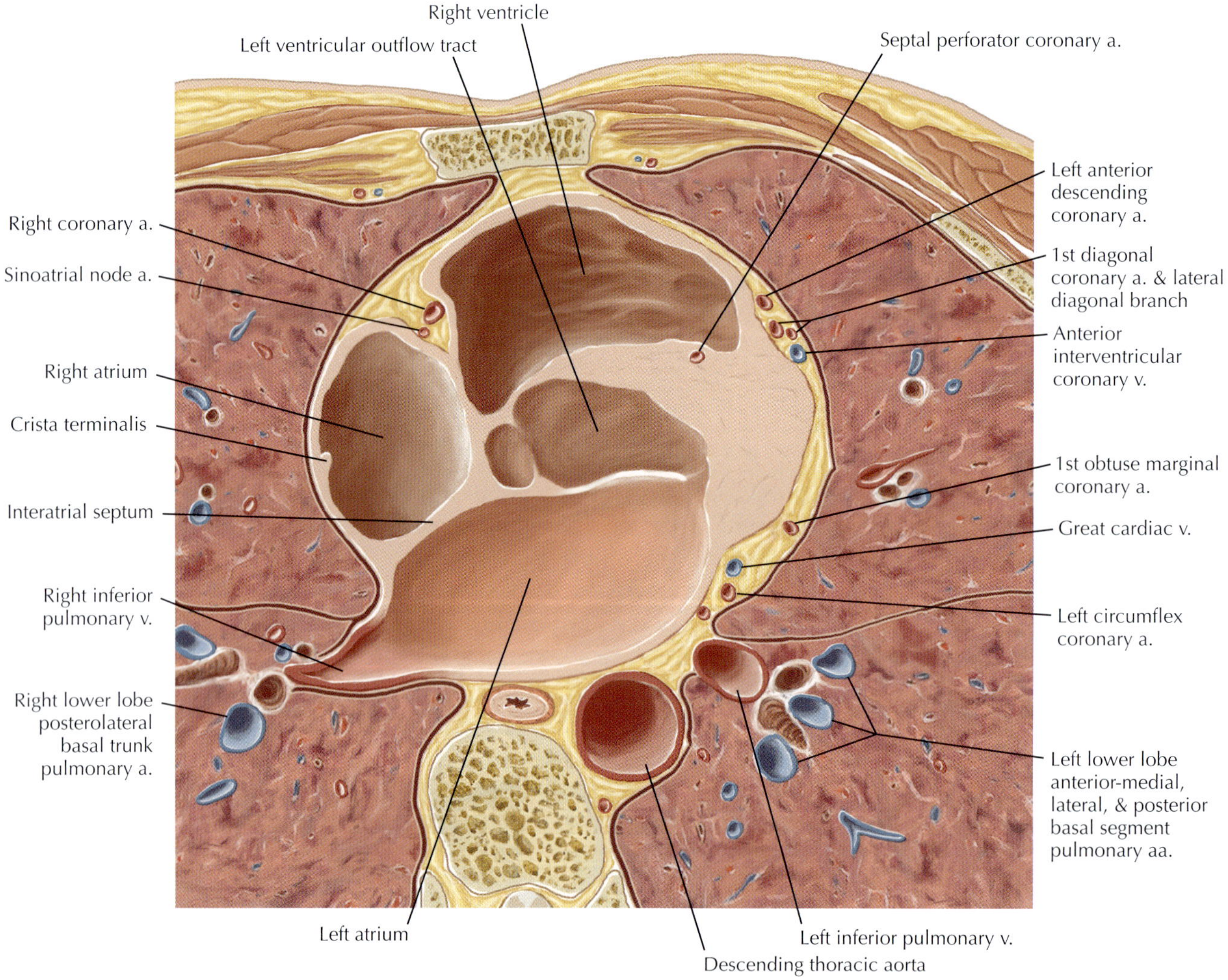

Right ventricle
Left ventricular outflow tract
Septal perforator coronary a.
Left anterior descending coronary a.
Right coronary a.
1st diagonal coronary a. & lateral diagonal branch
Sinoatrial node a.
Anterior interventricular coronary v.
Right atrium
Crista terminalis
1st obtuse marginal coronary a.
Interatrial septum
Great cardiac v.
Right inferior pulmonary v.
Left circumflex coronary a.
Right lower lobe posterolateral basal trunk pulmonary a.
Left lower lobe anterior-medial, lateral, & posterior basal segment pulmonary aa.
Left atrium
Left inferior pulmonary v.
Descending thoracic aorta

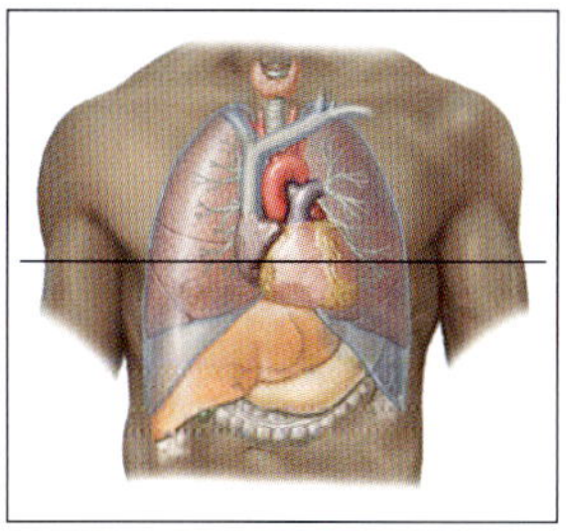

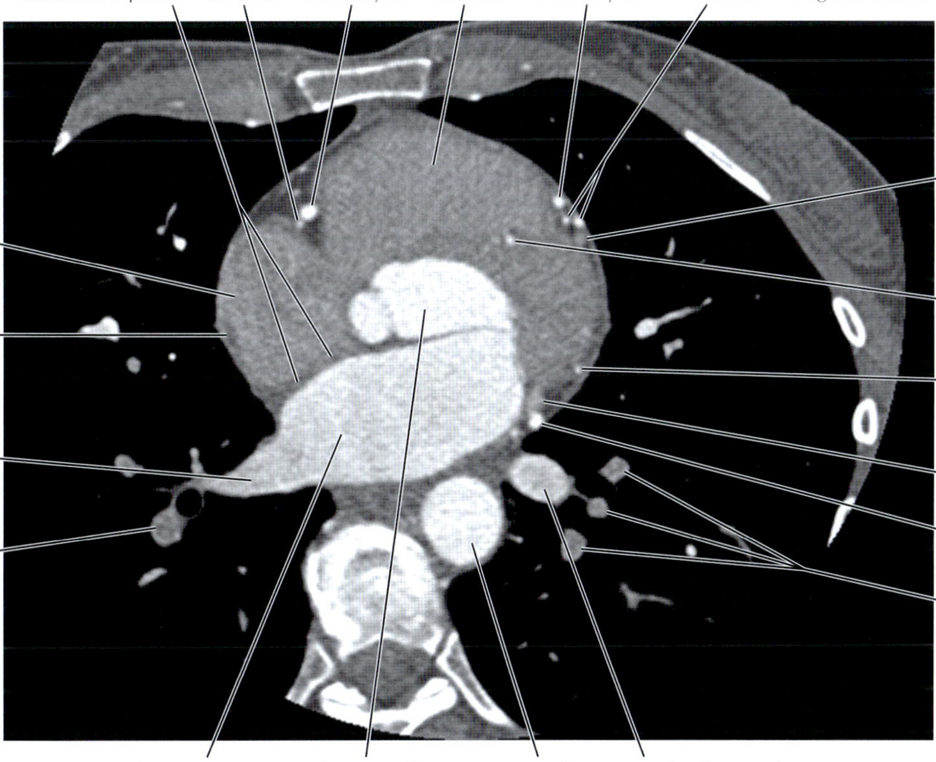
Interatrial septum
Sinoatrial node a.
Right coronary a.
Right ventricle
Left anterior descending coronary a.
1st diagonal coronary a. & lateral diagonal branch
Anterior interventricular coronary v.
Right atrium
Septal perforator coronary a.
Crista terminalis
1st obtuse marginal coronary a.
Right inferior pulmonary v.
Great cardiac v.
Left circumflex coronary a.
Right lower lobe posterolateral basal trunk pulmonary a.
Left lower lobe anterior-medial, lateral, & posterior basal segment pulmonary aa.
Left atrium
Left ventricular outflow tract
Descending thoracic aorta
Left inferior pulmonary v.

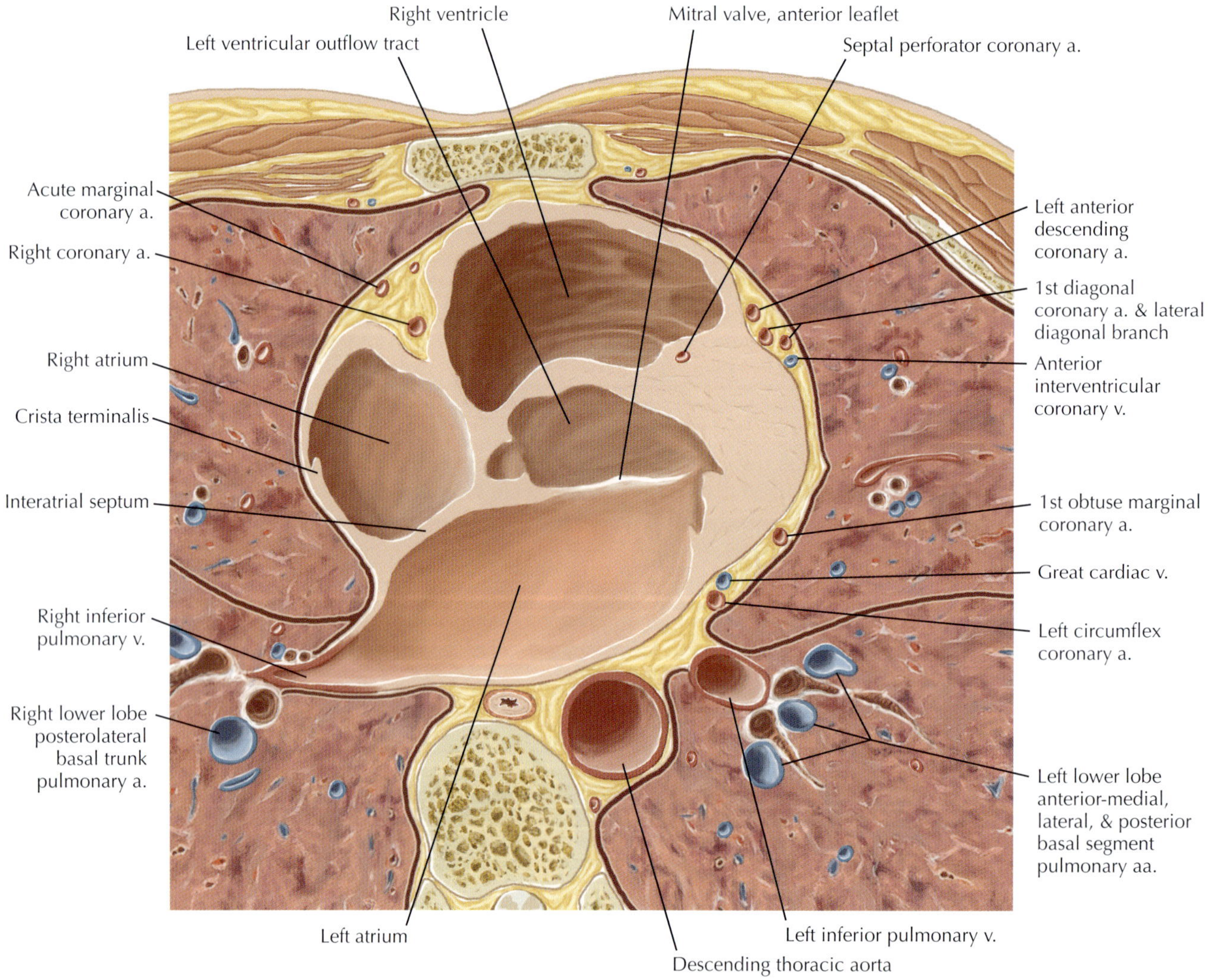
Right ventricle
Left ventricular outflow tract
Mitral valve, anterior leaflet
Septal perforator coronary a.
Acute marginal coronary a.
Right coronary a.
Right atrium
Crista terminalis
Interatrial septum
Right inferior pulmonary v.
Right lower lobe posterolateral basal trunk pulmonary a.
Left anterior descending coronary a.
1st diagonal coronary a. & lateral diagonal branch
Anterior interventricular coronary v.
1st obtuse marginal coronary a.
Great cardiac v.
Left circumflex coronary a.
Left lower lobe anterior-medial, lateral, & posterior basal segment pulmonary aa.
Left atrium
Left inferior pulmonary v.
Descending thoracic aorta

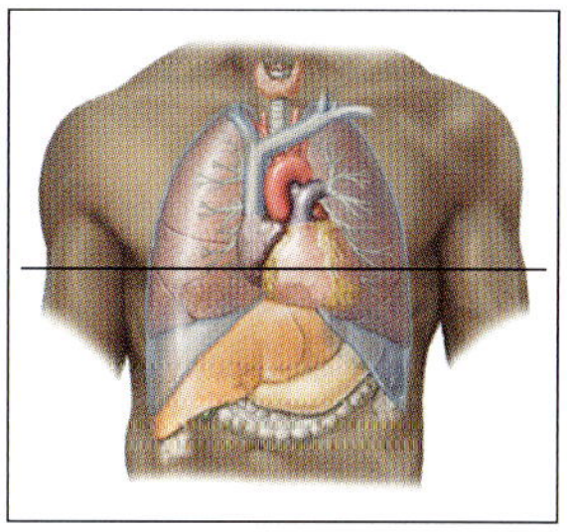

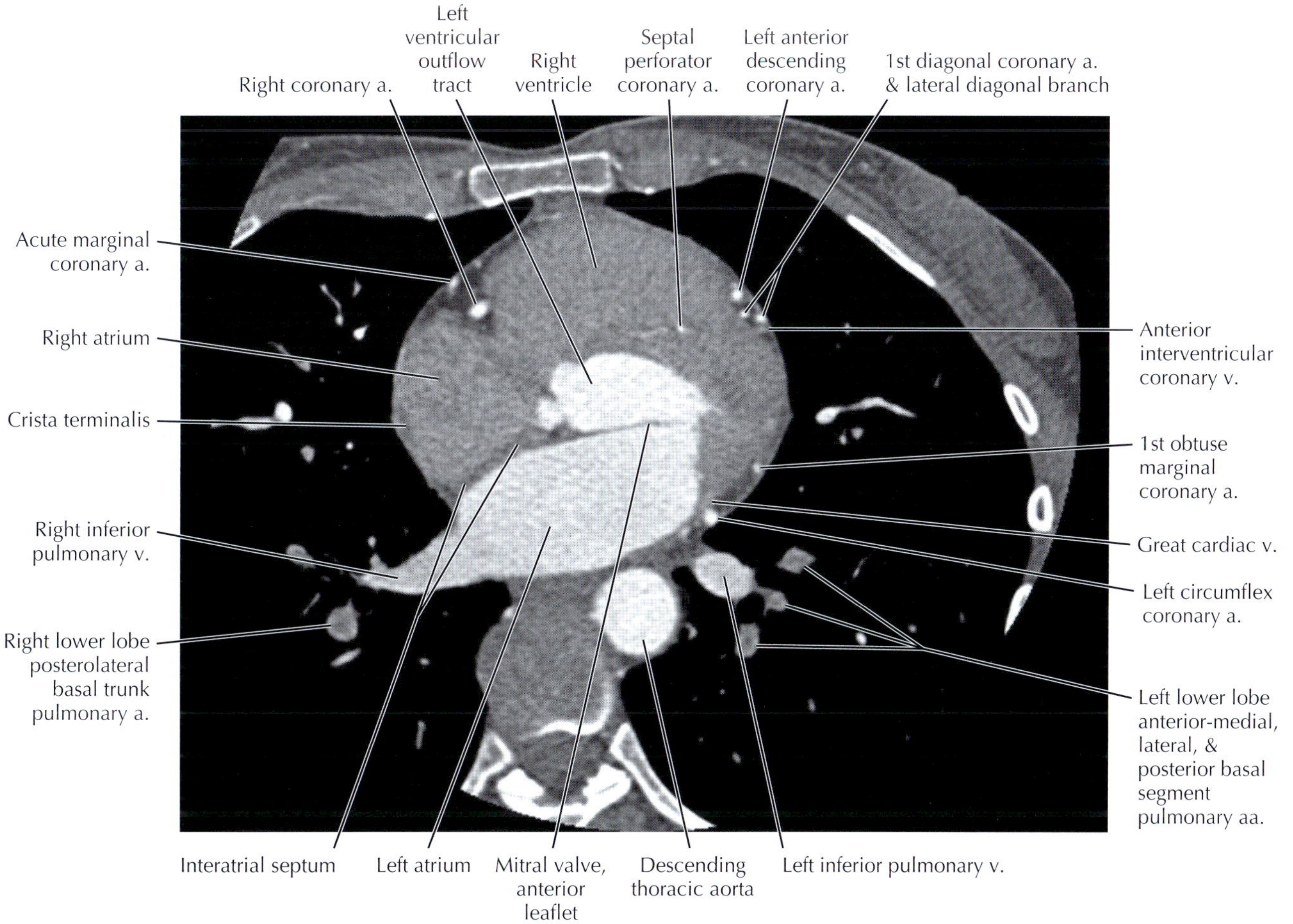
Left ventricular outflow tract
Right coronary a.
Right ventricle
Septal perforator coronary a.
Left anterior descending coronary a.
1st diagonal coronary a. & lateral diagonal branch
Acute marginal coronary a.
Right atrium
Crista terminalis
Right inferior pulmonary v.
Right lower lobe posterolateral basal trunk pulmonary a.
Anterior interventricular coronary v.
1st obtuse marginal coronary a.
Great cardiac v.
Left circumflex coronary a.
Left lower lobe anterior-medial, lateral, & posterior basal segment pulmonary aa.
Interatrial septum
Left atrium
Mitral valve, anterior leaflet
Descending thoracic aorta
Left inferior pulmonary v.

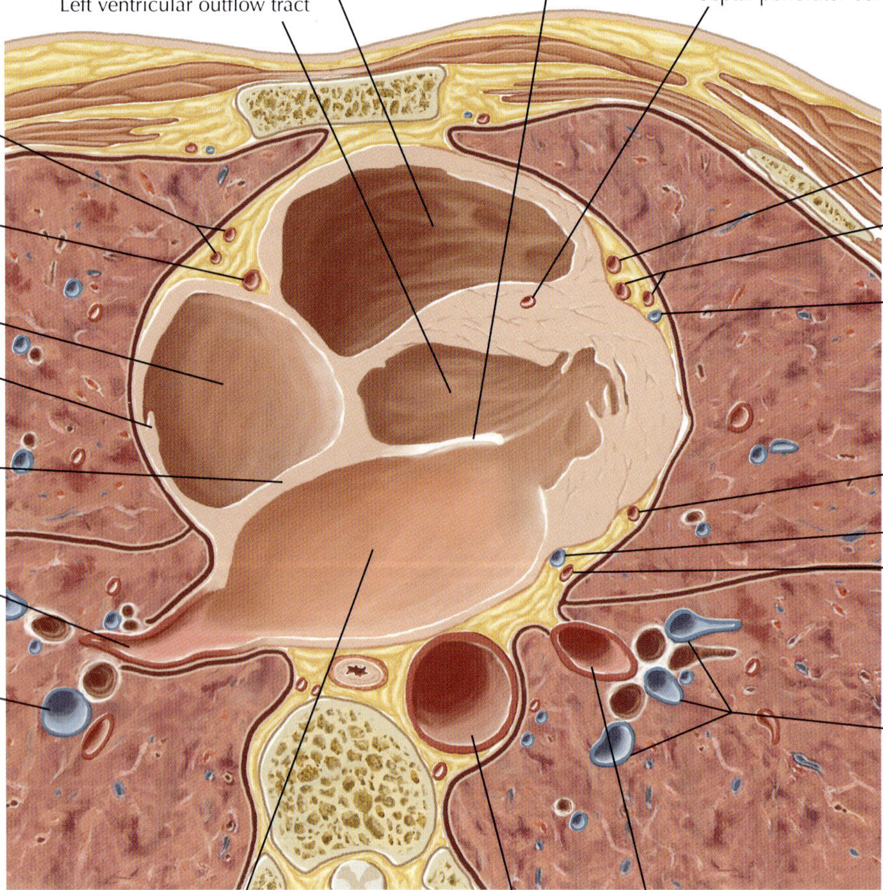
Right ventricle
Left ventricular outflow tract
Mitral valve, anterior leaflet
Septal perforator coronary a.
Acute marginal coronary aa.
Right coronary a.
Right atrium
Crista terminalis
Interatrial septum
Right inferior pulmonary v.
Right lower lobe posterolateral basal trunk pulmonary a.
Left descending coronary a.
1st diagonal coronary a. & lateral diagonal branch
Anterior interventricular coronary v.
1st obtuse marginal coronary a.
Great cardiac v.
Left circumflex coronary a.
Left lower lobe anterior-medial, lateral, & posterior basal segment pulmonary aa.
Left atrium
Left inferior pulmonary v.
Descending thoracic aorta

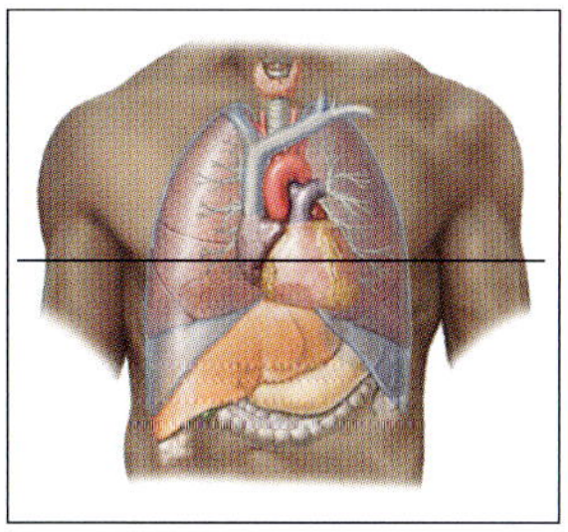

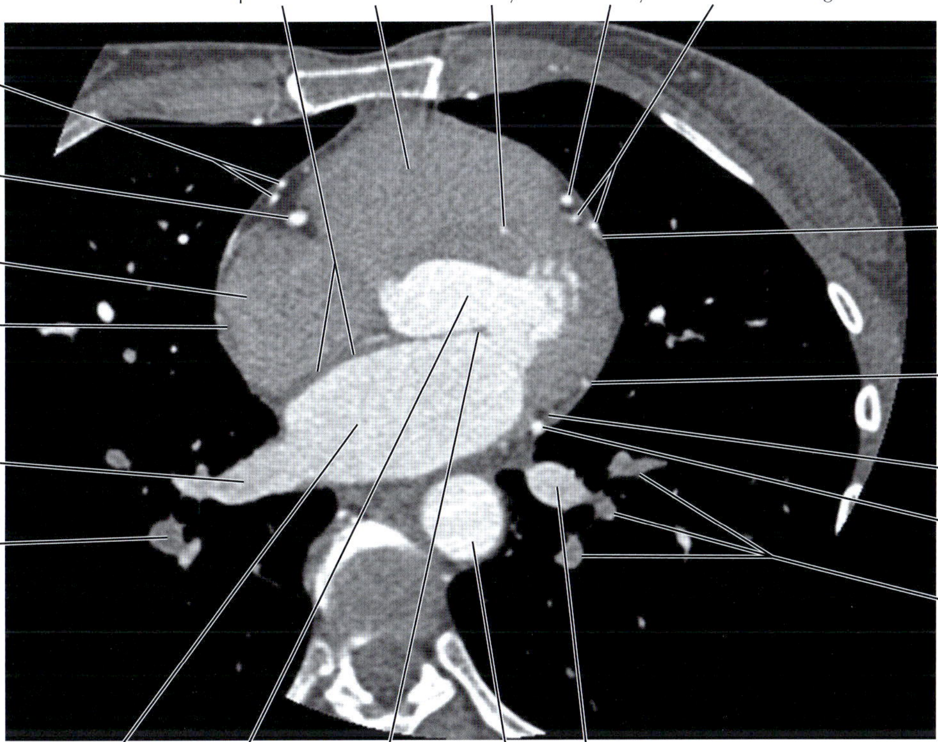
Interatrial septum
Right ventricle
Septal perforator coronary a.
Left anterior descending coronary a.
1st diagonal coronary a. & lateral diagonal branch
Acute marginal coronary aa.
Right coronary a.
Right atrium
Crista terminalis
Right inferior pulmonary v.
Right lower lobe posterolateral basal trunk pulmonary a.
Anterior interventricular coronary v.
1st obtuse marginal coronary a.
Great cardiac v.
Left circumflex coronary a.
Left lower lobe anterior-medial, lateral & posterior basal segment pulmonary aa.
Left atrium
Left ventricular outflow tract
Mitral valve, anterior leaflet
Descending thoracic aorta
Left inferior pulmonary v.

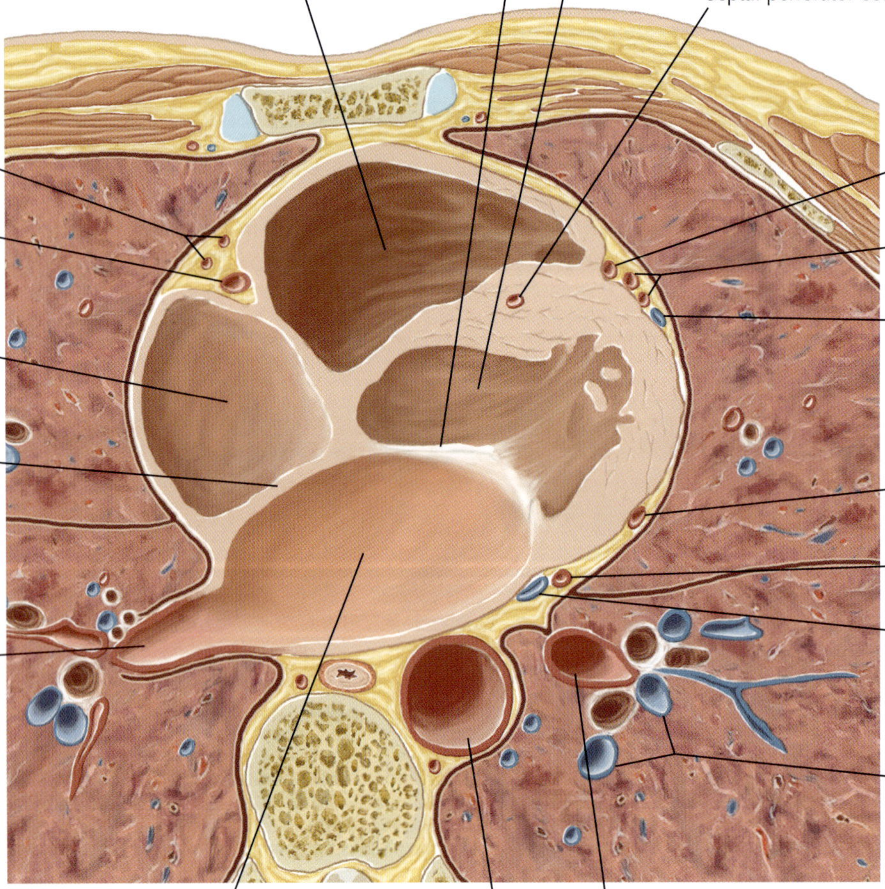
Mitral valve, anterior leaflet
Left ventricular outflow tract
Septal perforator coronary a.
Right ventricle
Acute marginal coronary aa.
Right coronary a.
Right atrium
Interatrial septum
Right inferior pulmonary v.
Left anterior descending coronary a.
1st diagonal coronary a. & lateral diagonal branch
Anterior interventricular coronary v.
1st obtuse marginal coronary a.
Left circumflex coronary a.
Great cardiac v.
Left lower lobe lateral, & posterior basal segment pulmonary aa.
Left atrium
Left inferior pulmonary v.
Descending thoracic aorta

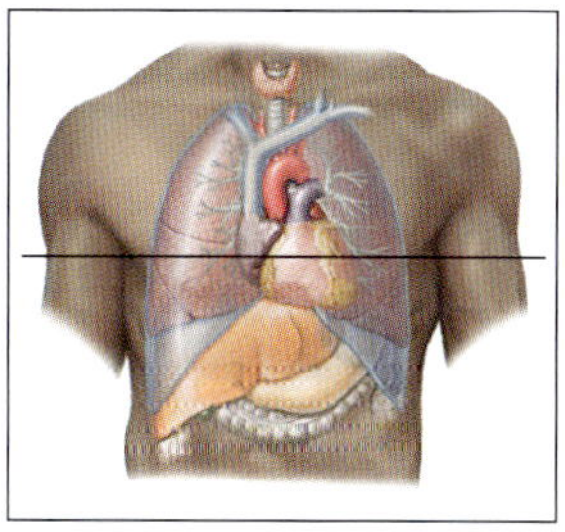

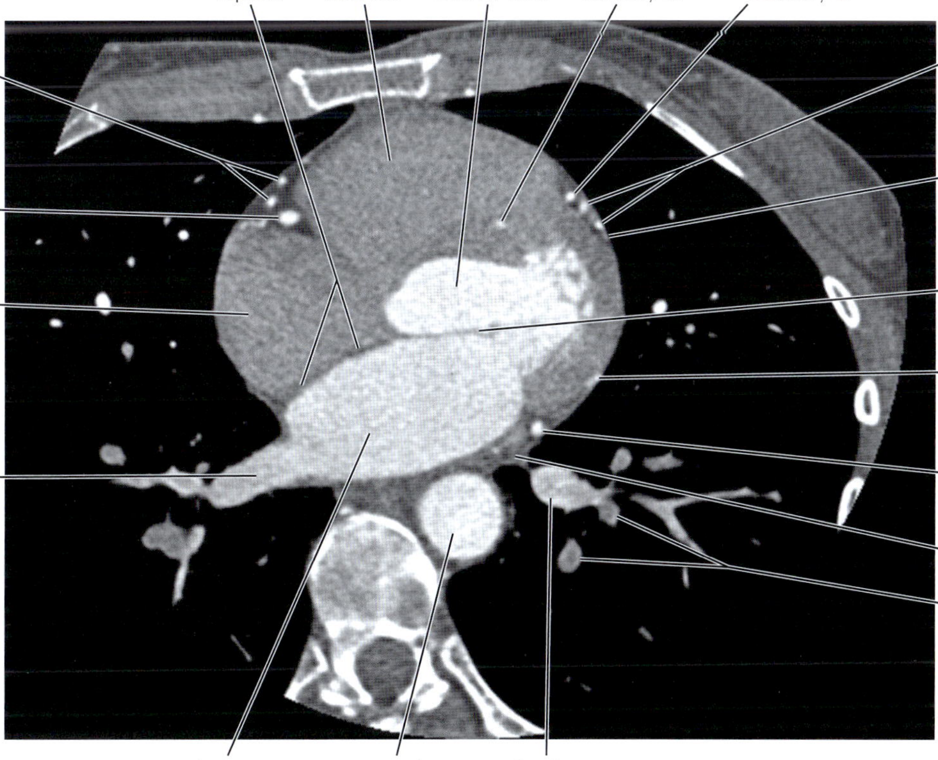
Interatrial septum
Right ventricle
Left ventricular outflow tract
Septal perforator coronary a.
Left anterior descending coronary a.
Acute marginal coronary aa.
1st diagonal coronary a. & lateral diagonal branch
Right coronary a.
Anterior interventricular coronary v.
Right atrium
Mitral valve, anterior leaflet
1st obtuse marginal coronary a.
Right inferior pulmonary v.
Left circumflex coronary a.
Great cardiac v.
Left lower lobe lateral & posterior basal segment pulmonary aa.
Left atrium
Descending thoracic aorta
Left inferior pulmonary v.

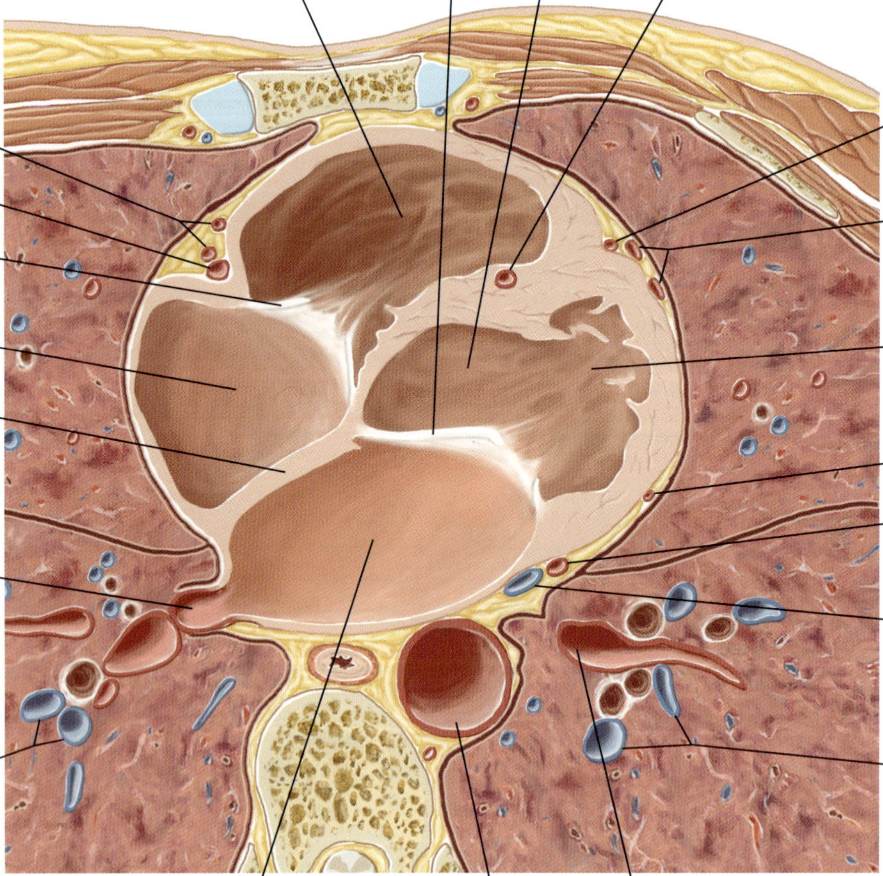

NORMAL ANATOMY

The left ventricular outflow tract is shown, demonstrating that the inflow (mitral valve) and outflow tracts of the left ventricle are closely related to one another. This contrasts with the right ventricle, in which the inflow portions (tricuspid valve) and outflow portions (right ventricular outflow tract, infundibulum, and pulmonic valve) are widely separated. Note that the left ventricular outflow tract is smooth, and that the anterior leaflet of the mitral valve is closely related to the aortic valvular apparatus (see Axials 22 to 25).

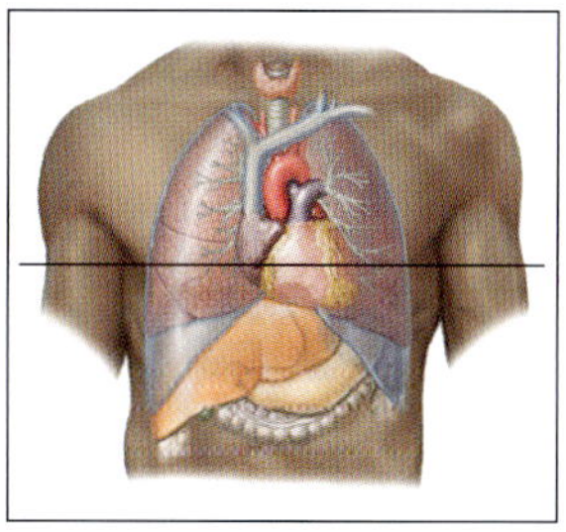

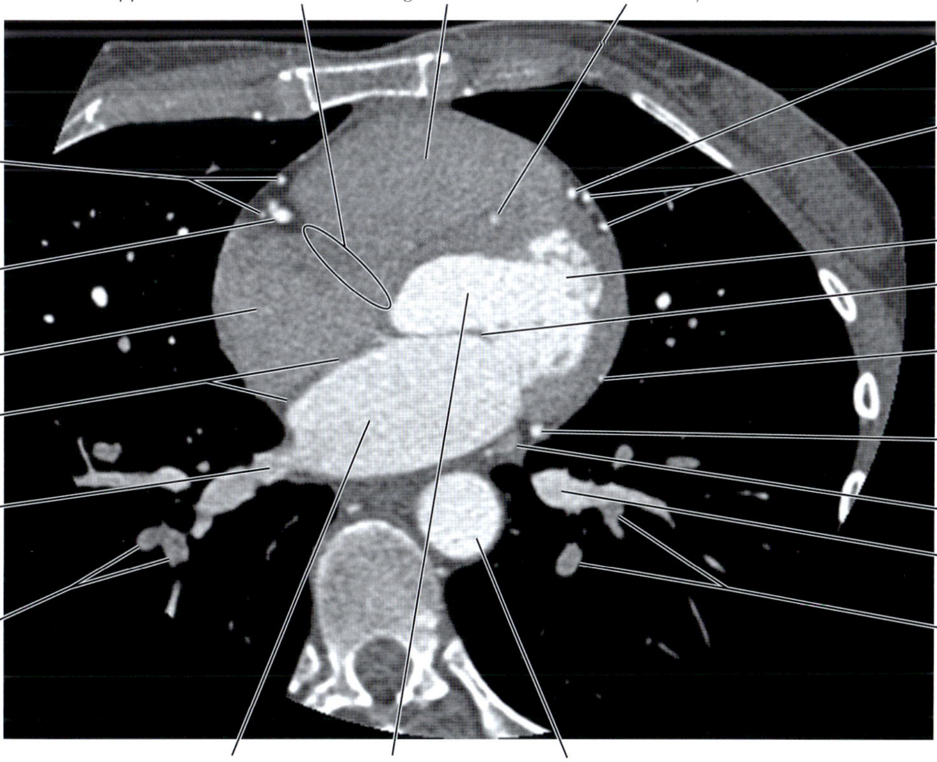
Tricuspid valve
(approximate location)
Right ventricle
Septal perforator
coronary a.
Left anterior
descending
coronary a.
1st diagonal
coronary a. &
lateral diagonal
branch
Left ventricle
Mitral valve,
anterior leaflet
1st obtuse
marginal
coronary a.
Left circumflex
coronary a.
Great cardiac v.
Left inferior
pulmonary v.
Left lower lobe
lateral &
posterior
basal segment
pulmonary aa.
Acute marginal
coronary aa.
Right
coronary a.
Right atrium
Interatrial
septum
Right inferior
pulmonary v.
Right lower lobe
lateral &
posterior basal
segment
pulmonary aa.
Left atrium
Left ventricular
outflow tract
Descending
thoracic aorta

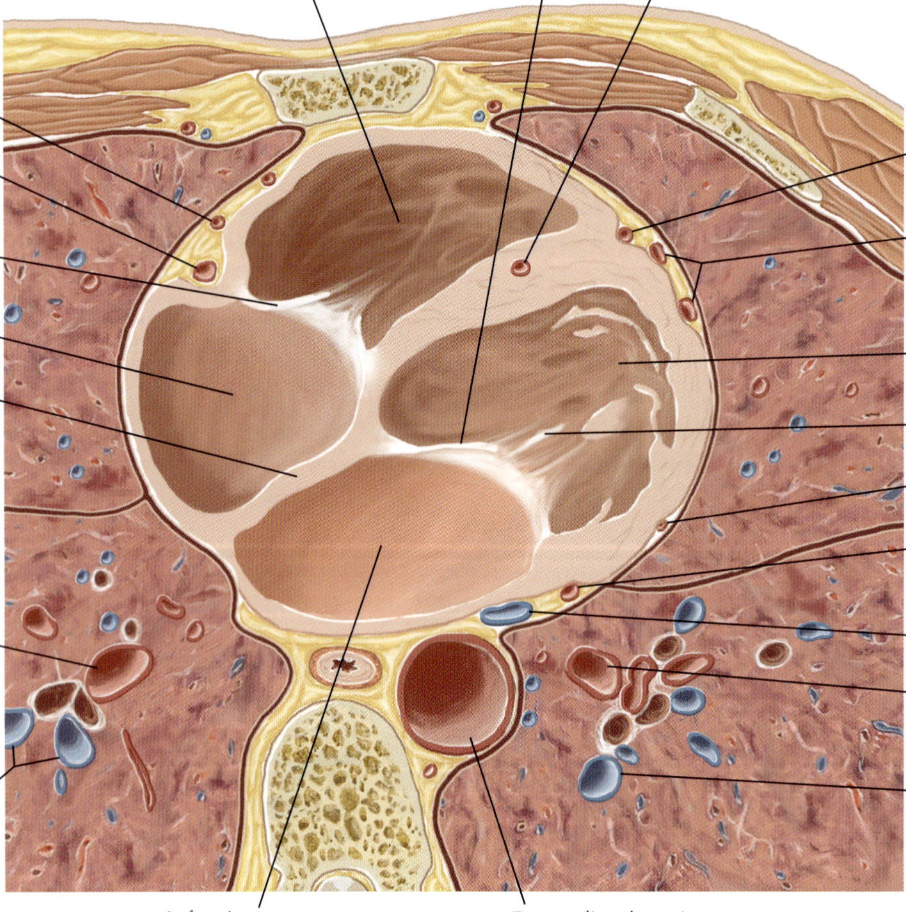
Mitral valve, anterior leaflet
Right ventricle
Septal perforator coronary a.
Acute marginal coronary a.
Right coronary a.
Tricuspid valve
Right atrium
Interatrial septum
Pulmonary v.
Right lower lobe lateral & posterior basal segment pulmonary aa.
Left atrium
Descending thoracic aorta
Left anterior descending coronary a.
1st diagonal coronary a. & lateral diagonal branch
Left ventricle
Chordae tendineae
1st obtuse marginal coronary a.
Left circumflex coronary a.
Great cardiac v.
Left inferior pulmonary v.
Left lower lobe posterior basal subsegmental pulmonary a.

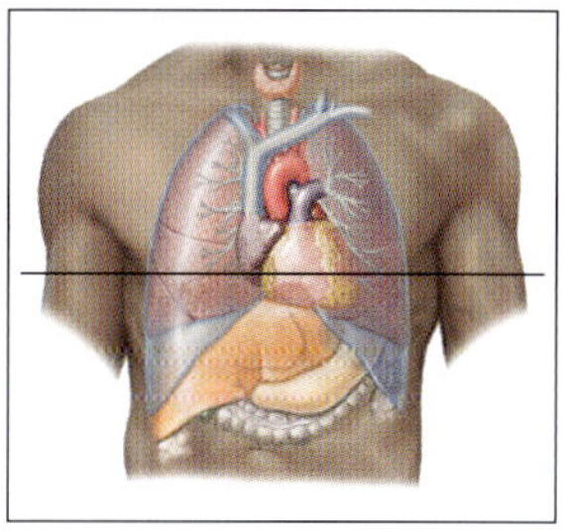

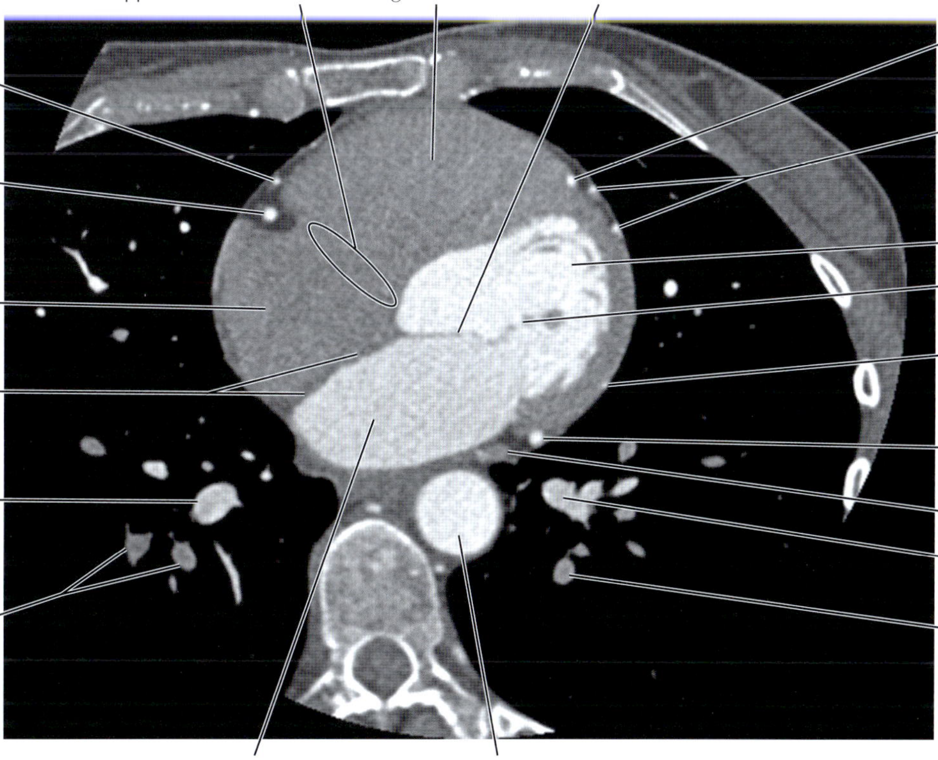

Tricuspid valve (approximate location)
Right ventricle
Mitral valve, anterior leaflet
Acute marginal coronary a.
Right coronary a.
Right atrium
Interatrial septum
Pulmonary v.
Right lower lobe lateral & posterior basal segment pulmonary aa.
Left atrium
Descending thoracic aorta
Left anterior descending coronary a.
1st diagonal coronary a. & lateral diagonal branch
Left ventricle
Chordae tendineae
1st obtuse marginal coronary a.
Left circumflex coronary a.
Great cardiac v.
Left inferior pulmonary v.
Left lower lobe posterior basal subsegmental pulmonary a.

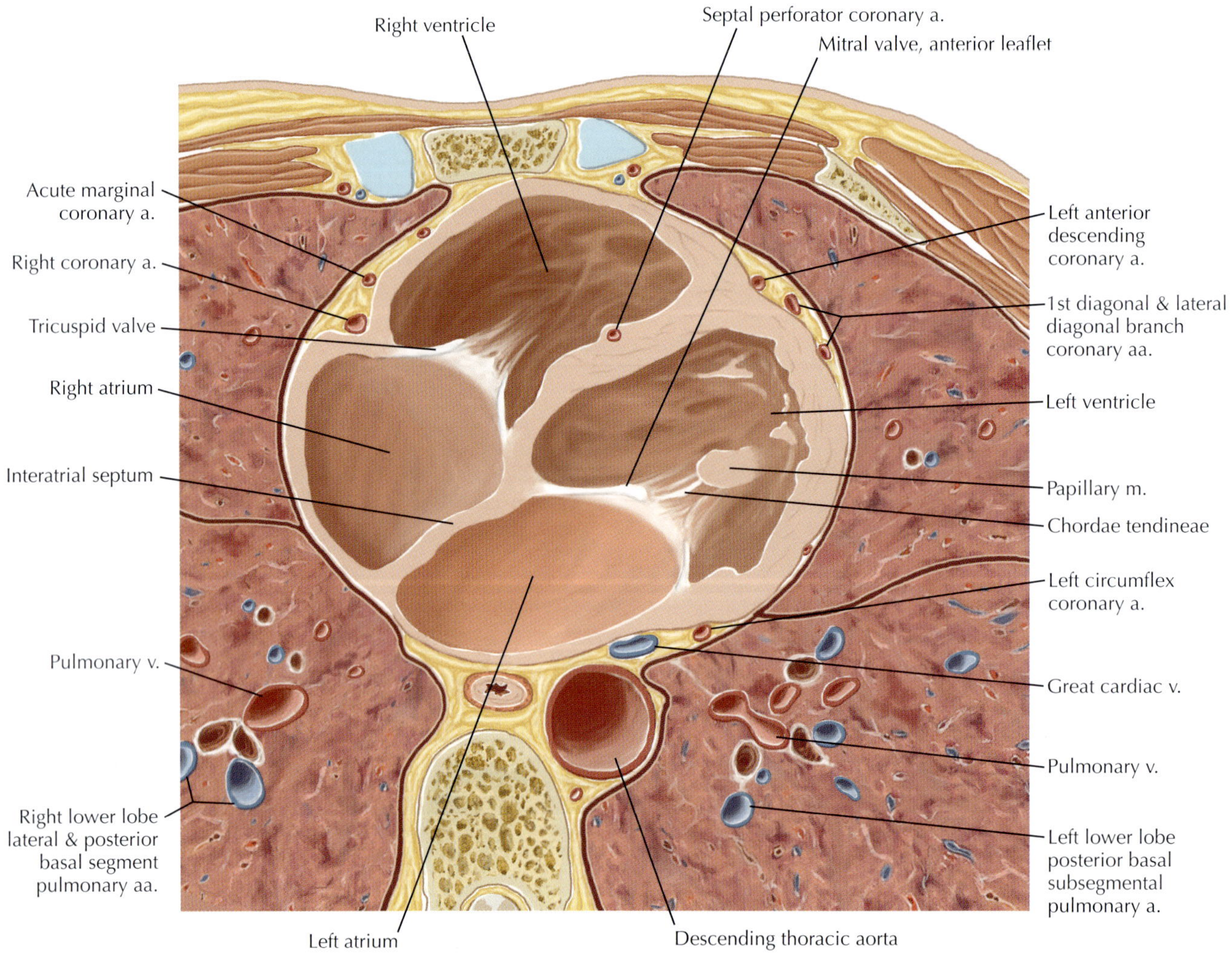
Right ventricle
Septal perforator coronary a.
Mitral valve, anterior leaflet
Acute marginal coronary a.
Right coronary a.
Tricuspid valve
Right atrium
Interatrial septum
Pulmonary v.
Right lower lobe lateral & posterior basal segment pulmonary aa.
Left atrium
Descending thoracic aorta
Left anterior descending coronary a.
1st diagonal & lateral diagonal branch coronary aa.
Left ventricle
Papillary m.
Chordae tendineae
Left circumflex coronary a.
Great cardiac v.
Pulmonary v.
Left lower lobe posterior basal subsegmental pulmonary a.

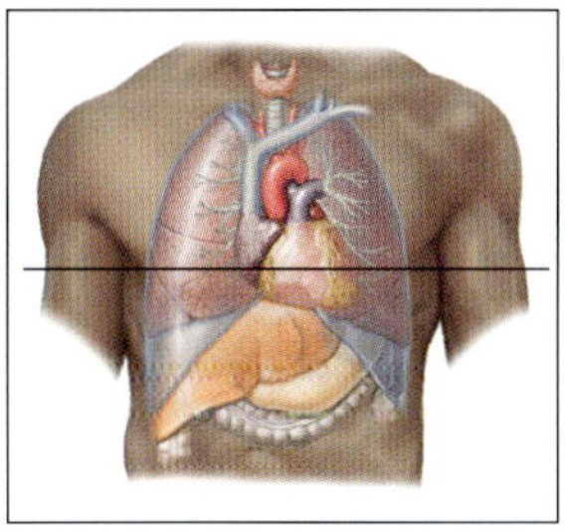

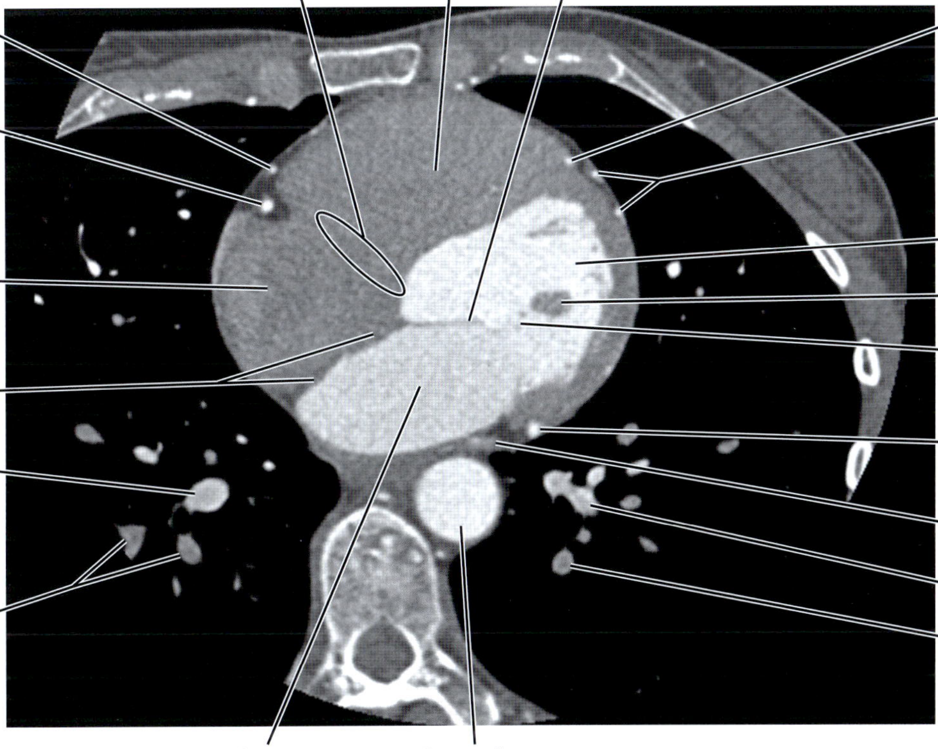
Tricuspid valve
(approximate location)
Right ventricle
Mitral valve,
anterior leaflet
Acute marginal
coronary a.
Right
coronary a.
Right atrium
Interatrial
septum
Pulmonary v.
Right lower lobe
lateral &
posterior basal
segment
pulmonary aa.
Left atrium
Descending
thoracic aorta
Left anterior
descending
coronary a.
1st diagonal
& lateral
diagonal branch
coronary aa.
Left ventricle
Papillary m.
Chordae
tendineae
Left circumflex
coronary a.
Great cardiac v.
Pulmonary v.
Left lower lobe
posterior basal
subsegmental
pulmonary a.

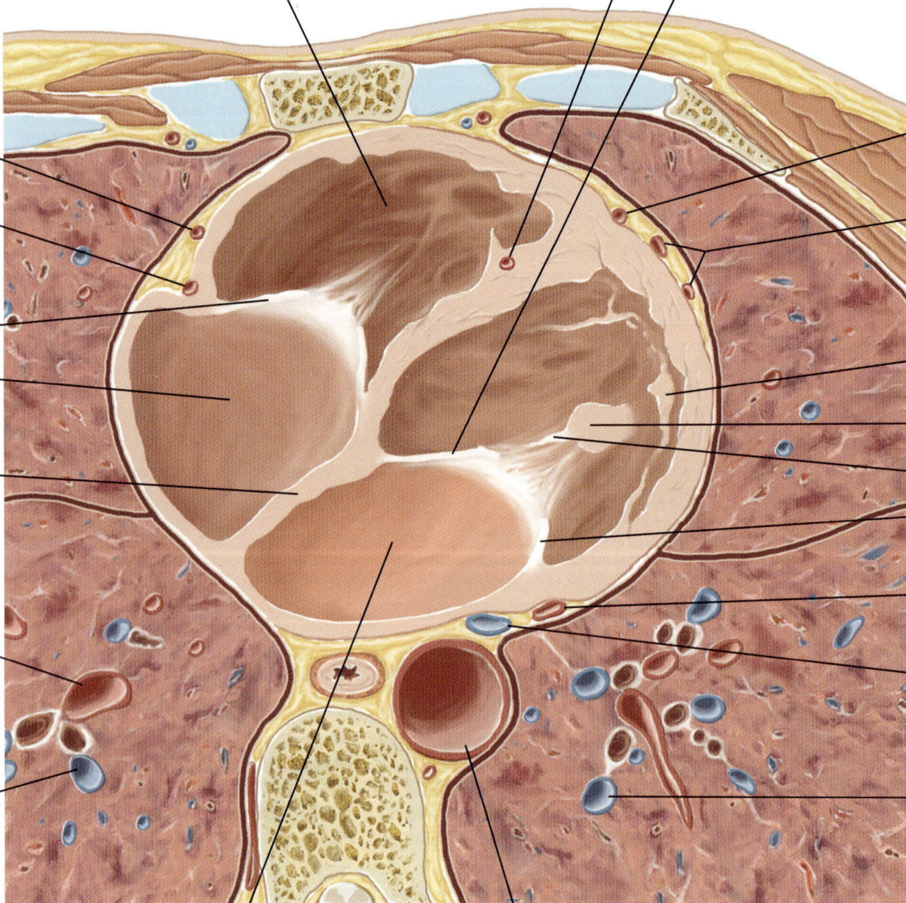
Septal perforator coronary a.
Mitral valve, anterior leaflet
Right ventricle
Acute marginal coronary a.
Right coronary a.
Tricuspid valve
Right atrium
Interatrial septum
Pulmonary v.
Right lower lobe posterior basal segment pulmonary a.
Left atrium
Descending thoracic aorta
Left anterior descending coronary a.
1st diagonal coronary a. & lateral diagonal branch
Left ventricle (trabeculae carneae)
Papillary m.
Chordae tendineae
Mitral valve, posterior leaflet
Left circumflex coronary a.
Great cardiac v.
Left lower lobe posterior basal subsegmental pulmonary a.

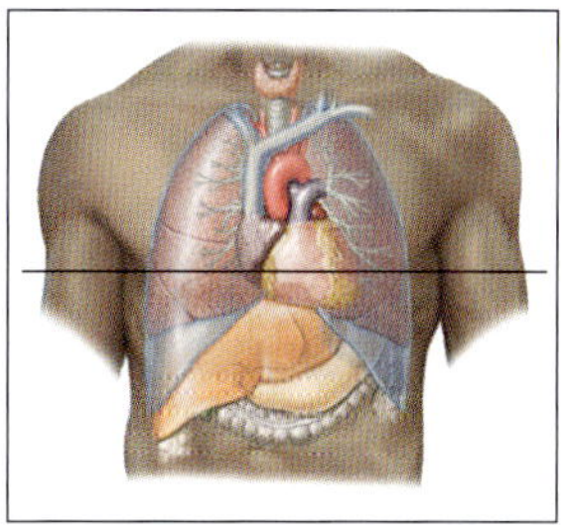

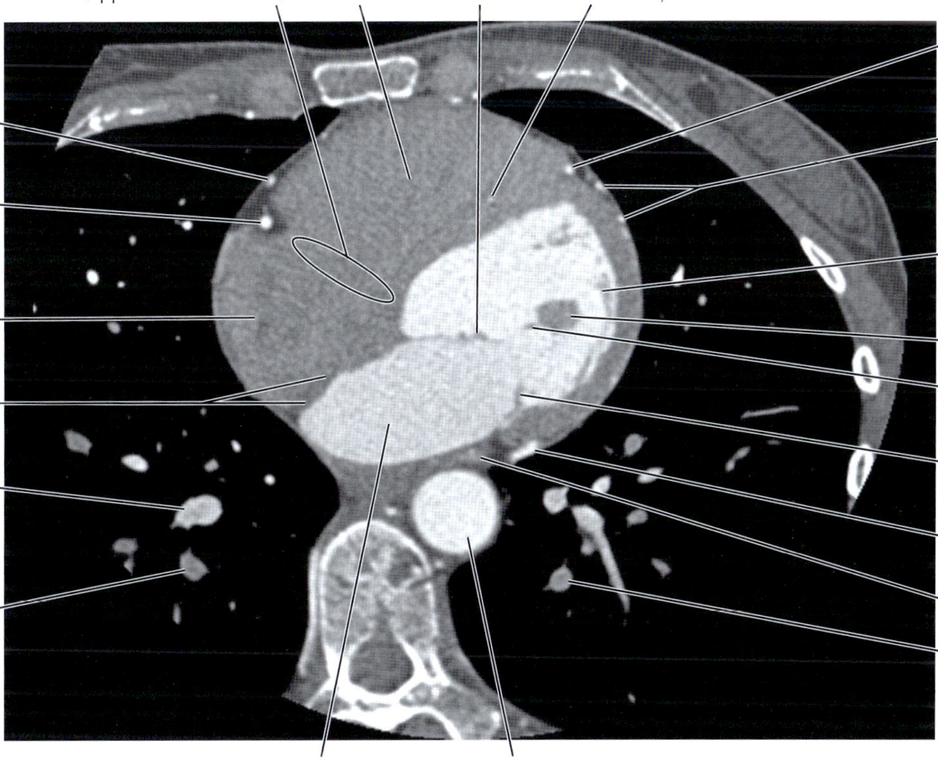
Tricuspid valve (approximate location)
Right ventricle
Mitral valve, anterior leaflet
Septal perforator coronary a.
Left anterior descending coronary a.
1st diagonal coronary a. & lateral diagonal branch
Left ventricle (trabeculae carneae)
Papillary m.
Chordae tendineae
Mitral valve, posterior leaflet
Left circumflex coronary a.
Great cardiac v.
Left lower lobe posterior basal subsegmental pulmonary a.
Acute marginal coronary a.
Right coronary a.
Right atrium
Interatrial septum
Pulmonary v.
Right lower lobe posterior basal segment pulmonary a.
Left atrium
Descending thoracic aorta

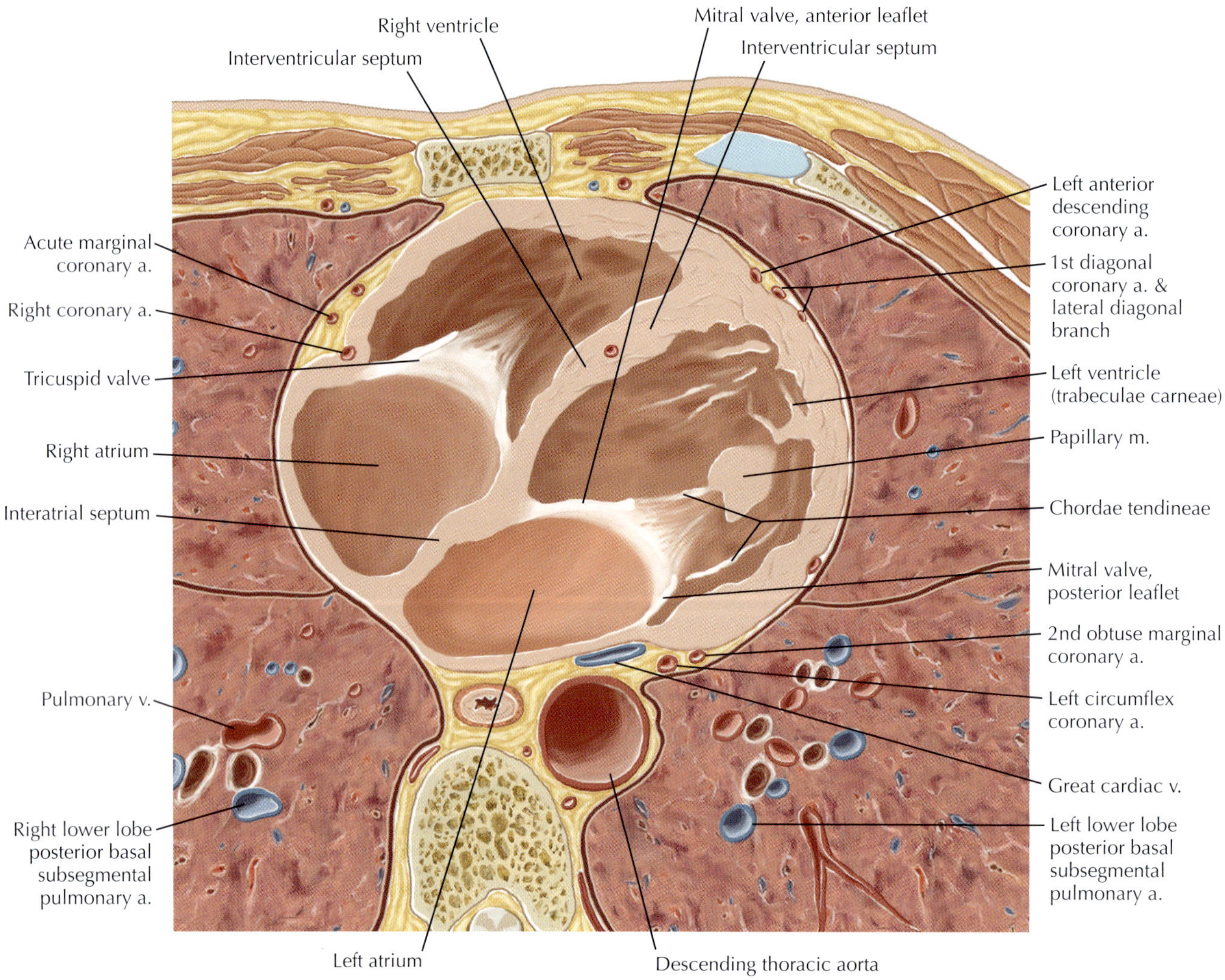
Right ventricle
Interventricular septum
Mitral valve, anterior leaflet
Interventricular septum
Acute marginal coronary a.
Right coronary a.
Tricuspid valve
Right atrium
Interatrial septum
Pulmonary v.
Right lower lobe posterior basal subsegmental pulmonary a.
Left atrium
Descending thoracic aorta
Left anterior descending coronary a.
1st diagonal coronary a. & lateral diagonal branch
Left ventricle (trabeculae carneae)
Papillary m.
Chordae tendineae
Mitral valve, posterior leaflet
2nd obtuse marginal coronary a.
Left circumflex coronary a.
Great cardiac v.
Left lower lobe posterior basal subsegmental pulmonary a.

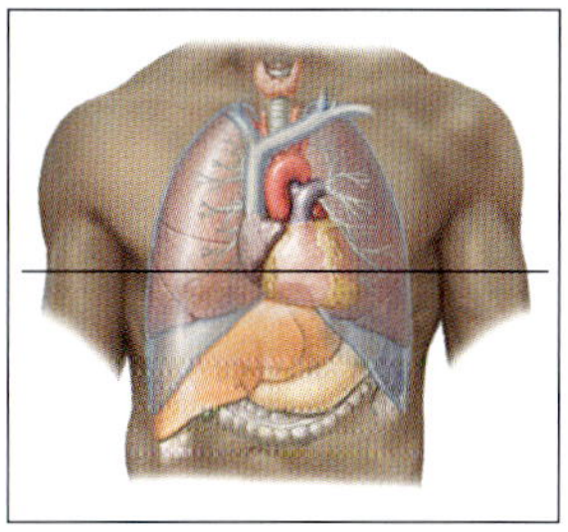

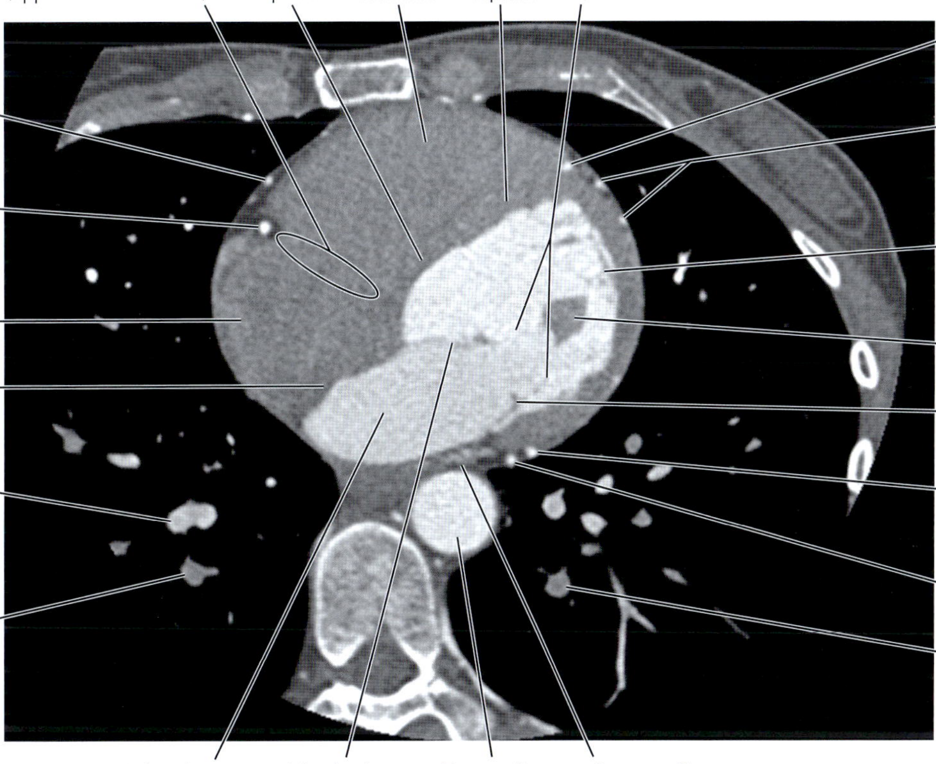
Tricuspid valve (approximate location)
Inter-ventricular septum
Right ventricle
Inter-ventricular septum
Chordae tendineae
Acute marginal coronary a.
Right coronary a.
Right atrium
Interatrial septum
Pulmonary v.
Right lower lobe posterior basal subsegmental pulmonary a.
Left anterior descending coronary a.
1st diagonal coronary a. & lateral diagonal branch
Left ventricle (trabeculae carneae)
Papillary m.
Mitral valve, posterior leaflet
2nd obtuse marginal coronary a.
Left circumflex coronary a.
Left lower lobe posterior basal subsegmental pulmonary a.
Left atrium
Mitral valve, anterior leaflet
Descending thoracic aorta
Great cardiac v.

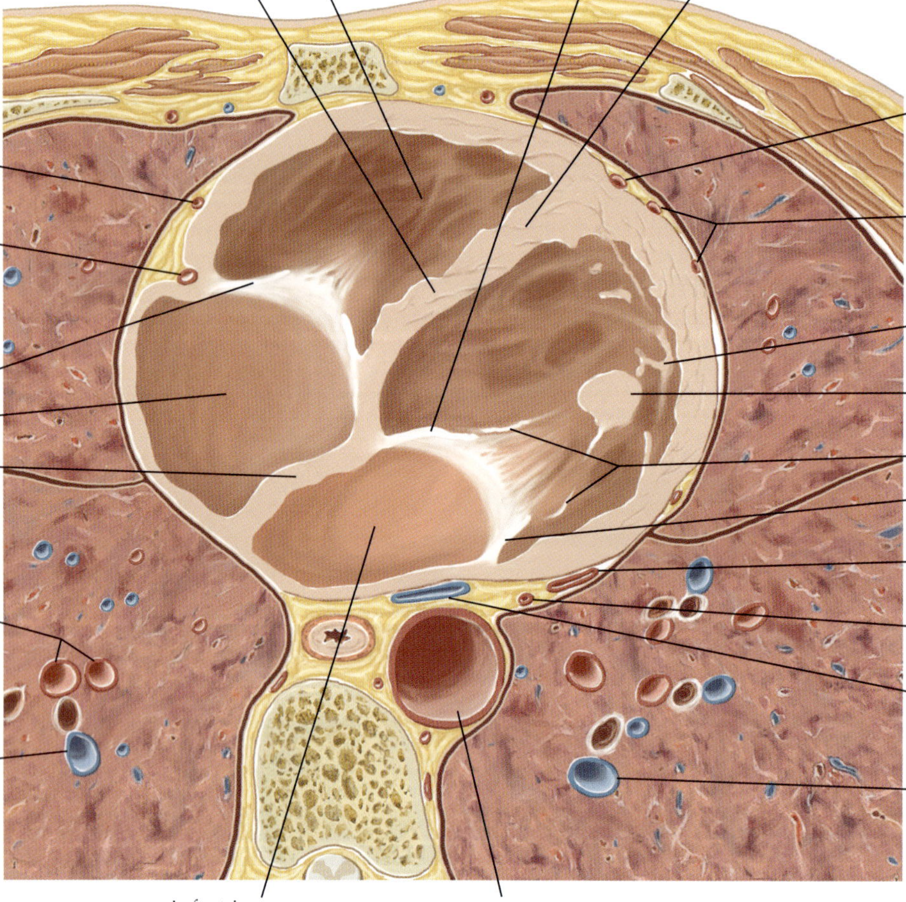

TECHNICAL CONSIDERATION

The mitral valve (left atrioventricular valve) is clearly open, indicating that this image was acquired during diastole. As discussed above in the Introduction, at lower heart rates, cardiac CT axial examinations are performed during diastole, when cardiac motion is minimal—this allows for nearly motion-free images.

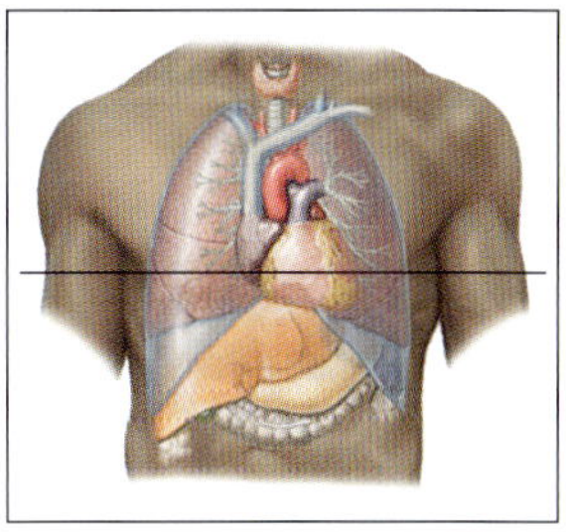

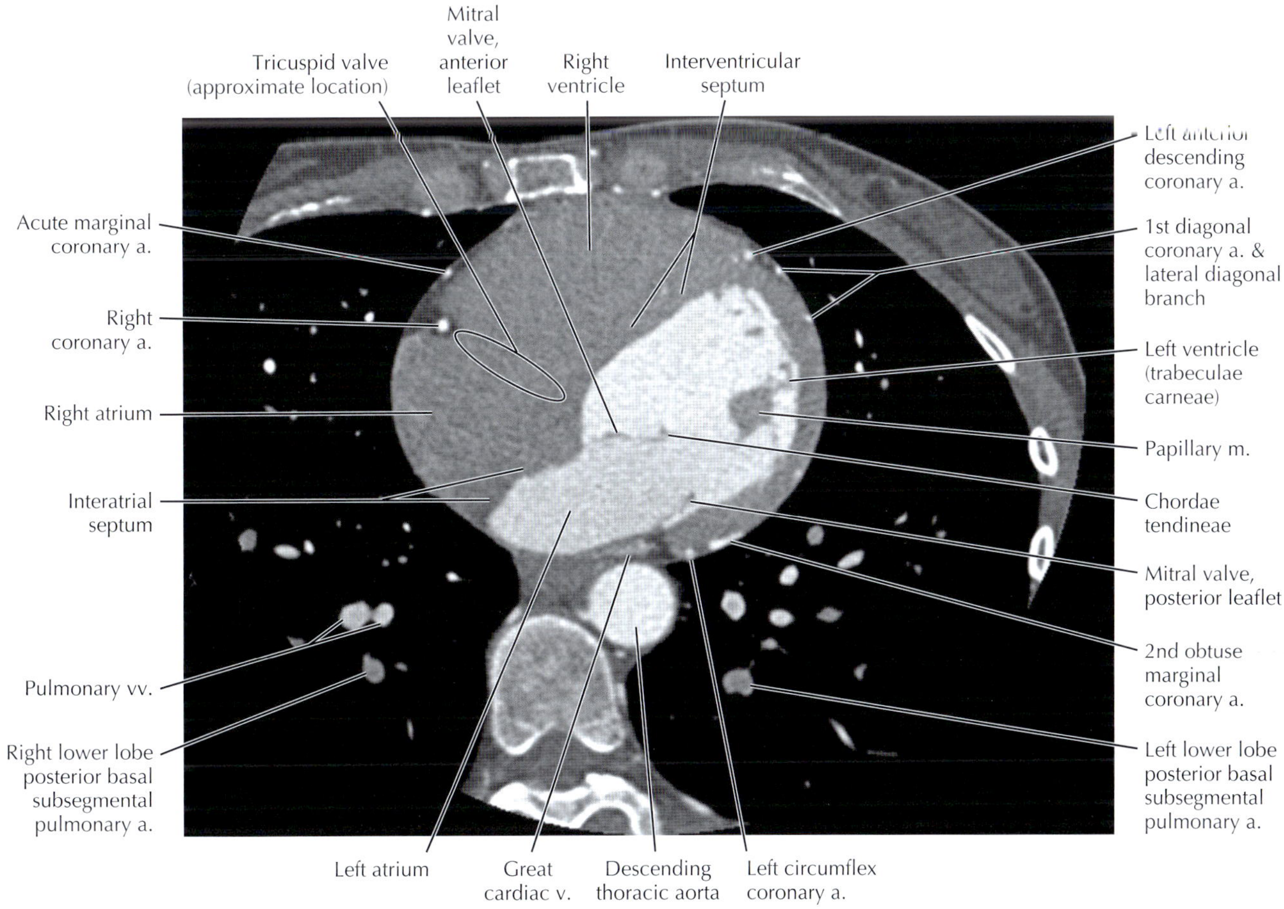
Tricuspid valve (approximate location)
Mitral valve, anterior leaflet
Right ventricle
Interventricular septum
Left anterior descending coronary a.
Acute marginal coronary a.
1st diagonal coronary a. & lateral diagonal branch
Right coronary a.
Left ventricle (trabeculae carneae)
Right atrium
Papillary m.
Interatrial septum
Chordae tendineae
Mitral valve, posterior leaflet
2nd obtuse marginal coronary a.
Pulmonary vv.
Right lower lobe posterior basal subsegmental pulmonary a.
Left lower lobe posterior basal subsegmental pulmonary a.
Left atrium
Great cardiac v.
Descending thoracic aorta
Left circumflex coronary a.

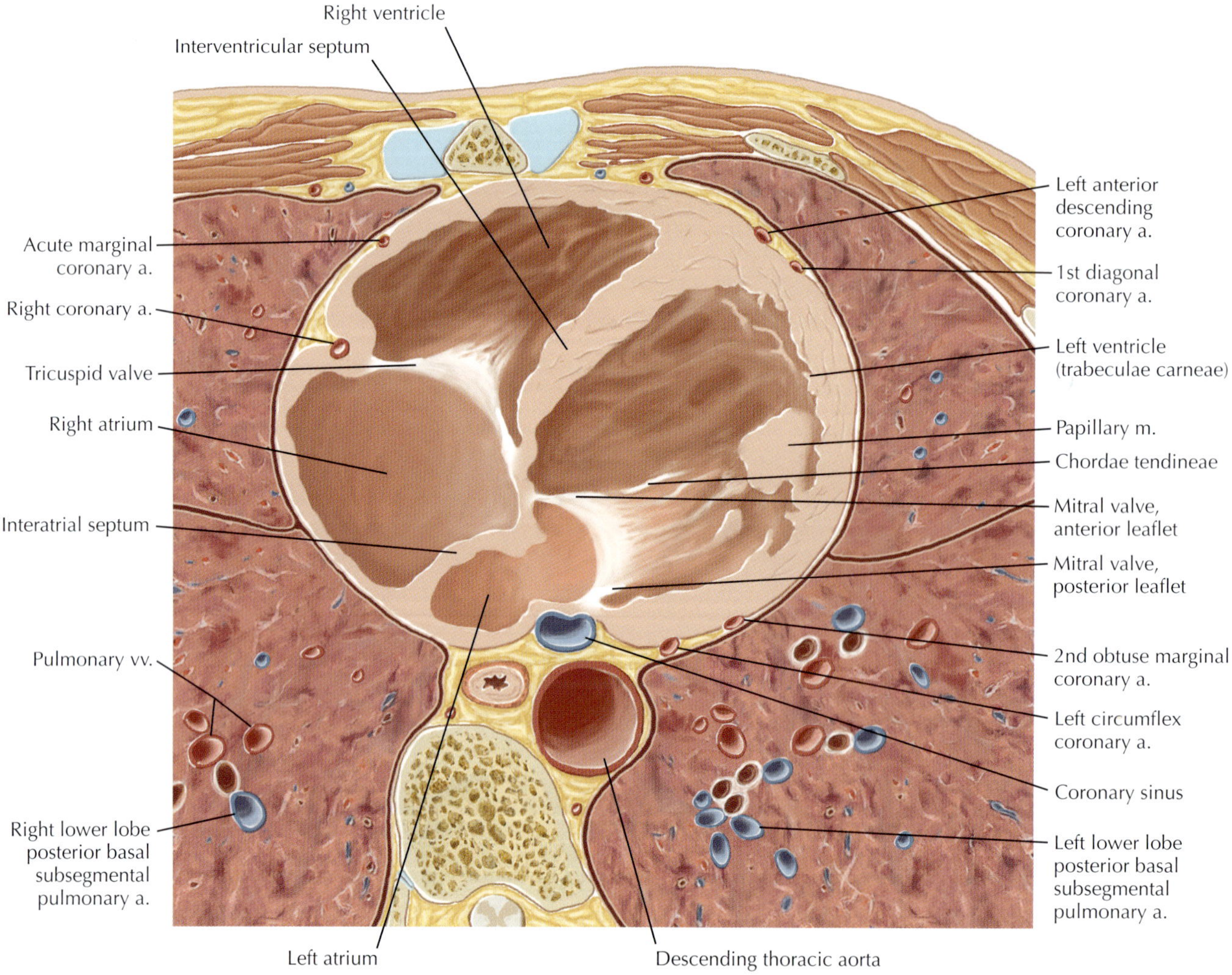
Right ventricle
Interventricular septum
Acute marginal coronary a.
Right coronary a.
Tricuspid valve
Right atrium
Interatrial septum
Pulmonary vv.
Right lower lobe posterior basal subsegmental pulmonary a.
Left atrium
Descending thoracic aorta
Left anterior descending coronary a.
1st diagonal coronary a.
Left ventricle (trabeculae carneae)
Papillary m.
Chordae tendineae
Mitral valve, anterior leaflet
Mitral valve, posterior leaflet
2nd obtuse marginal coronary a.
Left circumflex coronary a.
Coronary sinus
Left lower lobe posterior basal subsegmental pulmonary a.

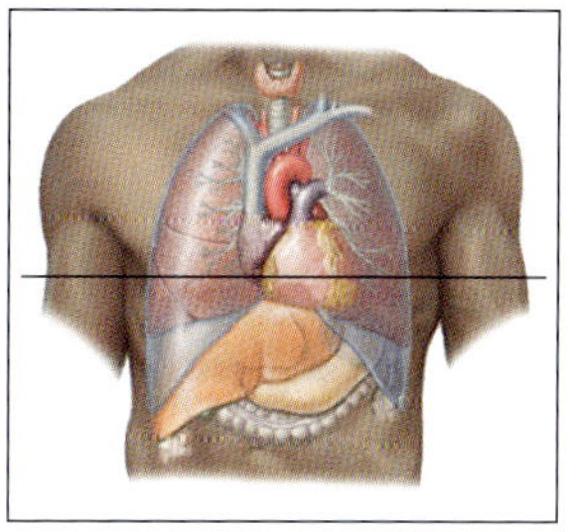

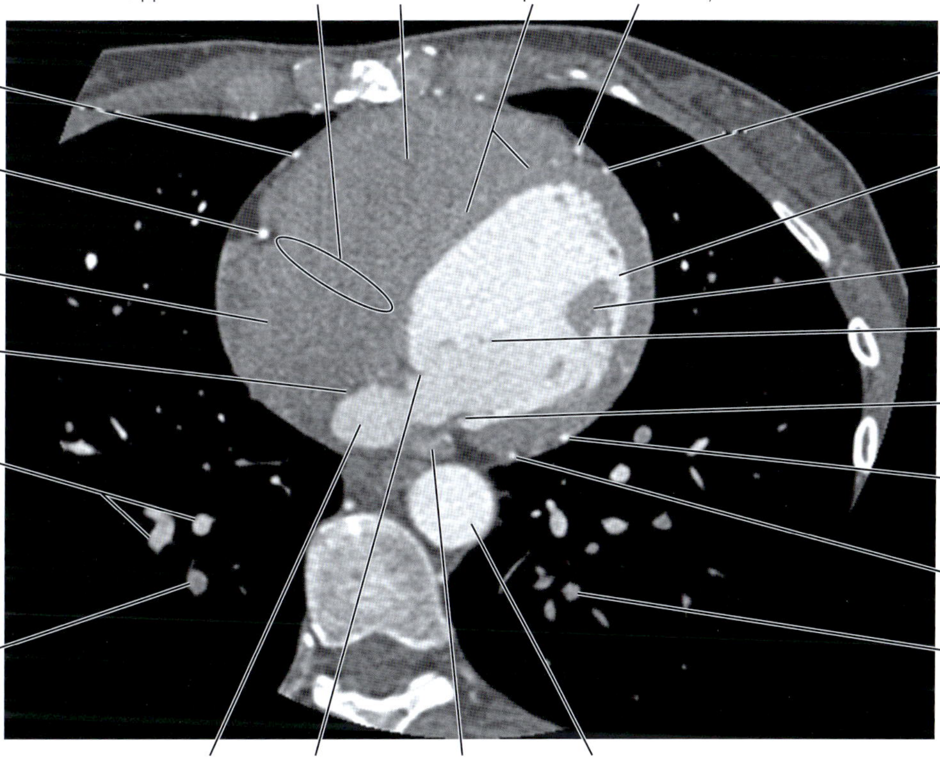
Tricuspid valve (approximate location)
Right ventricle
Interventricular septum
Left anterior descending coronary a.
Acute marginal coronary a.
Right coronary a.
Right atrium
Interatrial septum
Pulmonary vv.
Right lower lobe posterior basal subsegmental pulmonary a.
1st diagonal coronary a.
Left ventricle (trabeculae carneae)
Papillary m.
Chordae tendineae
Mitral valve, posterior leaflet
2nd obtuse marginal coronary a.
Left circumflex coronary a.
Left lower lobe posterior basal subsegmental pulmonary a.
Left atrium
Mitral valve, anterior leaflet
Coronary sinus
Descending thoracic aorta

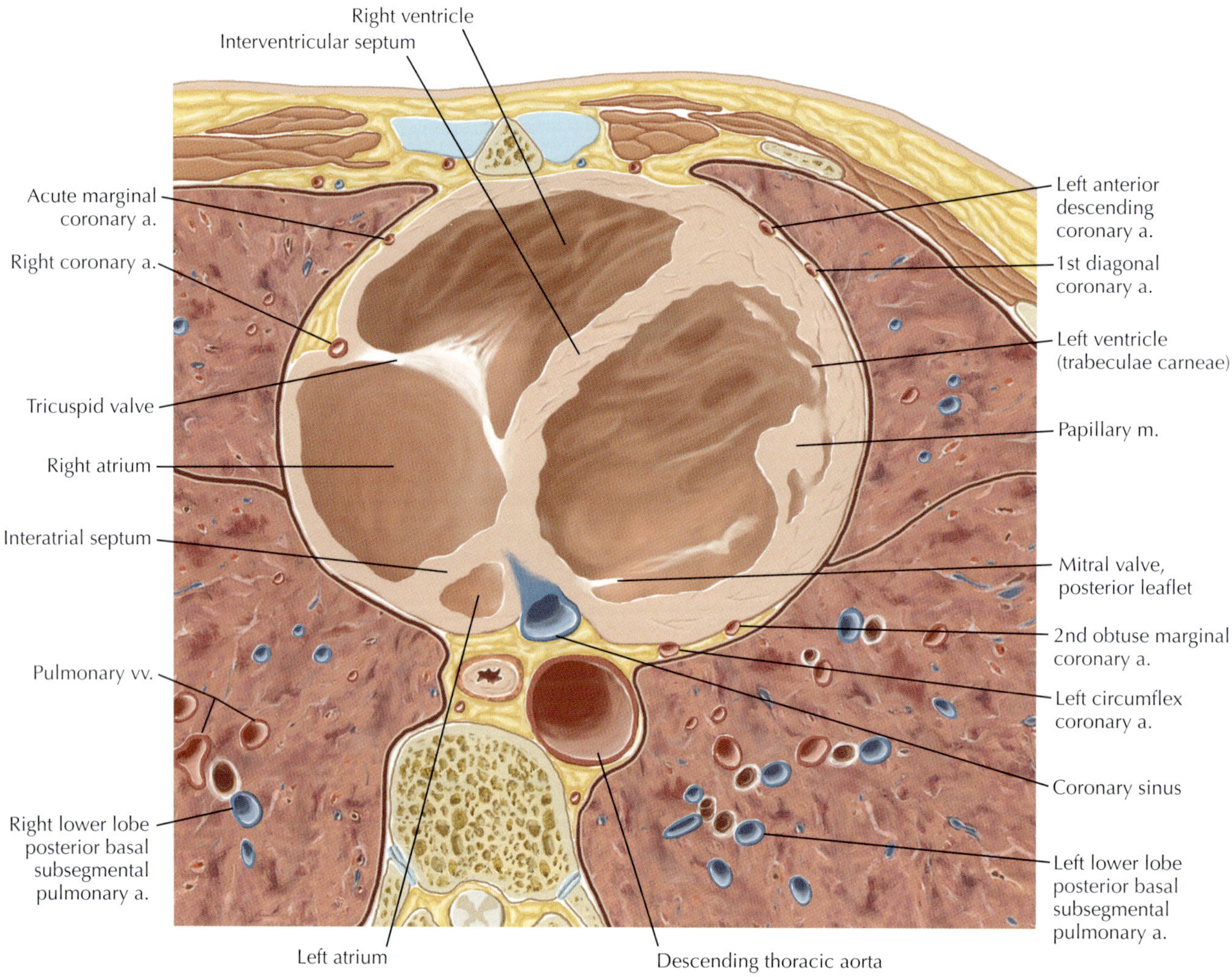
Right ventricle
Interventricular septum
Acute marginal coronary a.
Right coronary a.
Tricuspid valve
Right atrium
Interatrial septum
Pulmonary vv.
Right lower lobe posterior basal subsegmental pulmonary a.
Left atrium
Descending thoracic aorta
Left anterior descending coronary a.
1st diagonal coronary a.
Left ventricle (trabeculae carneae)
Papillary m.
Mitral valve, posterior leaflet
2nd obtuse marginal coronary a.
Left circumflex coronary a.
Coronary sinus
Left lower lobe posterior basal subsegmental pulmonary a.

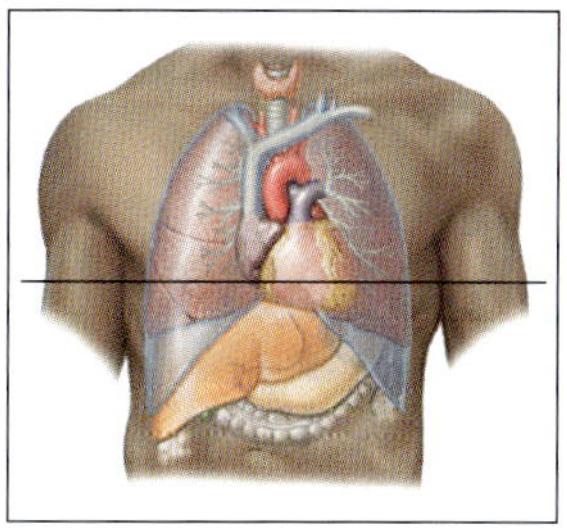

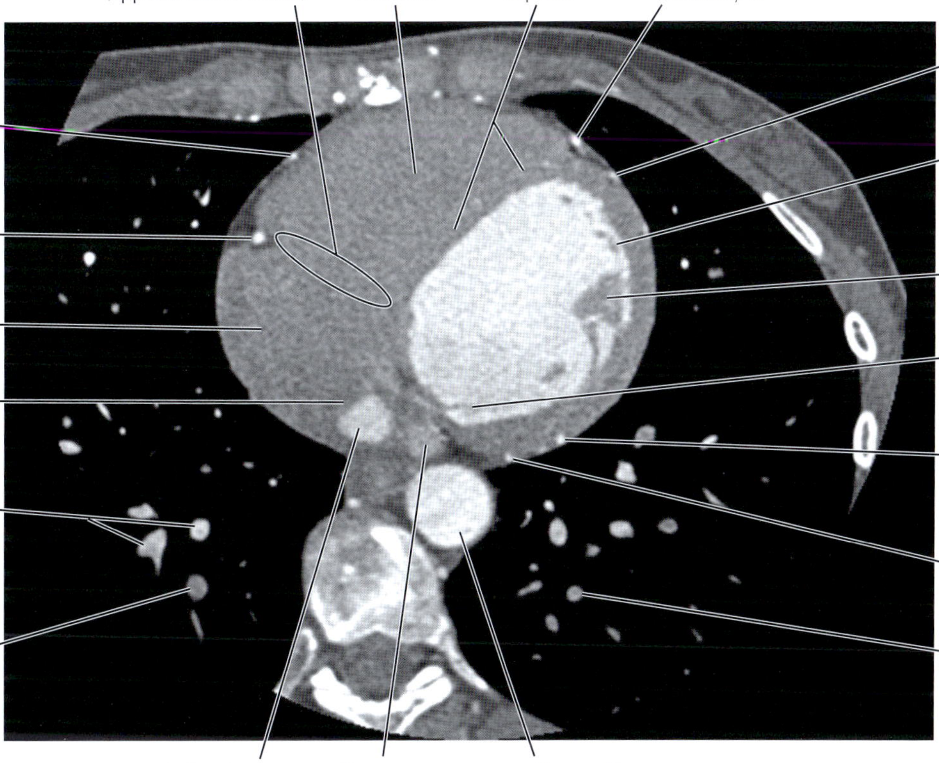
Tricuspid valve
(approximate location)
Right
ventricle
Interventricular
septum
Left anterior
descending
coronary a.
1st diagonal
coronary a.
Acute marginal
coronary a.
Left ventricle
(trabeculae
carneae)
Right
coronary a.
Papillary m.
Right atrium
Mitral valve,
posterior leaflet
Interatrial
septum
2nd obtuse
marginal
coronary a.
Pulmonary vv.
Left circumflex
coronary a.
Right lower lobe
posterior basal
subsegmental
pulmonary a.
Left lower lobe
posterior basal
subsegmental
pulmonary a.
Left atrium
Coronary
sinus
Descending
thoracic aorta

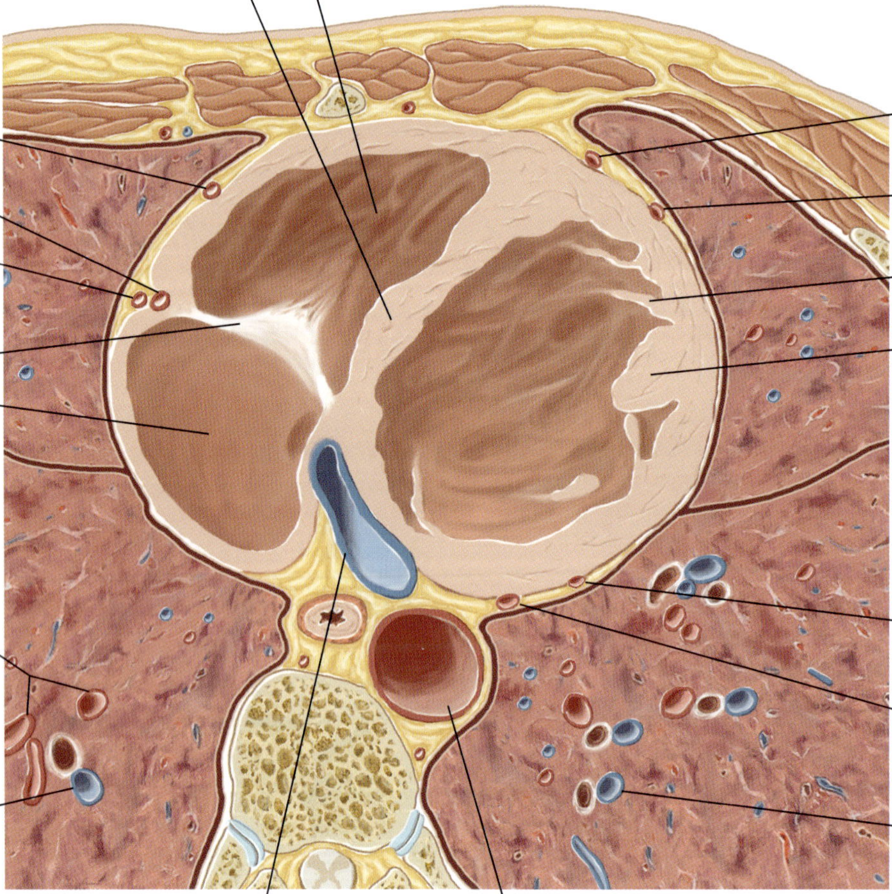
Right ventricle
Interventricular septum
1st acute marginal coronary a.
Right coronary a.
2nd acute marginal coronary a.
Tricuspid valve
Right atrium
Pulmonary vv.
Right lower lobe posterior basal subsegmental pulmonary a.
Coronary sinus
Descending thoracic aorta
Left anterior descending coronary a.
1st diagonal coronary a.
Left ventricle (trabeculae carneae)
Papillary m.
2nd obtuse marginal coronary a.
Left circumflex coronary a.
Left lower lobe posterior basal subsegmental pulmonary a.

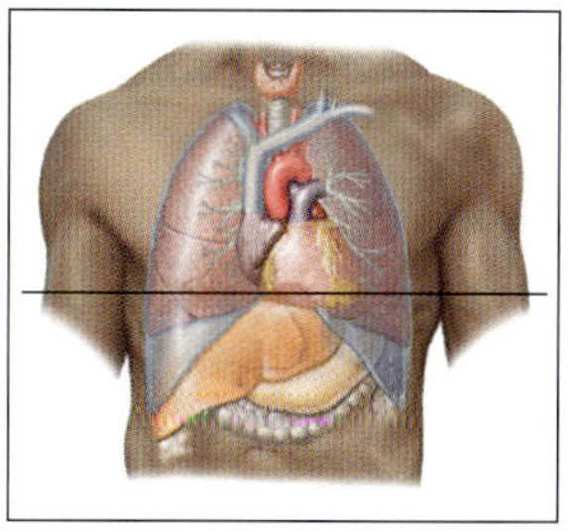

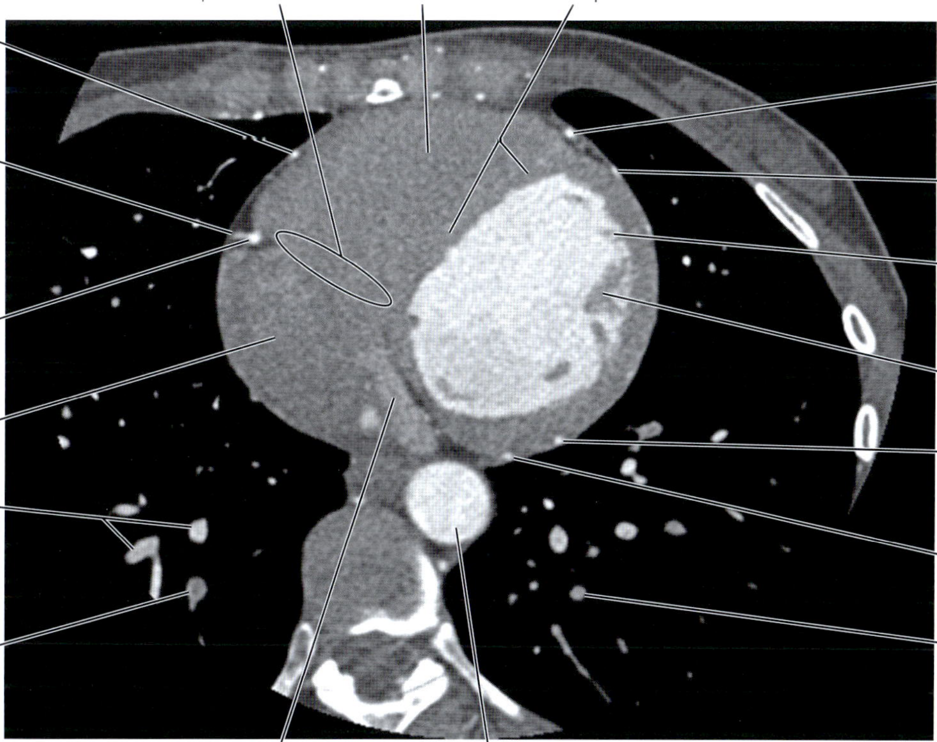
Tricuspid valve
Right ventricle
Interventricular septum
1st acute marginal coronary a.
2nd acute marginal coronary a.
Right coronary a.
Right atrium
Pulmonary vv.
Right lower lobe posterior basal subsegmental pulmonary a.
Coronary sinus
Descending thoracic aorta
Left anterior descending coronary a.
1st diagonal coronary a.
Left ventricle (trabeculae carneae)
Papillary m.
2nd obtuse marginal coronary a.
Left circumflex coronary a.
Left lower lobe posterior basal subsegmental pulmonary a.

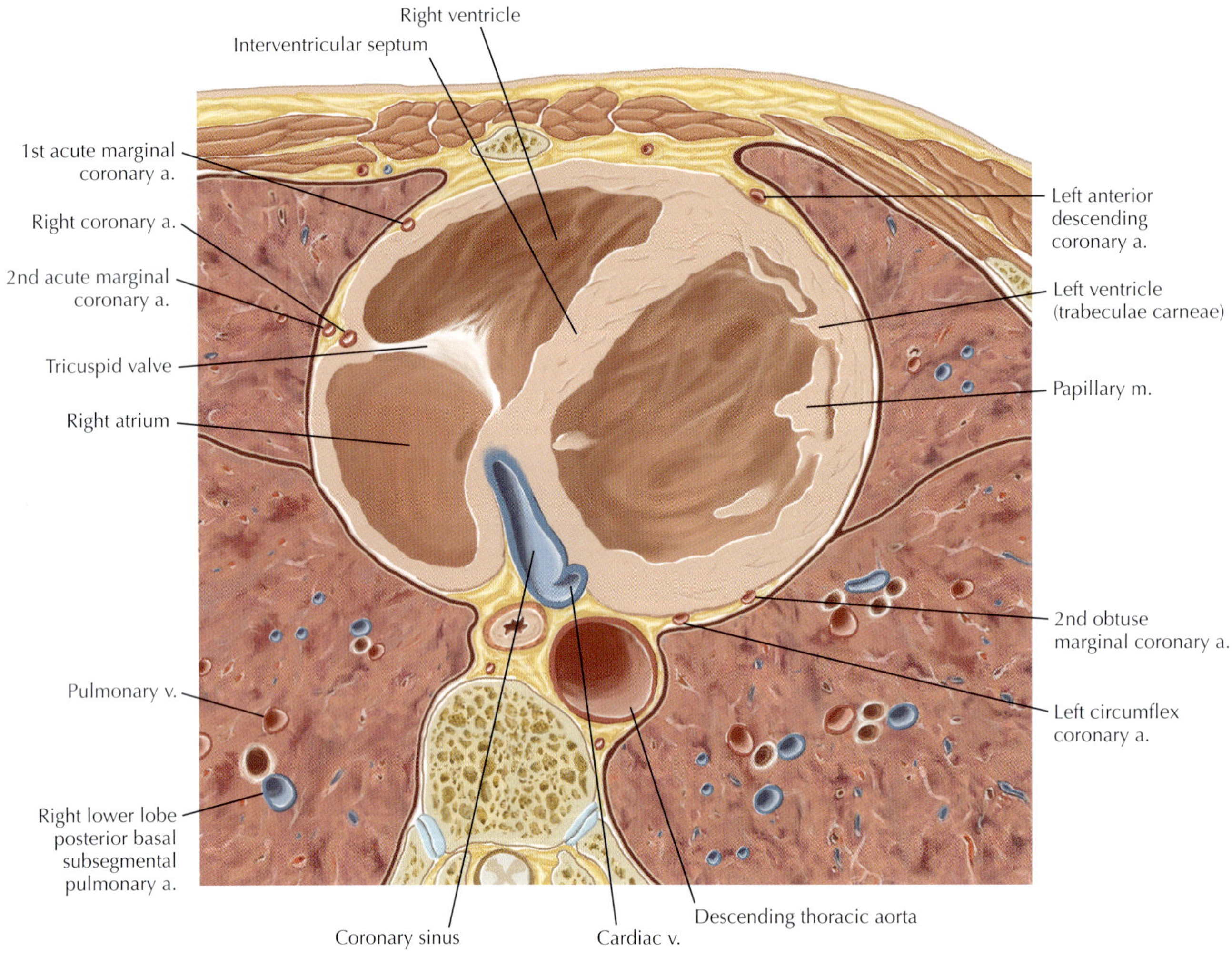
Right ventricle
Interventricular septum
1st acute marginal coronary a.
Right coronary a.
2nd acute marginal coronary a.
Tricuspid valve
Right atrium
Pulmonary v.
Right lower lobe posterior basal subsegmental pulmonary a.
Coronary sinus
Cardiac v.
Descending thoracic aorta
Left anterior descending coronary a.
Left ventricle (trabeculae carneae)
Papillary m.
2nd obtuse marginal coronary a.
Left circumflex coronary a.

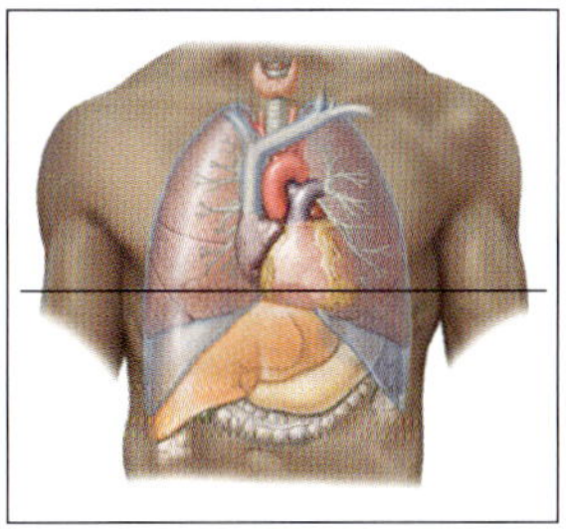

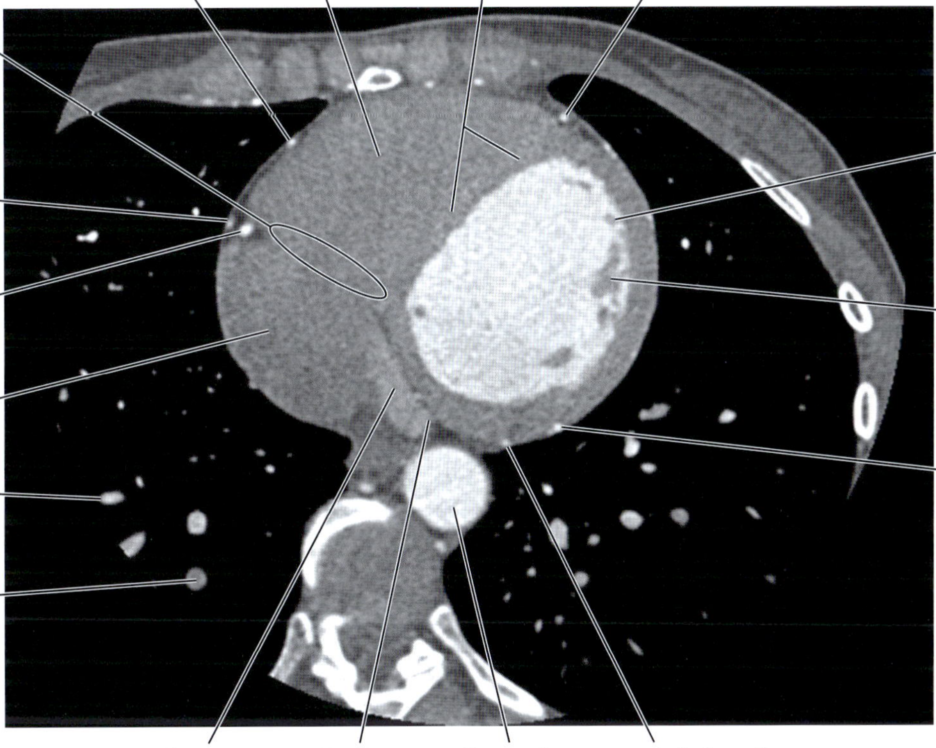

1st acute marginal coronary a.
Right ventricle
Interventricular septum
Left anterior descending coronary a.
Tricuspid valve (approximate location)
2nd acute marginal coronary a.
Right coronary a.
Right atrium
Pulmonary v.
Right lower lobe posterior basal subsegmental pulmonary a.
Left ventricle (trabeculae carneae)
Papillary m.
2nd obtuse marginal coronary a.
Coronary sinus
Cardiac v.
Descending thoracic aorta
Left circumflex coronary a.

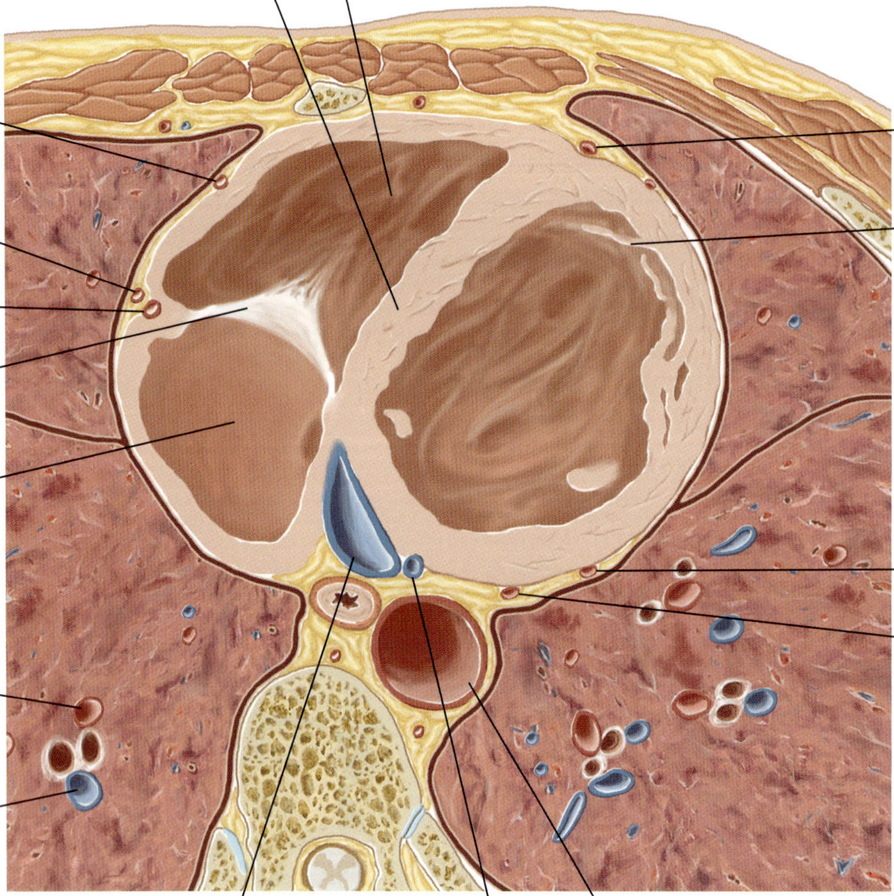

NORMAL ANATOMY

This view, and views located both cranial and caudal to this level, shows an irregular surface of the left ventricle, representing trabeculae carneae. Most of the left ventricle is covered by a mesh of trabeculae carneae, sparing only the left ventricular outflow tract (aortic vestibule). Trabeculae carneae are also present within the right ventricle but cannot be seen on this examination because the iodinated contrast has been "washed" from the right cardiac chambers by the use of a saline injection following the intravenous contrast injection (see Introduction above). See the section detailing cardiac MR anatomy for demonstration of right ventricular chamber anatomy.

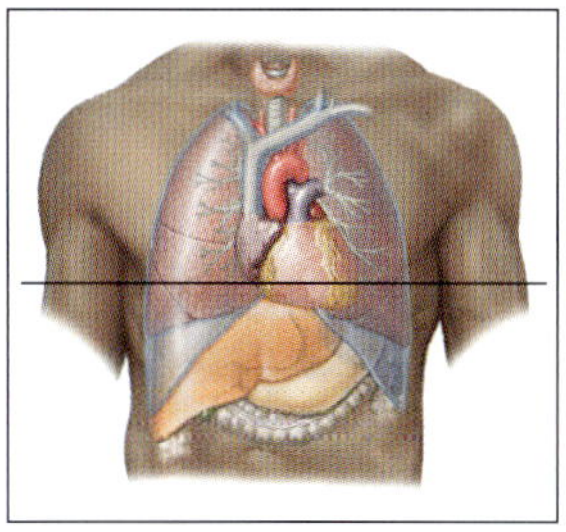

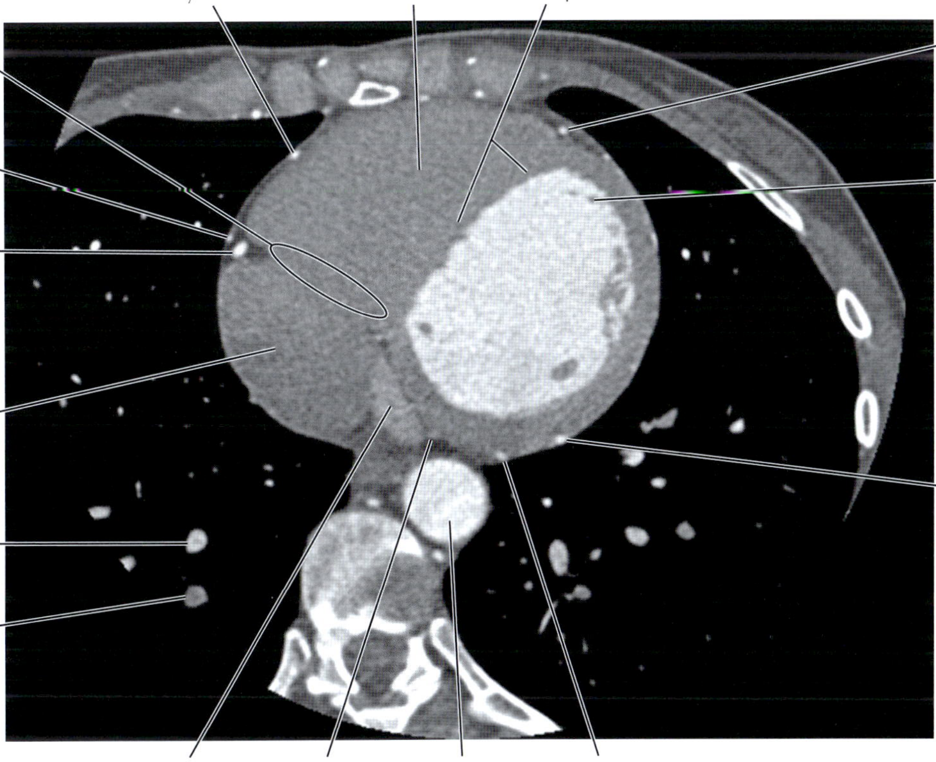
1st acute marginal coronary a.
Right ventricle
Interventricular septum
Tricuspid valve (approximate location)
Left anterior descending coronary a.
2nd acute marginal coronary a.
Left ventricle (trabeculae carneae)
Right coronary a.
Right atrium
2nd obtuse marginal coronary a.
Pulmonary v.
Right lower lobe posterior basal subsegmental pulmonary a.
Coronary sinus
Cardiac v.
Descending thoracic aorta
Left circumflex coronary a.

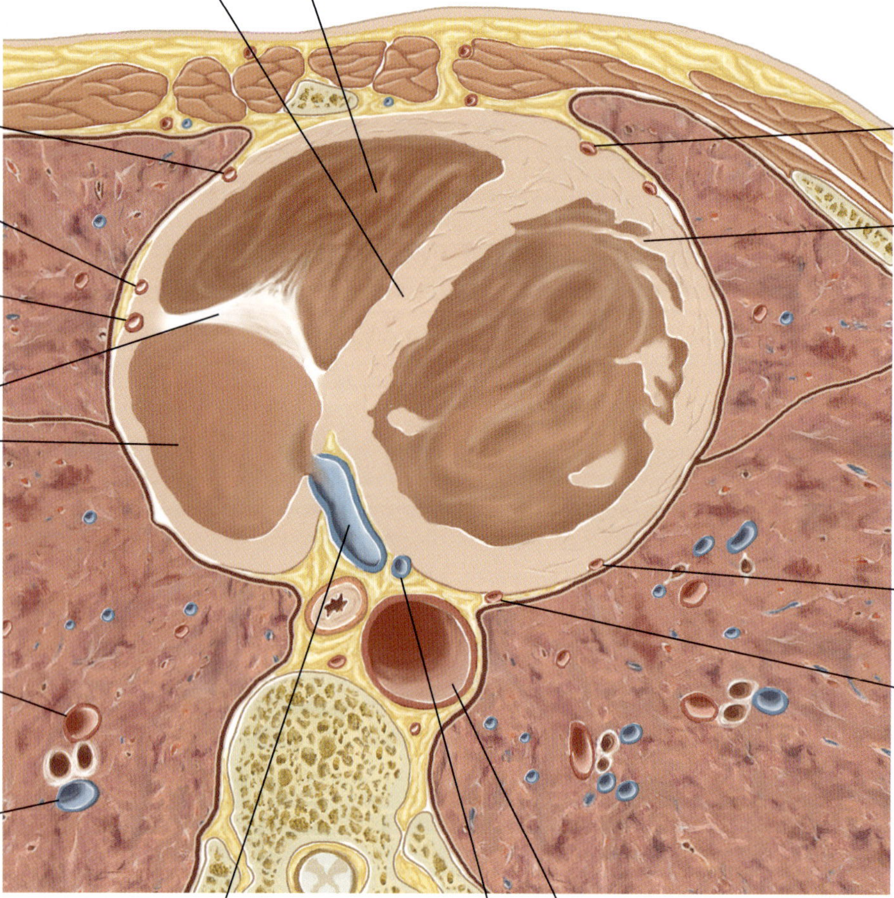

Right ventricle
Interventricular septum
1st acute marginal coronary a.
2nd acute marginal coronary a.
Right coronary a.
Tricuspid valve
Right atrium
Pulmonary v.
Right lower lobe posterior basal subsegmental pulmonary a.
Coronary sinus
Descending thoracic aorta
Cardiac v.
Left anterior descending coronary a.
Left ventricle (trabeculae carneae)
2nd obtuse marginal coronary a.
Left circumflex coronary a.

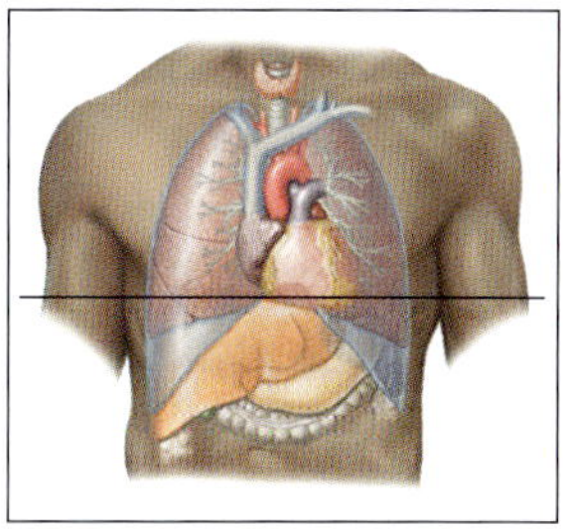

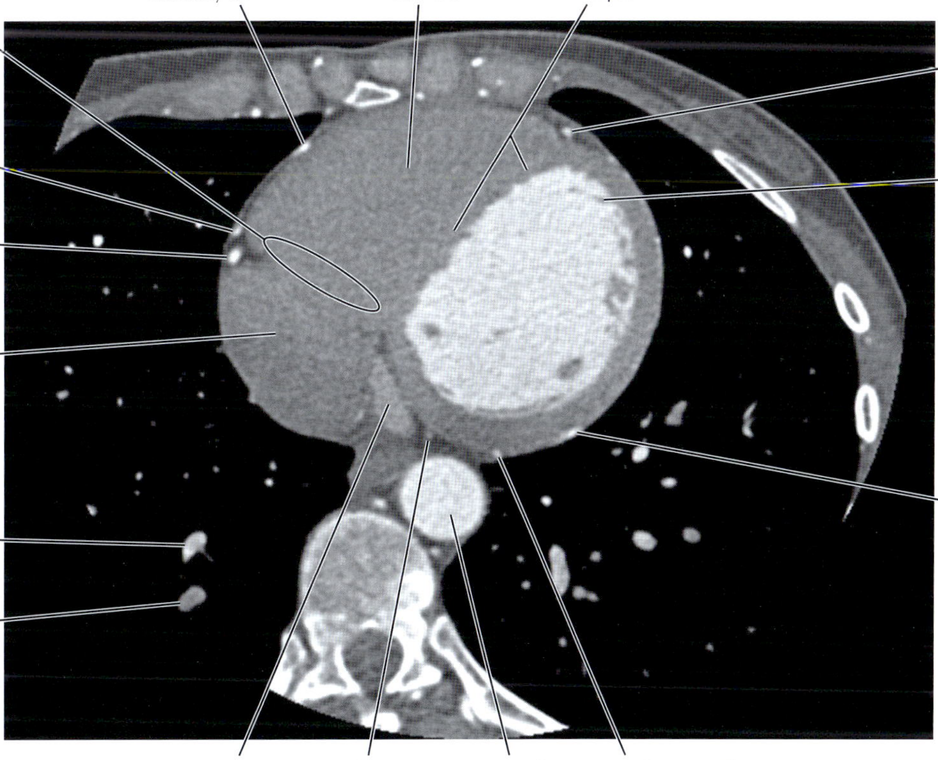
1st acute marginal coronary a.
Right ventricle
Interventricular septum
Tricuspid valve (approximate location)
Left anterior descending coronary a.
2nd acute marginal coronary a.
Left ventricle (trabeculae carneae)
Right coronary a.
Right atrium
2nd obtuse marginal coronary a.
Pulmonary v.
Right lower lobe posterior basal subsegmental pulmonary a.
Coronary sinus
Cardiac v.
Descending thoracic aorta
Left circumflex coronary a.

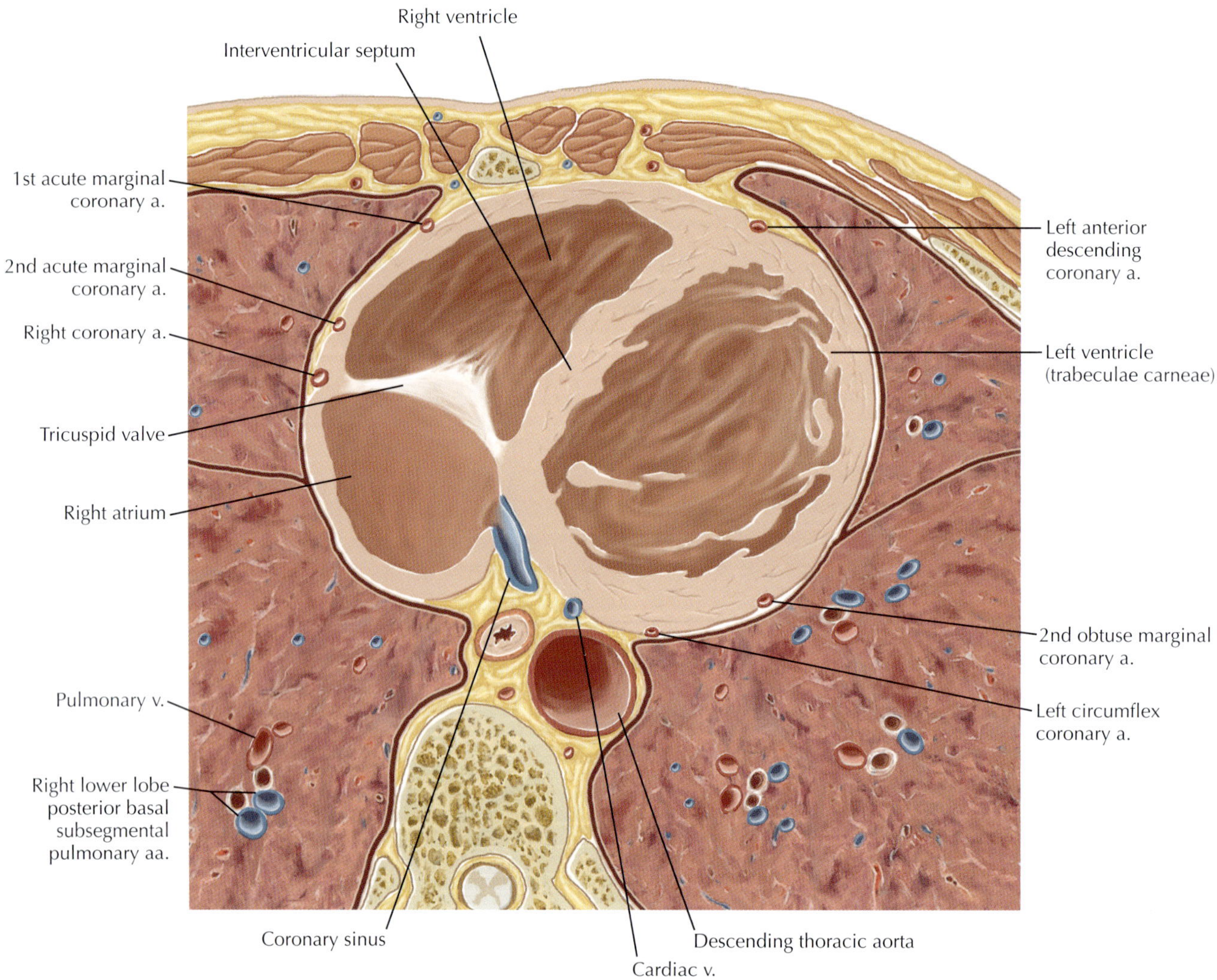
Right ventricle
Interventricular septum
1st acute marginal coronary a.
2nd acute marginal coronary a.
Right coronary a.
Tricuspid valve
Right atrium
Pulmonary v.
Right lower lobe posterior basal subsegmental pulmonary aa.
Coronary sinus
Cardiac v.
Descending thoracic aorta
Left anterior descending coronary a.
Left ventricle (trabeculae carneae)
2nd obtuse marginal coronary a.
Left circumflex coronary a.

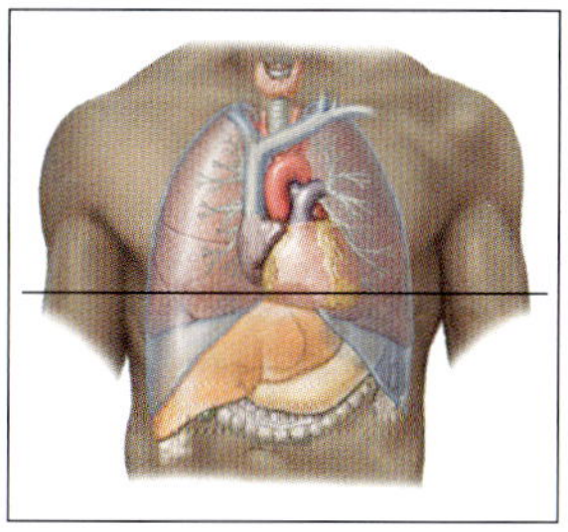

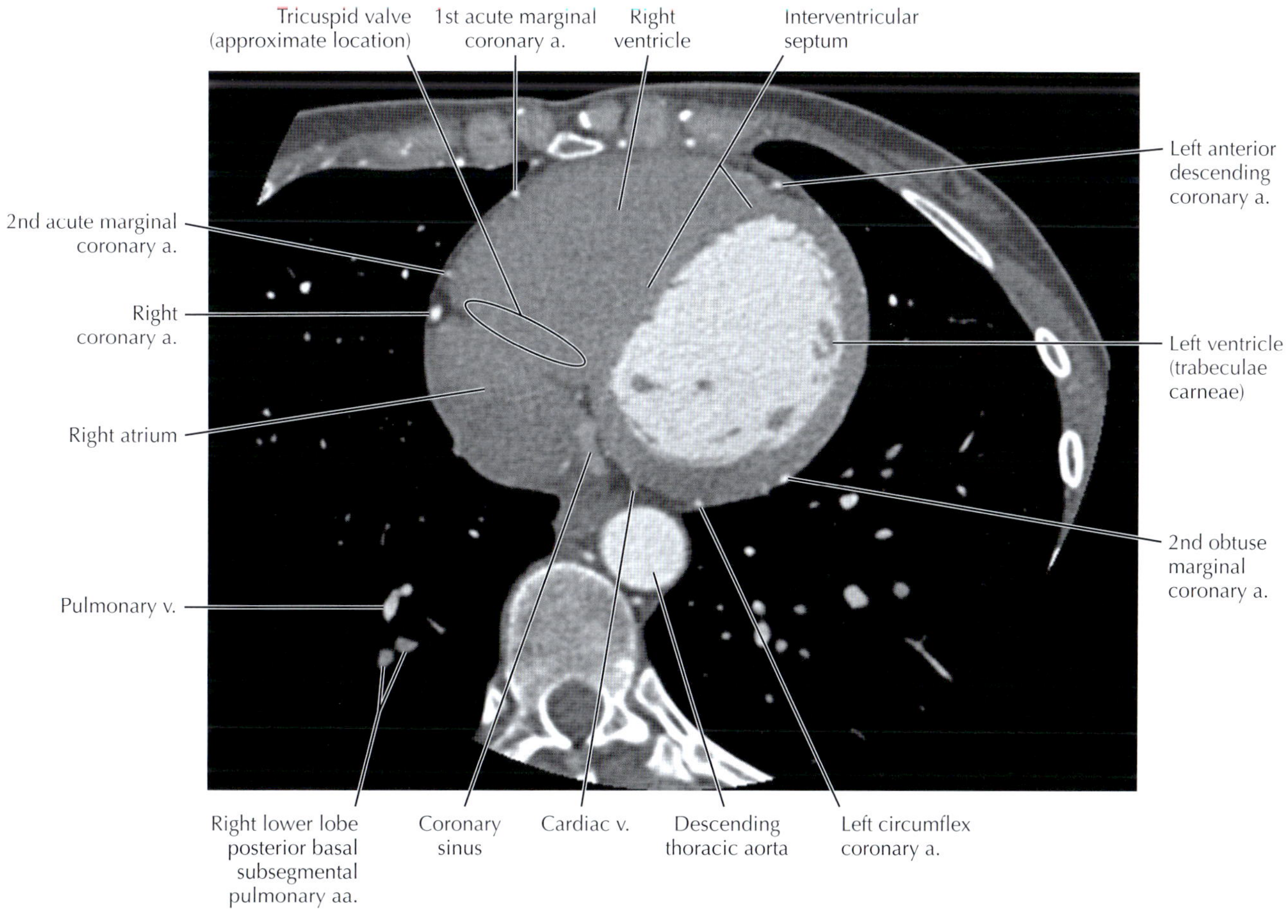
Tricuspid valve
(approximate location)
1st acute marginal
coronary a.
Right
ventricle
Interventricular
septum
Left anterior
descending
coronary a.
2nd acute marginal
coronary a.
Right
coronary a.
Left ventricle
(trabeculae
carneae)
Right atrium
2nd obtuse
marginal
coronary a.
Pulmonary v.
Right lower lobe
posterior basal
subsegmental
pulmonary aa.
Coronary
sinus
Cardiac v.
Descending
thoracic aorta
Left circumflex
coronary a.

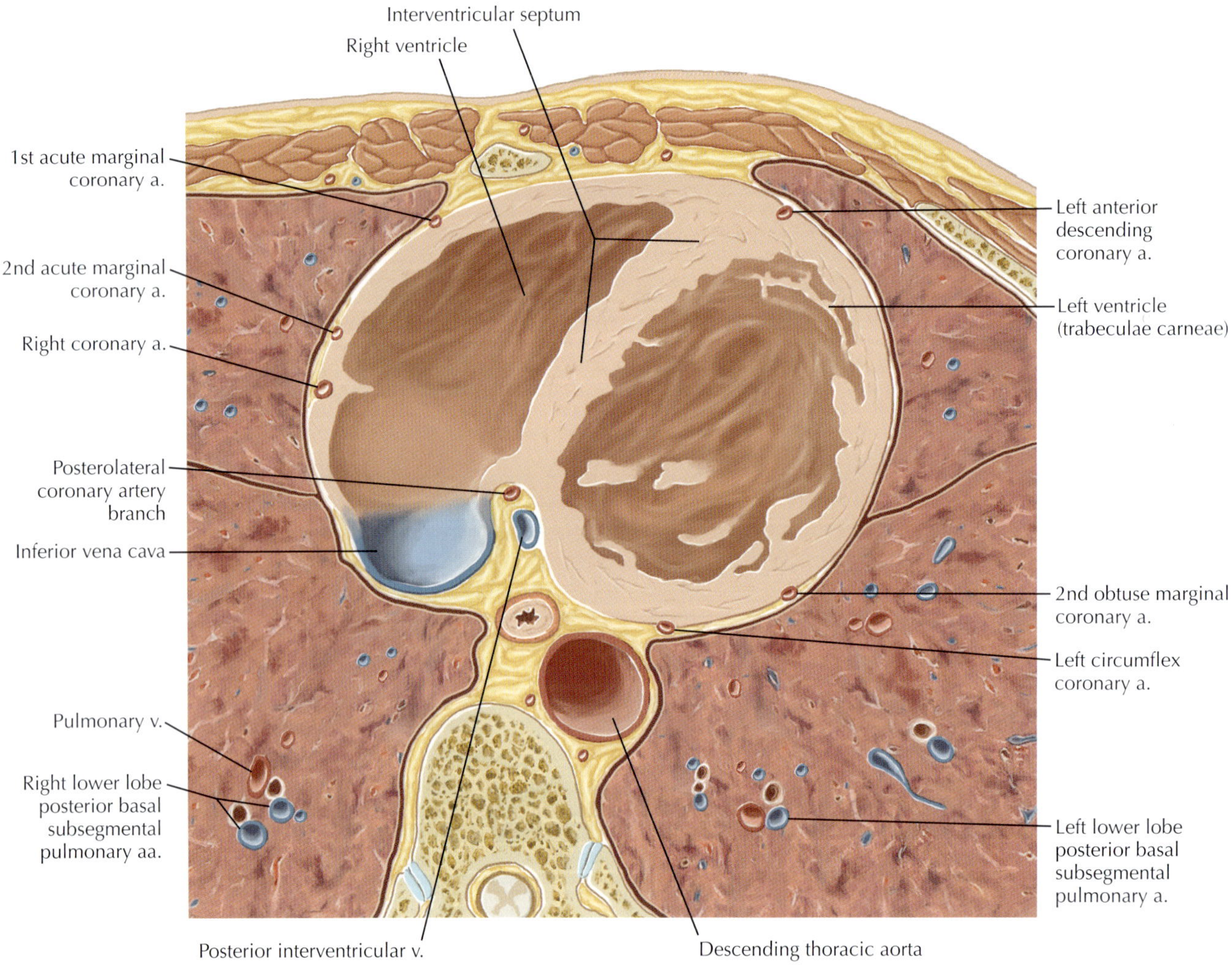
Interventricular septum
Right ventricle
1st acute marginal coronary a.
2nd acute marginal coronary a.
Right coronary a.
Posterolateral coronary artery branch
Inferior vena cava
Pulmonary v.
Right lower lobe posterior basal subsegmental pulmonary aa.
Posterior interventricular v.
Descending thoracic aorta
Left anterior descending coronary a.
Left ventricle (trabeculae carneae)
2nd obtuse marginal coronary a.
Left circumflex coronary a.
Left lower lobe posterior basal subsegmental pulmonary a.

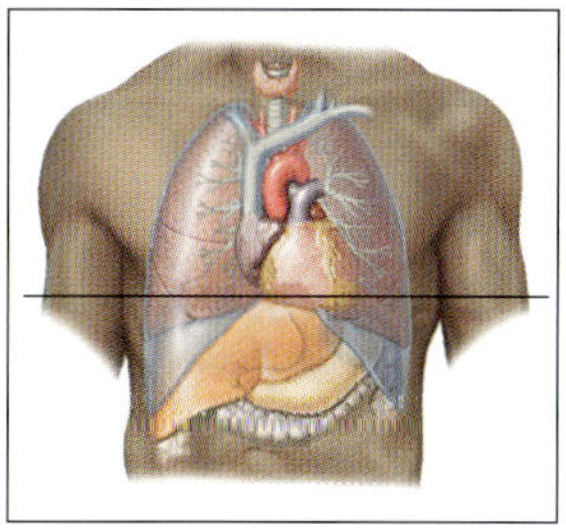

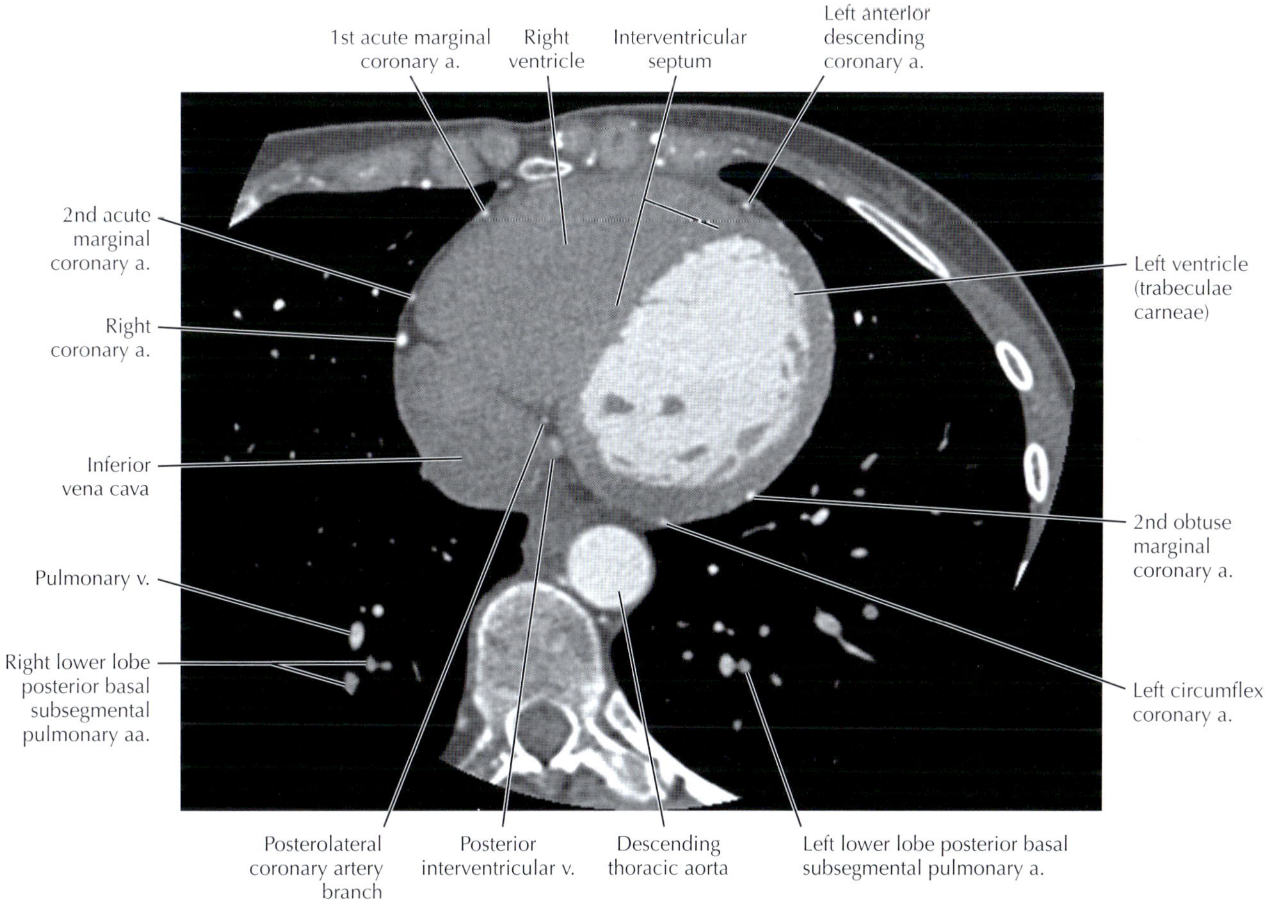
1st acute marginal coronary a.
Right ventricle
Interventricular septum
Left anterior descending coronary a.
2nd acute marginal coronary a.
Right coronary a.
Inferior vena cava
Pulmonary v.
Right lower lobe posterior basal subsegmental pulmonary aa.
Left ventricle (trabeculae carneae)
2nd obtuse marginal coronary a.
Left circumflex coronary a.
Posterolateral coronary artery branch
Posterior interventricular v.
Descending thoracic aorta
Left lower lobe posterior basal subsegmental pulmonary a.

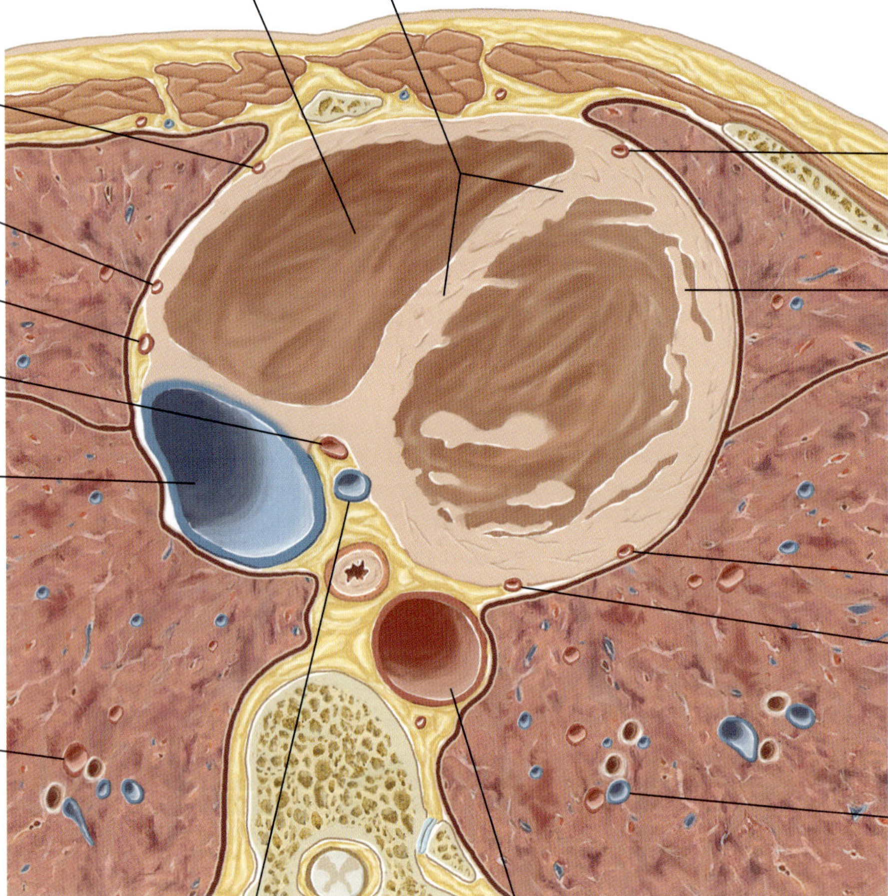
Interventricular septum
Right ventricle
1st acute marginal coronary a.
2nd acute marginal coronary a.
Right coronary a.
Posterolateral coronary artery branch
Inferior vena cava
Pulmonary v.
Posterior interventricular v.
Descending thoracic aorta
Left anterior descending coronary a.
Left ventricle (trabeculae carneae)
2nd obtuse marginal coronary a.
Left circumflex coronary a.
Left lower lobe posterior basal subsegmental pulmonary a.

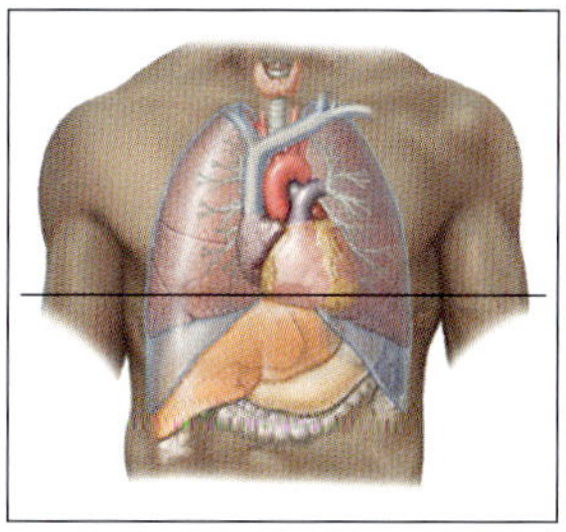

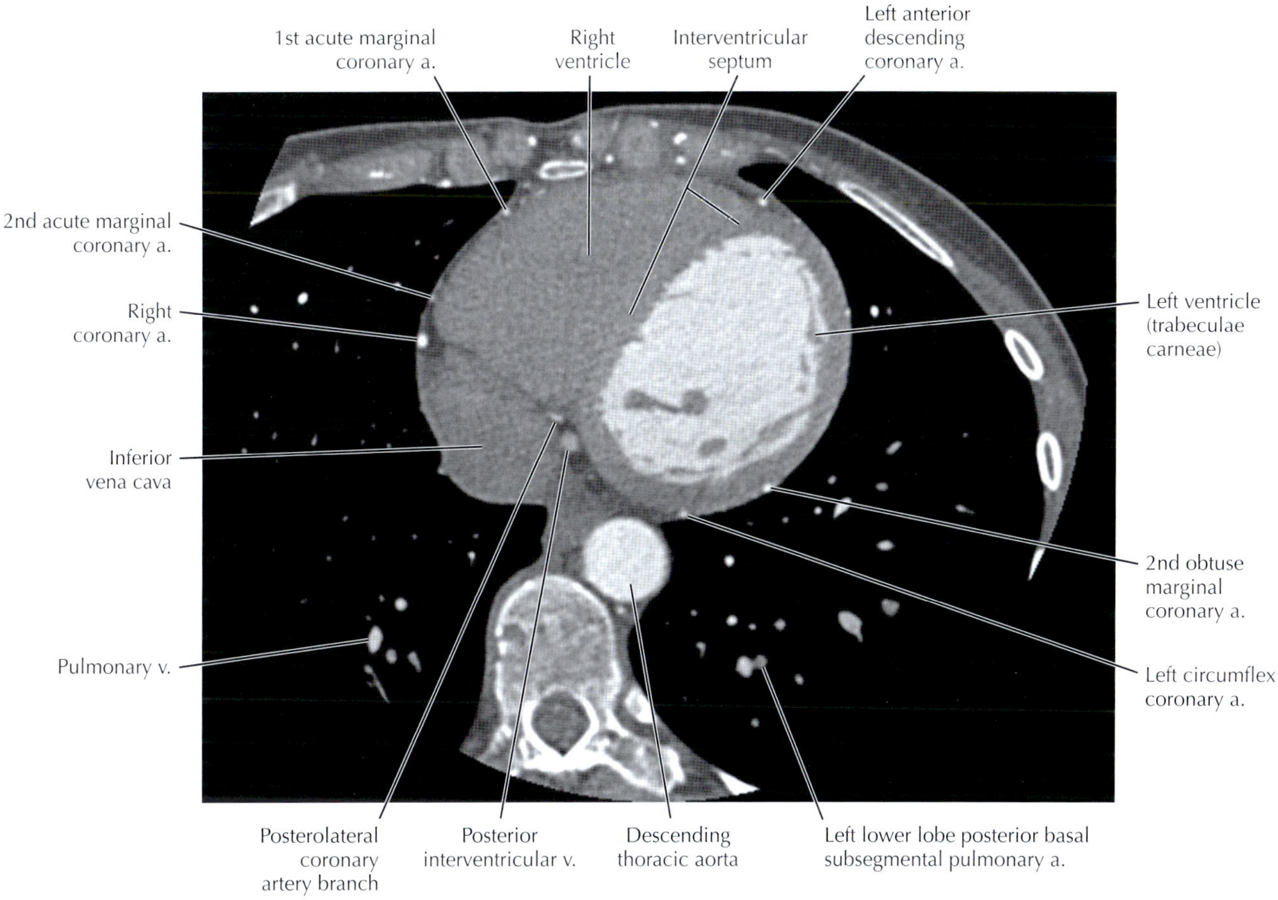

1st acute marginal coronary a.
Right ventricle
Interventricular septum
Left anterior descending coronary a.
2nd acute marginal coronary a.
Right coronary a.
Inferior vena cava
Pulmonary v.
Left ventricle (trabeculae carneae)
2nd obtuse marginal coronary a.
Left circumflex coronary a.
Posterolateral coronary artery branch
Posterior interventricular v.
Descending thoracic aorta
Left lower lobe posterior basal subsegmental pulmonary a.

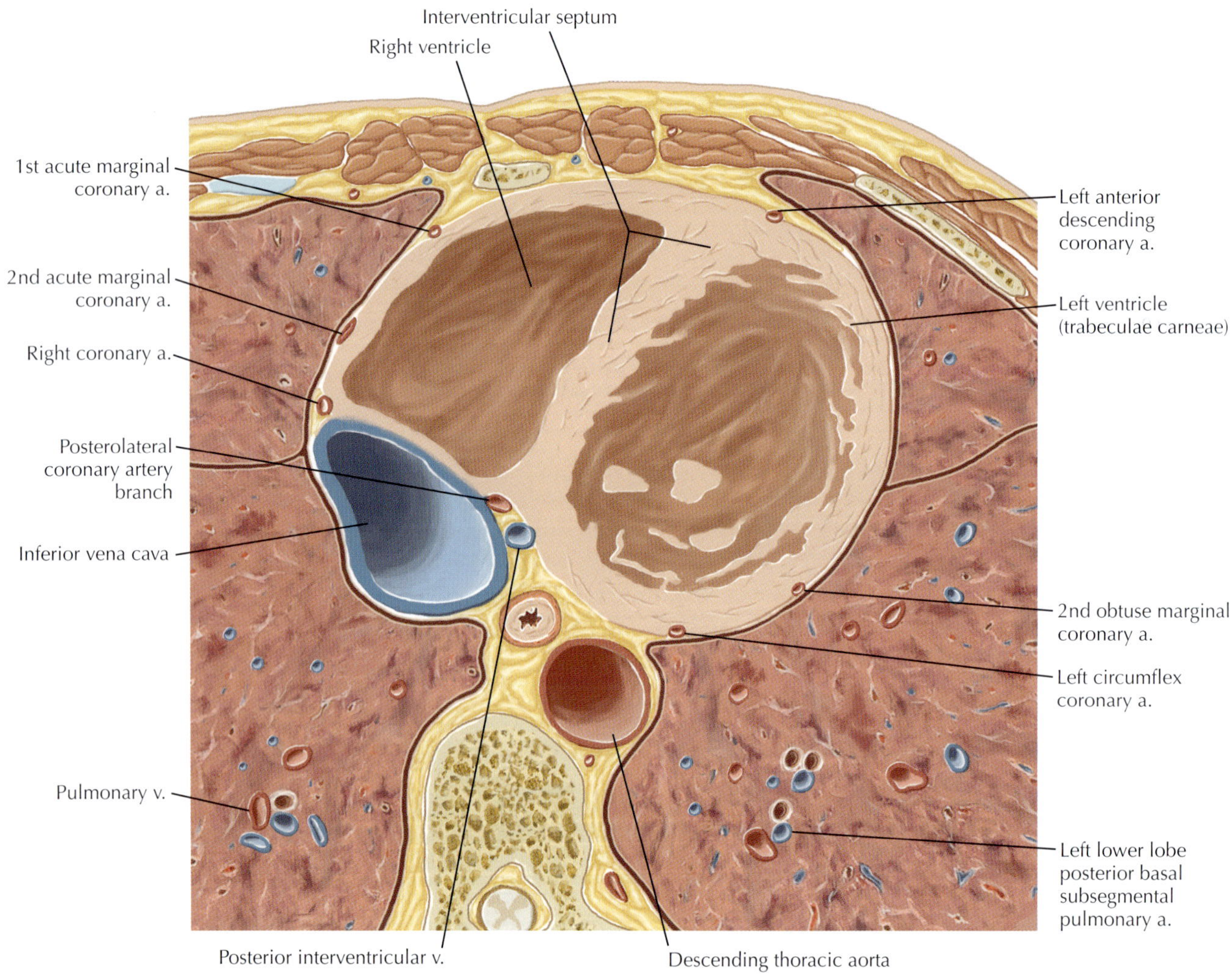
Interventricular septum
Right ventricle
1st acute marginal coronary a.
2nd acute marginal coronary a.
Right coronary a.
Posterolateral coronary artery branch
Inferior vena cava
Pulmonary v.
Posterior interventricular v.
Descending thoracic aorta
Left anterior descending coronary a.
Left ventricle (trabeculae carneae)
2nd obtuse marginal coronary a.
Left circumflex coronary a.
Left lower lobe posterior basal subsegmental pulmonary a.

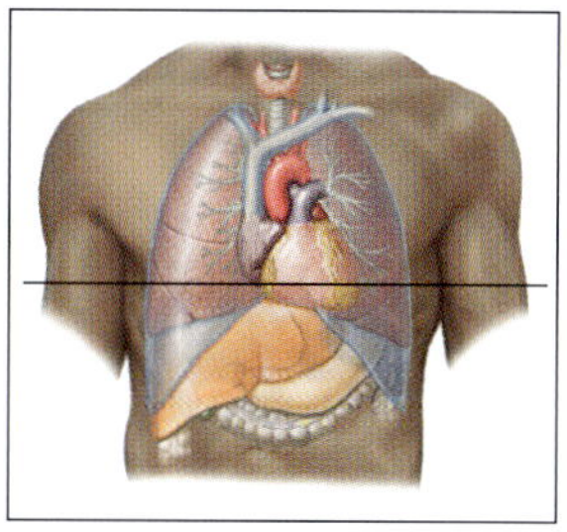

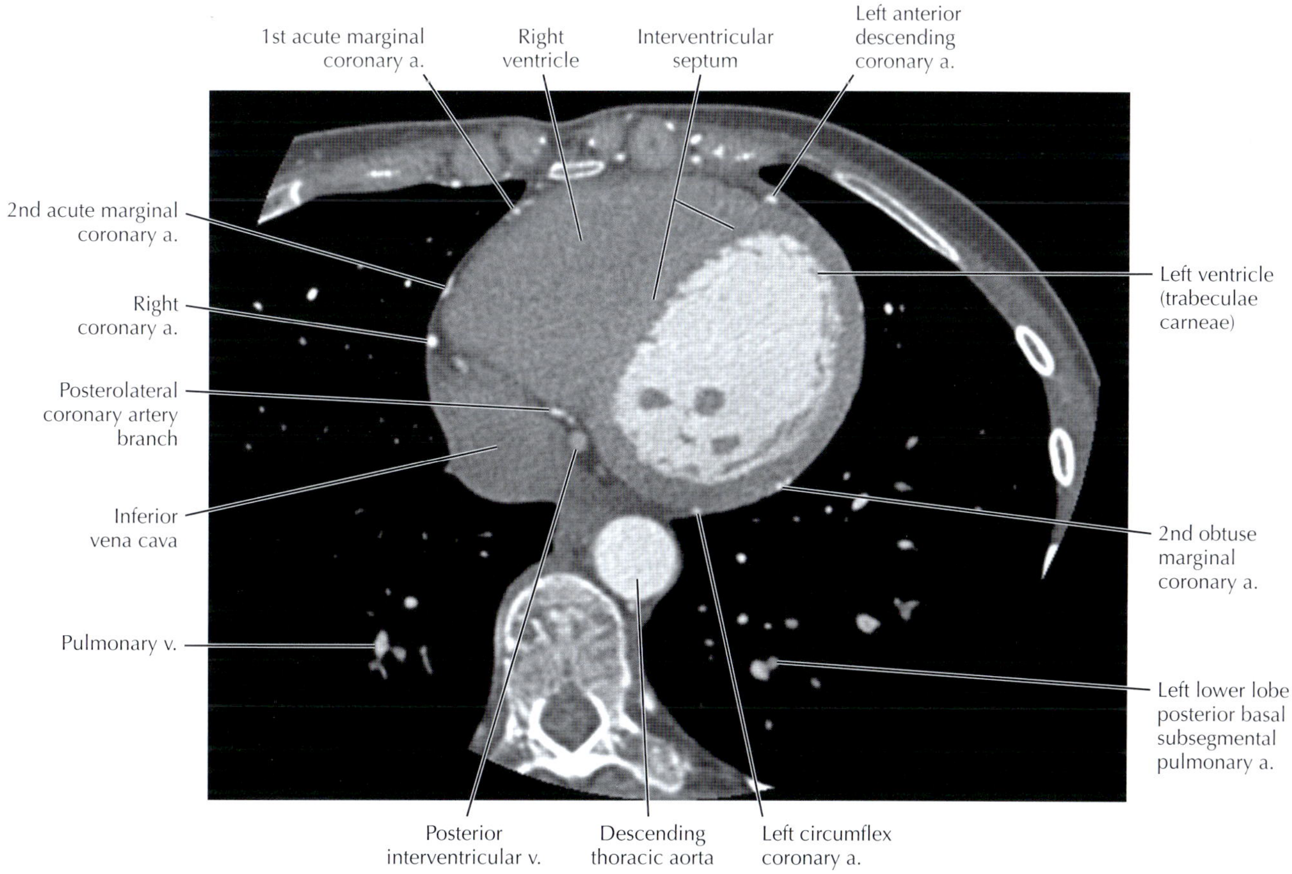
1st acute marginal coronary a.
Right ventricle
Interventricular septum
Left anterior descending coronary a.
2nd acute marginal coronary a.
Right coronary a.
Posterolateral coronary artery branch
Inferior vena cava
Pulmonary v.
Left ventricle (trabeculae carneae)
2nd obtuse marginal coronary a.
Left lower lobe posterior basal subsegmental pulmonary a.
Posterior interventricular v.
Descending thoracic aorta
Left circumflex coronary a.

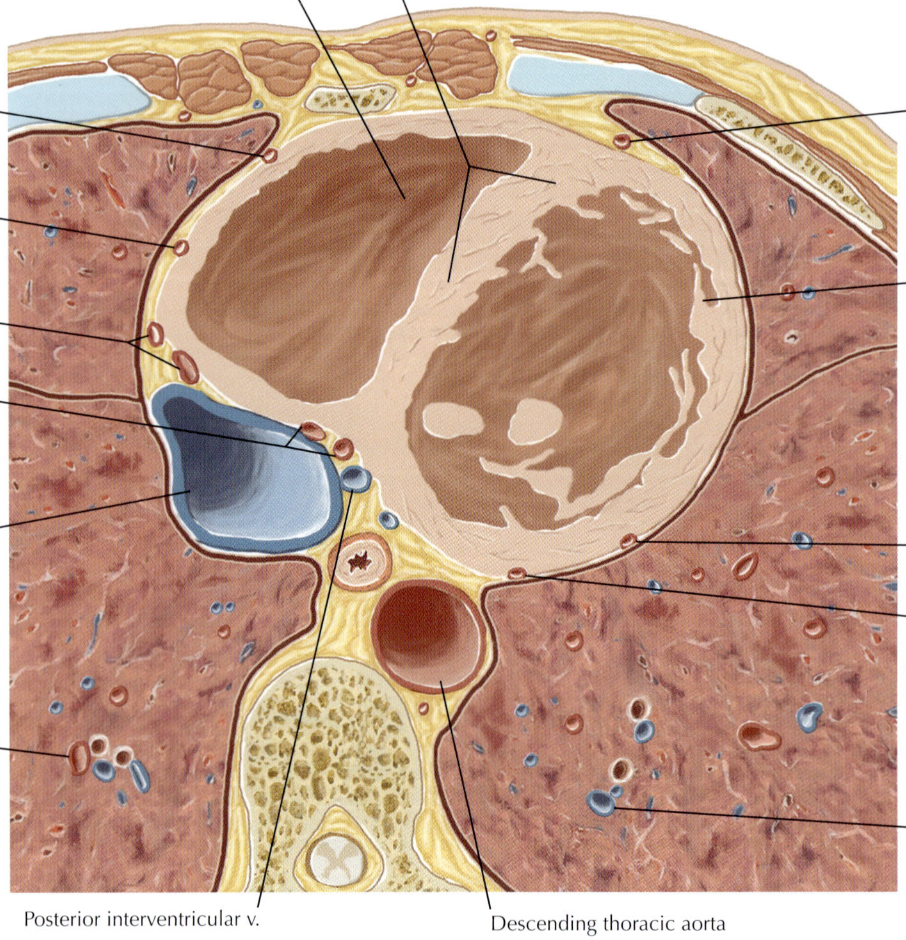
Interventricular septum
Right ventricle
1st acute marginal coronary a.
2nd acute marginal coronary a.
Right coronary a.
Posterolateral coronary artery branch
Inferior vena cava
Pulmonary v.
Posterior interventricular v.
Descending thoracic aorta
Left anterior descending coronary a.
Left ventricle (trabeculae carneae)
2nd obtuse marginal coronary a.
Left circumflex coronary a.
Left lower lobe posterior basal subsegmental pulmonary a.

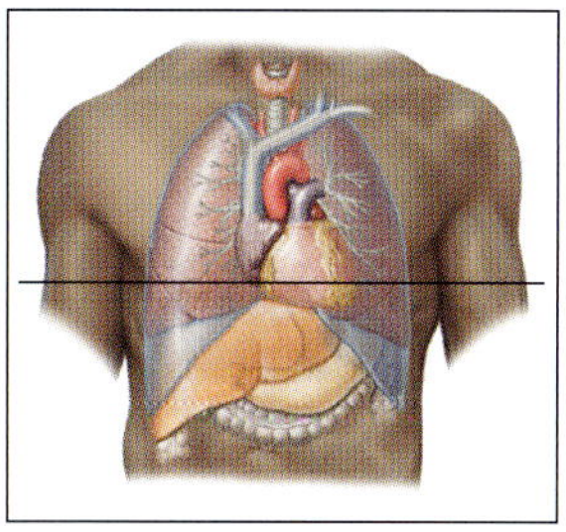

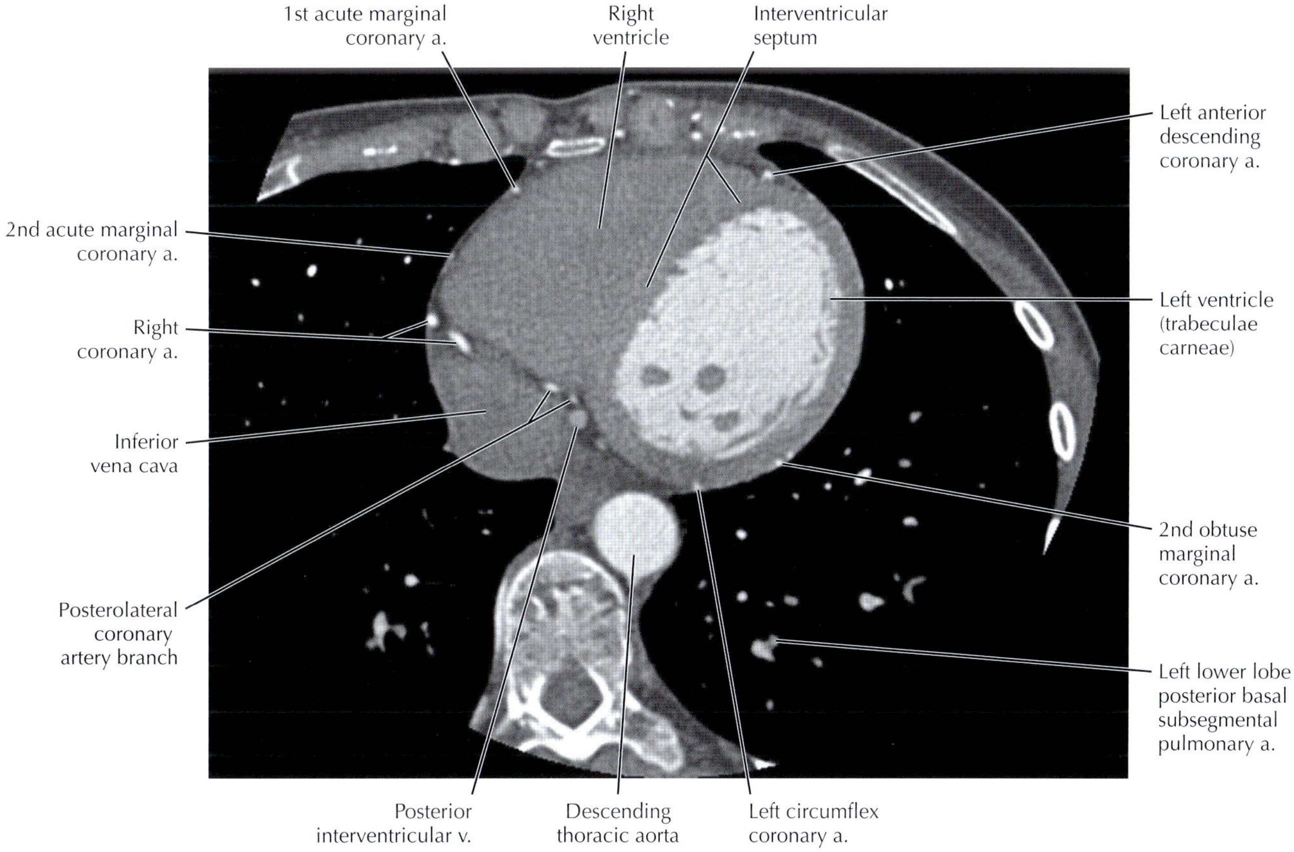
1st acute marginal coronary a.
Right ventricle
Interventricular septum
Left anterior descending coronary a.
2nd acute marginal coronary a.
Left ventricle (trabeculae carneae)
Right coronary a.
Inferior vena cava
2nd obtuse marginal coronary a.
Posterolateral coronary artery branch
Left lower lobe posterior basal subsegmental pulmonary a.
Posterior interventricular v.
Descending thoracic aorta
Left circumflex coronary a.

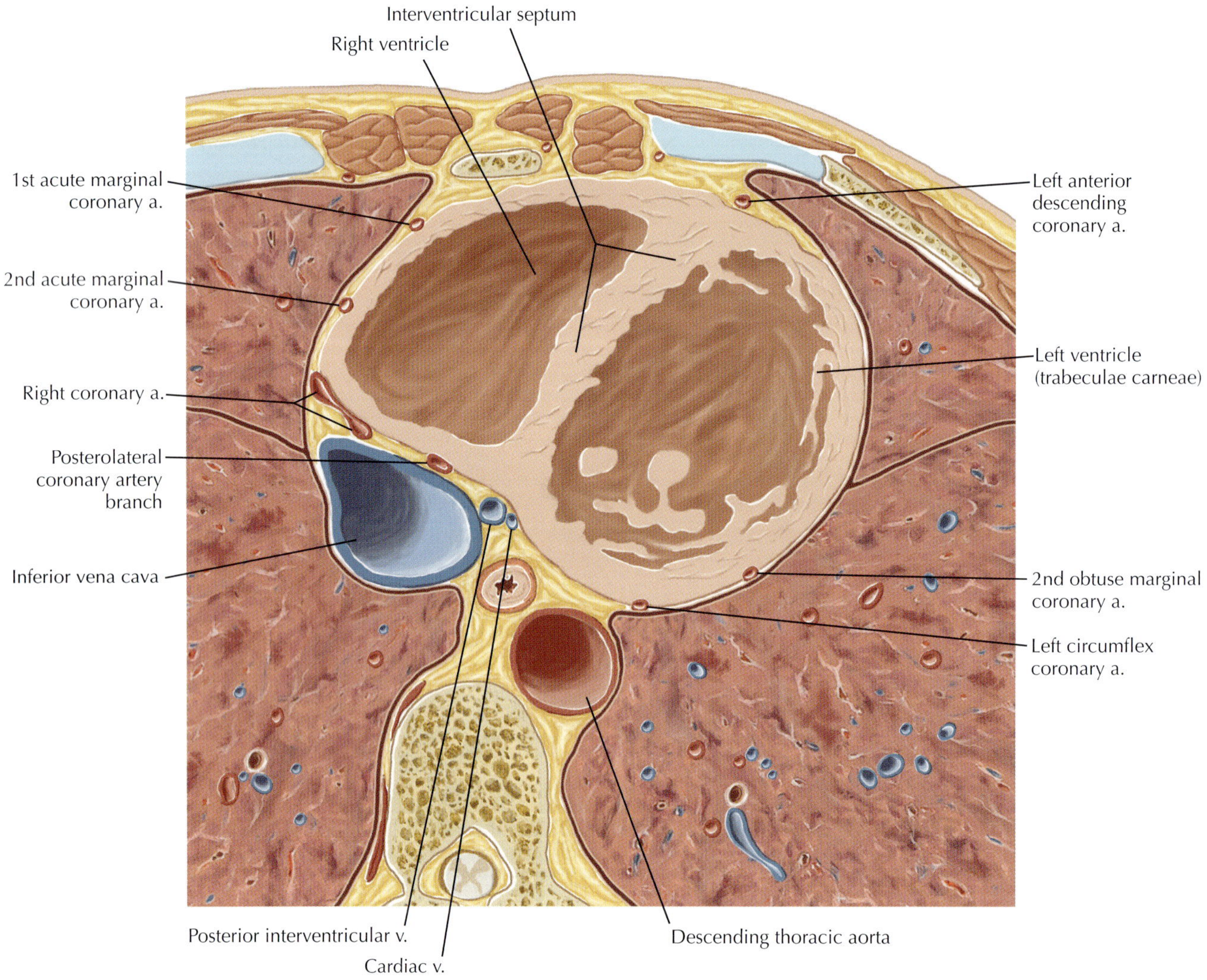
Interventricular septum
Right ventricle
1st acute marginal coronary a.
2nd acute marginal coronary a.
Right coronary a.
Posterolateral coronary artery branch
Inferior vena cava
Left anterior descending coronary a.
Left ventricle (trabeculae carneae)
2nd obtuse marginal coronary a.
Left circumflex coronary a.
Posterior interventricular v.
Cardiac v.
Descending thoracic aorta

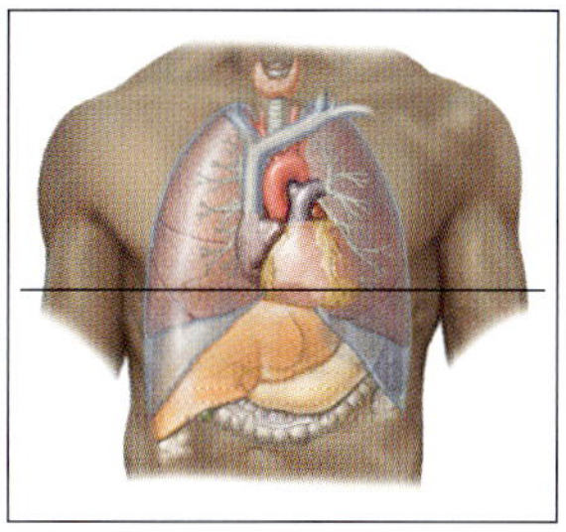

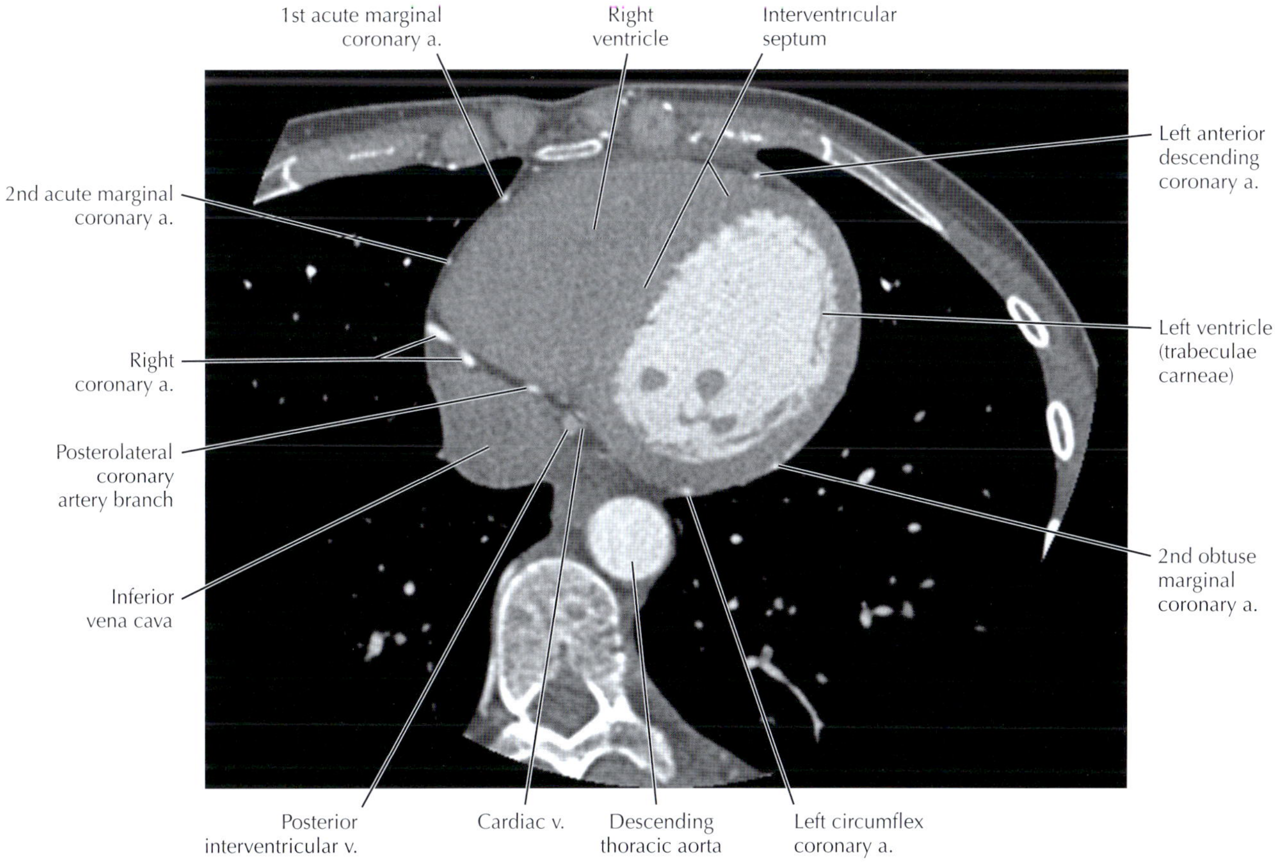
1st acute marginal coronary a.
Right ventricle
Interventricular septum
Left anterior descending coronary a.
2nd acute marginal coronary a.
Left ventricle (trabeculae carneae)
Right coronary a.
Posterolateral coronary artery branch
Inferior vena cava
2nd obtuse marginal coronary a.
Posterior interventricular v.
Cardiac v.
Descending thoracic aorta
Left circumflex coronary a.

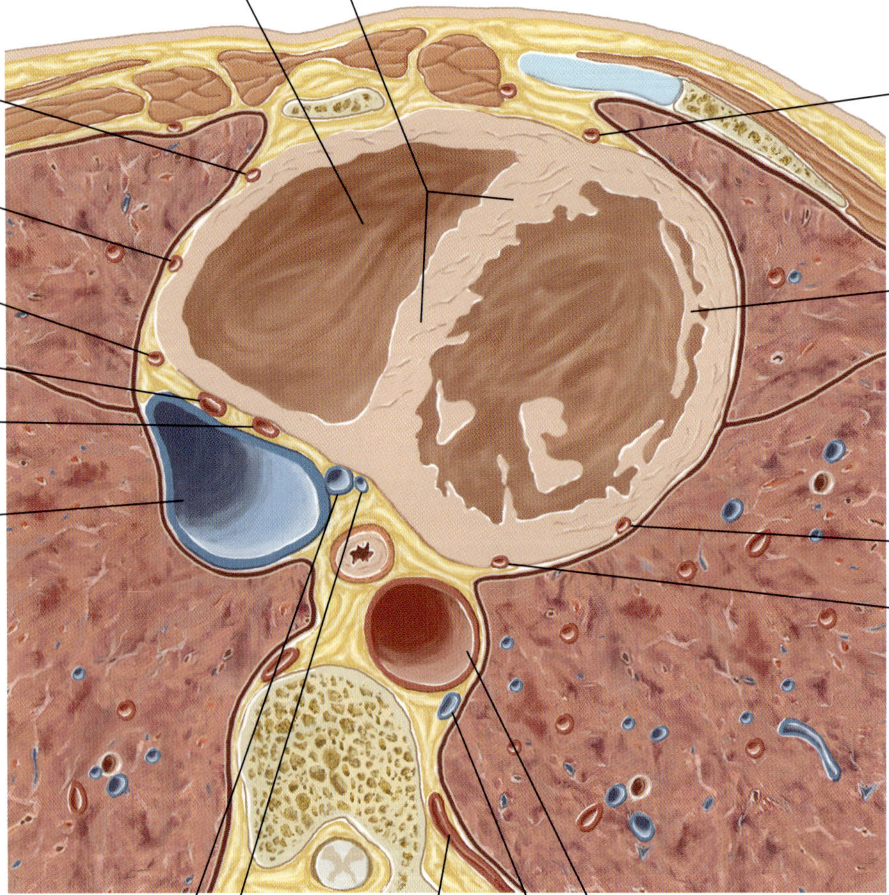

NORMAL ANATOMY

The atrioventricular nodal coronary artery arising from the right coronary artery is shown. The atrioventricular nodal coronary artery arises from the right coronary artery in 90% of patients.

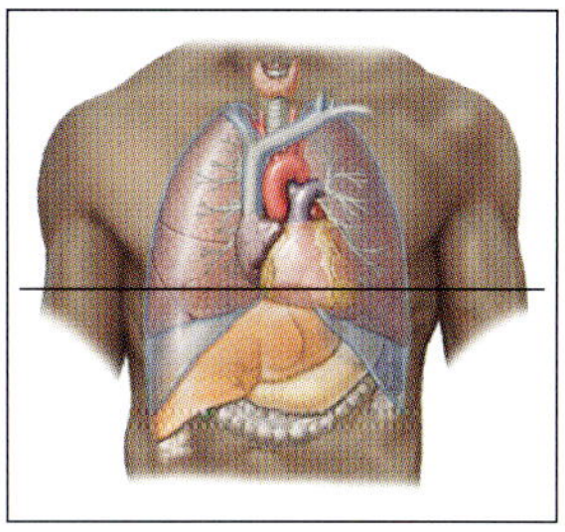

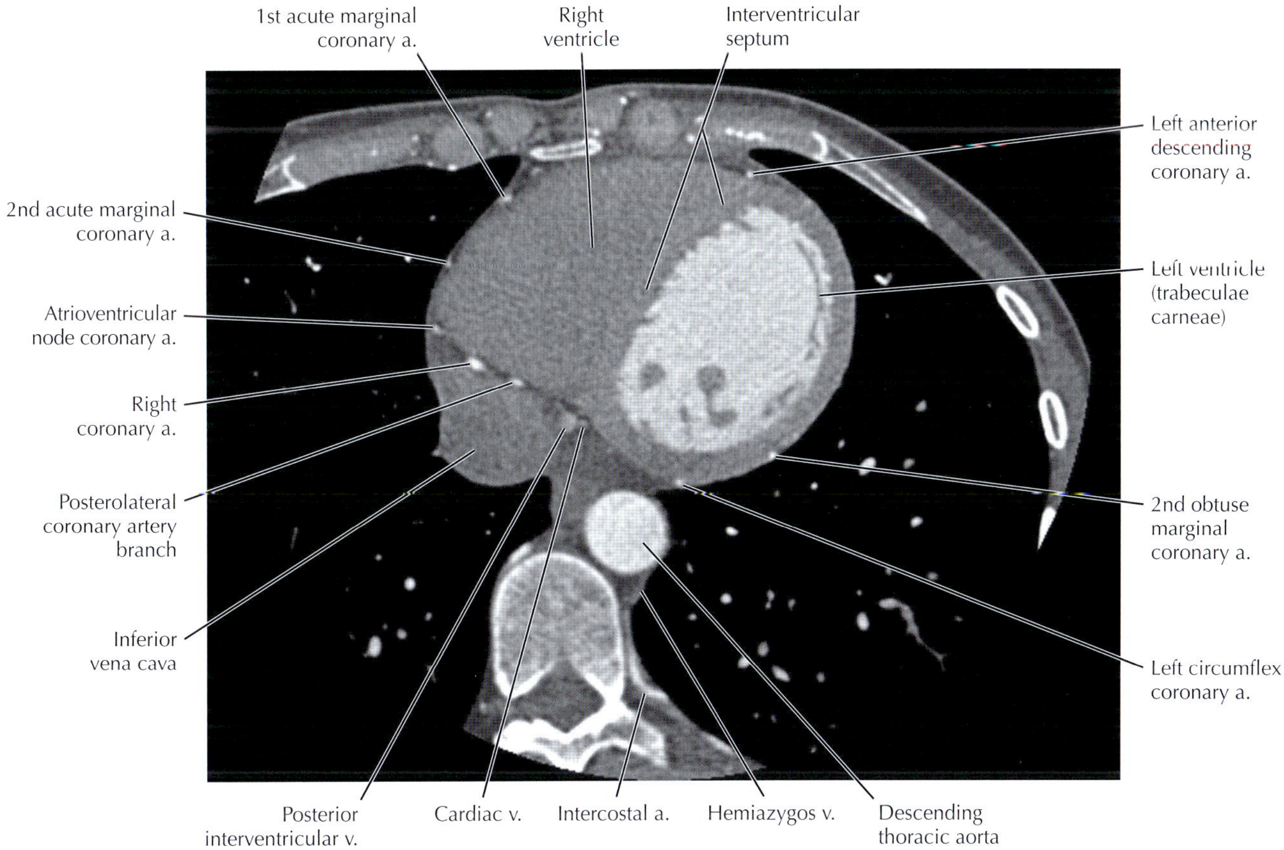
1st acute marginal coronary a.
Right ventricle
Interventricular septum
Left anterior descending coronary a.
2nd acute marginal coronary a.
Left ventricle (trabeculae carneae)
Atrioventricular node coronary a.
Right coronary a.
Posterolateral coronary artery branch
2nd obtuse marginal coronary a.
Inferior vena cava
Left circumflex coronary a.
Posterior interventricular v.
Cardiac v.
Intercostal a.
Hemiazygos v.
Descending thoracic aorta

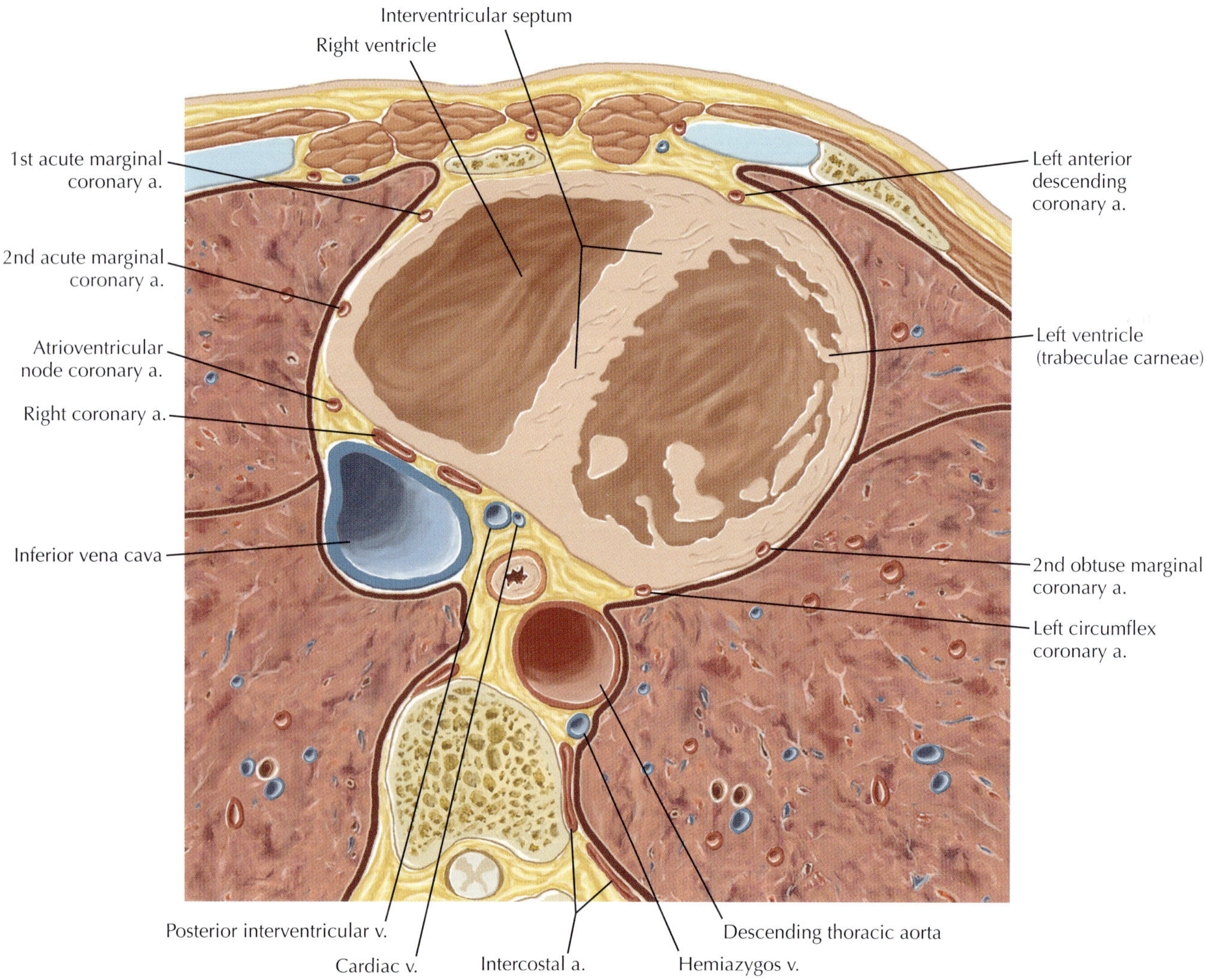
Interventricular septum
Right ventricle
1st acute marginal coronary a.
2nd acute marginal coronary a.
Atrioventricular node coronary a.
Right coronary a.
Inferior vena cava
Left anterior descending coronary a.
Left ventricle (trabeculae carneae)
2nd obtuse marginal coronary a.
Left circumflex coronary a.
Posterior interventricular v.
Cardiac v.
Intercostal a.
Descending thoracic aorta
Hemiazygos v.

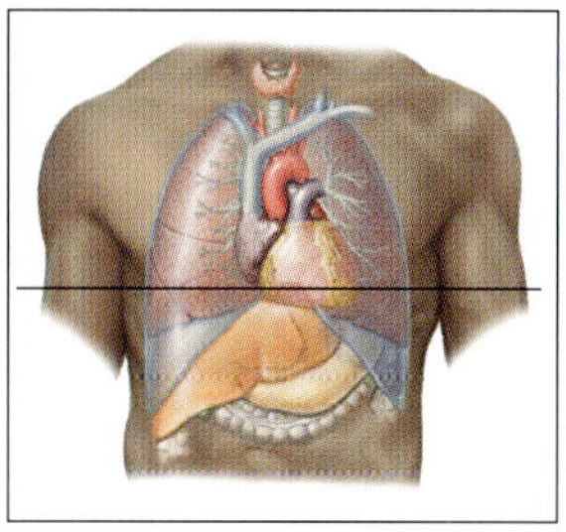

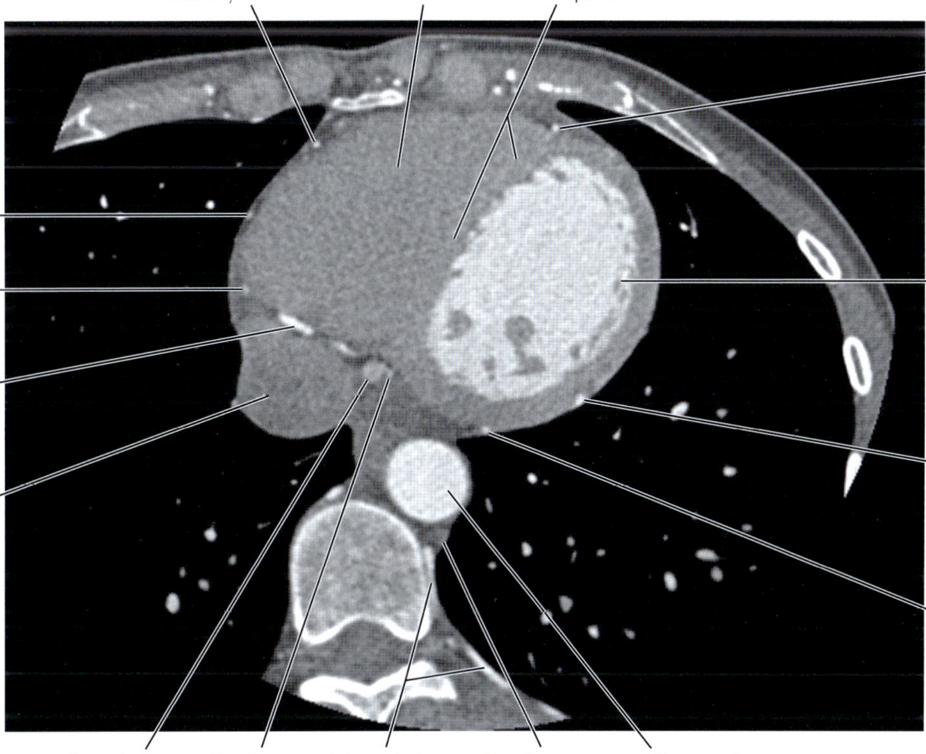
1st acute marginal coronary a.
Right ventricle
Interventricular septum
Left anterior descending coronary a.
2nd acute marginal coronary a.
Atrioventricular node coronary a.
Left ventricle (trabeculae carneae)
Right coronary a.
Inferior vena cava
2nd obtuse marginal coronary a.
Left circumflex coronary a.
Posterior interventricular v.
Cardiac v.
Intercostal a.
Hemiazygos v.
Descending thoracic aorta

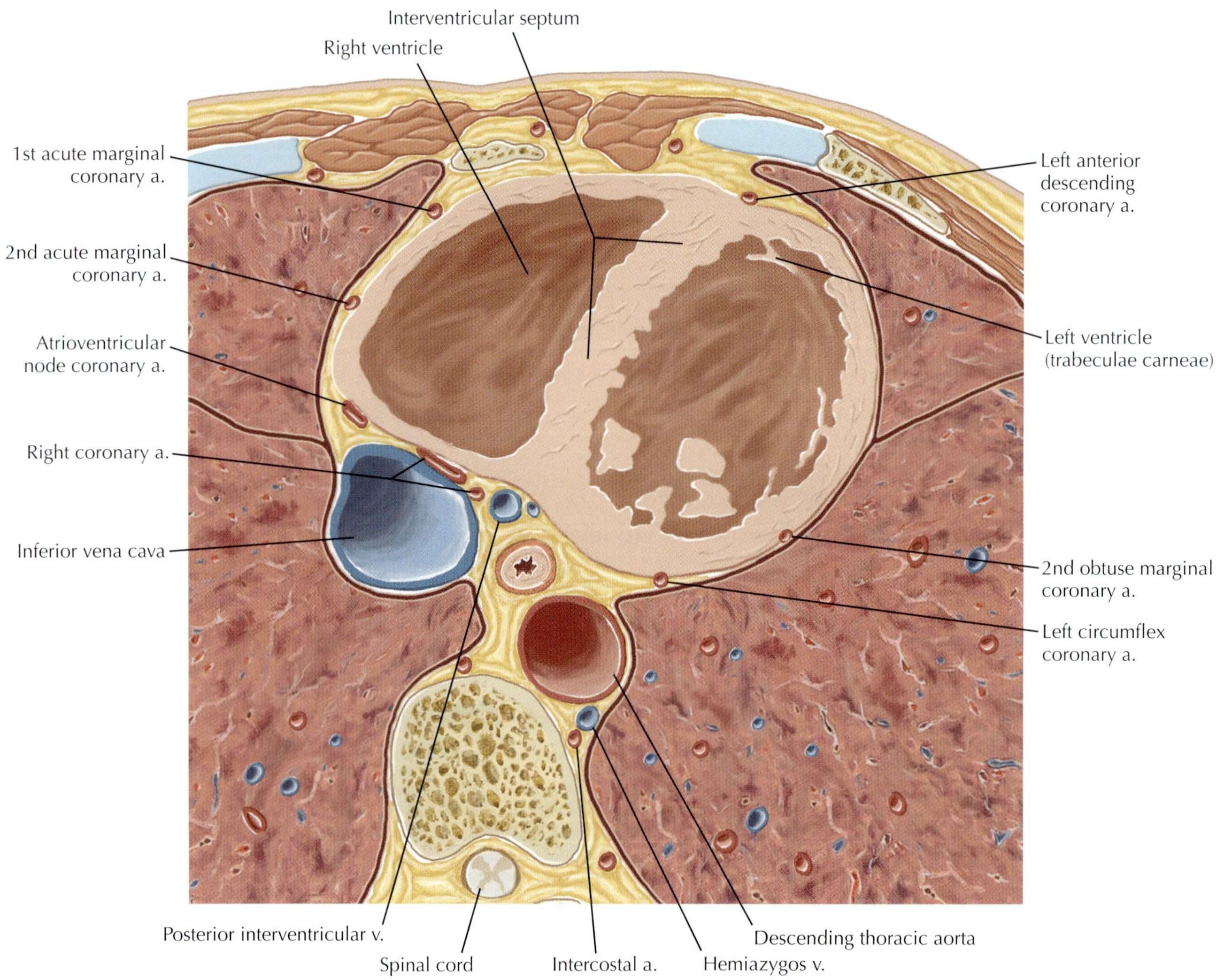
Interventricular septum
Right ventricle
1st acute marginal coronary a.
2nd acute marginal coronary a.
Atrioventricular node coronary a.
Right coronary a.
Inferior vena cava
Left anterior descending coronary a.
Left ventricle (trabeculae carneae)
2nd obtuse marginal coronary a.
Left circumflex coronary a.
Posterior interventricular v.
Spinal cord
Intercostal a.
Hemiazygos v.
Descending thoracic aorta

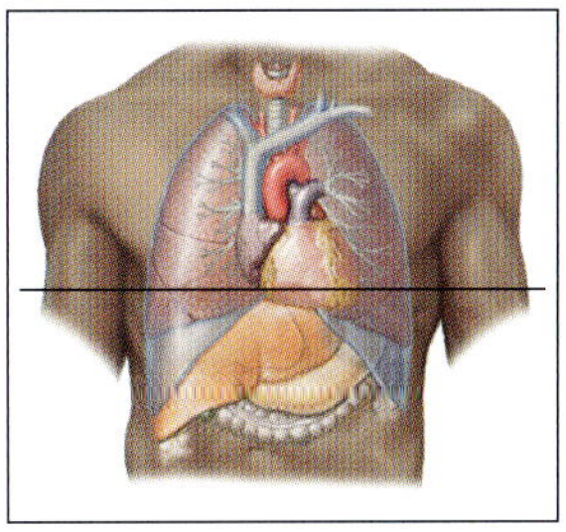

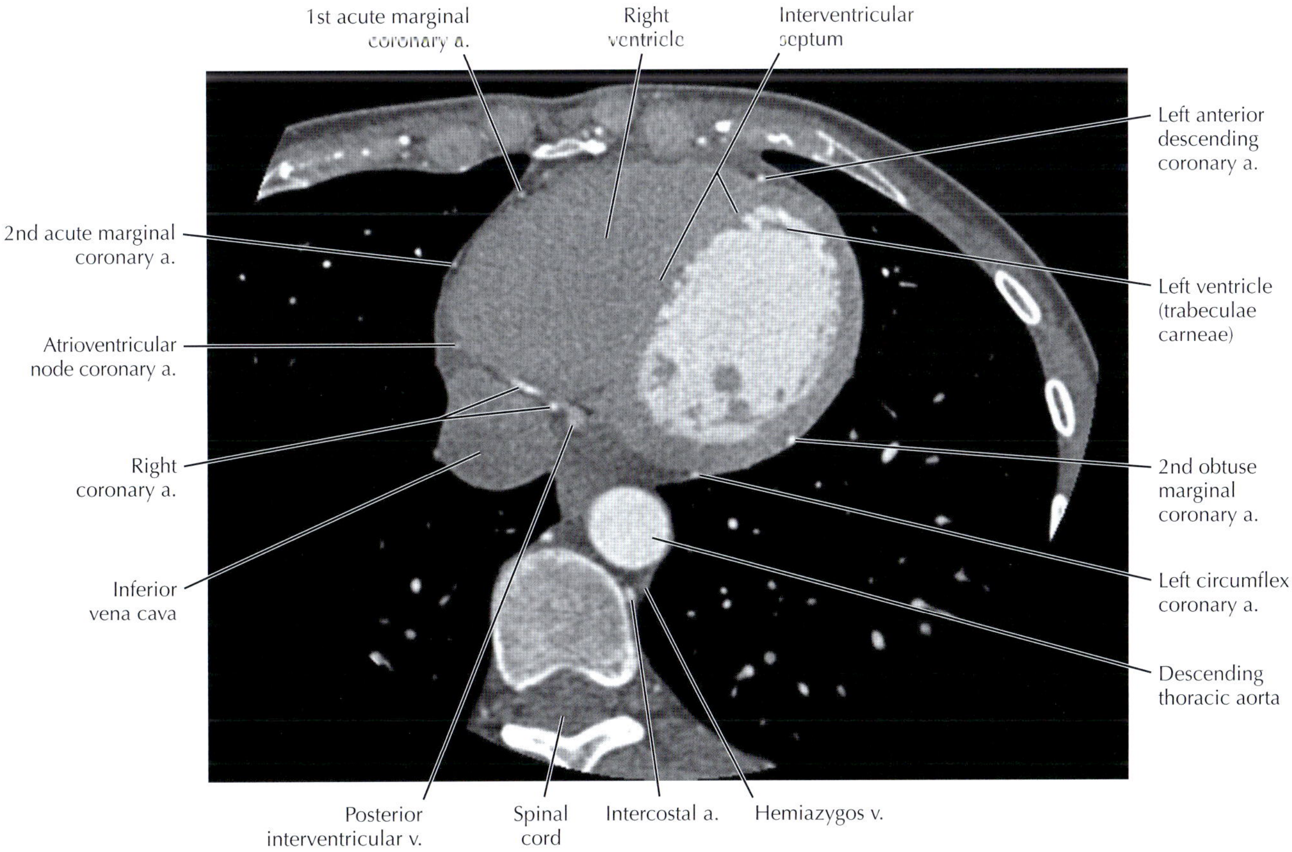
1st acute marginal coronary a.
Right ventricle
Interventricular septum
Left anterior descending coronary a.
2nd acute marginal coronary a.
Left ventricle (trabeculae carneae)
Atrioventricular node coronary a.
Right coronary a.
2nd obtuse marginal coronary a.
Inferior vena cava
Left circumflex coronary a.
Descending thoracic aorta
Posterior interventricular v.
Spinal cord
Intercostal a.
Hemiazygos v.

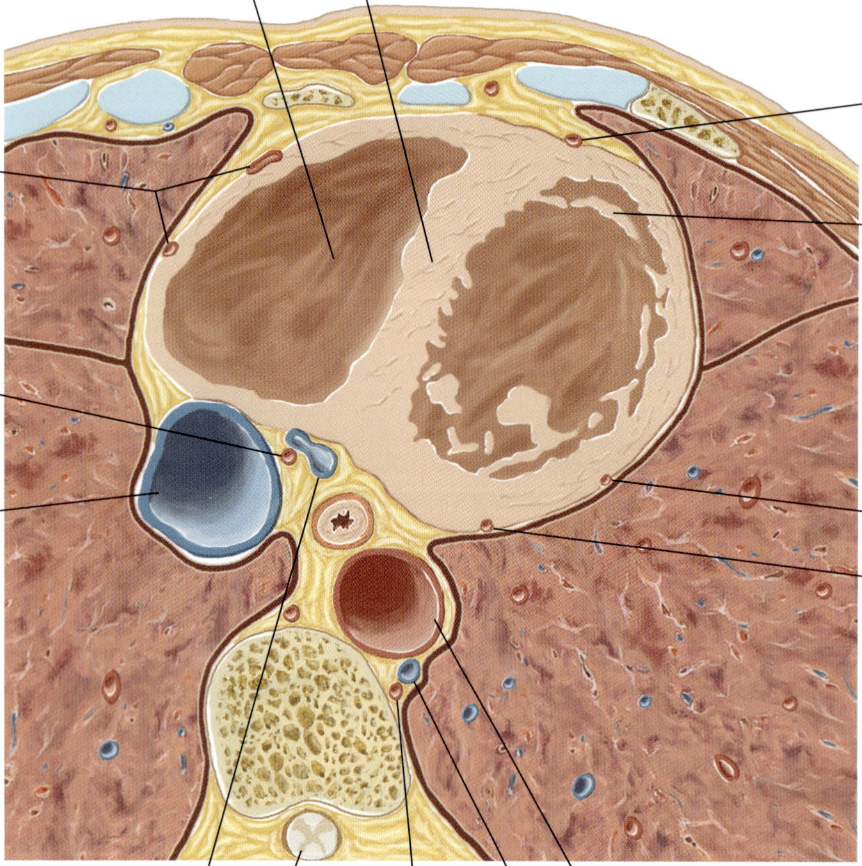
Interventricular septum
Right ventricle
1st & 2nd acute marginal coronary aa.
Left anterior descending coronary a.
Left ventricle (trabeculae carneae)
Right coronary a.
Inferior vena cava
2nd obtuse marginal coronary a.
Left circumflex coronary a.
Posterior interventricular v.
Spinal cord
Intercostal a.
Hemiazygos v.
Descending thoracic aorta

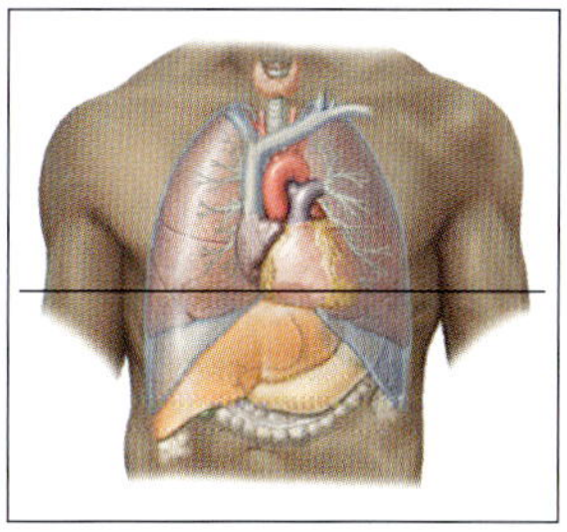

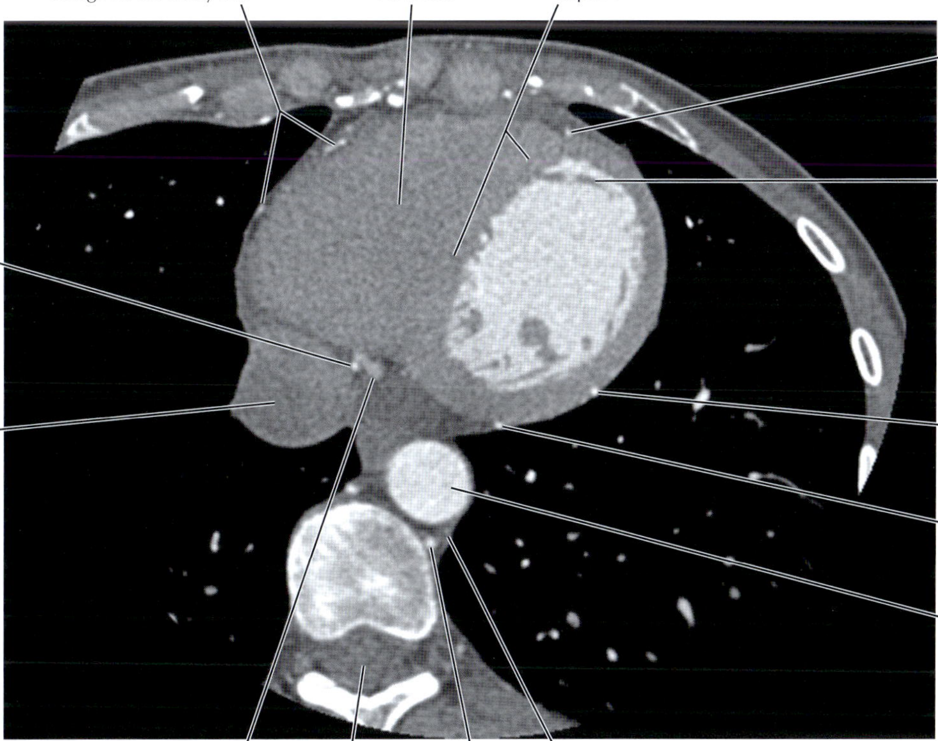
1st & 2nd acute
marginal coronary aa.
Right
ventricle
Interventricular
septum
Left anterior
descending
coronary a.
Left ventricle
(trabeculae
carneae)
Right
coronary a.
Inferior
vena cava
2nd obtuse
marginal
coronary a.
Left circumflex
coronary a.
Descending
thoracic aorta
Posterior
interventricular v.
Spinal
cord
Intercostal a.
Hemiazygos v.

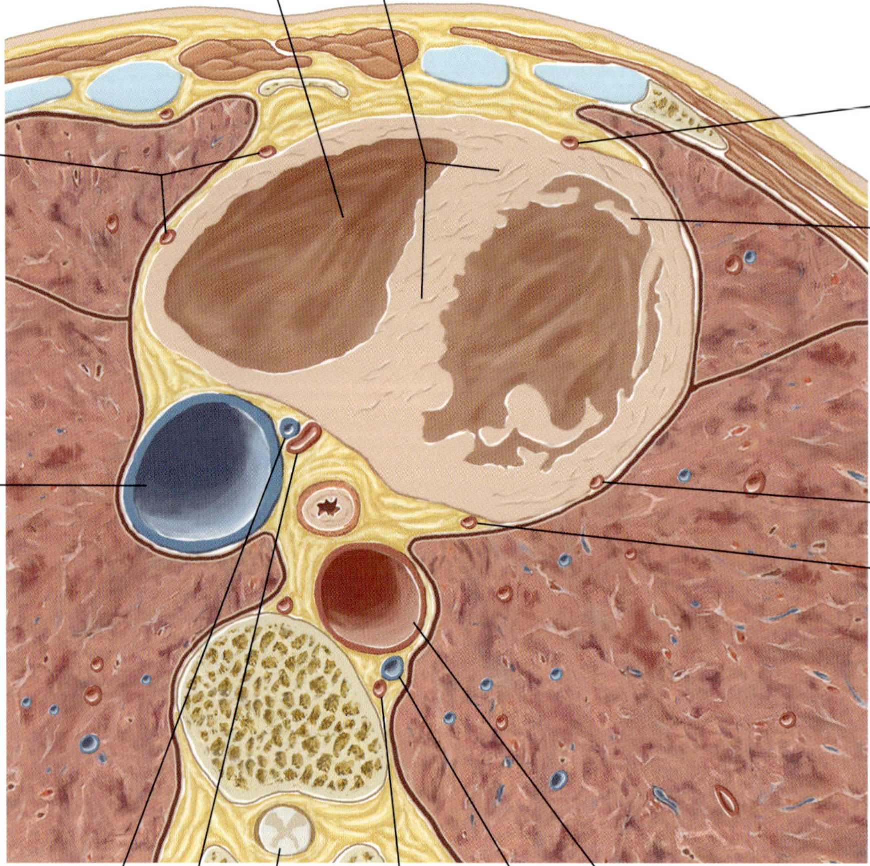

NORMAL ANATOMY

Coronary arterial dominance is variably defined by the vessel that gives rise to the posterior descending coronary artery (also known as the posterior interventricular coronary artery) or the atrioventricular nodal coronary artery. In approximately 85% of individuals, the right coronary artery is dominant, as is the case for this patient.

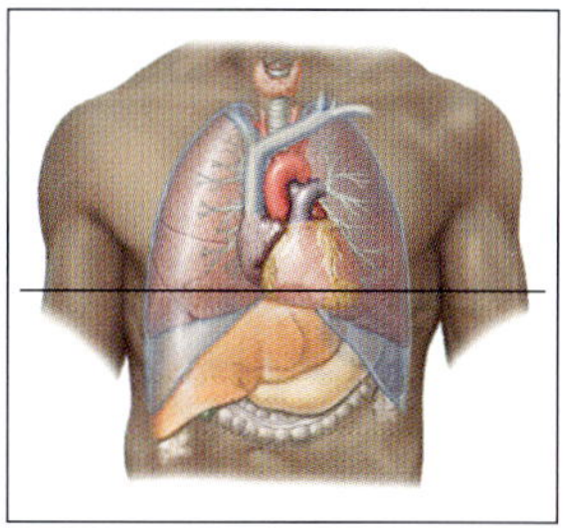

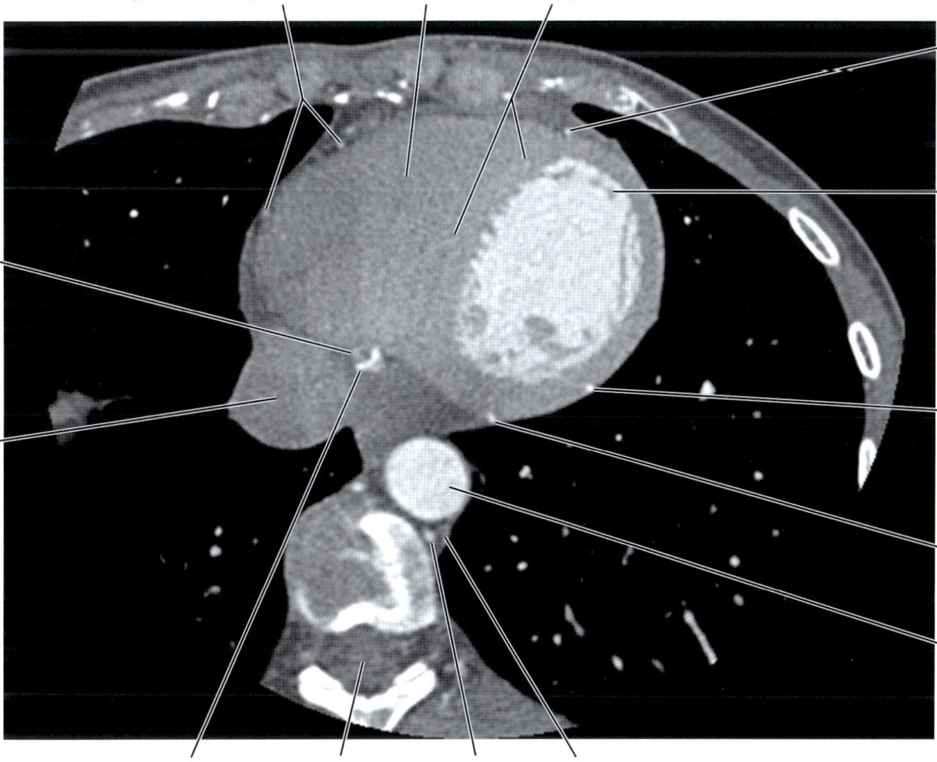
1st & 2nd acute
marginal coronary aa.
Right
ventricle
Interventricular
septum
Left anterior
descending
coronary a.
Left ventricle
(trabeculae
carneae)
Posterior inter-
ventricular v.
Inferior
vena cava
2nd obtuse
marginal
coronary a.
Left circumflex
coronary a.
Descending
thoracic aorta
Posterior descending
coronary a.
Spinal
cord
Intercostal a.
Hemiazygos v.

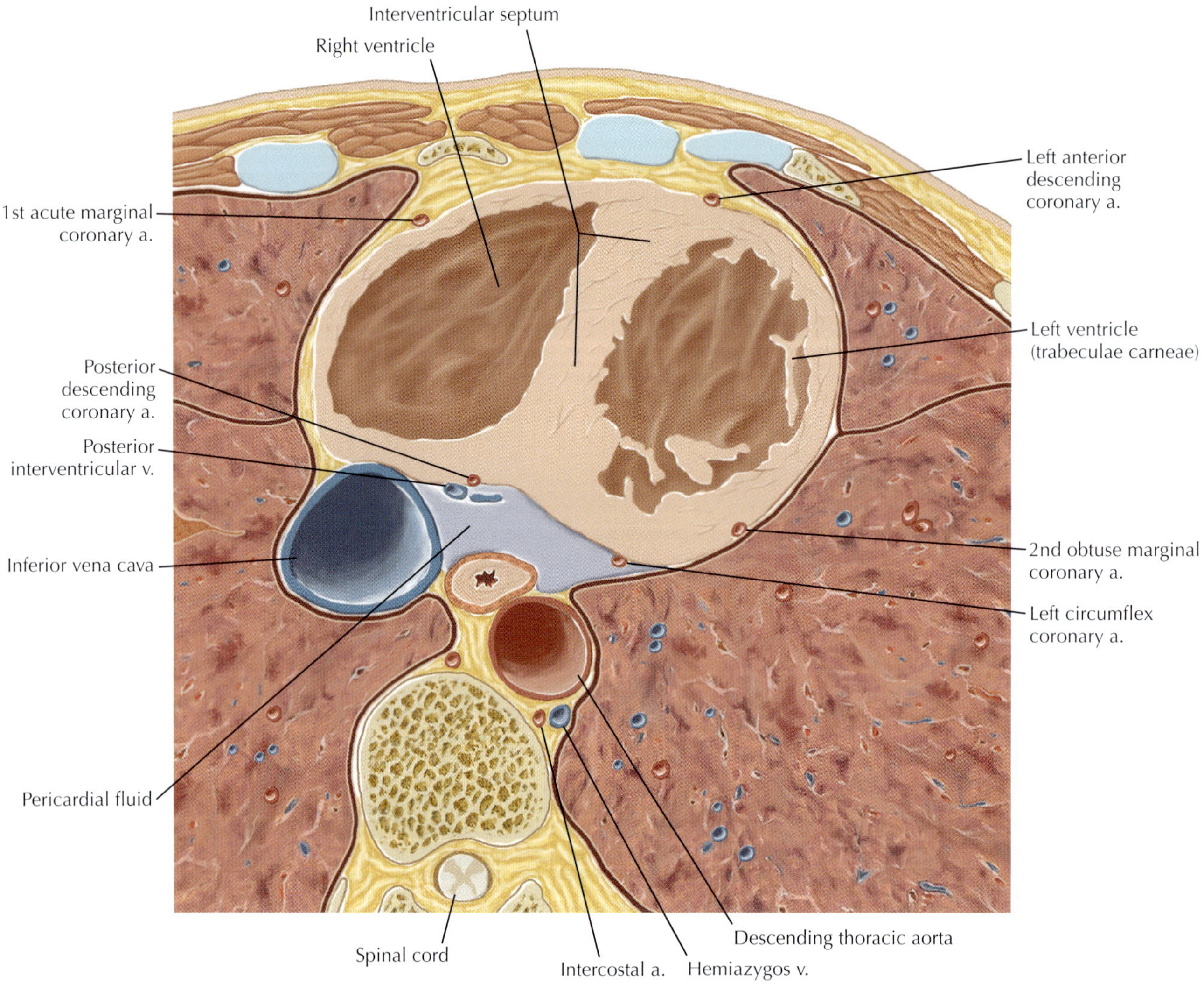
Interventricular septum
Right ventricle
Left anterior descending coronary a.
1st acute marginal coronary a.
Left ventricle (trabeculae carneae)
Posterior descending coronary a.
Posterior interventricular v.
Inferior vena cava
2nd obtuse marginal coronary a.
Left circumflex coronary a.
Pericardial fluid
Descending thoracic aorta
Spinal cord
Intercostal a.
Hemiazygos v.

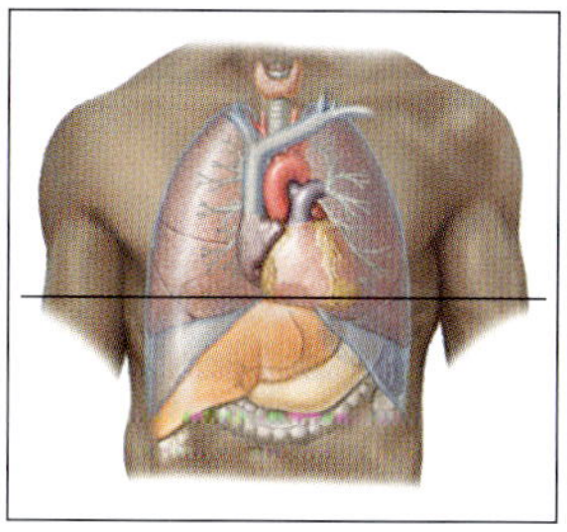

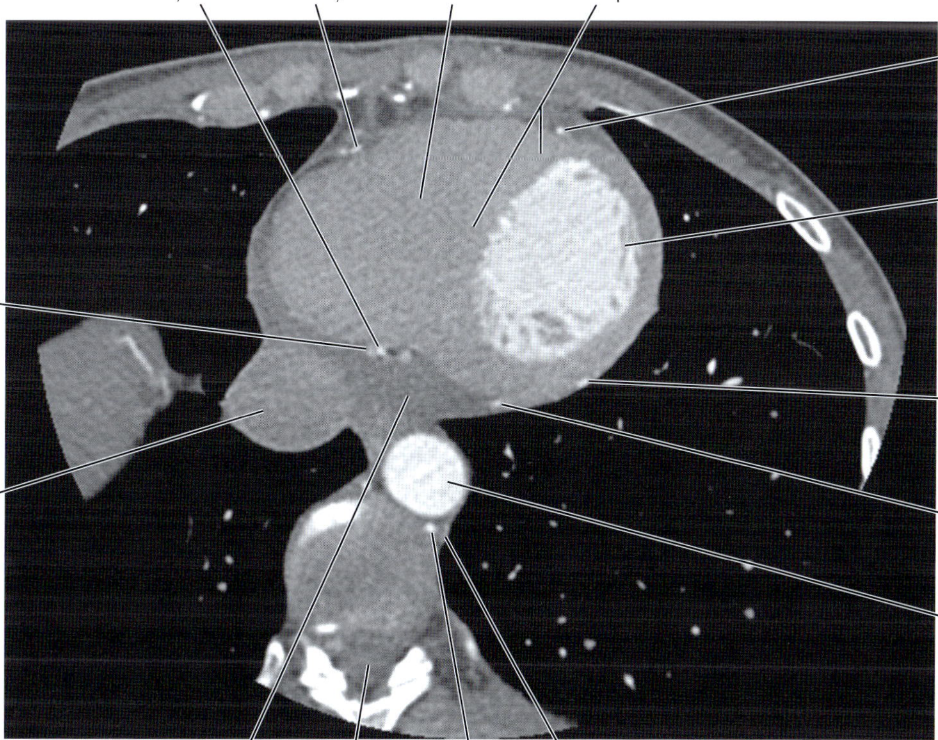

Posterior descending coronary a.
1st acute marginal coronary a.
Right ventricle
Interventricular septum
Left anterior descending coronary a.
Left ventricle (trabeculae carneae)
Posterior inter-ventricular v.
2nd obtuse marginal coronary a.
Inferior vena cava
Left circumflex coronary a.
Descending thoracic aorta
Pericardial fluid
Spinal cord
Intercostal a.
Hemiazygos v.

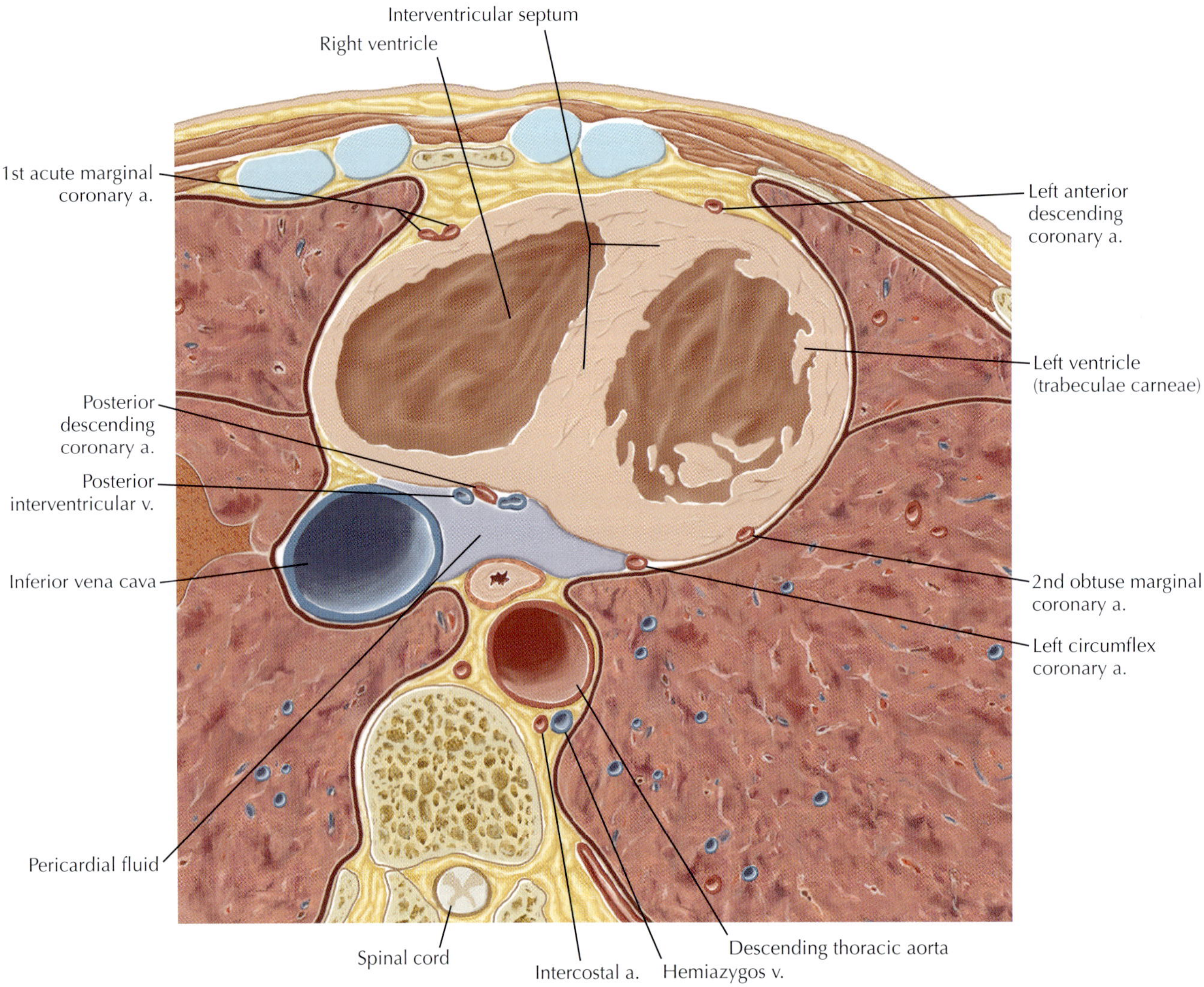
Interventricular septum
Right ventricle
1st acute marginal coronary a.
Left anterior descending coronary a.
Left ventricle (trabeculae carneae)
Posterior descending coronary a.
Posterior interventricular v.
Inferior vena cava
2nd obtuse marginal coronary a.
Left circumflex coronary a.
Pericardial fluid
Spinal cord
Intercostal a.
Hemiazygos v.
Descending thoracic aorta

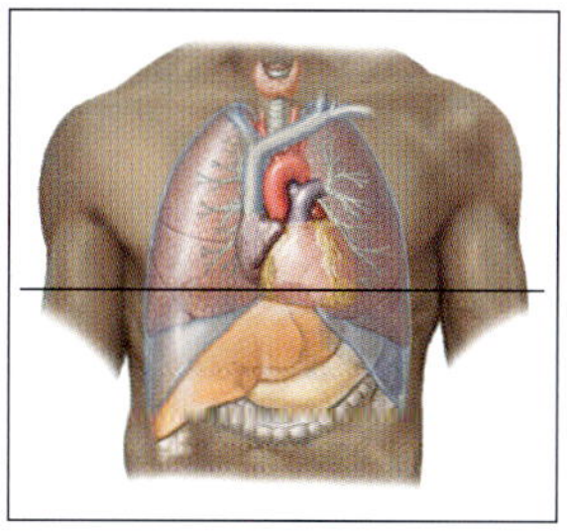

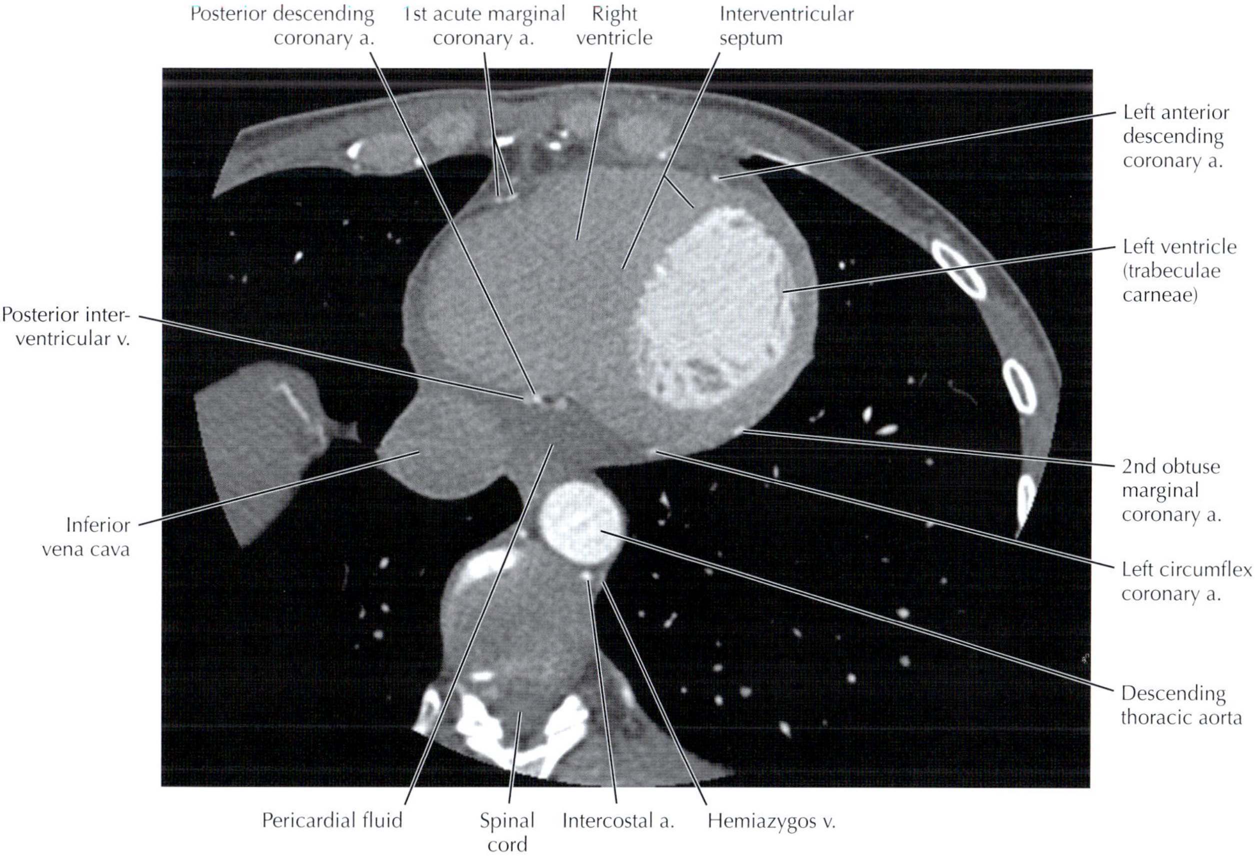
Posterior descending coronary a.
1st acute marginal coronary a.
Right ventricle
Interventricular septum
Left anterior descending coronary a.
Left ventricle (trabeculae carneae)
Posterior interventricular v.
Inferior vena cava
2nd obtuse marginal coronary a.
Left circumflex coronary a.
Descending thoracic aorta
Pericardial fluid
Spinal cord
Intercostal a.
Hemiazygos v.

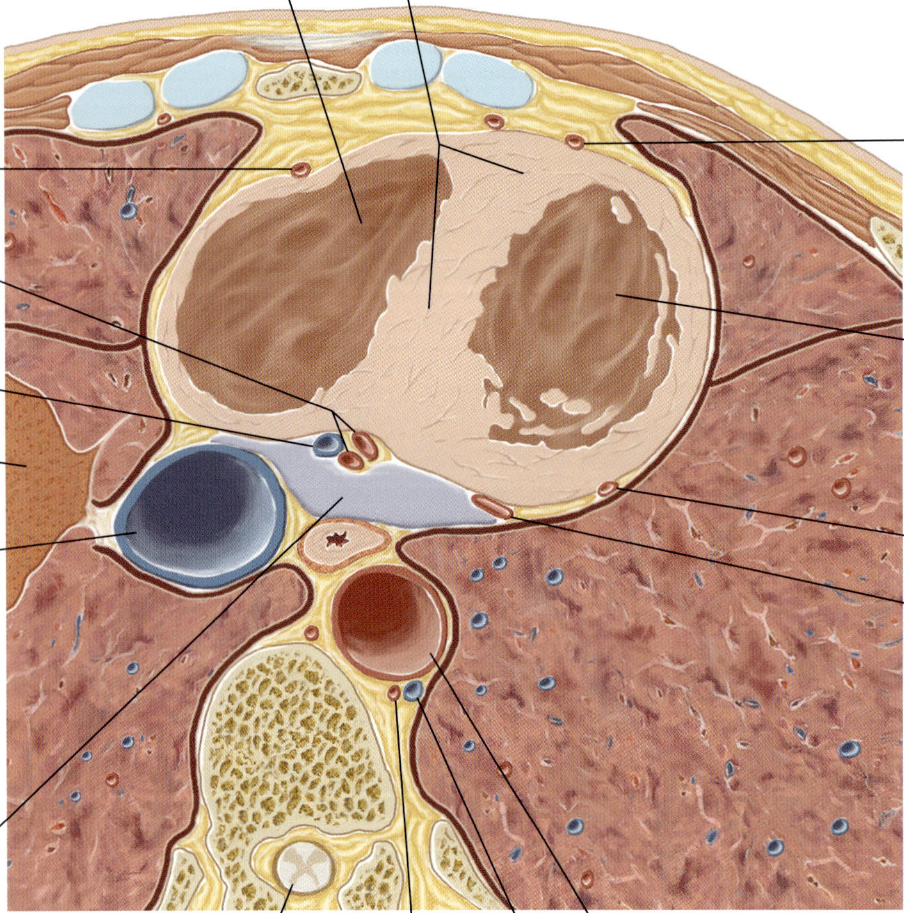
Interventricular septum
Right ventricle
1st acute marginal coronary a.
Left anterior descending coronary a.
Posterior descending coronary a.
Left ventricle
Posterior interventricular v.
Liver
Inferior vena cava
2nd obtuse marginal coronary a.
Left circumflex coronary a.
Pericardial fluid
Spinal cord
Intercostal a.
Hemiazygos v.
Descending thoracic aorta

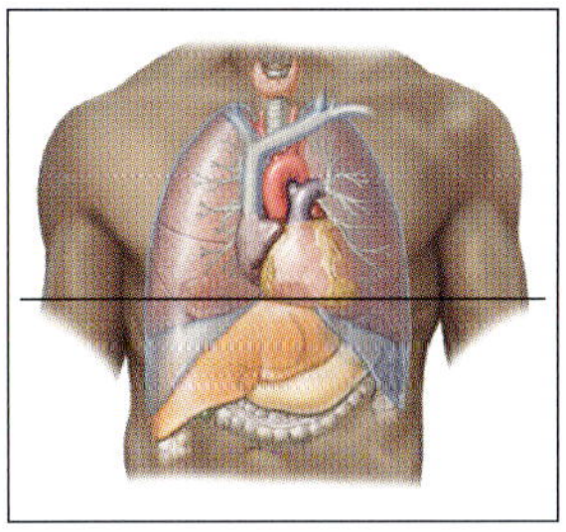

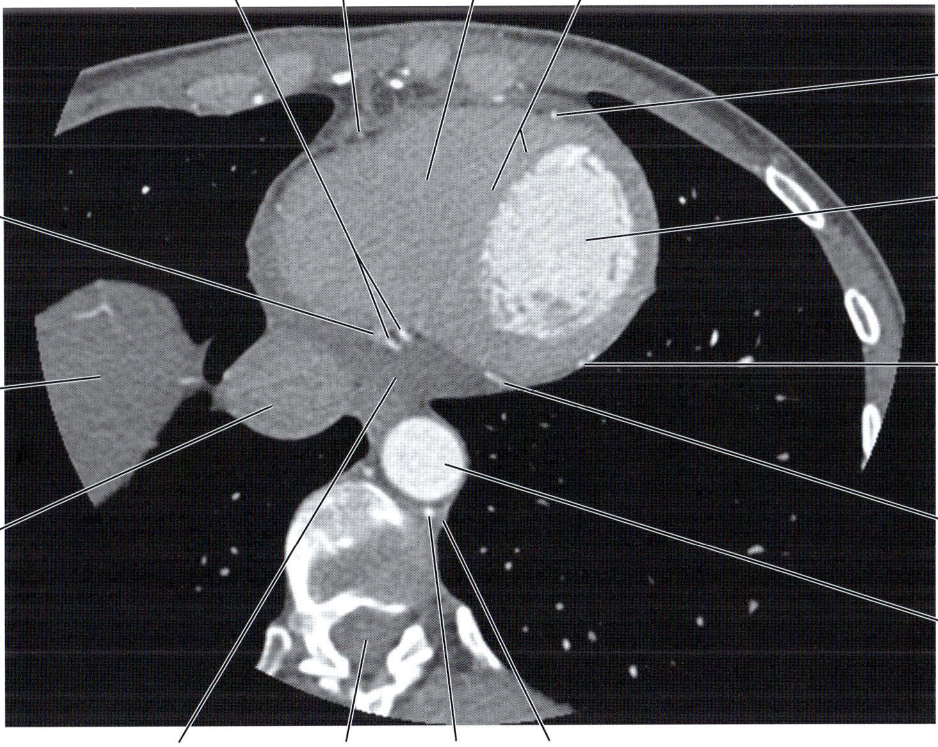
Posterior descending coronary a.
1st acute marginal coronary a.
Right ventricle
Interventricular septum
Left anterior descending coronary a.
Left ventricle
Posterior interventricular v.
Liver
2nd obtuse marginal coronary a.
Left circumflex coronary a.
Inferior vena cava
Descending thoracic aorta
Pericardial fluid
Spinal cord
Intercostal a.
Hemiazygos v.

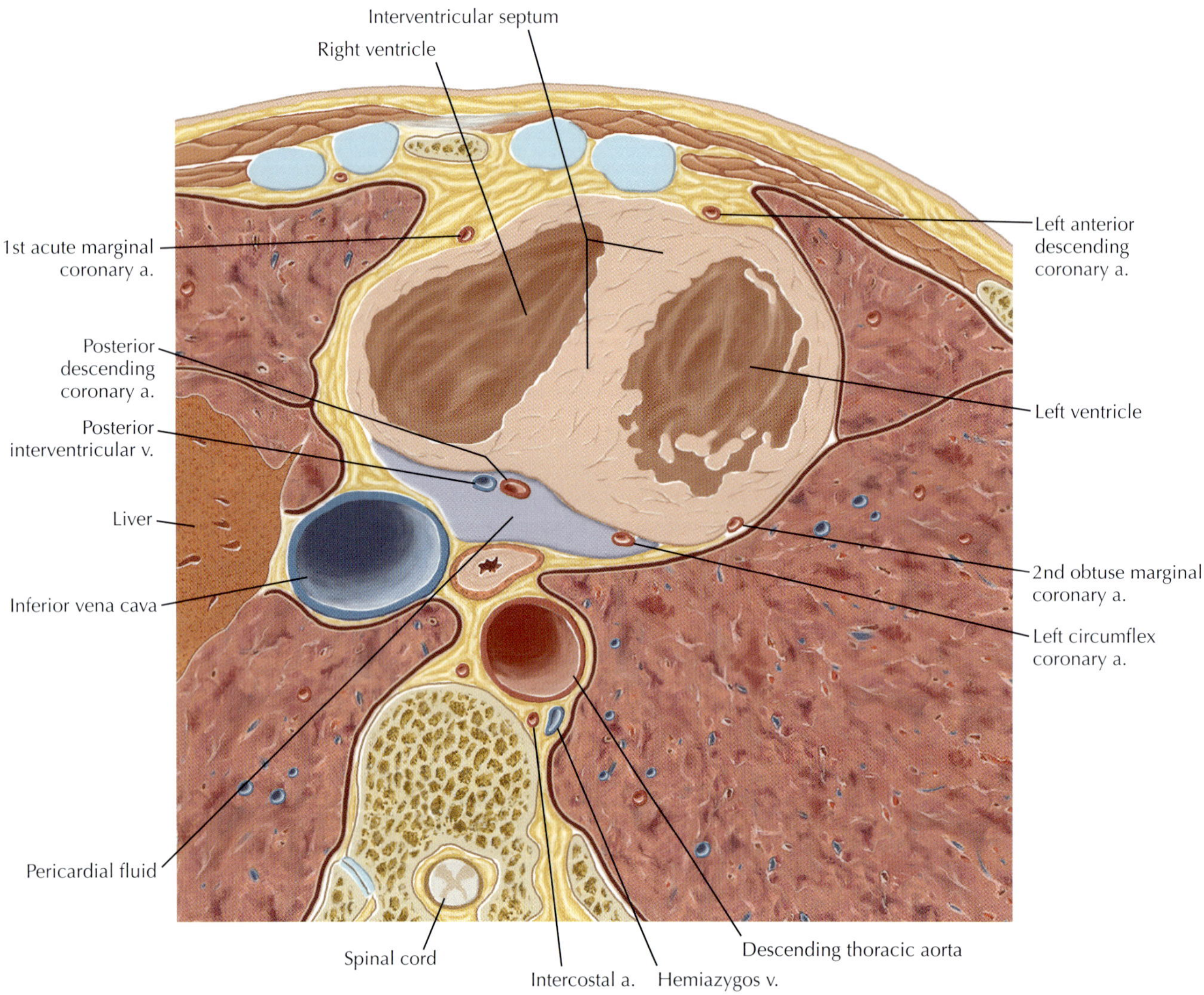
Interventricular septum
Right ventricle
1st acute marginal coronary a.
Posterior descending coronary a.
Posterior interventricular v.
Liver
Inferior vena cava
Pericardial fluid
Spinal cord
Intercostal a.
Hemiazygos v.
Descending thoracic aorta
Left anterior descending coronary a.
Left ventricle
2nd obtuse marginal coronary a.
Left circumflex coronary a.

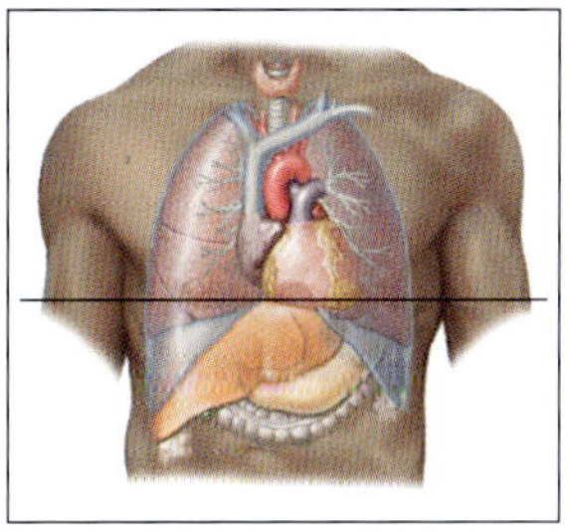

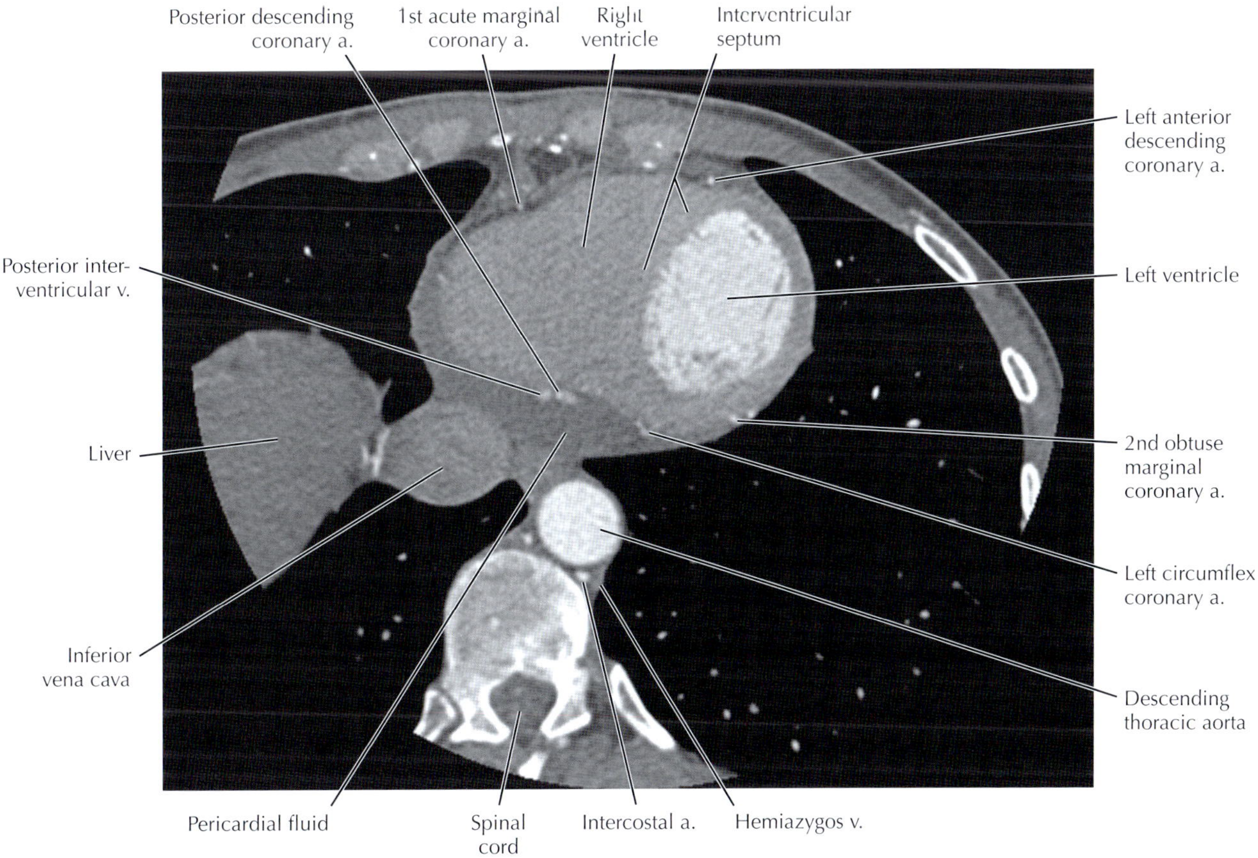
Posterior descending coronary a.
1st acute marginal coronary a.
Right ventricle
Interventricular septum
Left anterior descending coronary a.
Posterior interventricular v.
Left ventricle
Liver
2nd obtuse marginal coronary a.
Left circumflex coronary a.
Inferior vena cava
Descending thoracic aorta
Pericardial fluid
Spinal cord
Intercostal a.
Hemiazygos v.

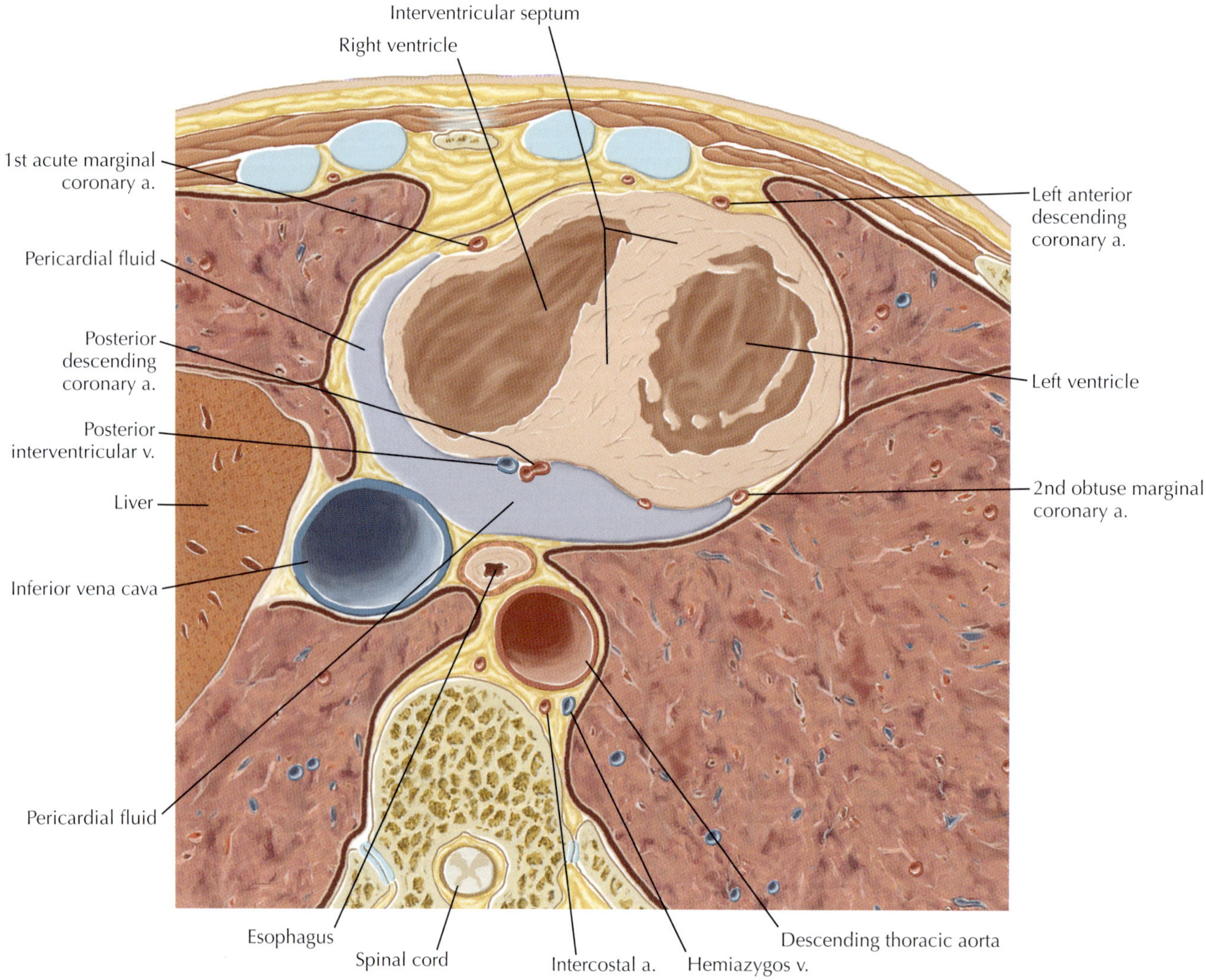
Interventricular septum
Right ventricle
1st acute marginal coronary a.
Pericardial fluid
Posterior descending coronary a.
Posterior interventricular v.
Liver
Inferior vena cava
Pericardial fluid
Left anterior descending coronary a.
Left ventricle
2nd obtuse marginal coronary a.
Esophagus
Spinal cord
Intercostal a.
Hemiazygos v.
Descending thoracic aorta

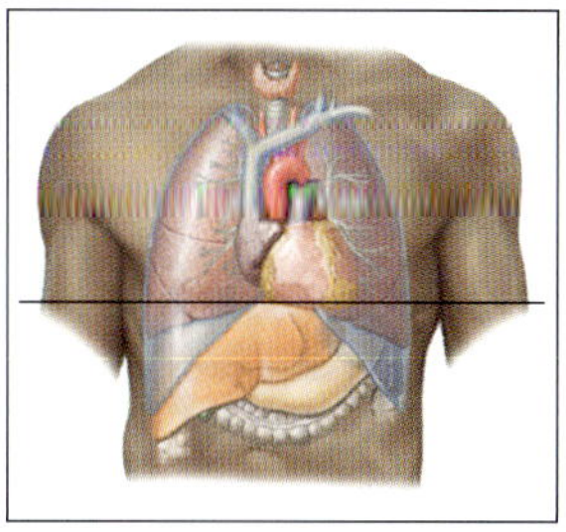

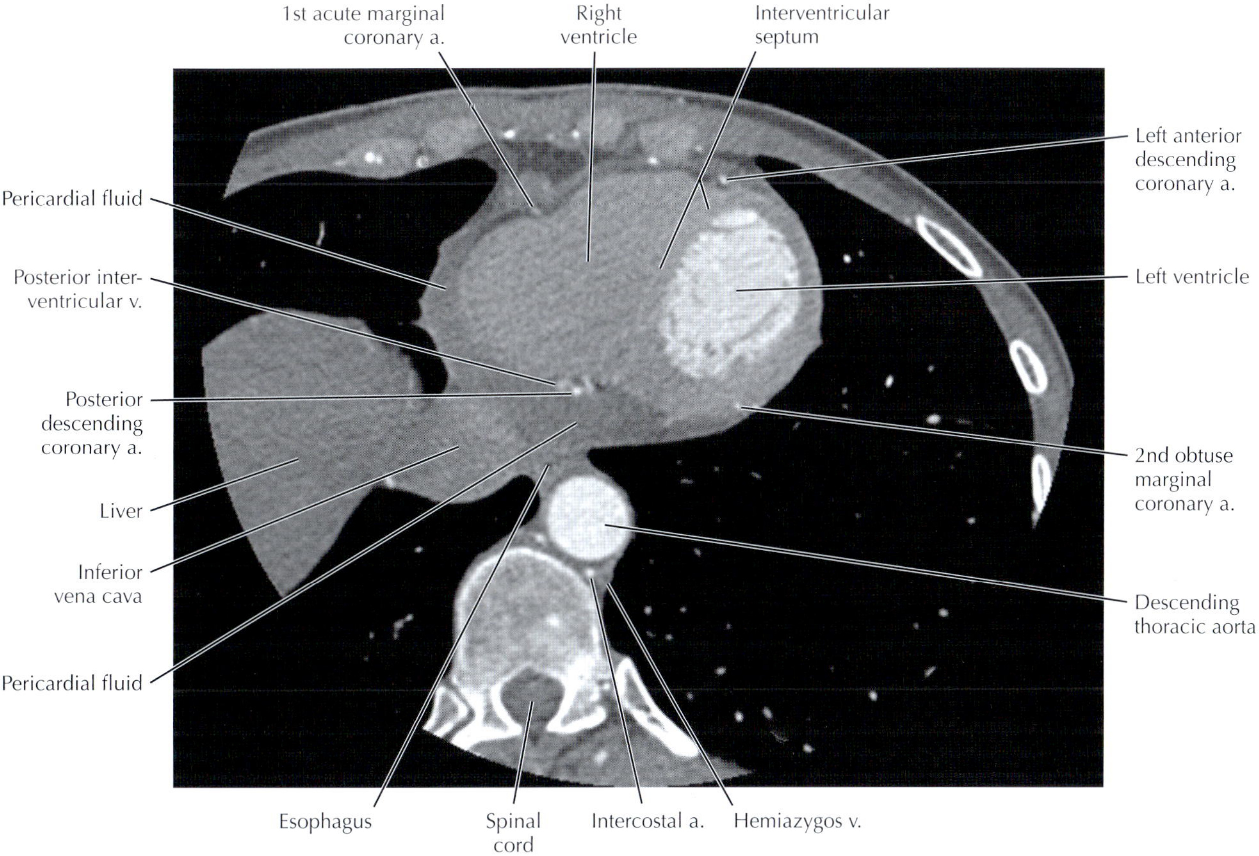
1st acute marginal coronary a.
Right ventricle
Interventricular septum
Left anterior descending coronary a.
Pericardial fluid
Posterior inter-ventricular v.
Left ventricle
Posterior descending coronary a.
2nd obtuse marginal coronary a.
Liver
Inferior vena cava
Descending thoracic aorta
Pericardial fluid
Esophagus
Spinal cord
Intercostal a.
Hemiazygos v.

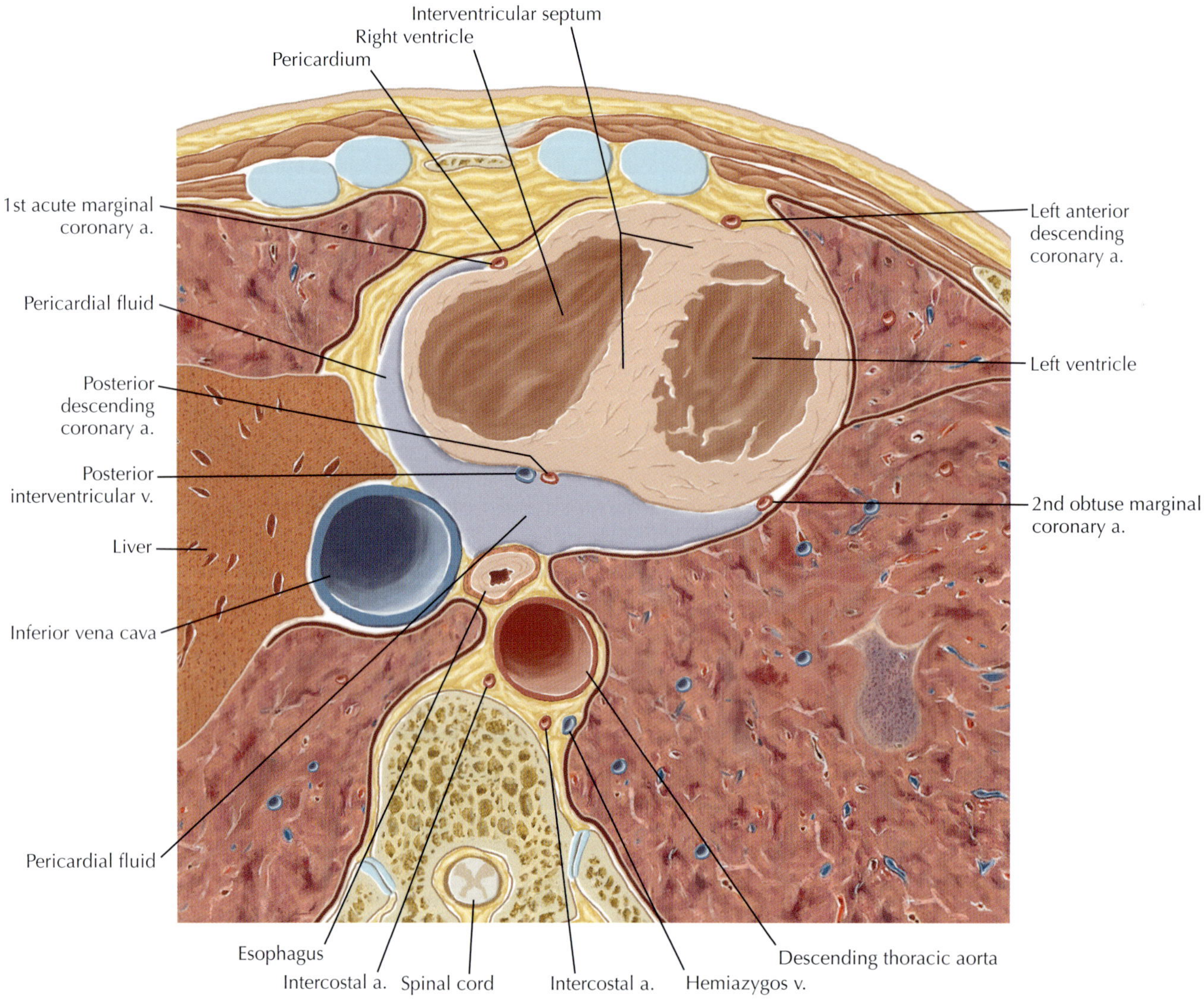
Interventricular septum
Right ventricle
Pericardium
1st acute marginal coronary a.
Pericardial fluid
Posterior descending coronary a.
Posterior interventricular v.
Liver
Inferior vena cava
Pericardial fluid
Left anterior descending coronary a.
Left ventricle
2nd obtuse marginal coronary a.
Esophagus
Intercostal a.
Spinal cord
Intercostal a.
Hemiazygos v.
Descending thoracic aorta

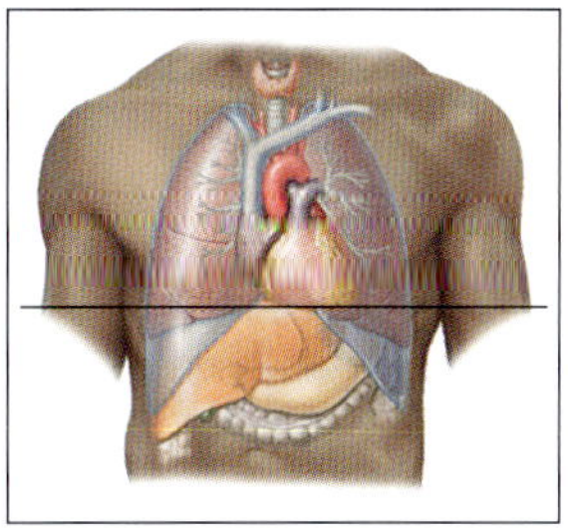

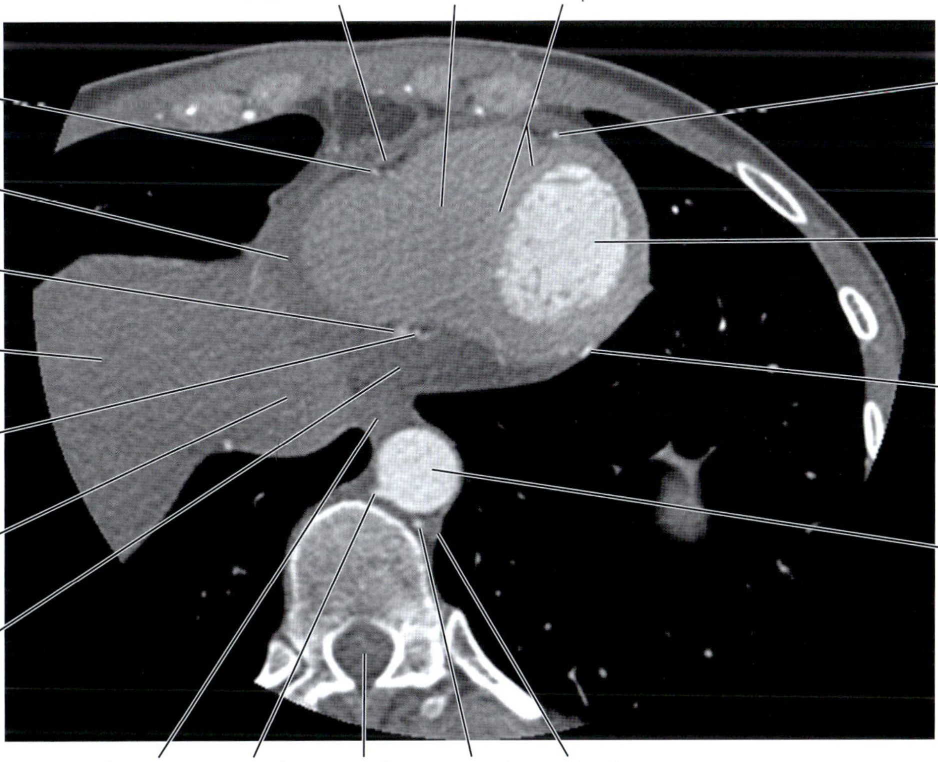
Pericardium
Right ventricle
Interventricular septum
1st acute marginal coronary a.
Pericardial fluid
Posterior interventricular v.
Liver
Posterior descending coronary a.
Inferior vena cava
Pericardial fluid
Left anterior descending coronary a.
Left ventricle
2nd obtuse marginal coronary a.
Descending thoracic aorta
Esophagus
Intercostal a.
Spinal cord
Intercostal a.
Hemiazygos v.

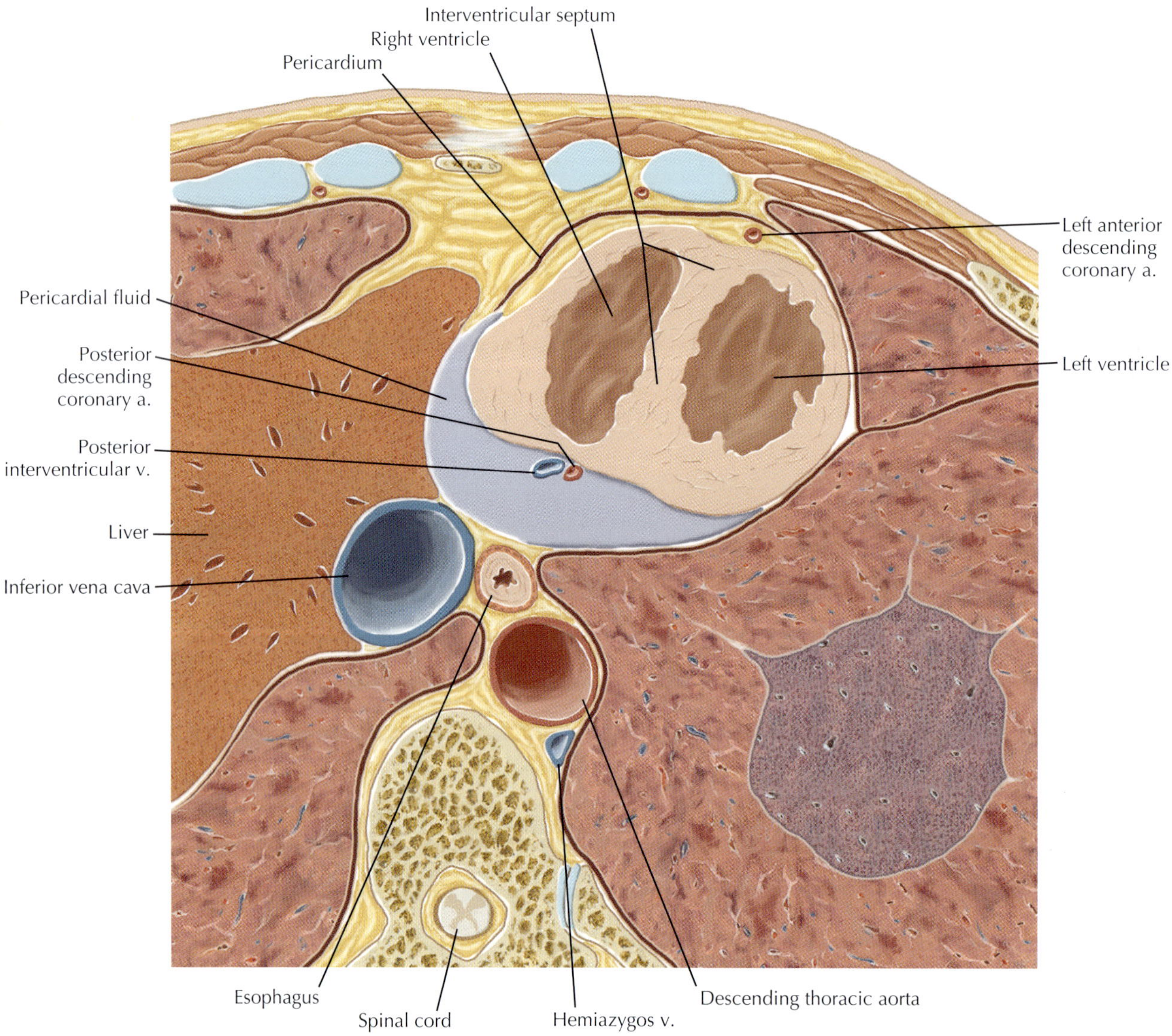
Interventricular septum
Right ventricle
Pericardium
Left anterior descending coronary a.
Pericardial fluid
Posterior descending coronary a.
Left ventricle
Posterior interventricular v.
Liver
Inferior vena cava
Esophagus
Spinal cord
Hemiazygos v.
Descending thoracic aorta

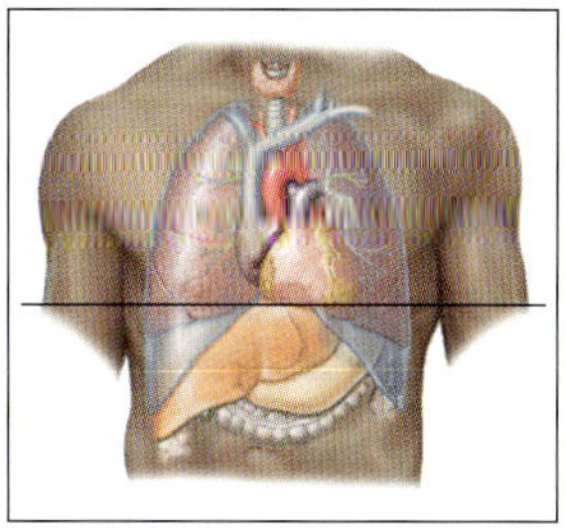

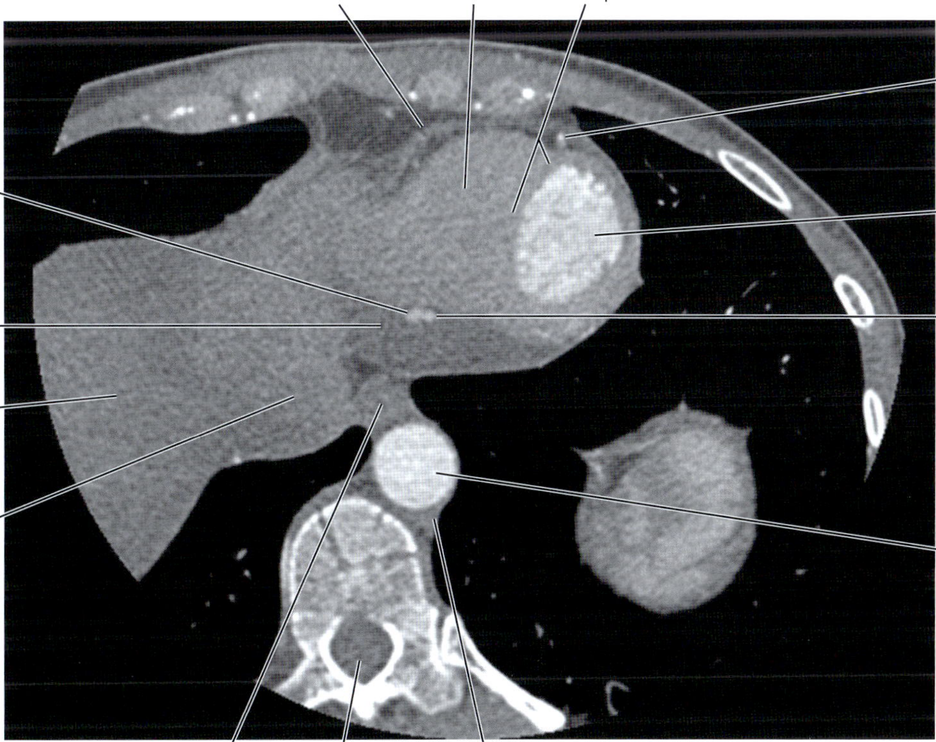
Pericardium
Right ventricle
Interventricular septum
Left anterior descending coronary a.
Posterior inter-ventricular v.
Left ventricle
Pericardial fluid
Posterior descending coronary a.
Liver
Inferior vena cava
Descending thoracic aorta
Esophagus
Spinal cord
Hemiazygos v.

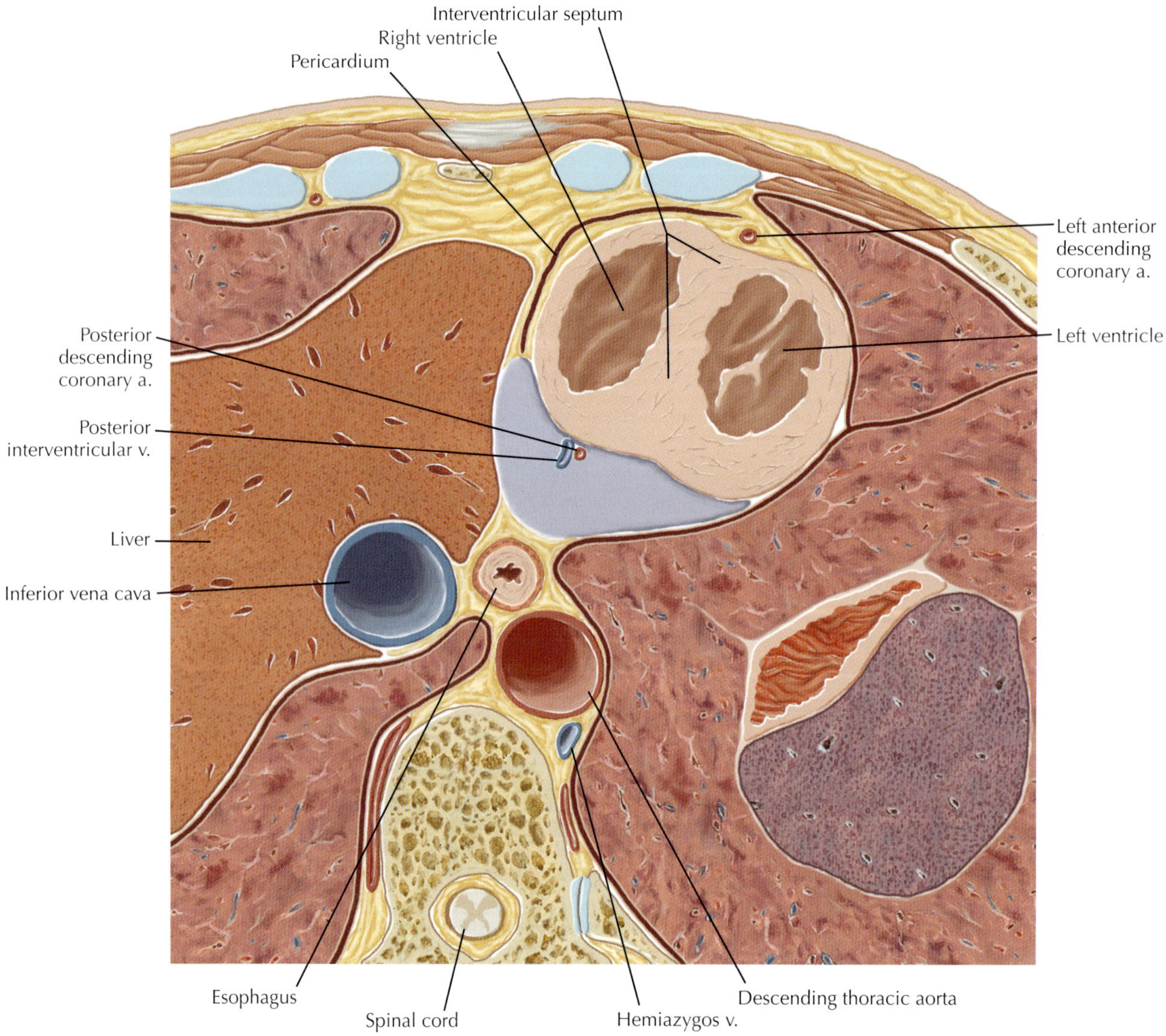
Interventricular septum
Right ventricle
Pericardium
Left anterior descending coronary a.
Left ventricle
Posterior descending coronary a.
Posterior interventricular v.
Liver
Inferior vena cava
Esophagus
Spinal cord
Hemiazygos v.
Descending thoracic aorta

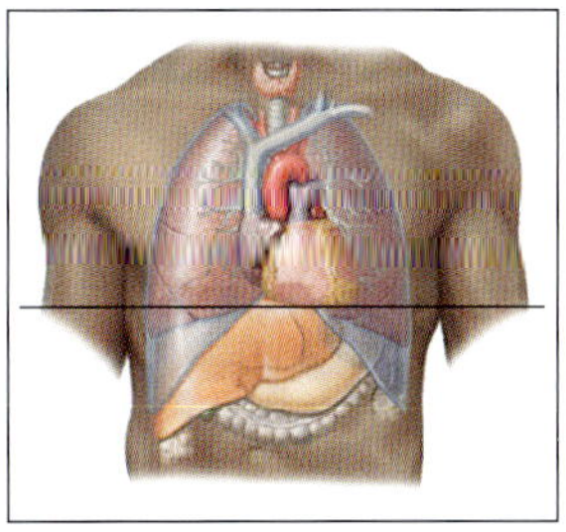

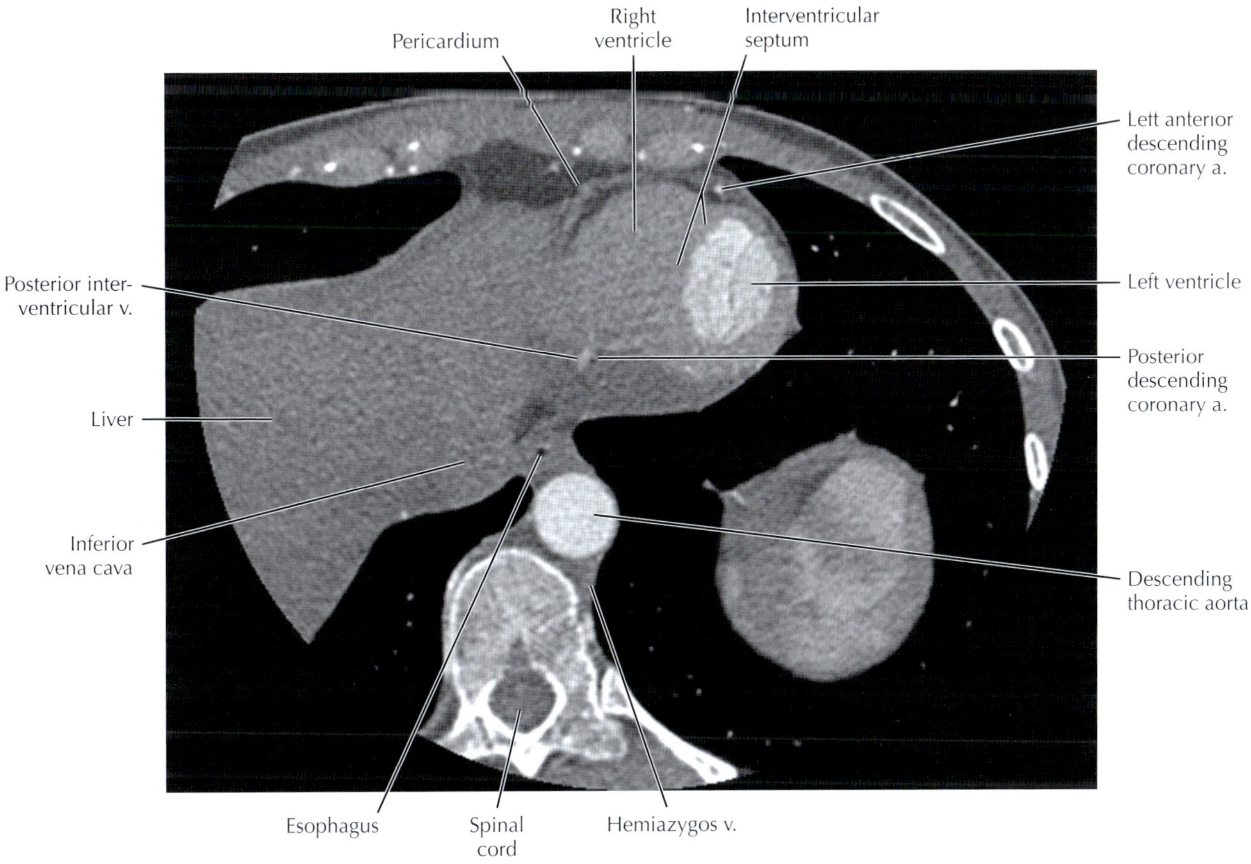
Pericardium
Right ventricle
Interventricular septum
Left anterior descending coronary a.
Left ventricle
Posterior descending coronary a.
Descending thoracic aorta
Posterior interventricular v.
Liver
Inferior vena cava
Esophagus
Spinal cord
Hemiazygos v.

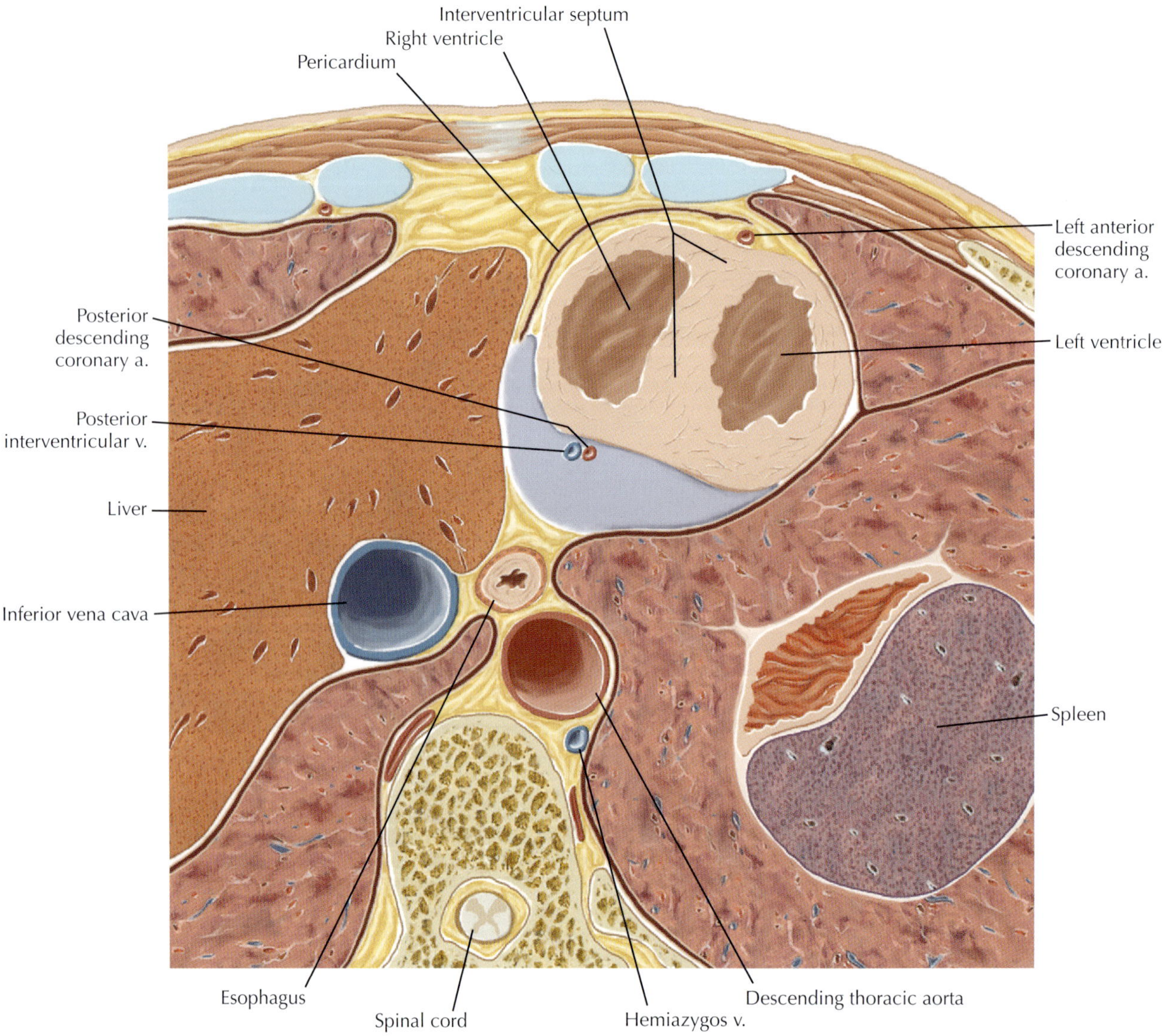
Interventricular septum
Right ventricle
Pericardium
Left anterior descending coronary a.
Posterior descending coronary a.
Left ventricle
Posterior interventricular v.
Liver
Inferior vena cava
Spleen
Esophagus
Spinal cord
Hemiazygos v.
Descending thoracic aorta

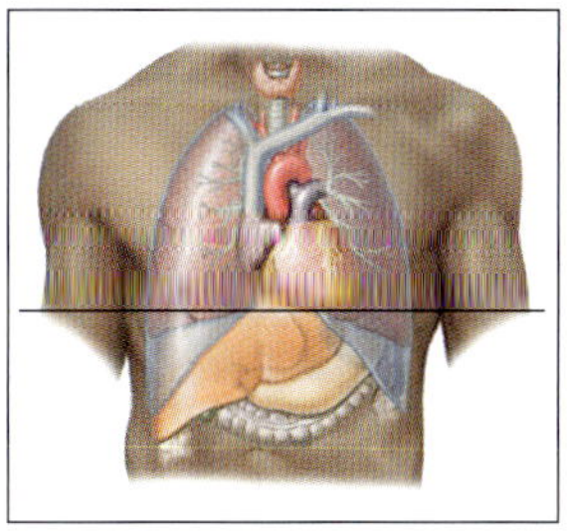

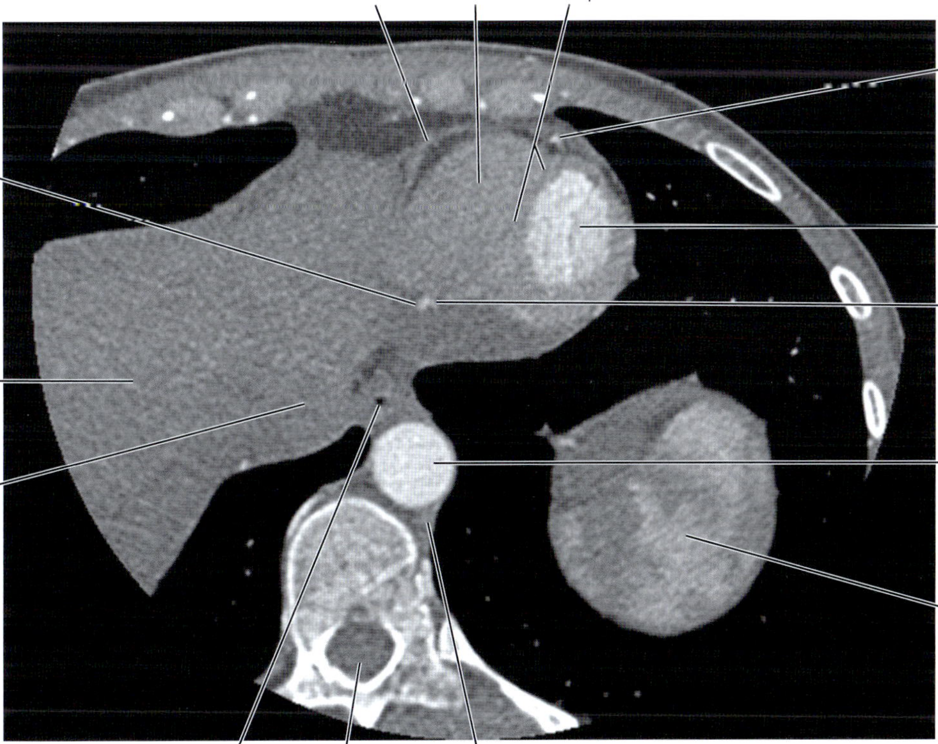
Pericardium
Right ventricle
Interventricular septum
Left anterior descending coronary a.
Posterior interventricular v.
Left ventricle
Posterior descending coronary a.
Liver
Inferior vena cava
Descending thoracic aorta
Spleen
Esophagus
Spinal cord
Hemiazygos v.

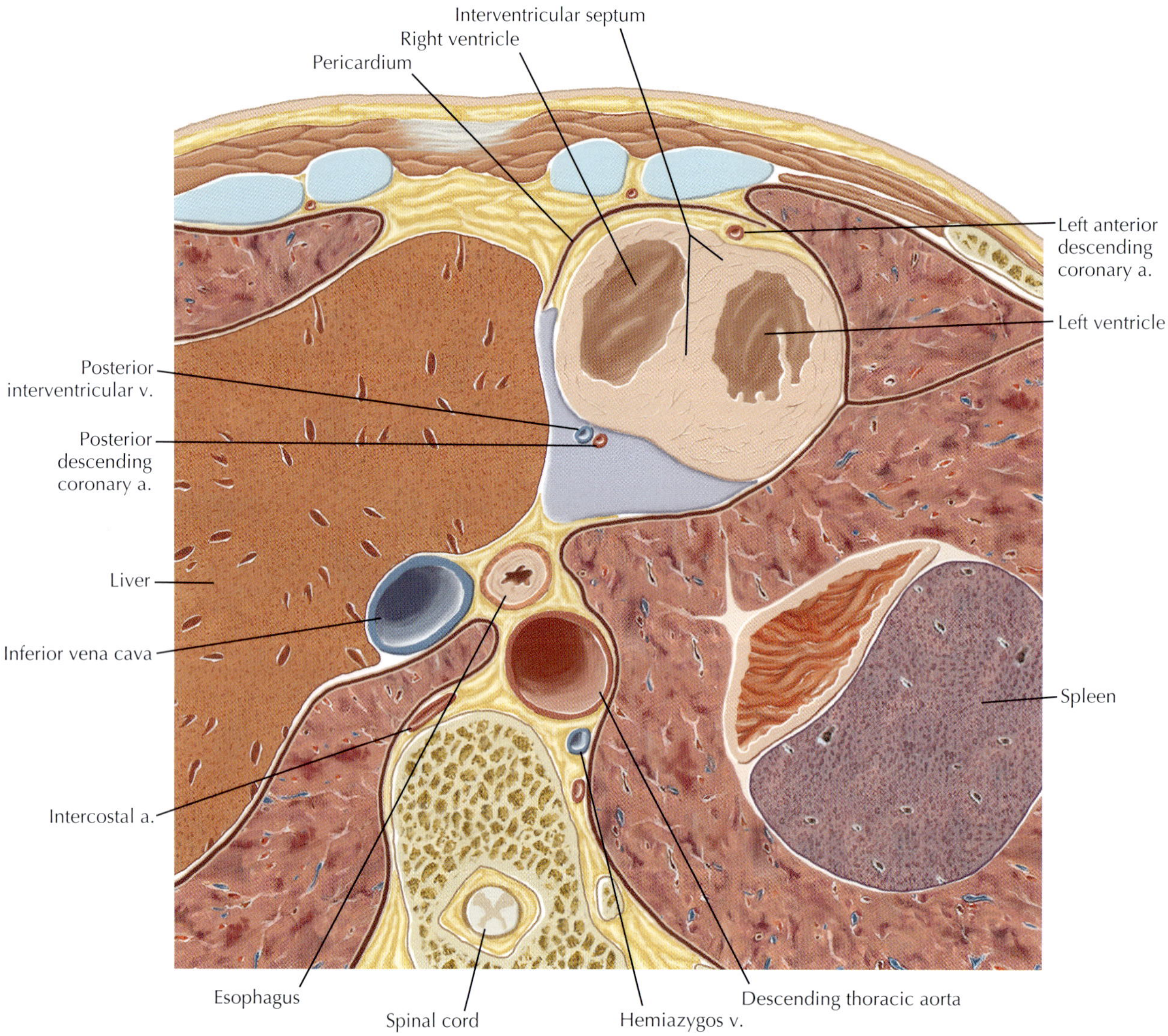
Interventricular septum
Right ventricle
Pericardium
Left anterior descending coronary a.
Left ventricle
Posterior interventricular v.
Posterior descending coronary a.
Liver
Inferior vena cava
Spleen
Intercostal a.
Esophagus
Spinal cord
Hemiazygos v.
Descending thoracic aorta

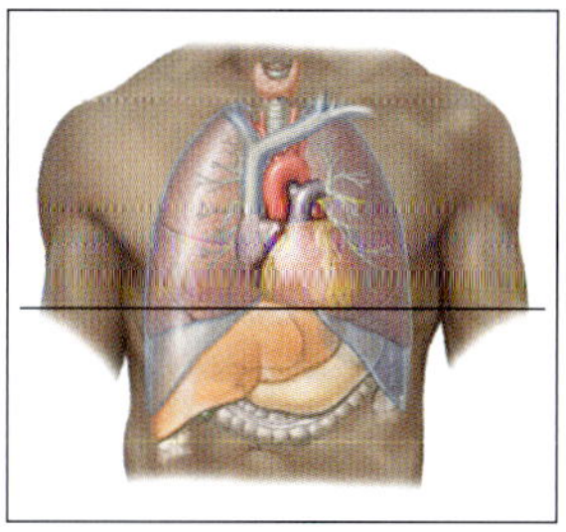

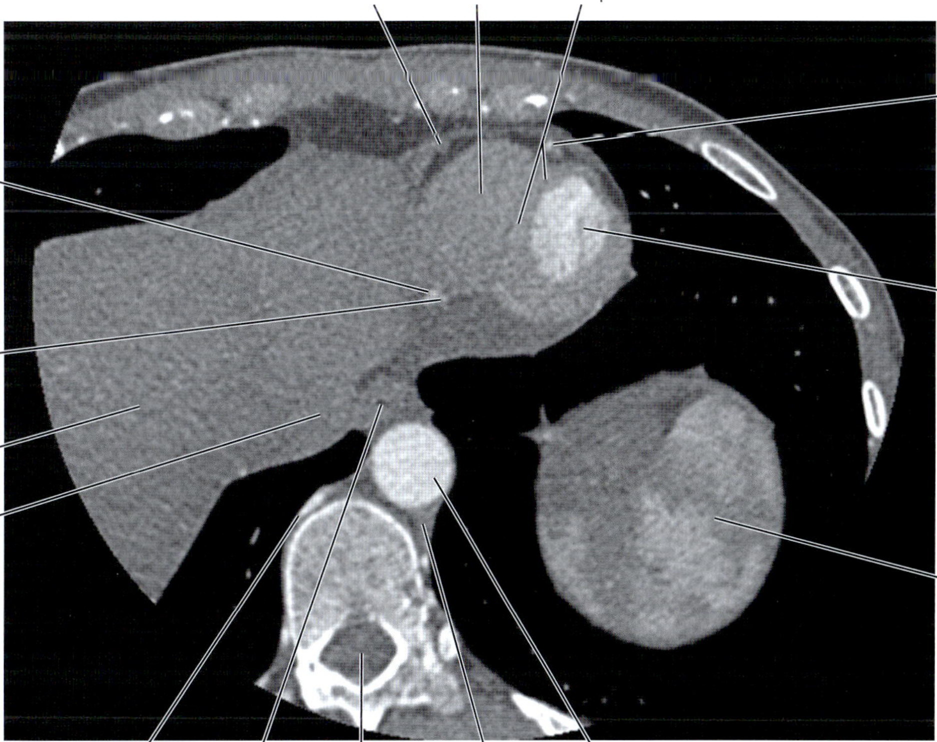

Pericardium
Right ventricle
Interventricular septum
Left anterior descending coronary a.
Posterior interventricular v.
Left ventricle
Posterior descending coronary a.
Liver
Inferior vena cava
Spleen
Intercostal a.
Esophagus
Spinal cord
Hemiazygos v.
Descending thoracic aorta

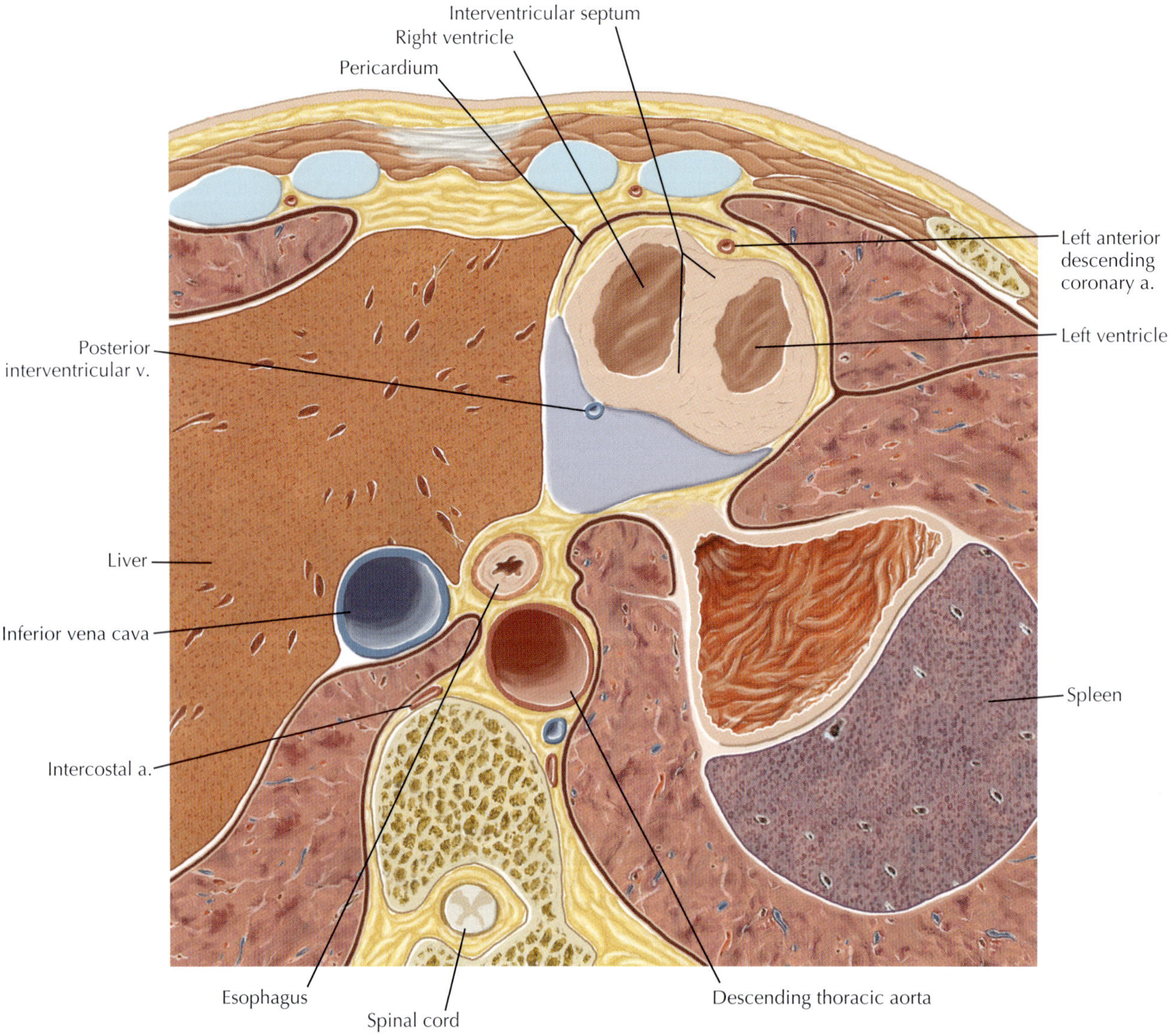
Interventricular septum
Right ventricle
Pericardium
Left anterior descending coronary a.
Posterior interventricular v.
Left ventricle
Liver
Inferior vena cava
Spleen
Intercostal a.
Esophagus
Spinal cord
Descending thoracic aorta

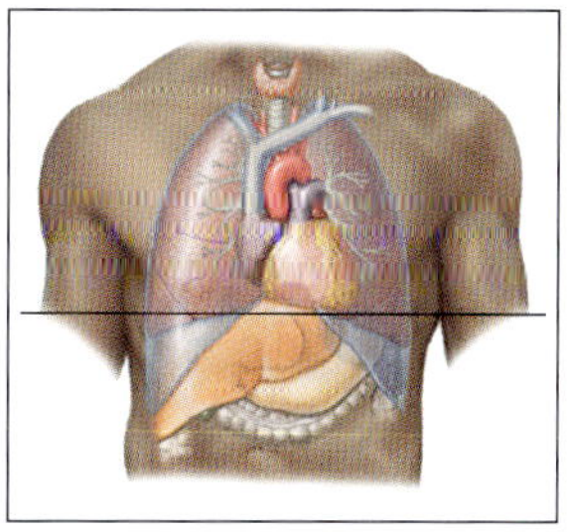

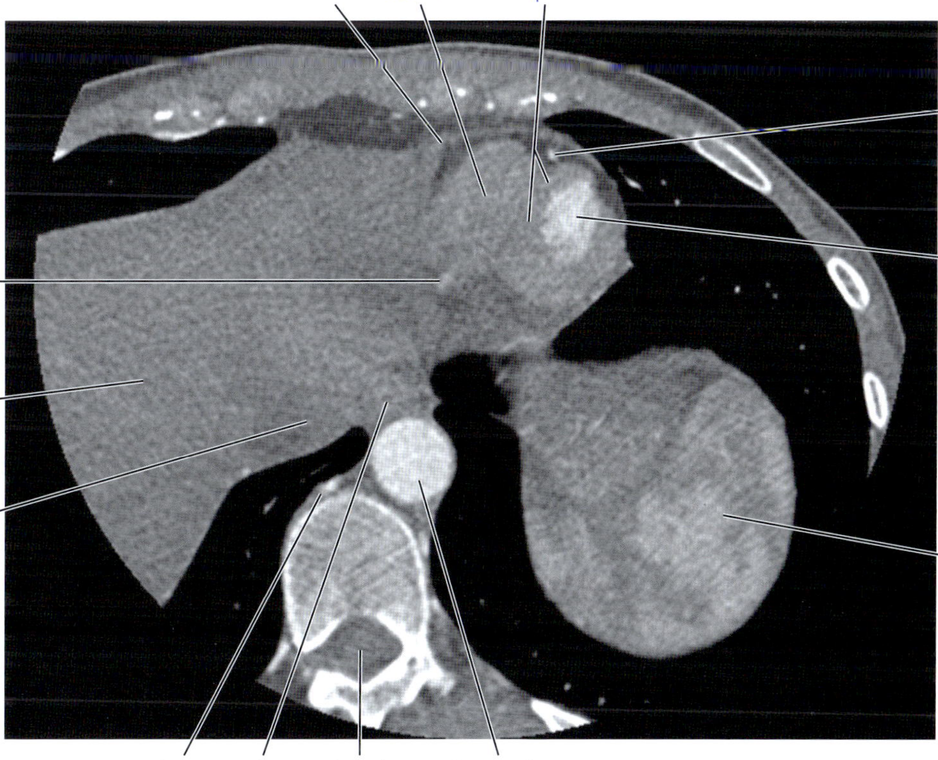
Pericardium
Right ventricle
Interventricular septum
Left anterior descending coronary a.
Left ventricle
Posterior interventricular v.
Liver
Inferior vena cava
Spleen
Intercostal a.
Esophagus
Spinal cord
Descending thoracic aorta

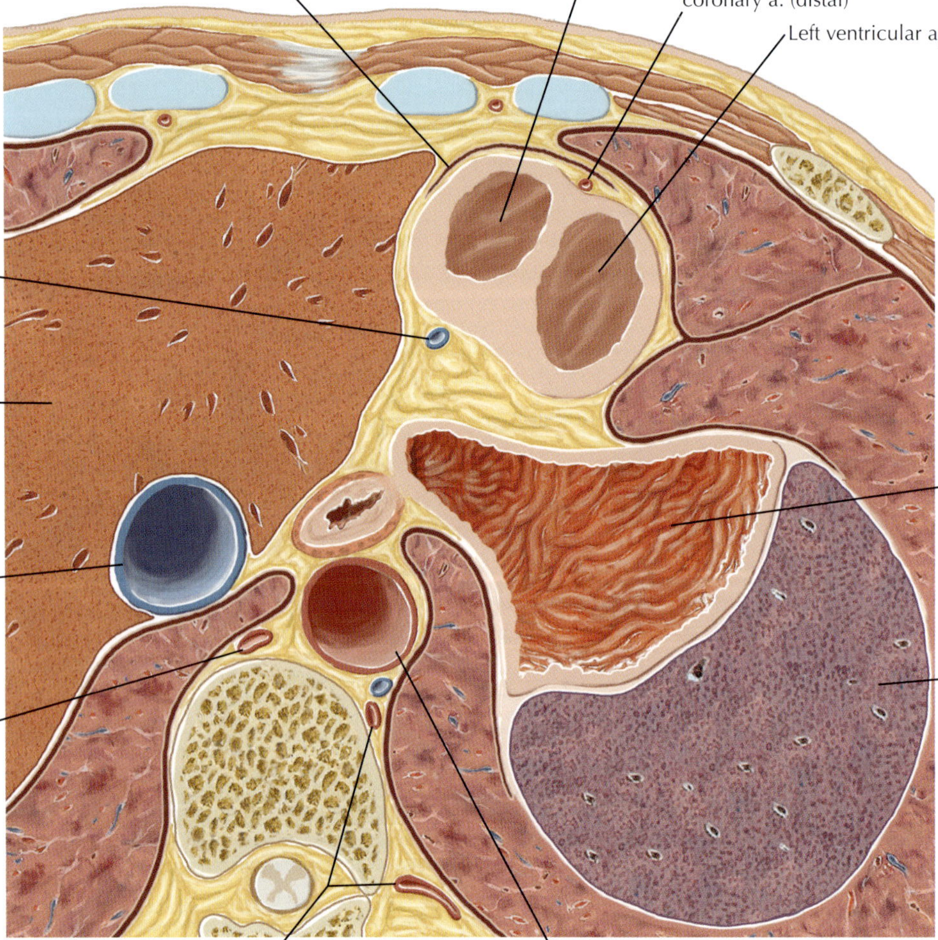
Right ventricular apex
Pericardium
Left anterior descending coronary a. (distal)
Left ventricular apex
Posterior interventricular v.
Liver
Stomach
Inferior vena cava
Spleen
Intercostal a.
Intercostal a.
Descending thoracic aorta

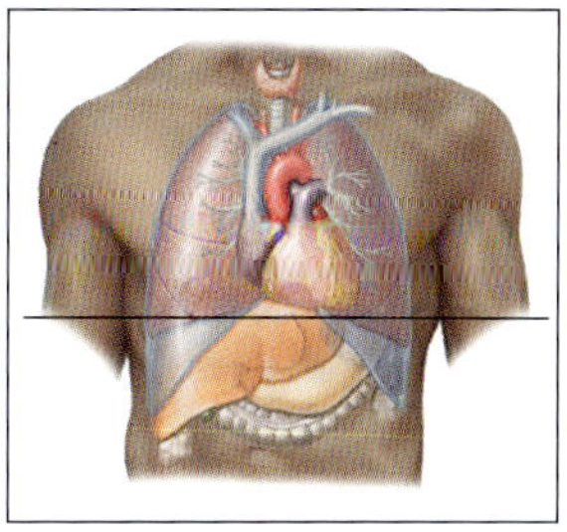

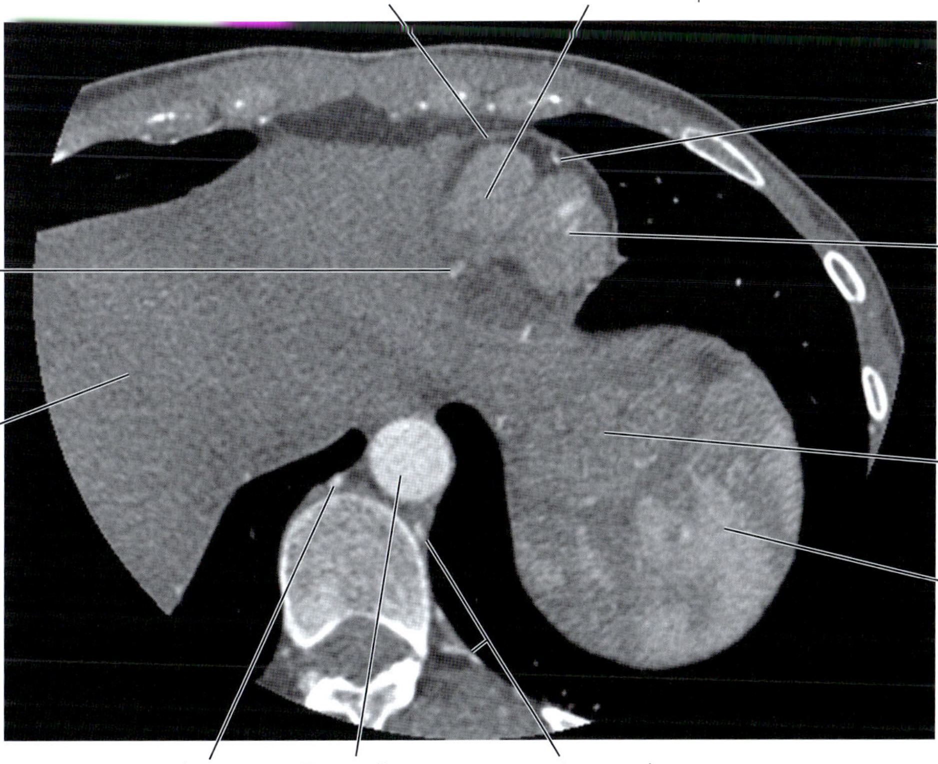
Pericardium
Right ventricular apex
Left anterior descending coronary a. (distal)
Left ventricular apex
Posterior interventricular v.
Liver
Stomach
Spleen
Intercostal a.
Descending thoracic aorta
Intercostal a.

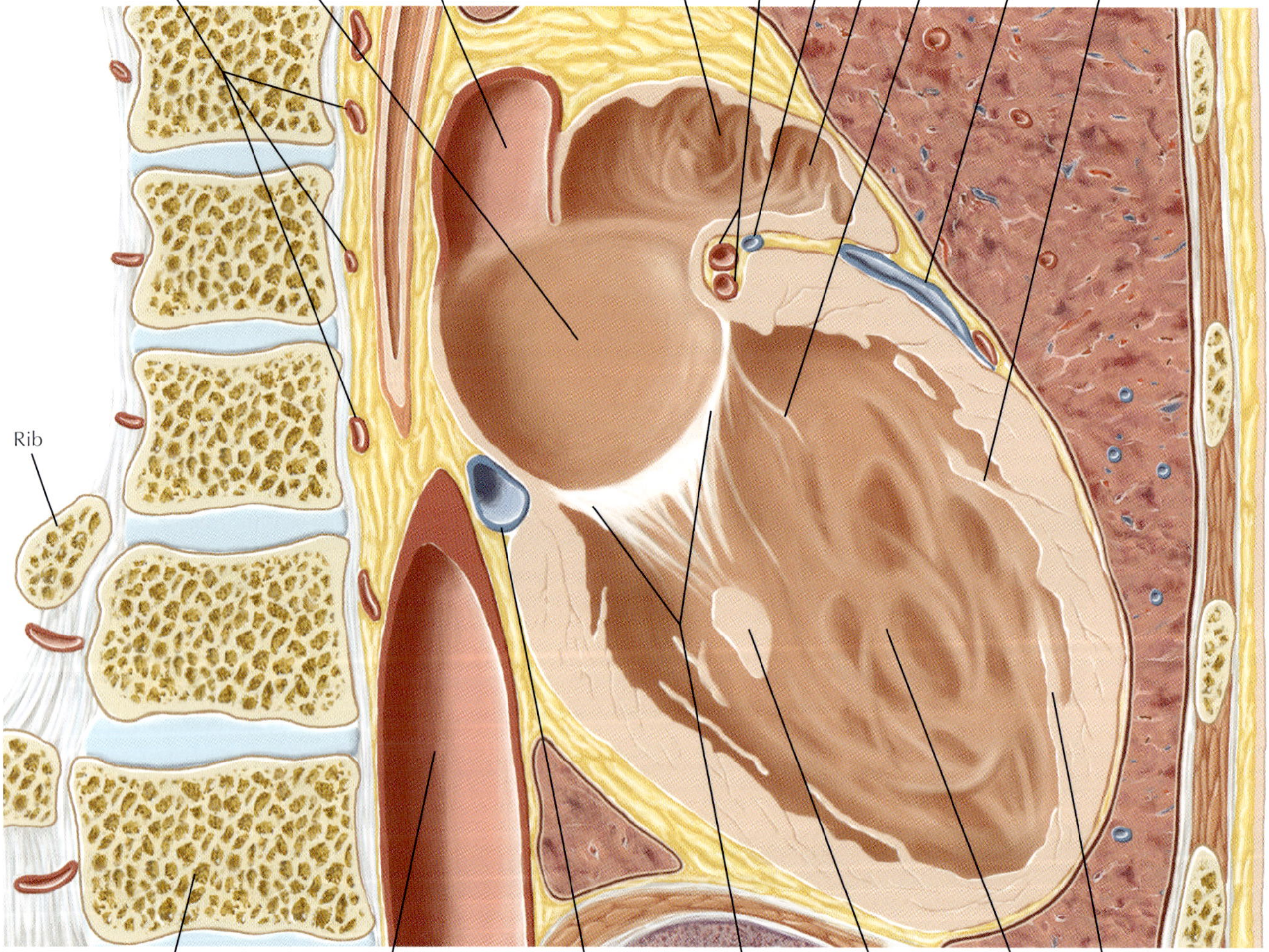

TECHNICAL CONSIDERATION

Cardiac imaging is often interpreted with images displayed in planes oriented with reference to the cardiac axis, as opposed to the axes of the body as is typical for most imaging applications (the axial, coronal, and sagittal planes). Cardiac imaging planes typically include "two-chamber," "three-chamber," "four-chamber," and "short axis" planes, and are commonly used for cardiac CT, MRI, nuclear medicine, and echocardiography. This "two-chamber" or "vertical long axis" view of the heart is useful for assessing the left ventricular cavity, left ventricular inferior and anterior wall motion, the mitral valve, and the left atrial appendage.

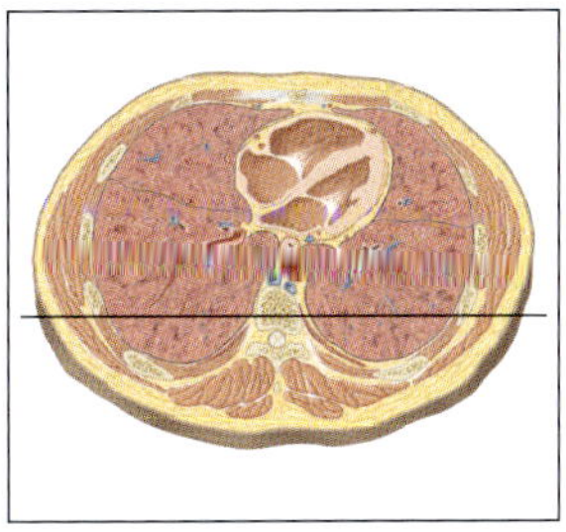

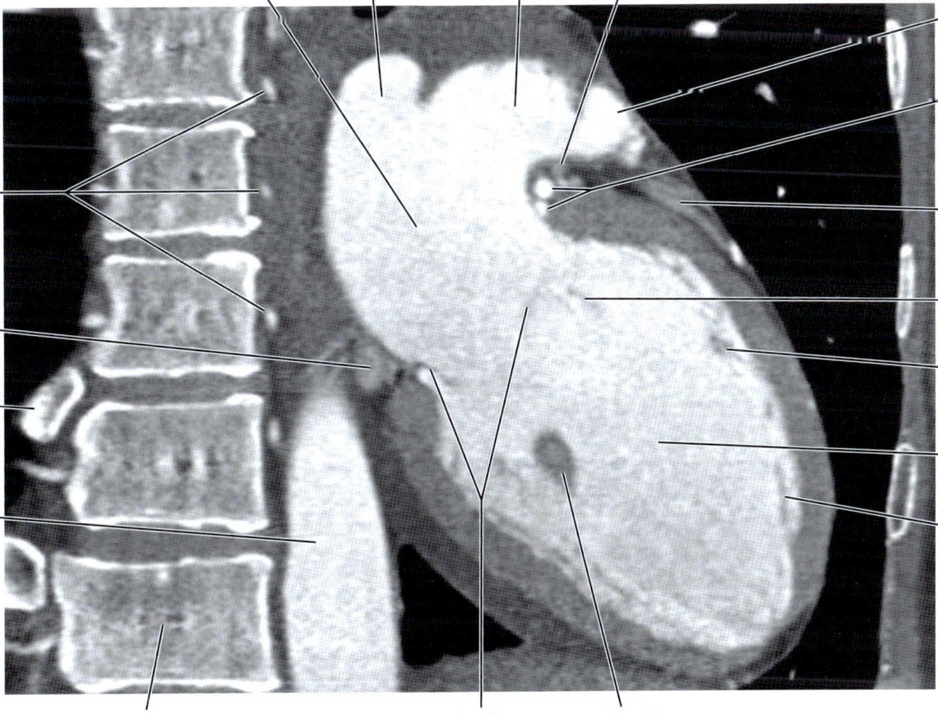
Left atrium
Left superior pulmonary v.
Left atrial appendage
Great cardiac v.
Left atrial appendage
Left circumflex & obtuse marginal coronary aa.
Anterior interventricular coronary v.
Chordae tendineae
Trabeculae carnae
Left ventricle
Trabeculae carneae
Intercostal aa.
Coronary sinus
Rib
Descending thoracic aorta
Vertebral body
Mitral valve
Papillary m.

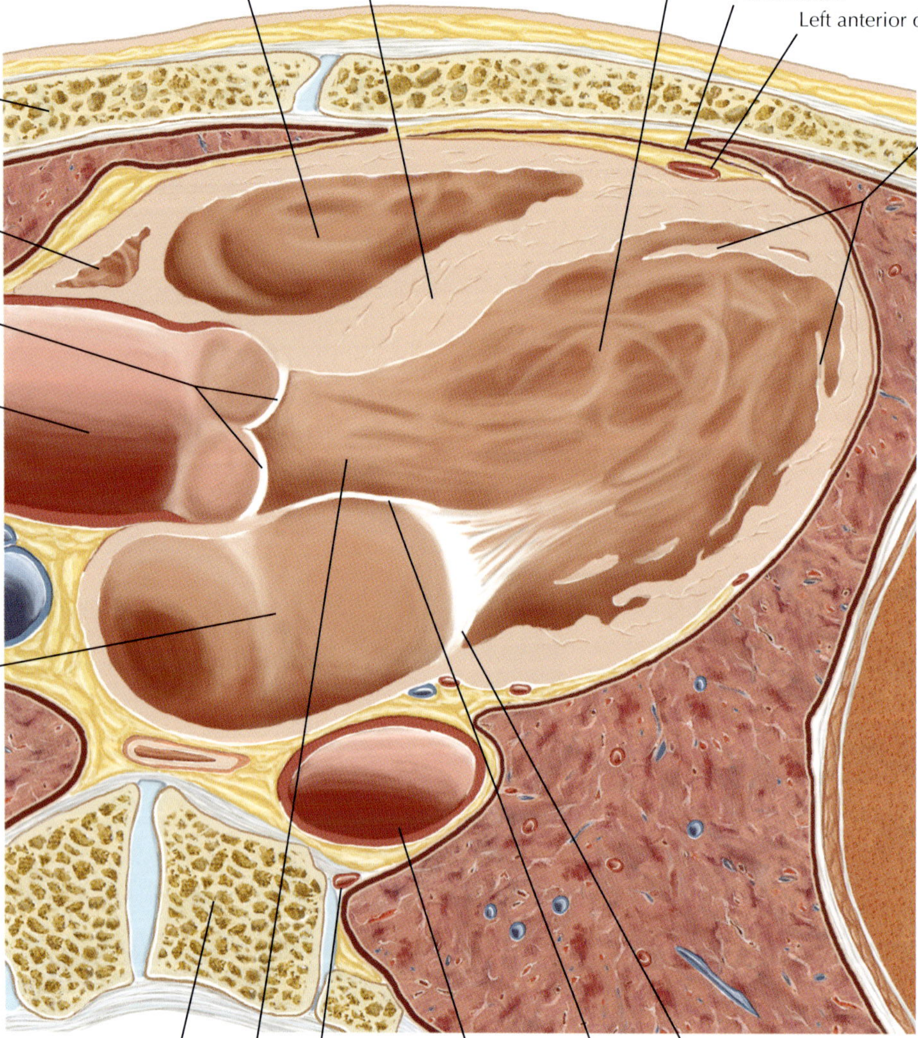

TECHNICAL CONSIDERATION

This "three-chamber" view of the heart is useful for displaying the left ventricular outflow tract, left atrium, and mitral and aortic valves. The anteroseptal and inferolateral walls of the left ventricle are also well demonstrated. Note how the continuity between the aortic valve apparatus and anterior mitral valve are well shown in this view.

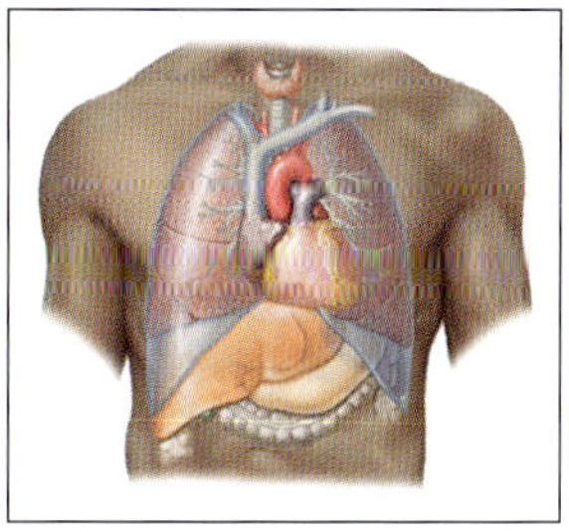

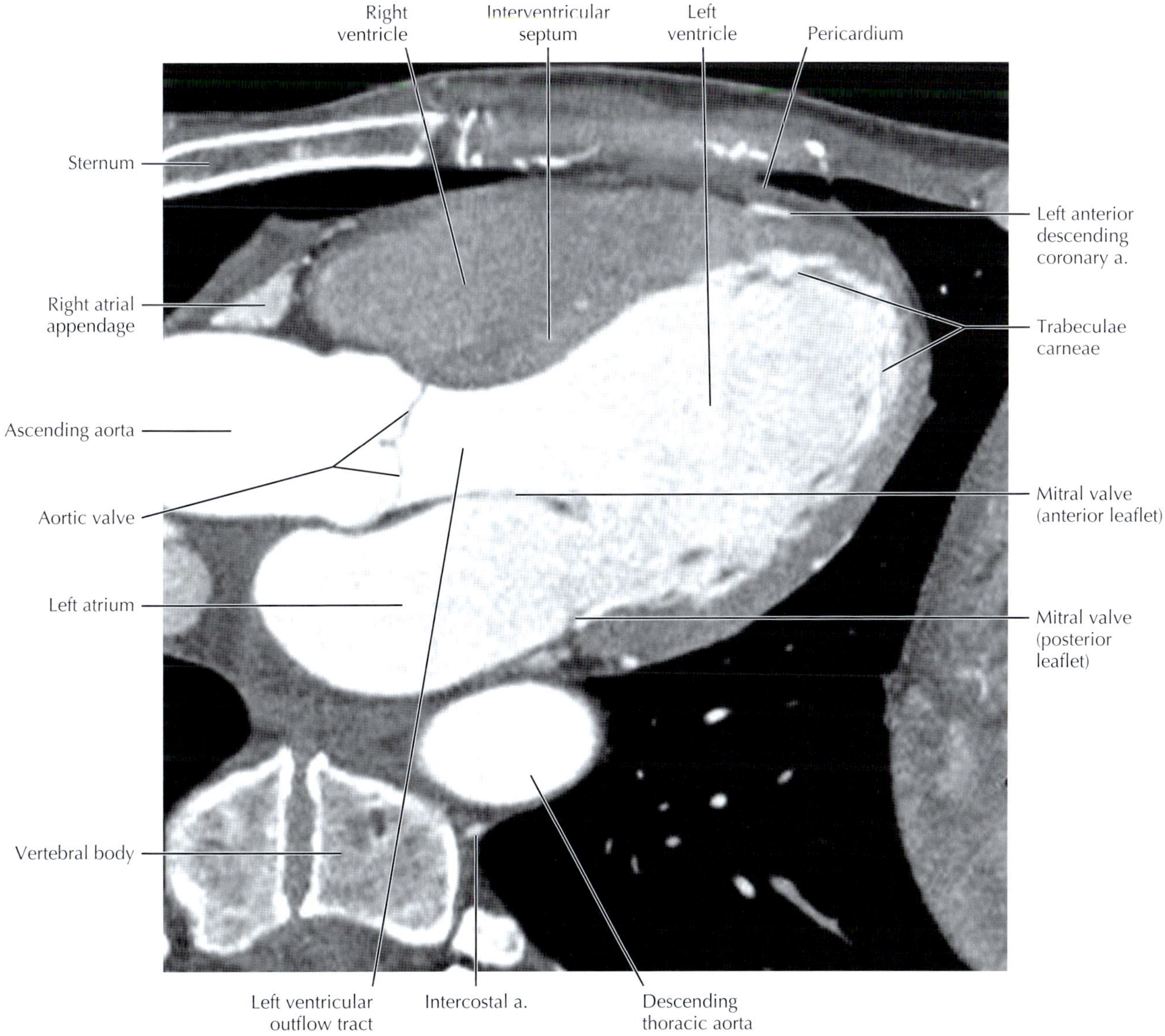
Right ventricle
Interventricular septum
Left ventricle
Pericardium
Sternum
Left anterior descending coronary a.
Right atrial appendage
Trabeculae carneae
Ascending aorta
Aortic valve
Mitral valve (anterior leaflet)
Left atrium
Mitral valve (posterior leaflet)
Vertebral body
Left ventricular outflow tract
Intercostal a.
Descending thoracic aorta

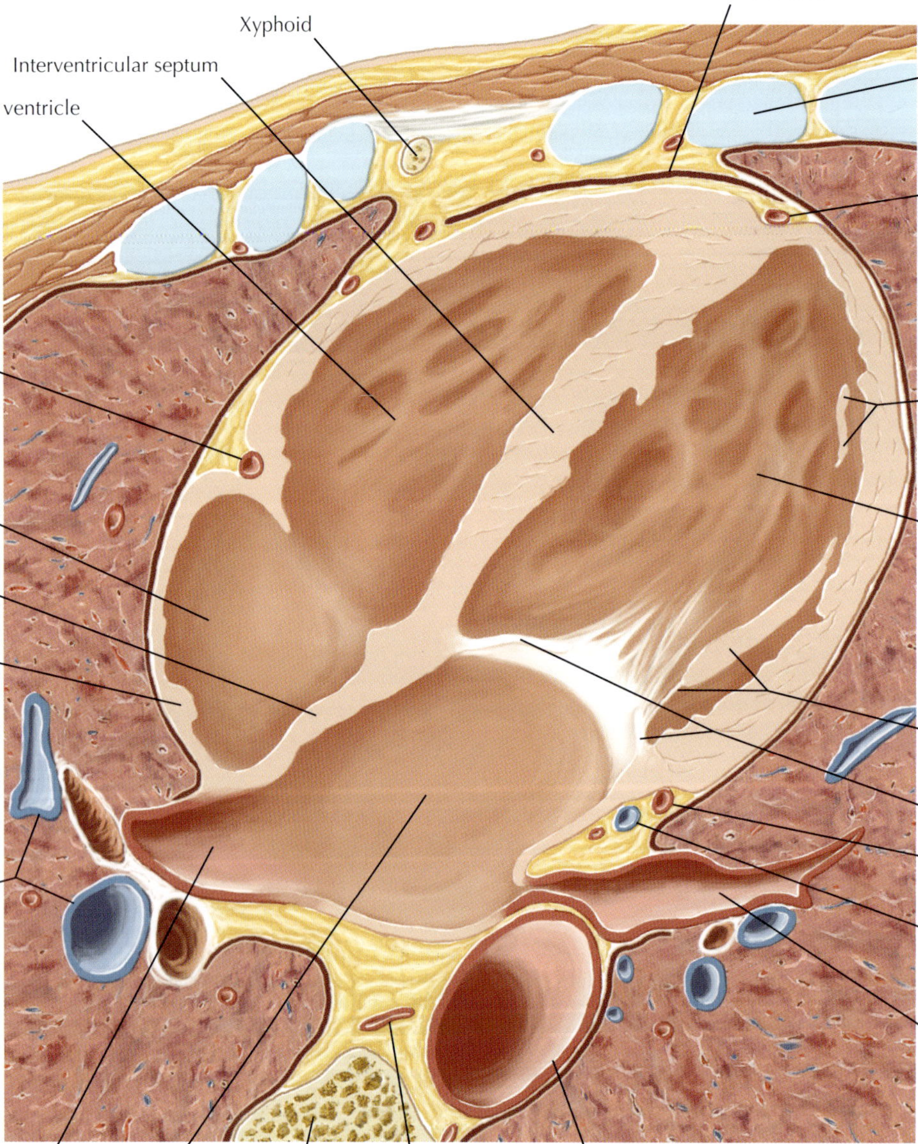

TECHNICAL CONSIDERATION

This "four-chamber" or "horizontal long axis" view is oriented through the mid portions of the right and left ventricles, along a plane extending through the mitral valve to the apex of the heart. This projection provides a more precise analysis of ventricular size and morphology than standard axial, coronal, or sagittal imaging and is useful for assessing the function of the mitral and tricuspid valves. Left ventricular septal and lateral wall motion is also evaluable in this view.

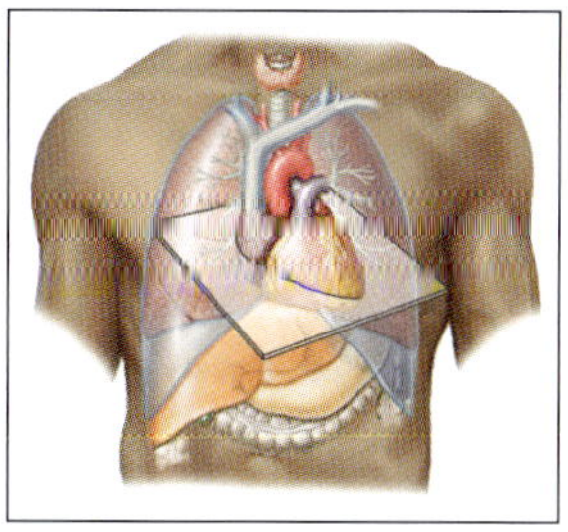

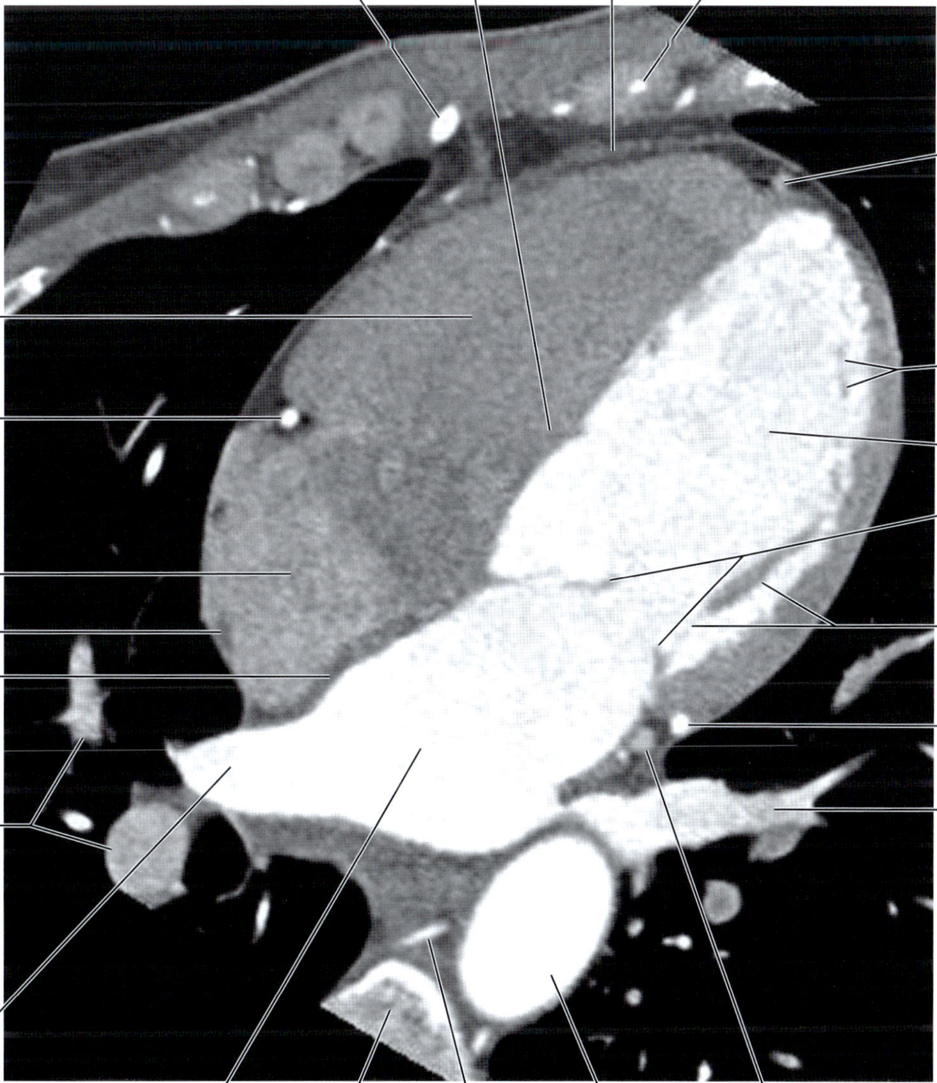
Xyphoid
Interventricular septum
Pericardium
Costochondral junction
Left anterior descending coronary a.
Right ventricle
Trabeculae carneae
Right coronary a.
Left ventricle
Mitral valve
Right atrium
Crista terminalis
Papillary m. & chordae tendineae
Interatrial septum
Left circumflex coronary a.
Pulmonary aa.
Pulmonary v.
Pulmonary v.
Left atrium
Vertebral body
Intercostal a.
Descending thoracic aorta
Great cardiac v.

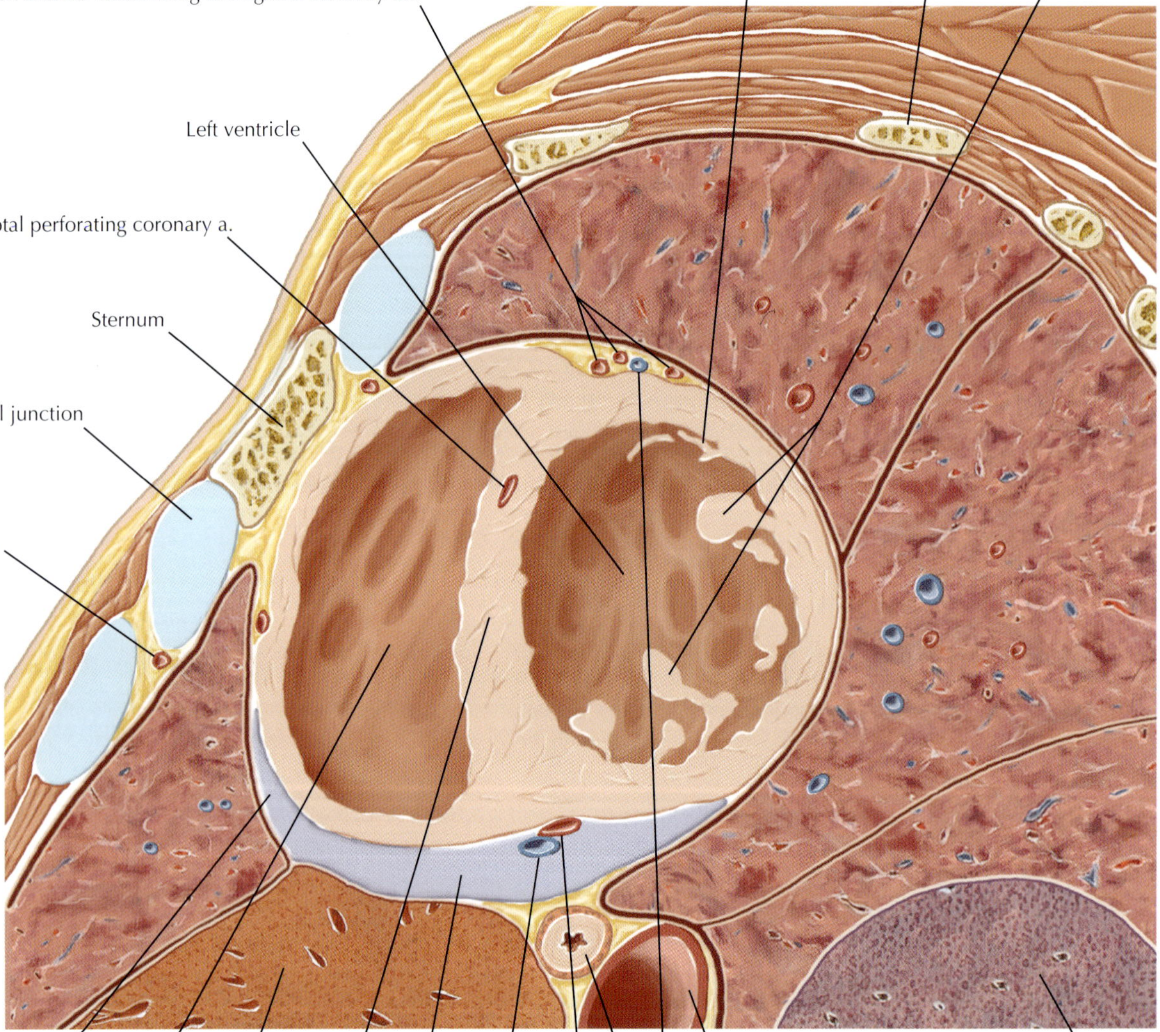

TECHNICAL CONSIDERATION

This "short axis" view is oriented orthogonal to the four-chamber view, perpendicular to the long axis of the left ventricle from the mitral valve to the apex of the heart. This view is used for calculation of ventricular volumes and ejection fraction as well as assessment of left ventricular wall motion.

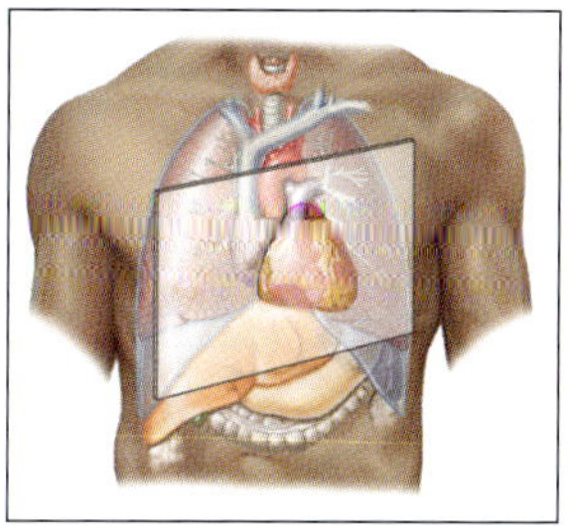

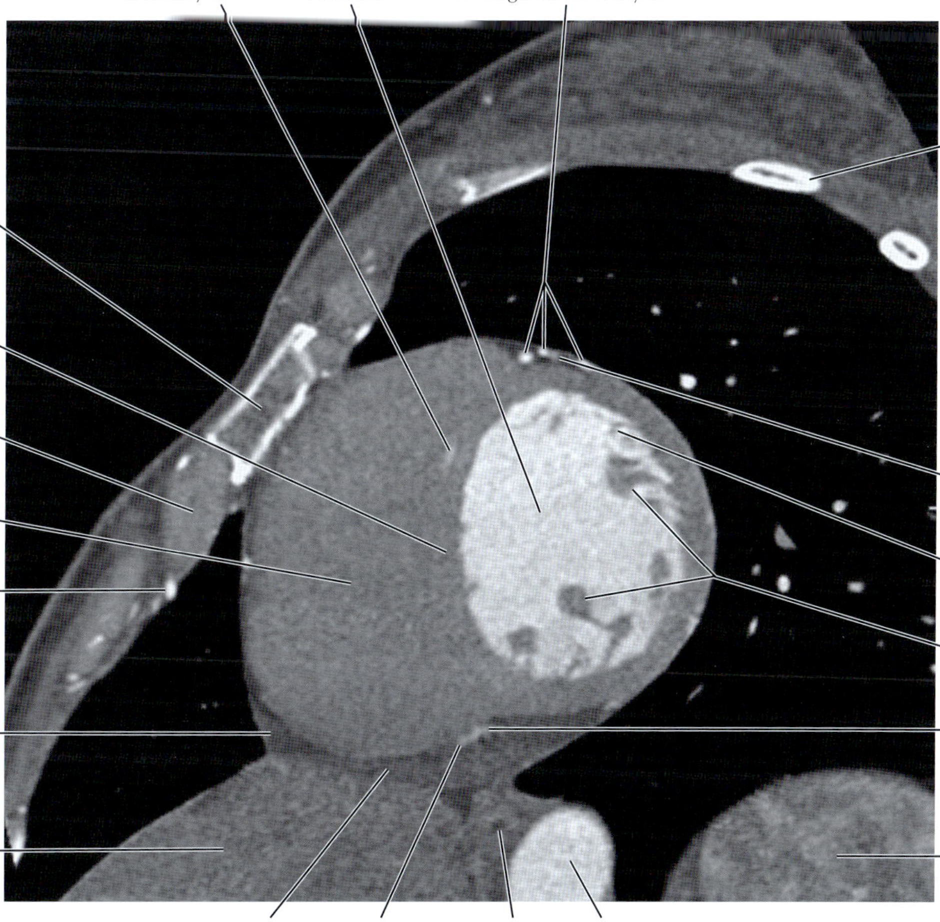
Septal perforating coronary a.
Left ventricle
Left anterior descending & diagonal coronary aa.
Rib
Sternum
Interventricular septum
Costochondral junction
Right ventricle
Left internal mammary a.
Pericardial fluid
Liver
Anterior interventricular coronary v.
Trabeculae carneae
Papillary mm.
Posterior descending coronary a.
Spleen
Pericardial fluid
Posterior interventricular coronary v. (middle cardiac v.)
Esophagus
Descending thoracic aorta

Chapter 9 CARDIAC ANATOMY USING MR

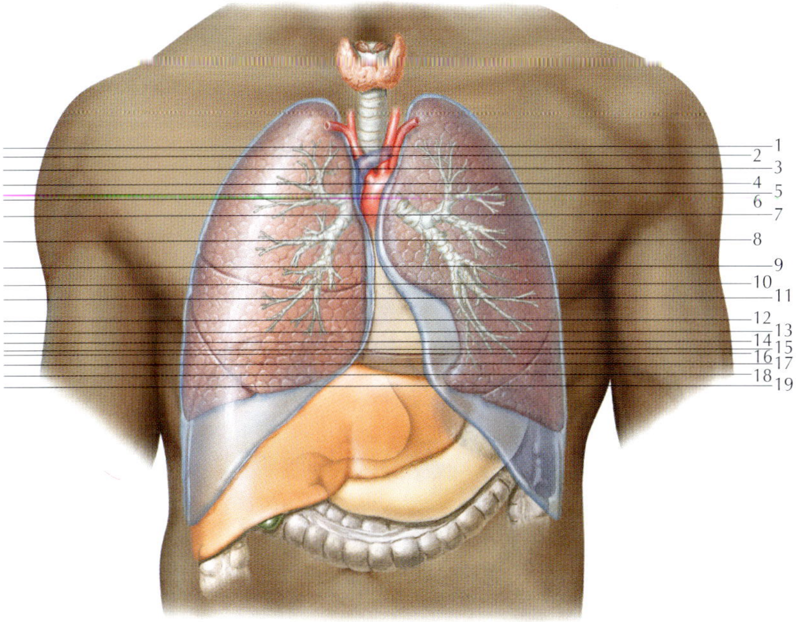

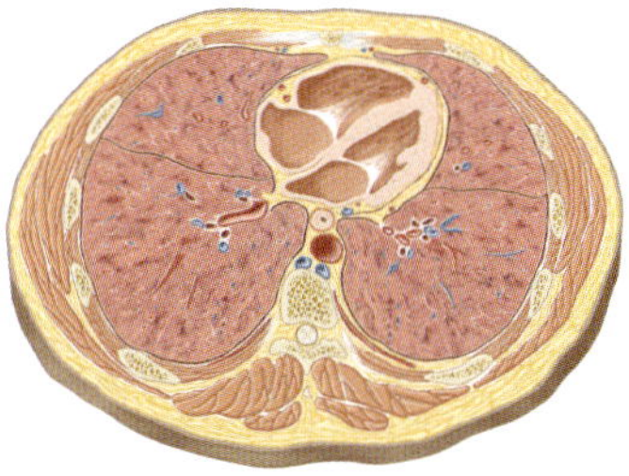

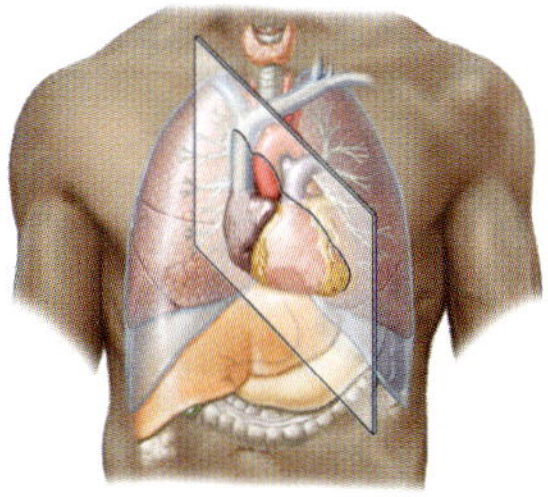

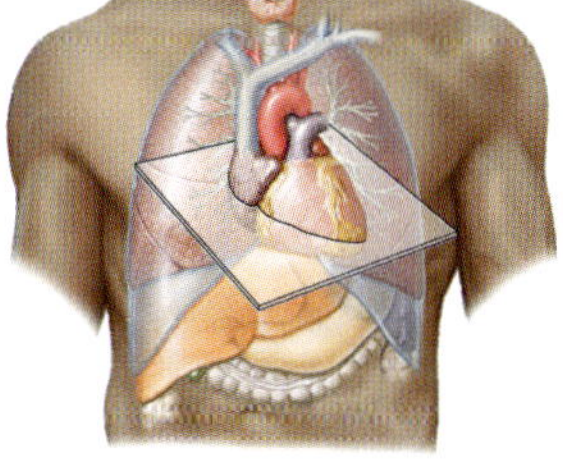

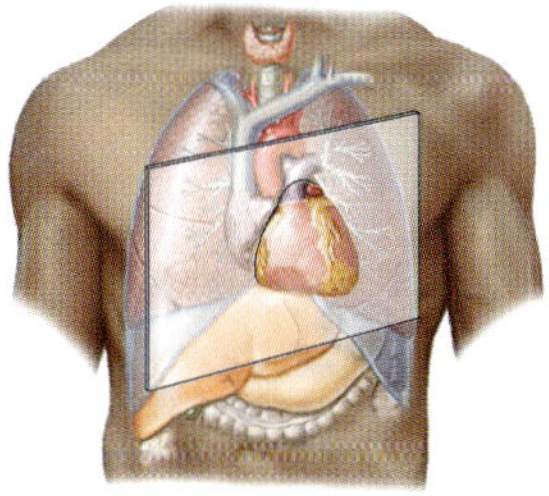

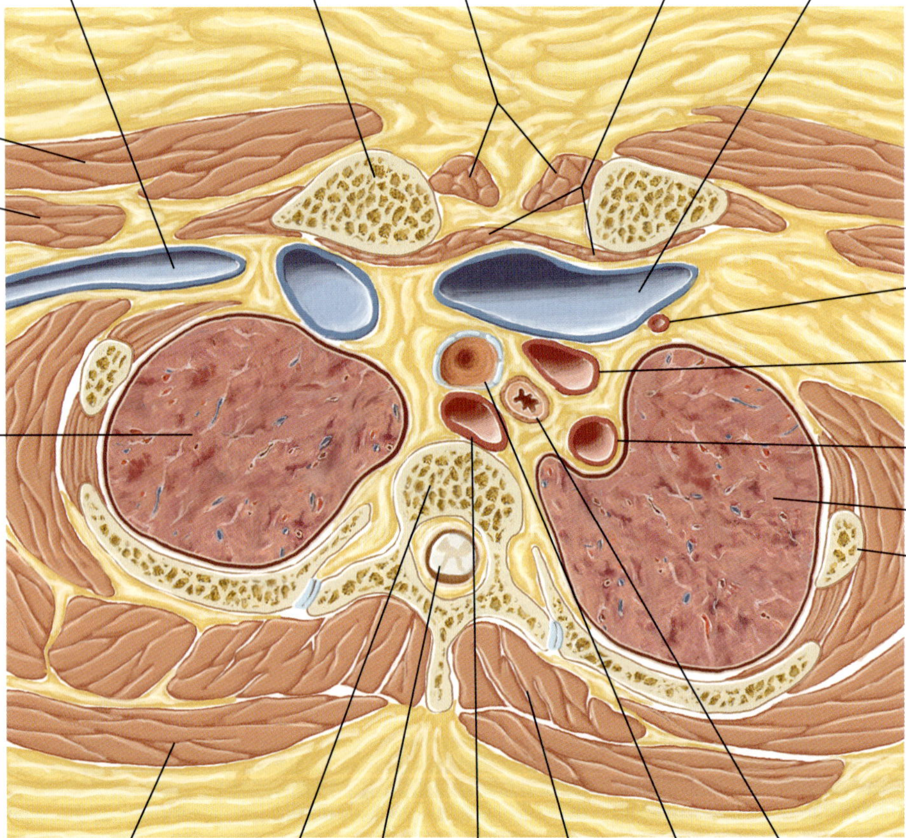

NORMAL VARIANT

This axial MR image shows a common vascular variation—an aberrant right subclavian artery. Thoracic CT Soft Tissue Axial Plates 1 to 5 show the normal origin and course of the right subclavian artery. The aberrant right subclavian artery is one of the most common congenital vascular anomalies affecting the aortic arch and great vessels. Normally the right subclavian artery arises from the right brachiocephalic artery and courses into the right upper extremity (see Thoracic CT Soft Tissue Axial Plates 1 to 5). In contrast, the aberrant right subclavian artery typically arises from the distal aspect of the aortic arch or proximal descending thoracic aorta and courses through the mediastinum, posterior to the esophagus, to reach the right upper extremity.

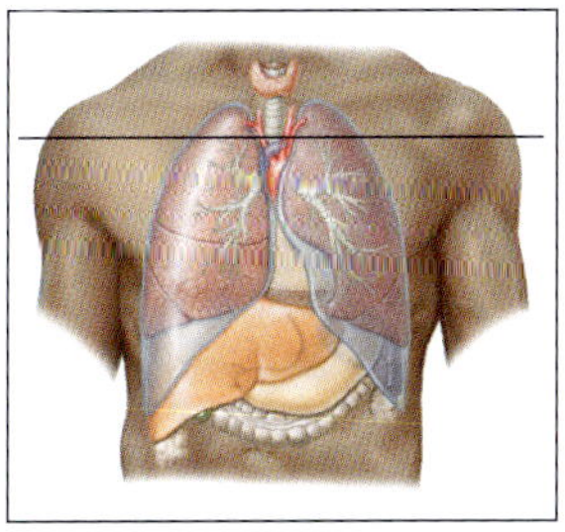

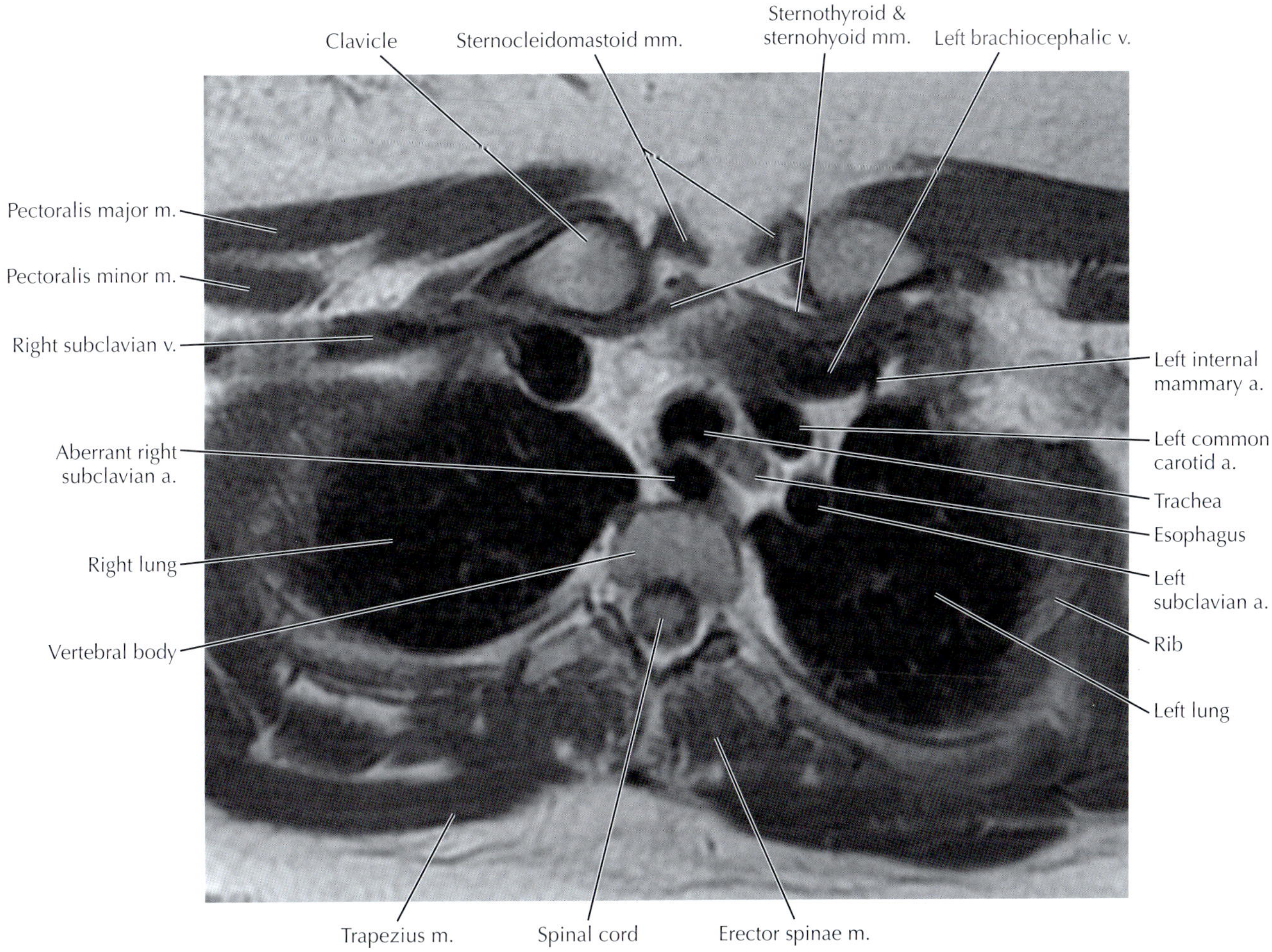
Clavicle
Sternocleidomastoid mm.
Sternothyroid & sternohyoid mm.
Left brachiocephalic v.
Pectoralis major m.
Pectoralis minor m.
Right subclavian v.
Left internal mammary a.
Left common carotid a.
Aberrant right subclavian a.
Trachea
Esophagus
Right lung
Left subclavian a.
Vertebral body
Rib
Left lung
Trapezius m.
Spinal cord
Erector spinae m.

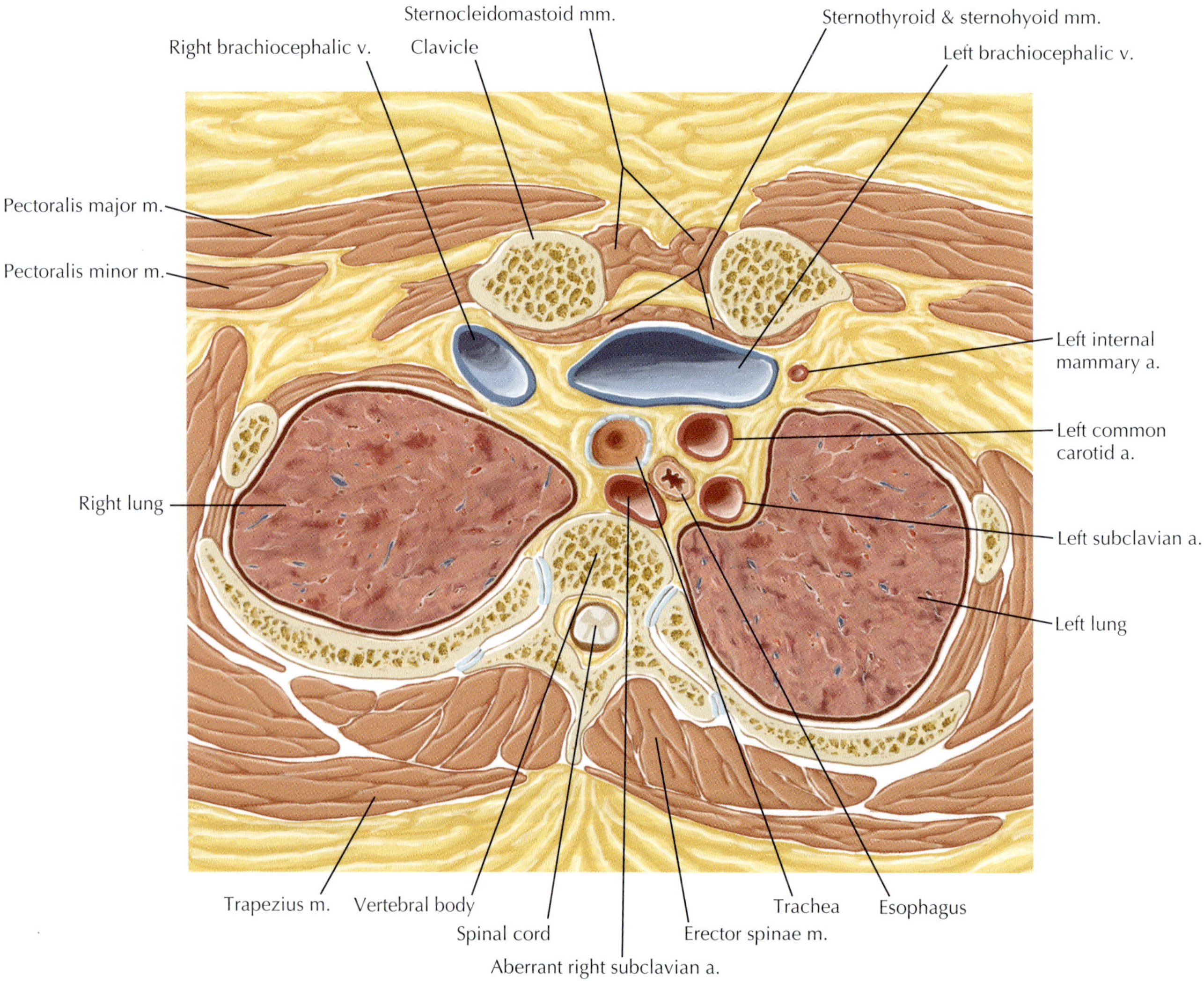
Sternocleidomastoid mm.
Sternothyroid & sternohyoid mm.
Right brachiocephalic v.
Clavicle
Left brachiocephalic v.
Pectoralis major m.
Pectoralis minor m.
Left internal mammary a.
Left common carotid a.
Right lung
Left subclavian a.
Left lung
Trapezius m.
Vertebral body
Trachea
Esophagus
Spinal cord
Erector spinae m.
Aberrant right subclavian a.

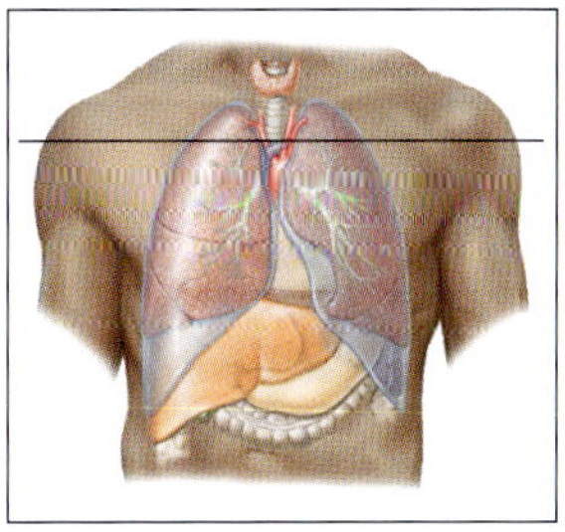

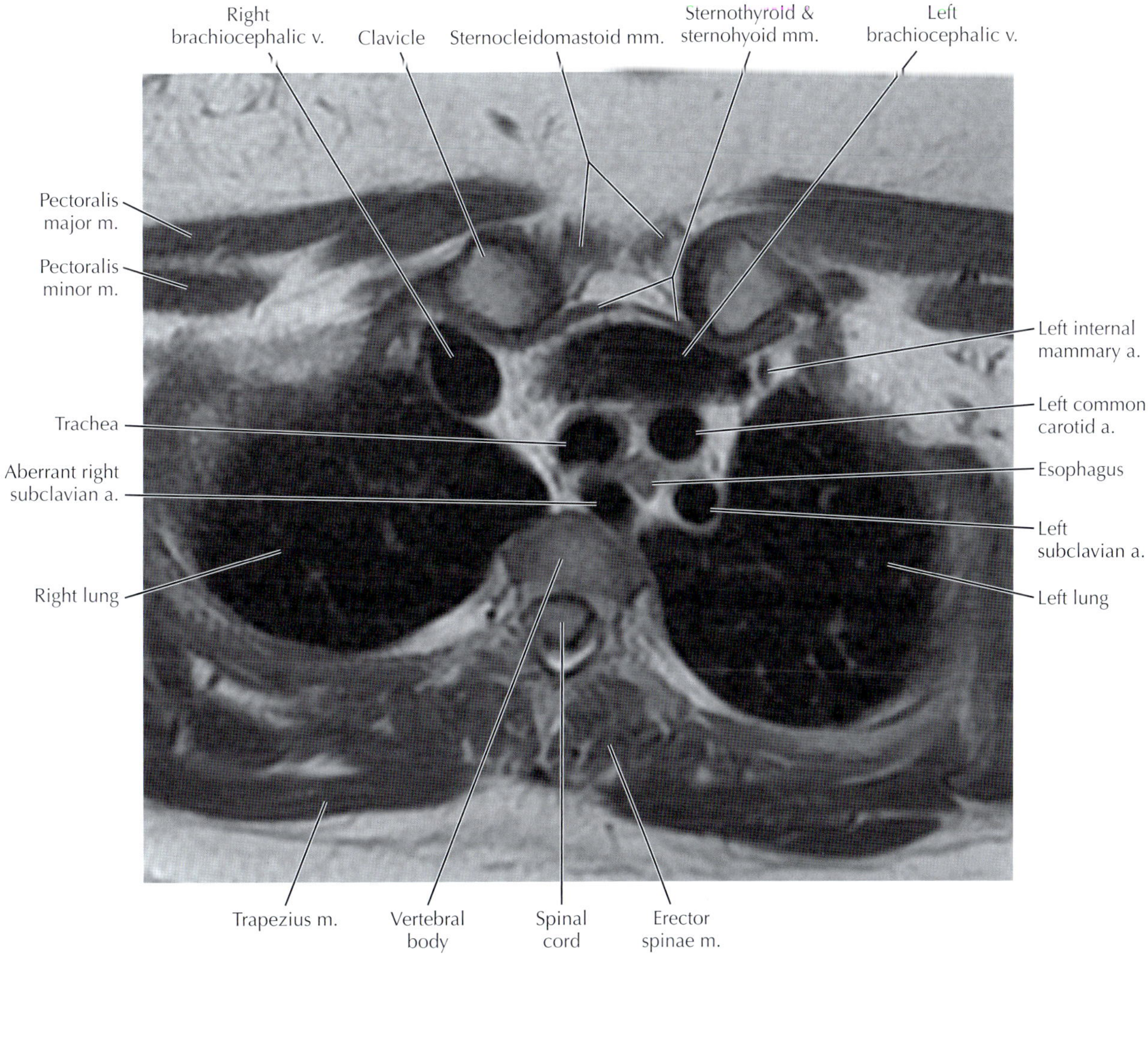
Right brachiocephalic v.
Clavicle
Sternocleidomastoid mm.
Sternothyroid & sternohyoid mm.
Left brachiocephalic v.
Pectoralis major m.
Pectoralis minor m.
Left internal mammary a.
Trachea
Left common carotid a.
Esophagus
Aberrant right subclavian a.
Left subclavian a.
Right lung
Left lung
Trapezius m.
Vertebral body
Spinal cord
Erector spinae m.

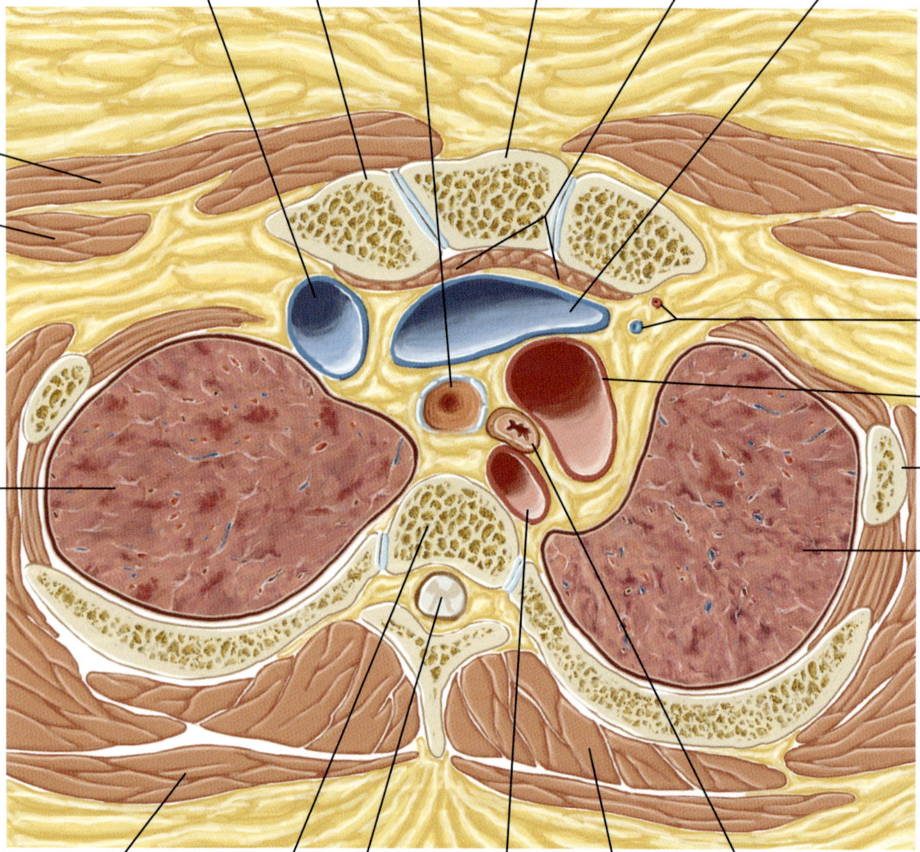
Right brachiocephalic v.
Clavicle
Trachea
Manubrium
Sternothyroid & sternohyoid mm.
Left brachiocephalic v.
Pectoralis major m.
Pectoralis minor m.
Left internal mammary a. & v.
Aortic arch
Rib
Right lung
Left lung
Trapezius m.
Vertebral body
Spinal cord
Aberrant right subclavian a.
Erector spinae m.
Esophagus

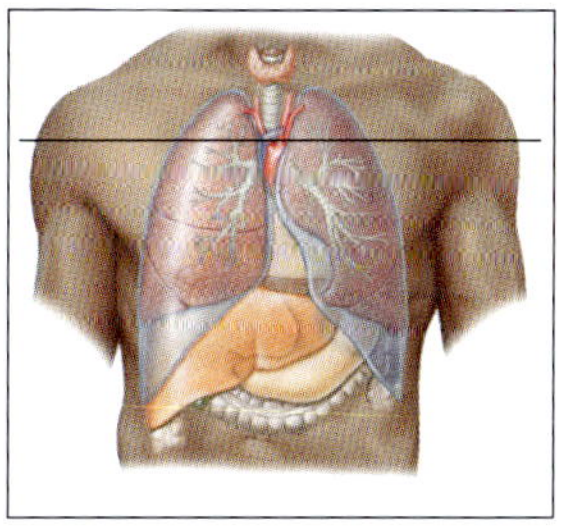

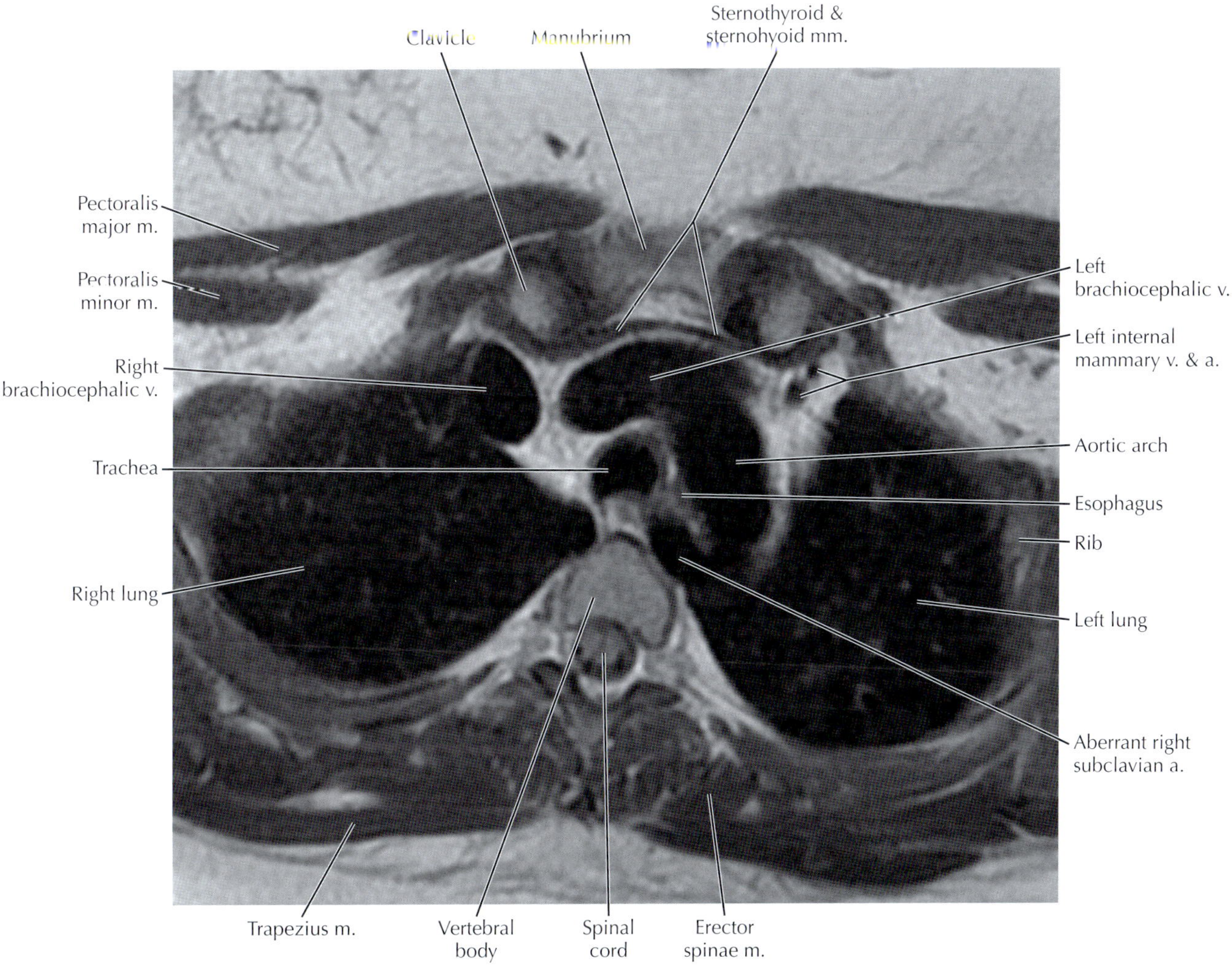

Clavicle
Manubrium
Sternothyroid & sternohyoid mm.
Pectoralis major m.
Pectoralis minor m.
Right brachiocephalic v.
Trachea
Right lung
Left brachiocephalic v.
Left internal mammary v. & a.
Aortic arch
Esophagus
Rib
Left lung
Aberrant right subclavian a.
Trapezius m.
Vertebral body
Spinal cord
Erector spinae m.

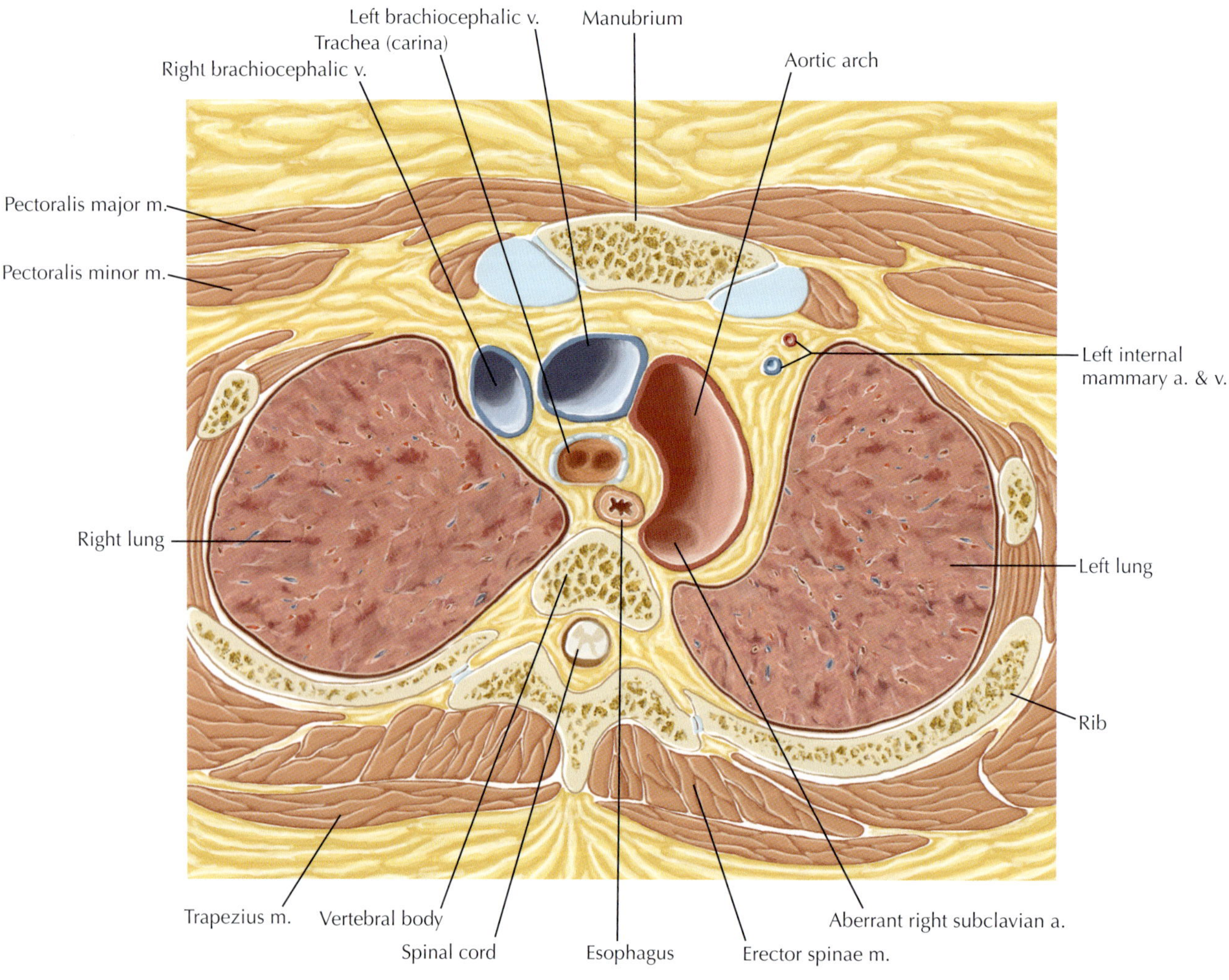
Left brachiocephalic v.
Manubrium
Trachea (carina)
Right brachiocephalic v.
Aortic arch
Pectoralis major m.
Pectoralis minor m.
Left internal mammary a. & v.
Right lung
Left lung
Rib
Trapezius m.
Vertebral body
Spinal cord
Esophagus
Erector spinae m.
Aberrant right subclavian a.

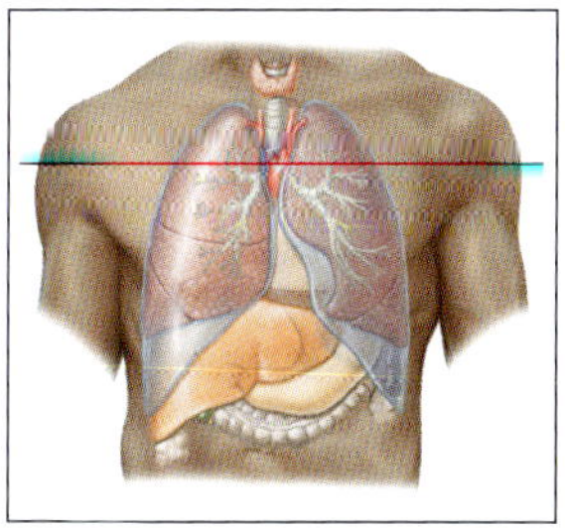

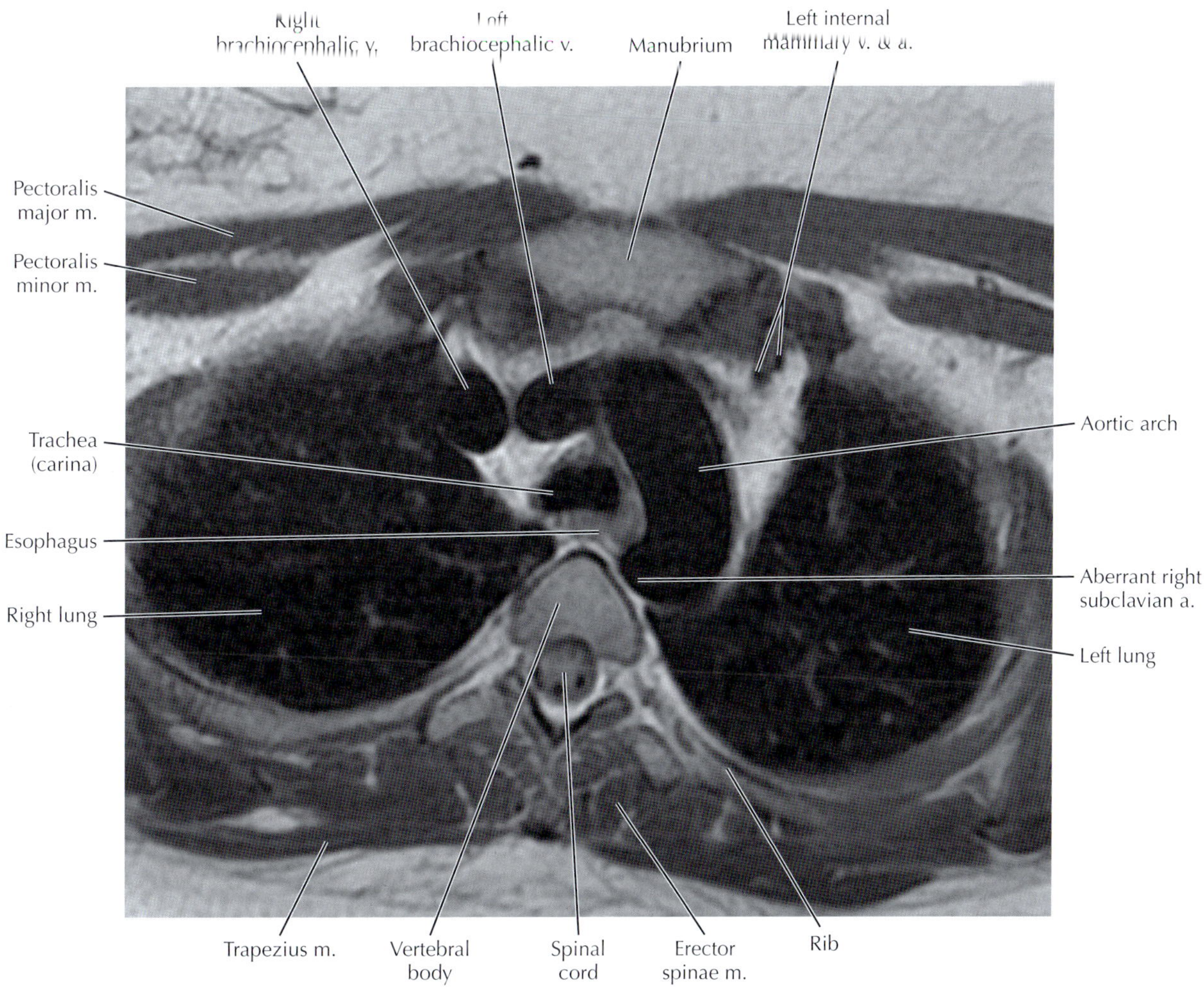
Right brachiocephalic v.
Left brachiocephalic v.
Manubrium
Left internal mammary v. & a.
Pectoralis major m.
Pectoralis minor m.
Trachea (carina)
Esophagus
Right lung
Aortic arch
Aberrant right subclavian a.
Left lung
Trapezius m.
Vertebral body
Spinal cord
Erector spinae m.
Rib

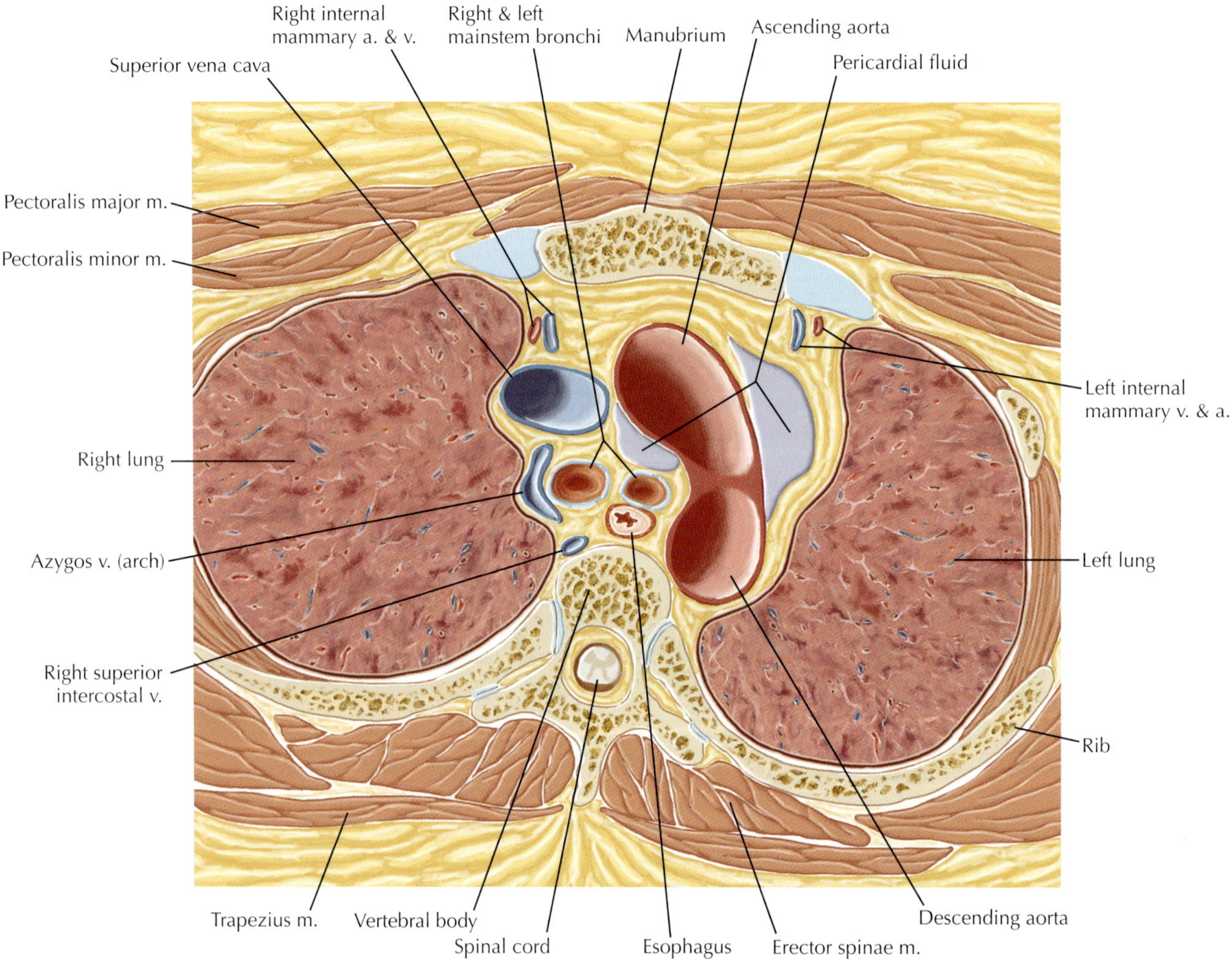

TECHNICAL CONSIDERATION

These two MR images illustrate two of the many MR techniques used to examine the thoracic and cardiovascular system: "black blood" and "white blood" imaging techniques, named for the appearance of flowing blood on the image. There are a number of ways in which "black blood" images may be created, but these techniques have in common the lack of significant signal associated with flowing blood—hence, the vessels and cardiac chambers appear black. "White blood" sequences are often used for functional analysis and, although the bright signal within the vessels and cardiac chambers gives the impression that intravenous contrast has been injected, these imaging sequences do not require the use of intravenous contrast to generate signal within the vascular system.

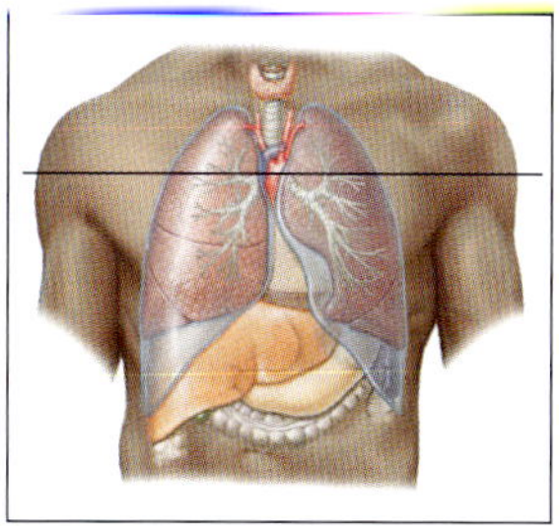

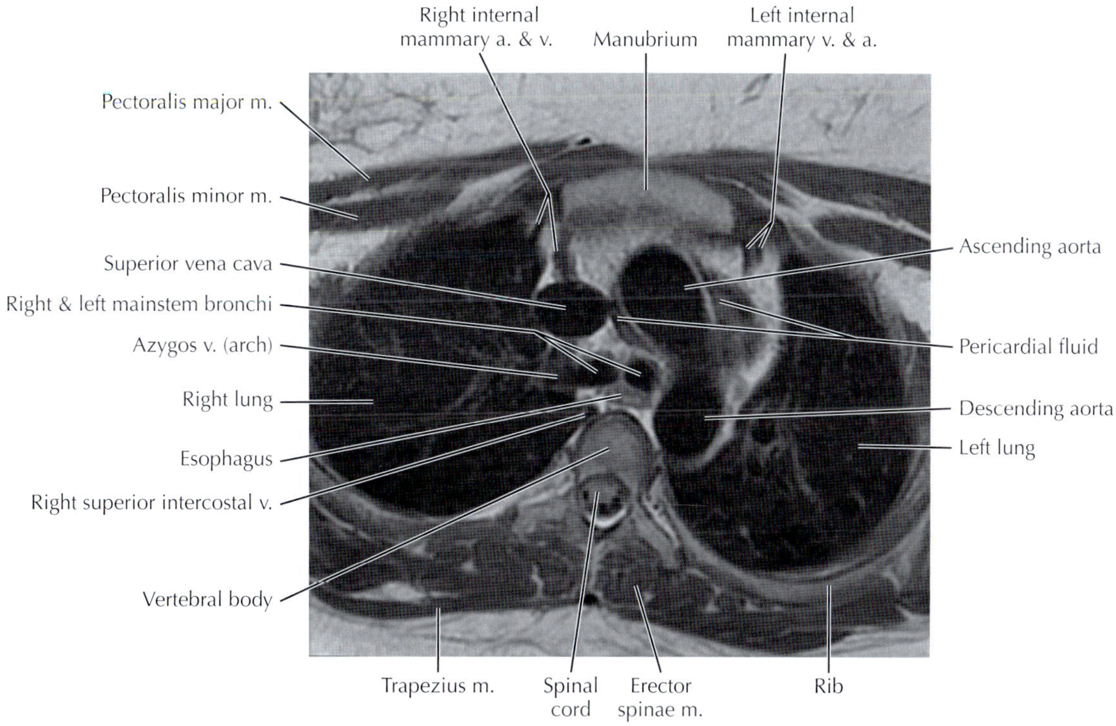
Right internal mammary a. & v.
Manubrium
Left internal mammary v. & a.
Pectoralis major m.
Pectoralis minor m.
Superior vena cava
Right & left mainstem bronchi
Azygos v. (arch)
Right lung
Esophagus
Right superior intercostal v.
Vertebral body
Ascending aorta
Pericardial fluid
Descending aorta
Left lung
Trapezius m.
Spinal cord
Erector spinae m.
Rib

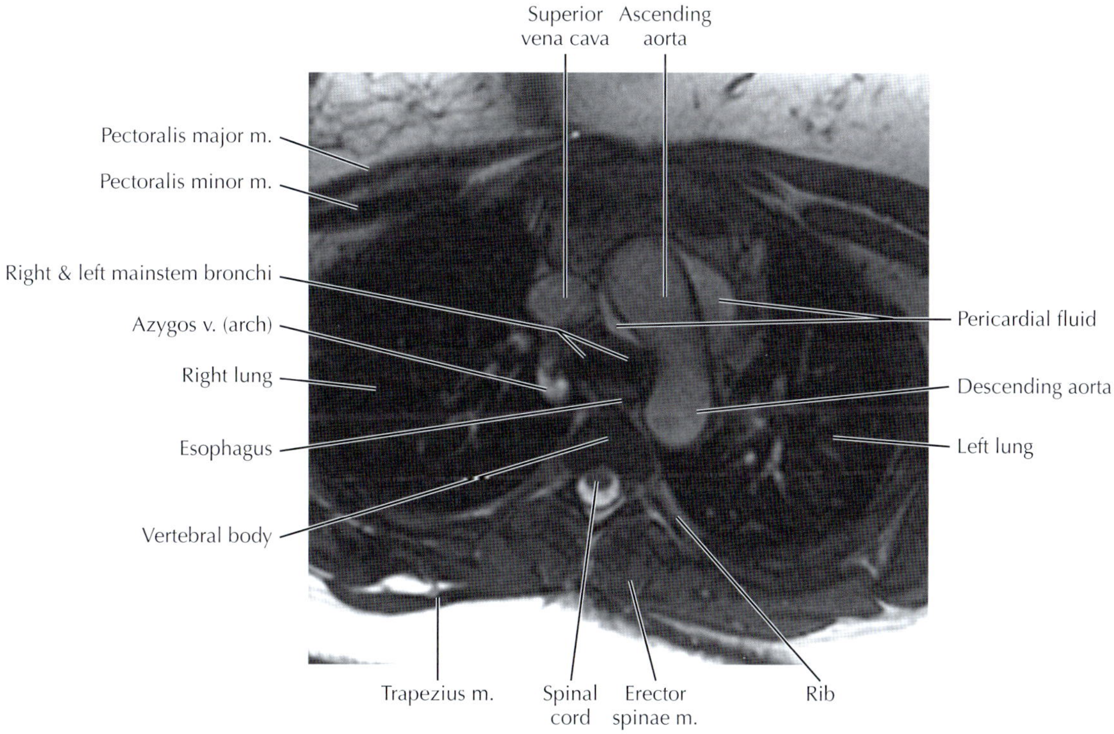
Superior vena cava
Ascending aorta
Pectoralis major m.
Pectoralis minor m.
Right & left mainstem bronchi
Azygos v. (arch)
Right lung
Esophagus
Vertebral body
Pericardial fluid
Descending aorta
Left lung
Trapezius m.
Spinal cord
Erector spinae m.
Rib

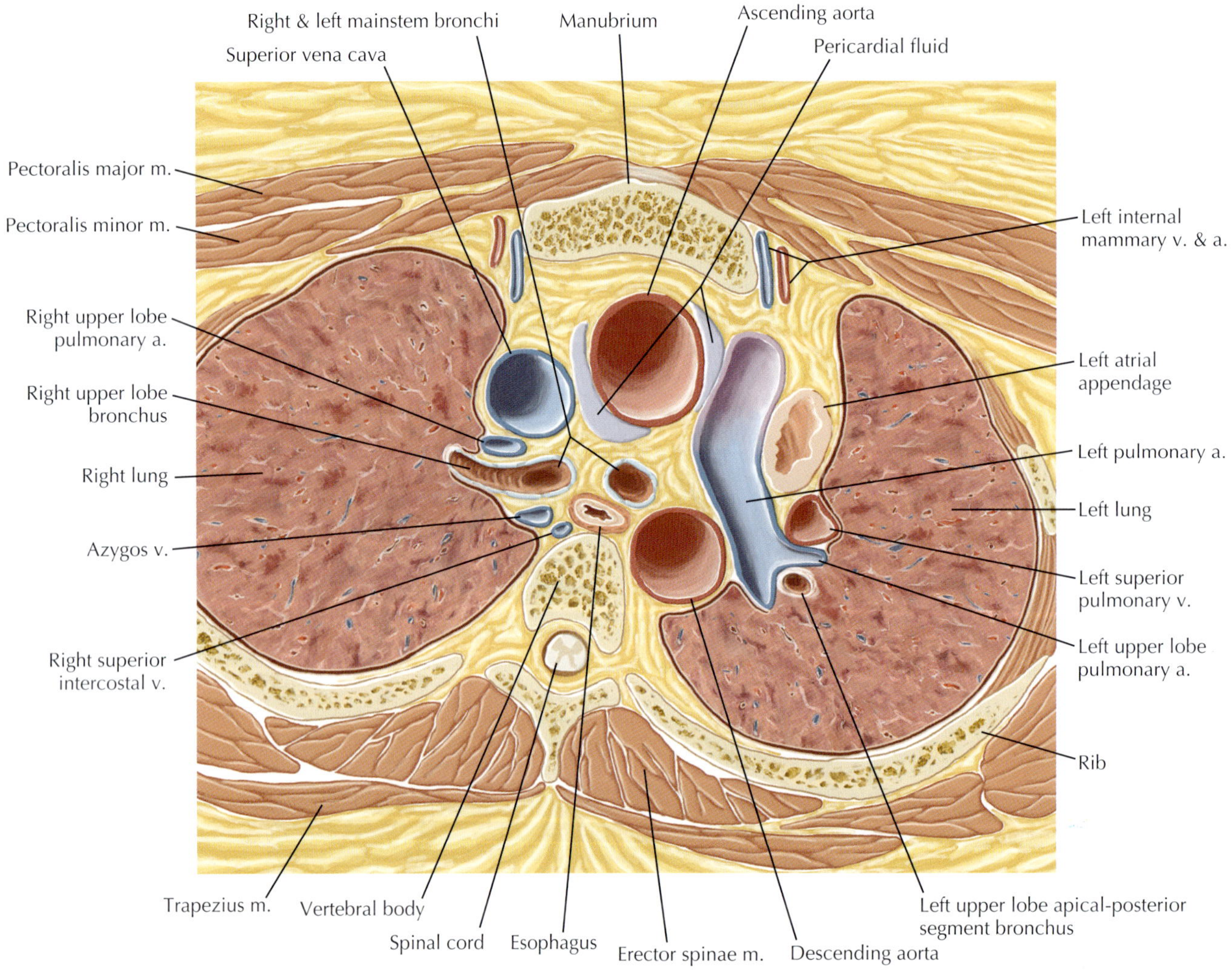

Right & left mainstem bronchi
Manubrium
Ascending aorta
Pericardial fluid
Superior vena cava
Pectoralis major m.
Pectoralis minor m.
Left internal mammary v. & a.
Right upper lobe pulmonary a.
Left atrial appendage
Right upper lobe bronchus
Left pulmonary a.
Right lung
Left lung
Azygos v.
Left superior pulmonary v.
Left upper lobe pulmonary a.
Right superior intercostal v.
Rib
Trapezius m.
Vertebral body
Spinal cord
Esophagus
Erector spinae m.
Descending aorta
Left upper lobe apical-posterior segment bronchus

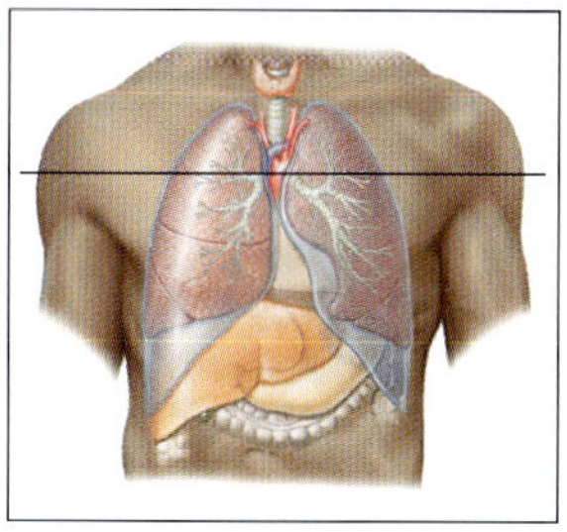

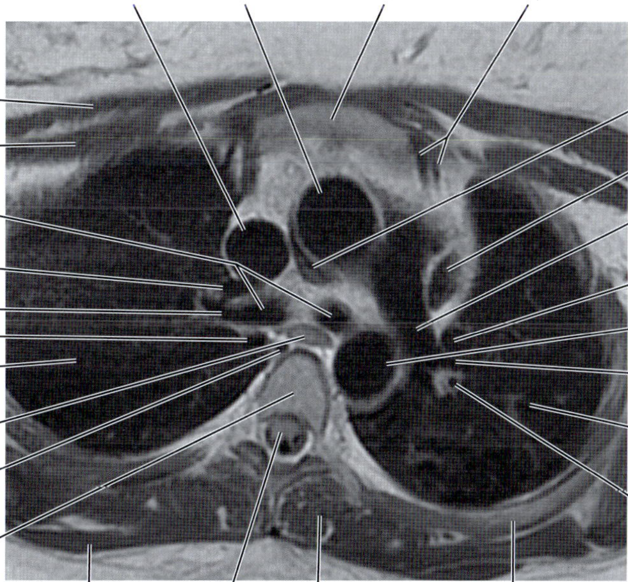
Superior vena cava
Ascending aorta
Manubrium
Left internal mammary v. & a.
Pectoralis major m.
Pectoralis minor m.
Right & left mainstem bronchi
Right upper lobe pulmonary a.
Right upper lobe bronchus
Azygos v.
Right lung
Esophagus
Right superior intercostal v.
Vertebral body
Pericardial fluid
Left atrial appendage
Left pulmonary a.
Left superior pulmonary v.
Descending aorta
Left upper lobe pulmonary a.
Left lung
Left upper lobe apical-posterior segment bronchus
Trapezius m.
Spinal cord
Erector spinae m.
Rib

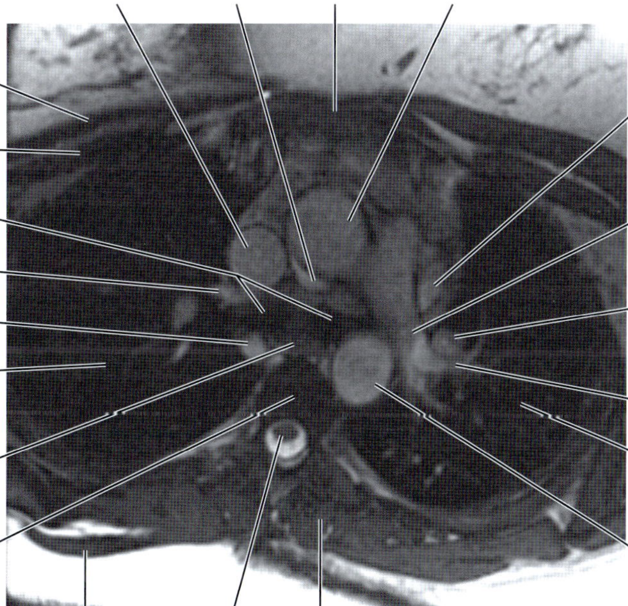
Superior vena cava
Pericardial fluid
Manubrium
Ascending aorta
Pectoralis major m.
Pectoralis minor m.
Right & left mainstem bronchi
Right upper lobe pulmonary a.
Azygos v.
Right lung
Esophagus
Vertebral body
Left atrial appendage
Left pulmonary a.
Left superior pulmonary v.
Left upper lobe pulmonary a.
Left lung
Descending aorta
Trapezius m.
Spinal cord
Erector spinae m.

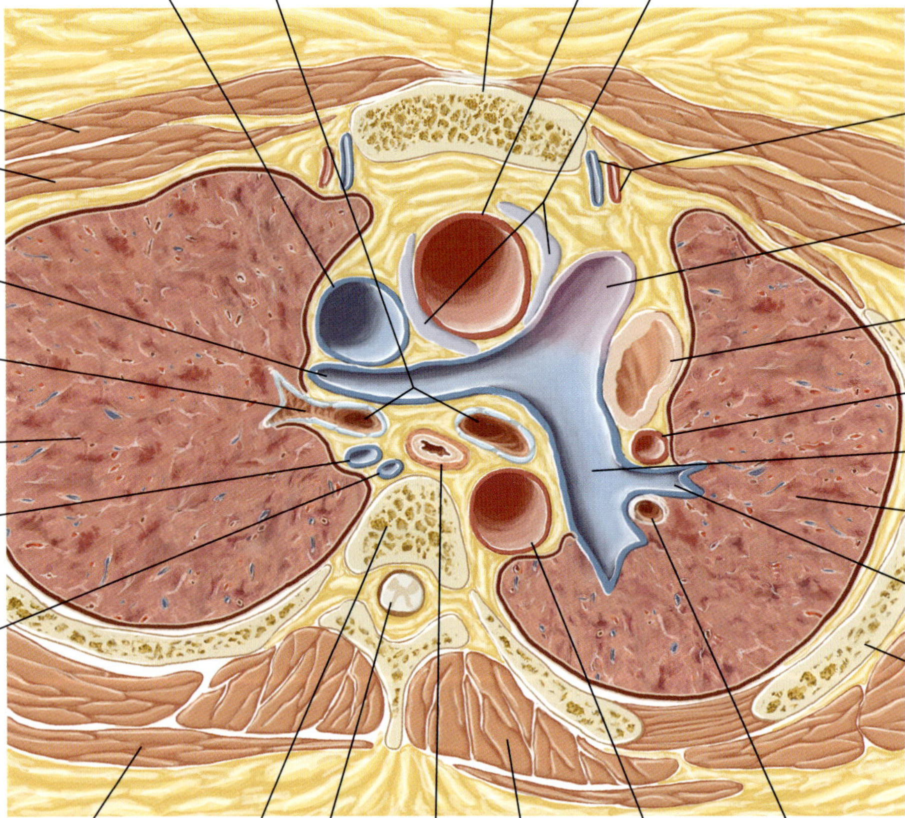

DIAGNOSTIC CONSIDERATION

A small amount of pericardial fluid is shown surrounding the ascending aorta. The normal pericardial sac is composed of an outer fibrous layer and an inner serous pericardial sac. The serous pericardium consists of an inner visceral layer (the epicardium), which is intimately adherent to the heart and epicardial fat, and an outer parietal layer, which lines the inner surface of the fibrous pericardium. The pericardial sac is divided into the pericardium proper and a number of sinuses and recesses. Up to 25 mL of fluid may be present within the pericardial sac under normal conditions. On MR and CT, normal pericardium is often seen, and the thickness of normal pericardium typically does not exceed 2 mm.

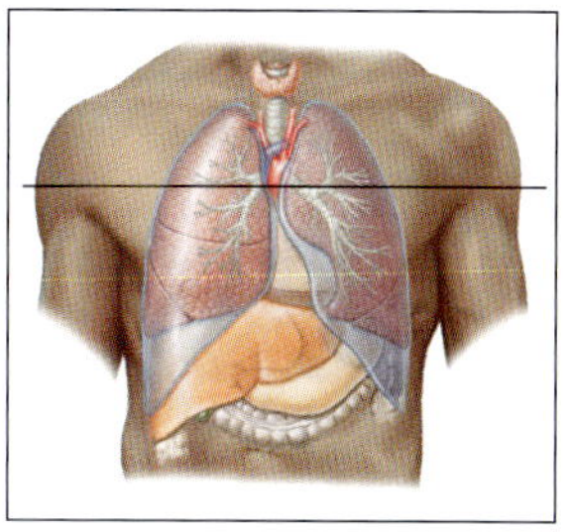

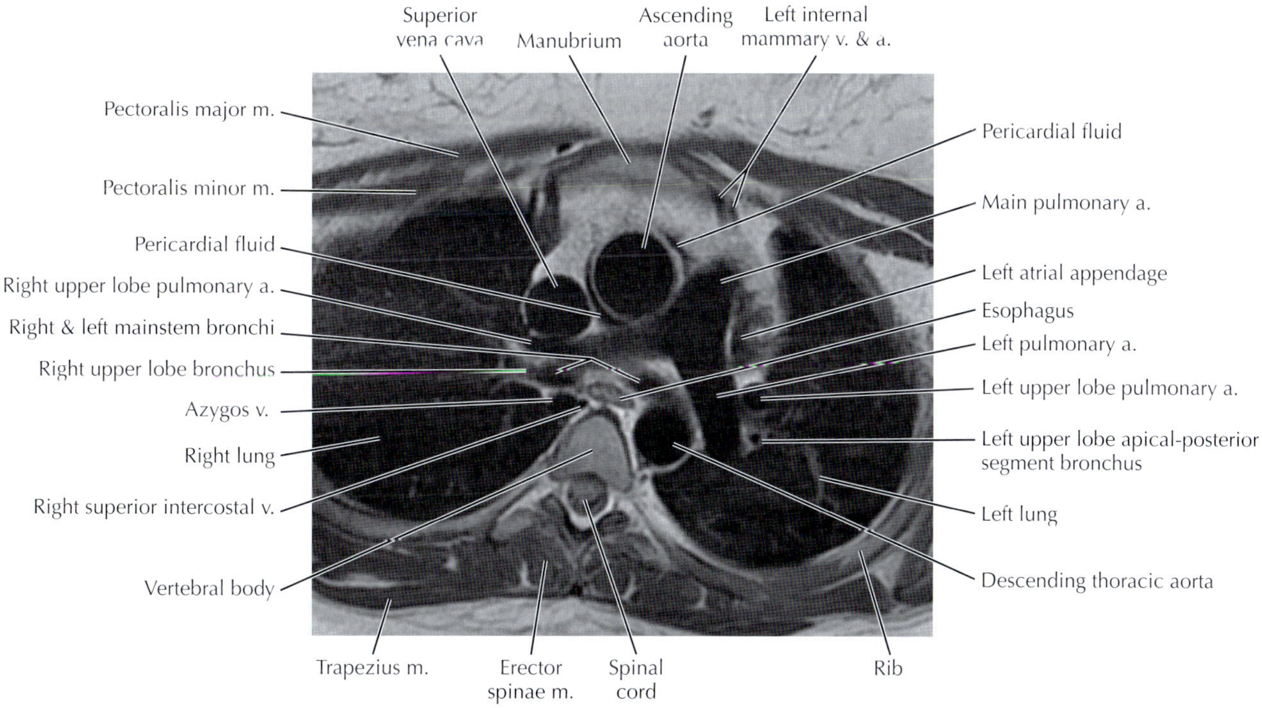
Superior vena cava
Manubrium
Ascending aorta
Left internal mammary v. & a.
Pectoralis major m.
Pectoralis minor m.
Pericardial fluid
Right upper lobe pulmonary a.
Right & left mainstem bronchi
Right upper lobe bronchus
Azygos v.
Right lung
Right superior intercostal v.
Vertebral body
Pericardial fluid
Main pulmonary a.
Left atrial appendage
Esophagus
Left pulmonary a.
Left upper lobe pulmonary a.
Left upper lobe apical-posterior segment bronchus
Left lung
Descending thoracic aorta
Trapezius m.
Erector spinae m.
Spinal cord
Rib

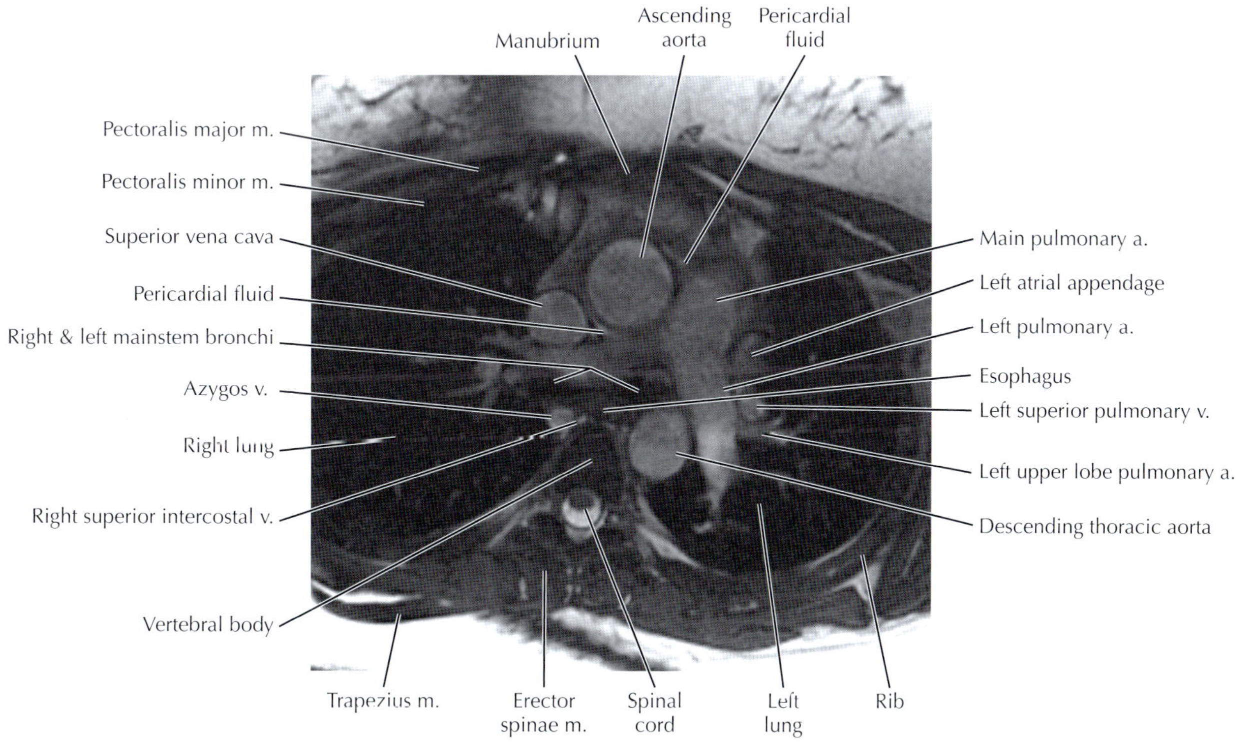
Manubrium
Ascending aorta
Pericardial fluid
Pectoralis major m.
Pectoralis minor m.
Superior vena cava
Pericardial fluid
Right & left mainstem bronchi
Azygos v.
Right lung
Right superior intercostal v.
Vertebral body
Main pulmonary a.
Left atrial appendage
Left pulmonary a.
Esophagus
Left superior pulmonary v.
Left upper lobe pulmonary a.
Descending thoracic aorta
Trapezius m.
Erector spinae m.
Spinal cord
Left lung
Rib

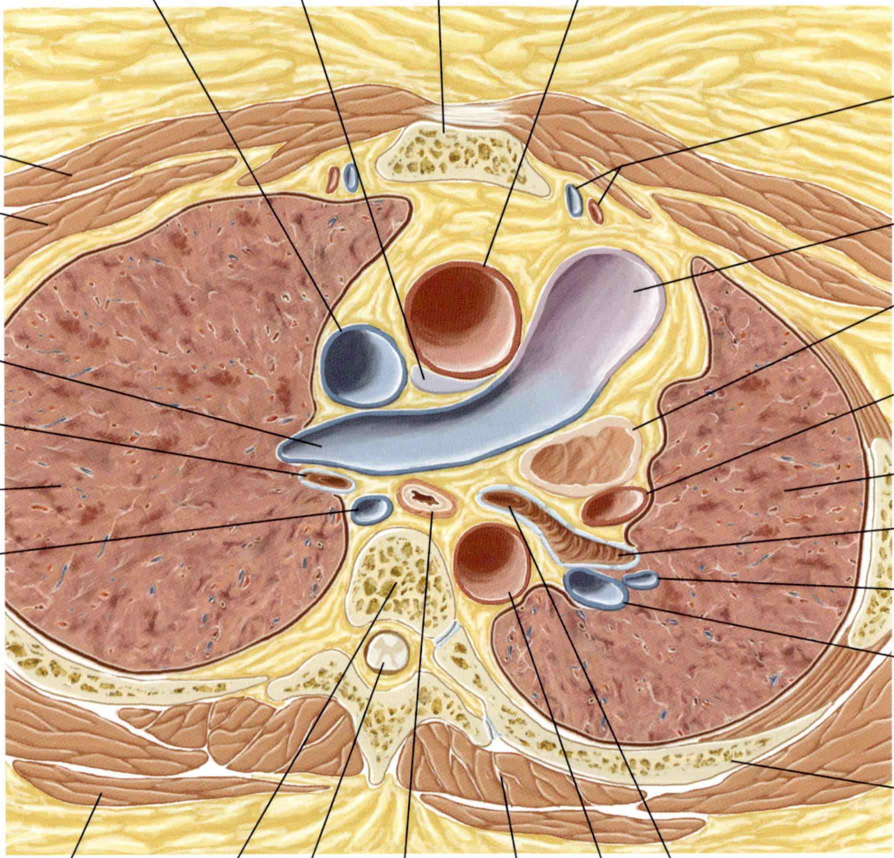
Pericardial fluid
Manubrium
Superior vena cava
Ascending aorta
Left internal mammary v. & a.
Pectoralis major m.
Pectoralis minor m.
Main pulmonary a.
Left atrial appendage
Right pulmonary a.
Left superior pulmonary v.
Bronchus intermedius
Left lung
Right lung
Left upper lobe bronchus
Azygos v.
Lingular pulmonary a.
Left interlobar pulmonary a.
Rib
Left mainstem bronchus
Trapezius m.
Vertebral body
Erector spinae m.
Descending aorta
Spinal cord
Esophagus

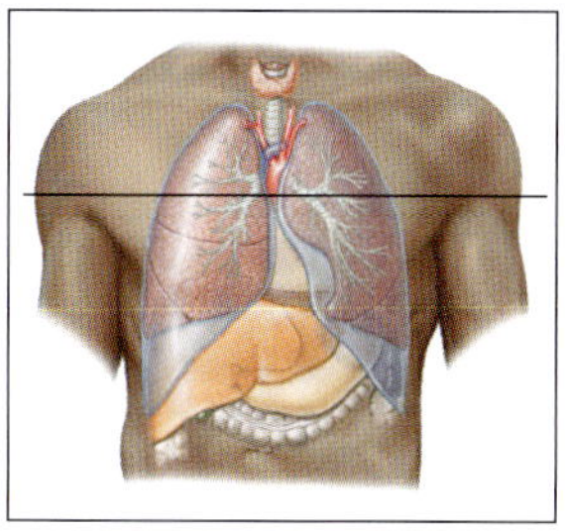

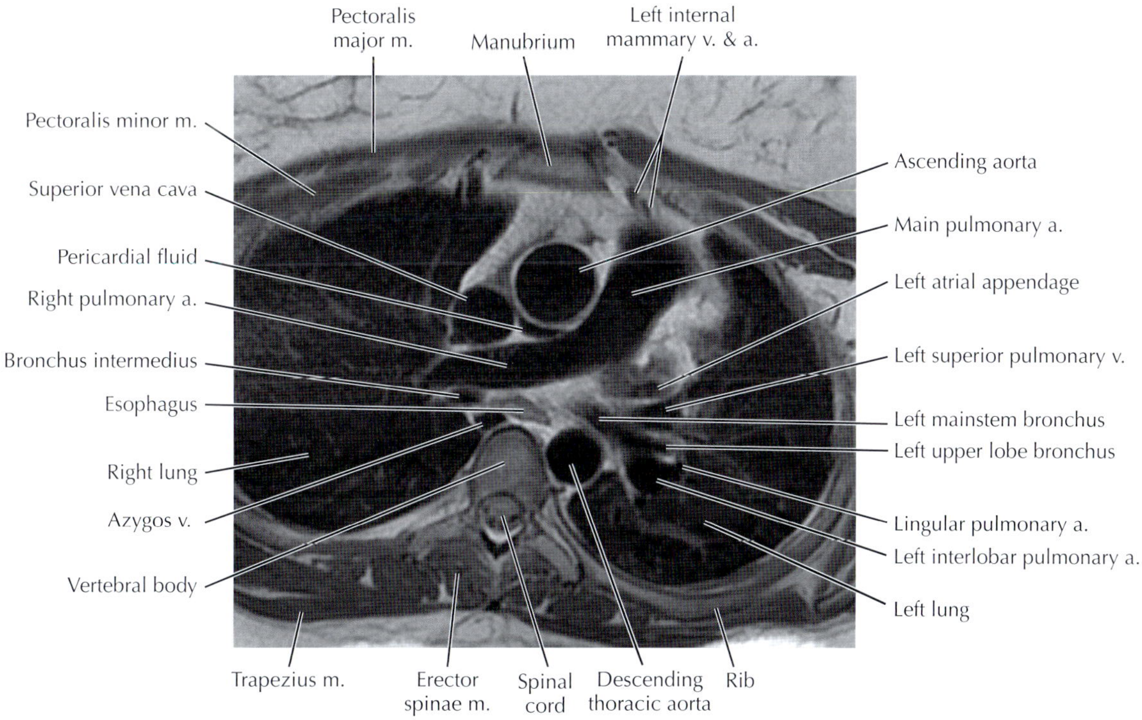
Pectoralis major m.
Manubrium
Left internal mammary v. & a.
Pectoralis minor m.
Superior vena cava
Pericardial fluid
Right pulmonary a.
Bronchus intermedius
Esophagus
Right lung
Azygos v.
Vertebral body
Ascending aorta
Main pulmonary a.
Left atrial appendage
Left superior pulmonary v.
Left mainstem bronchus
Left upper lobe bronchus
Lingular pulmonary a.
Left interlobar pulmonary a.
Left lung
Trapezius m.
Erector spinae m.
Spinal cord
Descending thoracic aorta
Rib

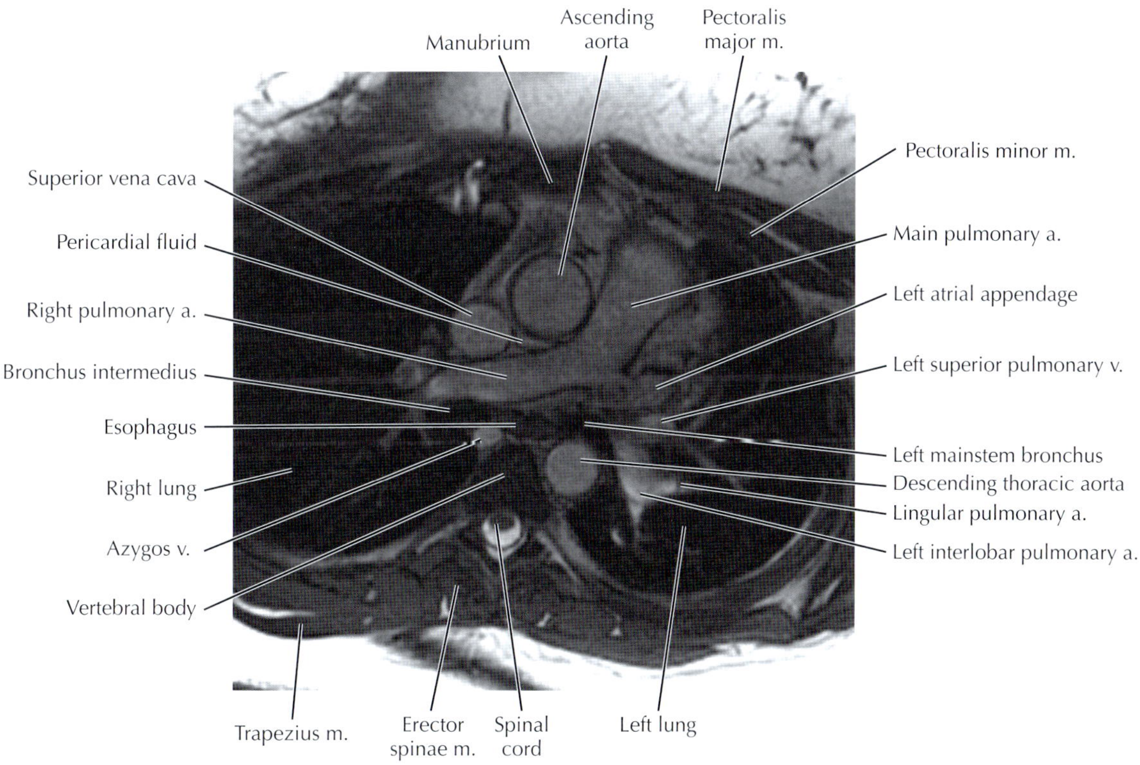
Manubrium
Ascending aorta
Pectoralis major m.
Superior vena cava
Pericardial fluid
Right pulmonary a.
Bronchus intermedius
Esophagus
Right lung
Azygos v.
Vertebral body
Pectoralis minor m.
Main pulmonary a.
Left atrial appendage
Left superior pulmonary v.
Left mainstem bronchus
Descending thoracic aorta
Lingular pulmonary a.
Left interlobar pulmonary a.
Trapezius m.
Erector spinae m.
Spinal cord
Left lung

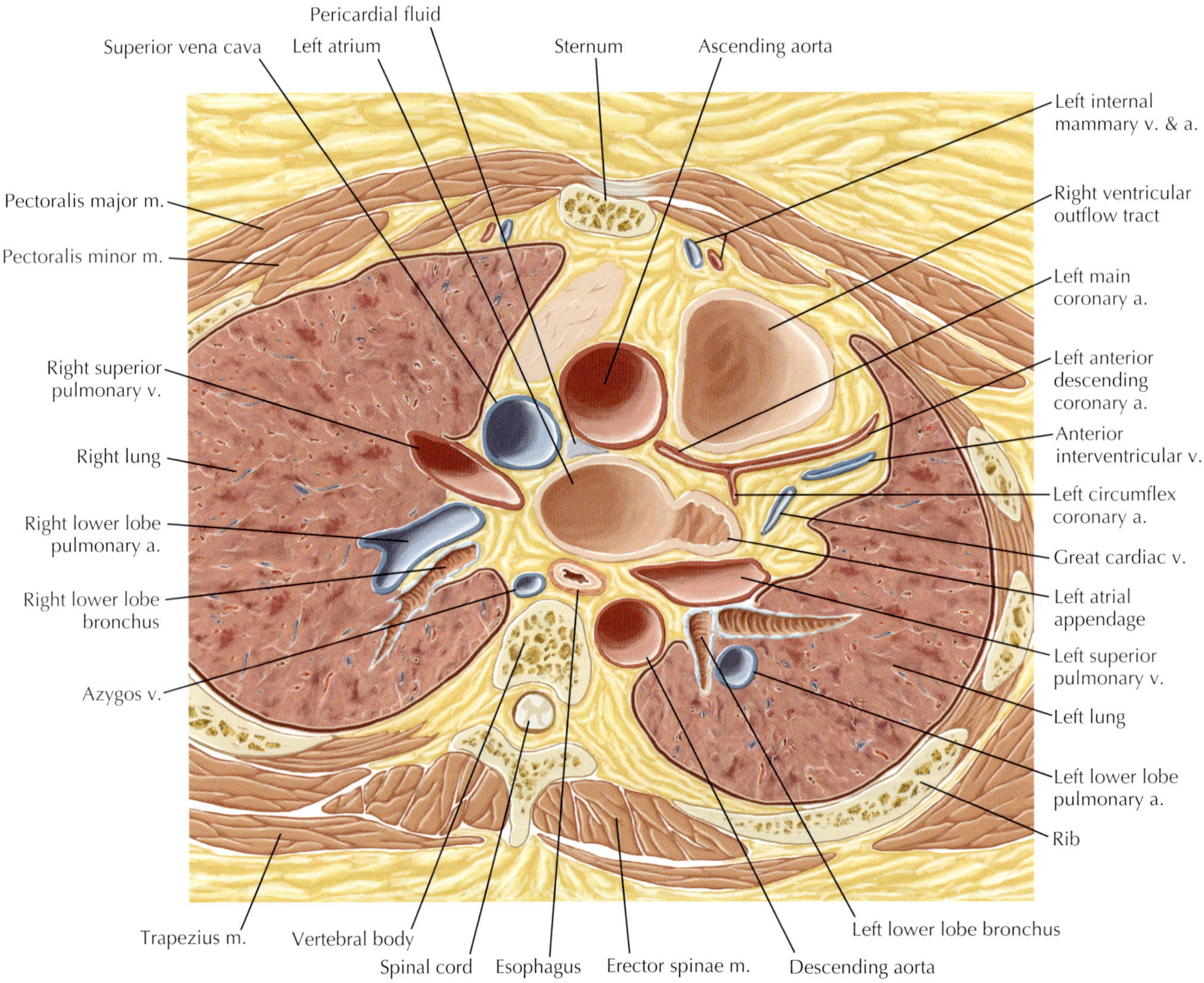
Pericardial fluid
Superior vena cava
Left atrium
Sternum
Ascending aorta
Left internal mammary v. & a.
Pectoralis major m.
Right ventricular outflow tract
Pectoralis minor m.
Left main coronary a.
Left anterior descending coronary a.
Right superior pulmonary v.
Anterior interventricular v.
Right lung
Left circumflex coronary a.
Right lower lobe pulmonary a.
Great cardiac v.
Left atrial appendage
Right lower lobe bronchus
Left superior pulmonary v.
Azygos v.
Left lung
Left lower lobe pulmonary a.
Rib
Left lower lobe bronchus
Trapezius m.
Vertebral body
Spinal cord
Esophagus
Erector spinae m.
Descending aorta

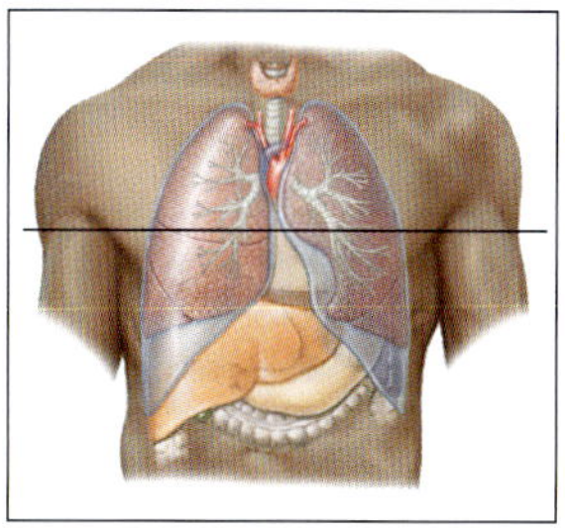

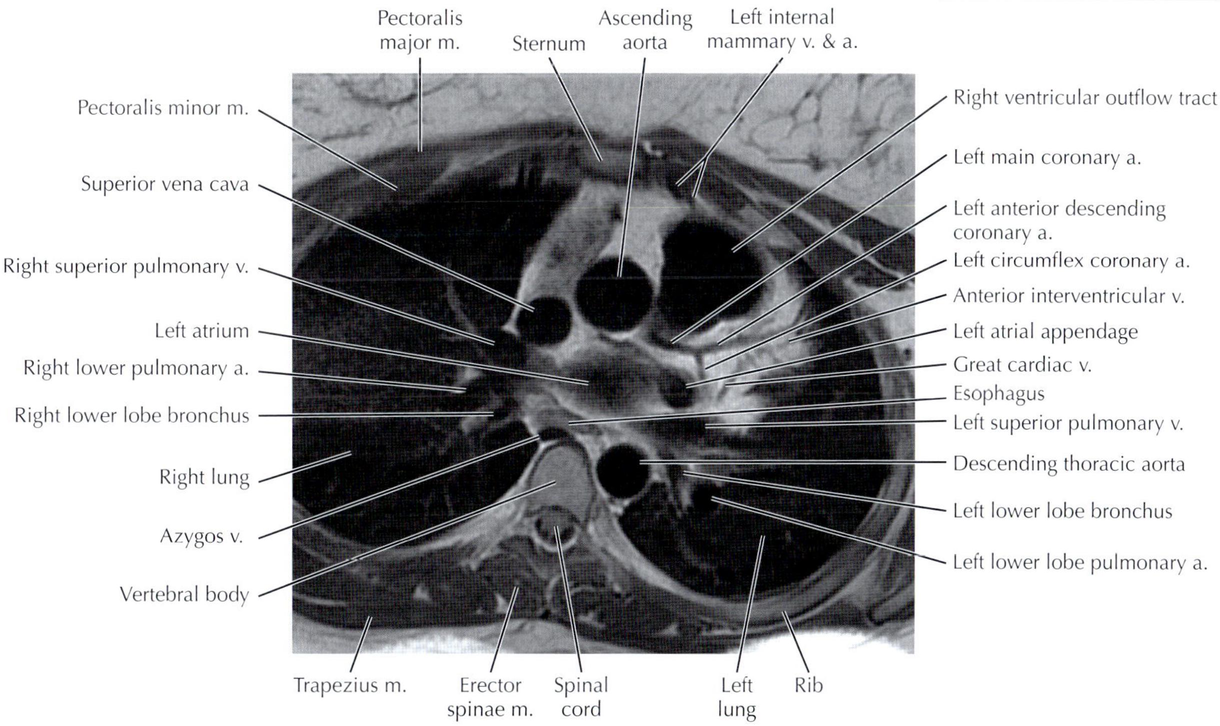
Pectoralis major m.
Sternum
Ascending aorta
Left internal mammary v. & a.
Pectoralis minor m.
Superior vena cava
Right superior pulmonary v.
Left atrium
Right lower pulmonary a.
Right lower lobe bronchus
Right lung
Azygos v.
Vertebral body
Right ventricular outflow tract
Left main coronary a.
Left anterior descending coronary a.
Left circumflex coronary a.
Anterior interventricular v.
Left atrial appendage
Great cardiac v.
Esophagus
Left superior pulmonary v.
Descending thoracic aorta
Left lower lobe bronchus
Left lower lobe pulmonary a.
Trapezius m.
Erector spinae m.
Spinal cord
Left lung
Rib

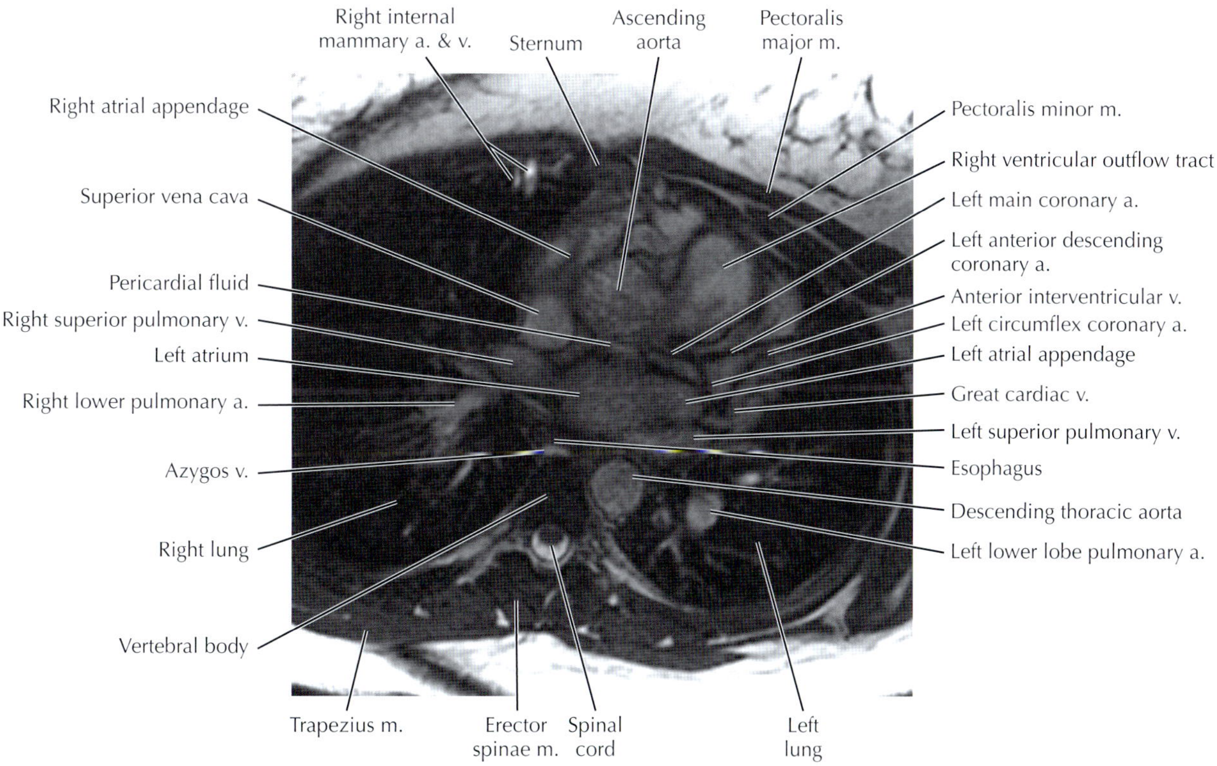
Right internal mammary a. & v.
Sternum
Ascending aorta
Pectoralis major m.
Right atrial appendage
Superior vena cava
Pericardial fluid
Right superior pulmonary v.
Left atrium
Right lower pulmonary a.
Azygos v.
Right lung
Vertebral body
Pectoralis minor m.
Right ventricular outflow tract
Left main coronary a.
Left anterior descending coronary a.
Anterior interventricular v.
Left circumflex coronary a.
Left atrial appendage
Great cardiac v.
Left superior pulmonary v.
Esophagus
Descending thoracic aorta
Left lower lobe pulmonary a.
Trapezius m.
Erector spinae m.
Spinal cord
Left lung

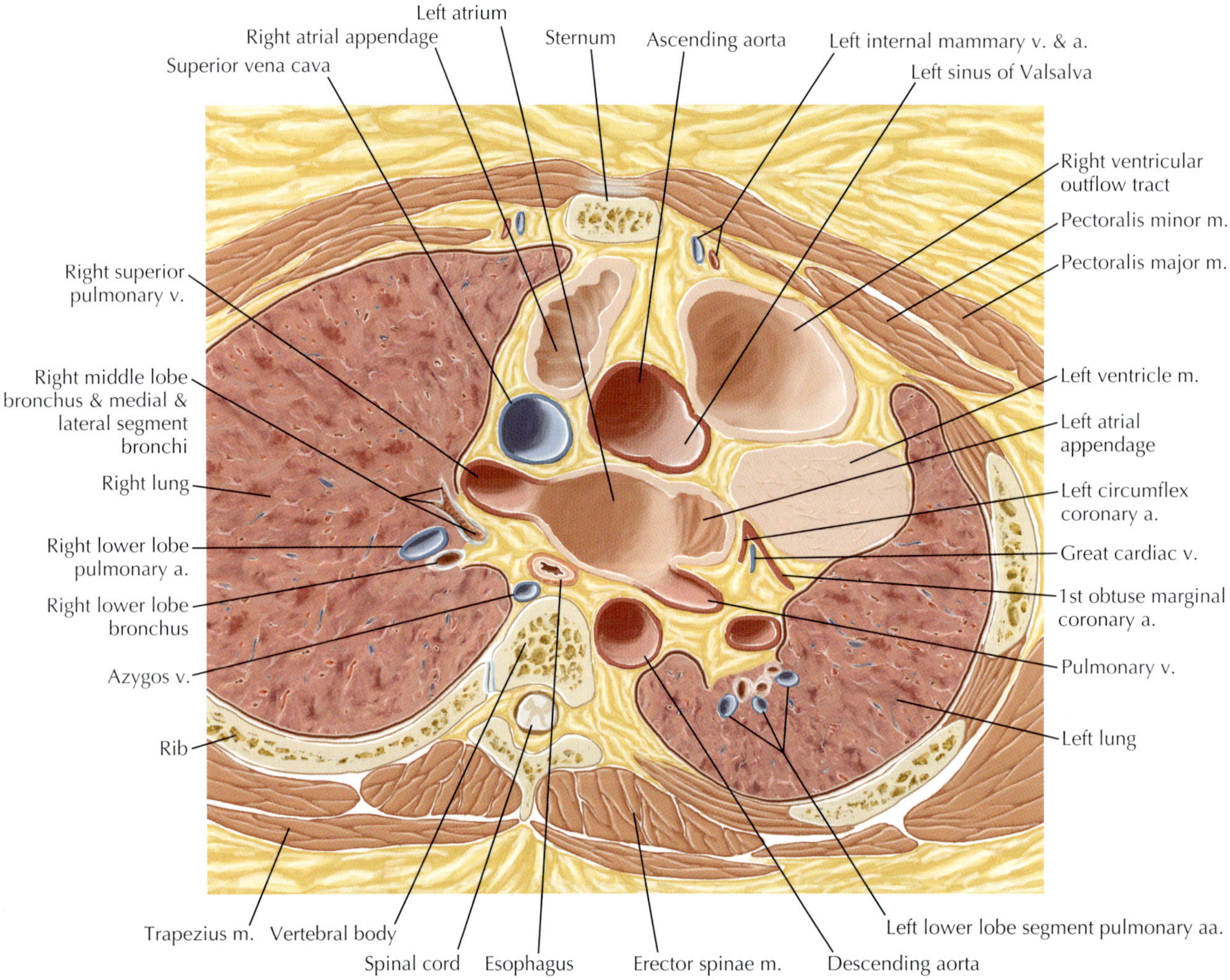
Left atrium
Right atrial appendage
Sternum
Ascending aorta
Left internal mammary v. & a.
Superior vena cava
Left sinus of Valsalva
Right ventricular outflow tract
Pectoralis minor m.
Pectoralis major m.
Right superior pulmonary v.
Right middle lobe bronchus & medial & lateral segment bronchi
Left ventricle m.
Left atrial appendage
Right lung
Left circumflex coronary a.
Right lower lobe pulmonary a.
Great cardiac v.
Right lower lobe bronchus
1st obtuse marginal coronary a.
Azygos v.
Pulmonary v.
Rib
Left lung
Trapezius m.
Vertebral body
Left lower lobe segment pulmonary aa.
Spinal cord
Esophagus
Erector spinae m.
Descending aorta

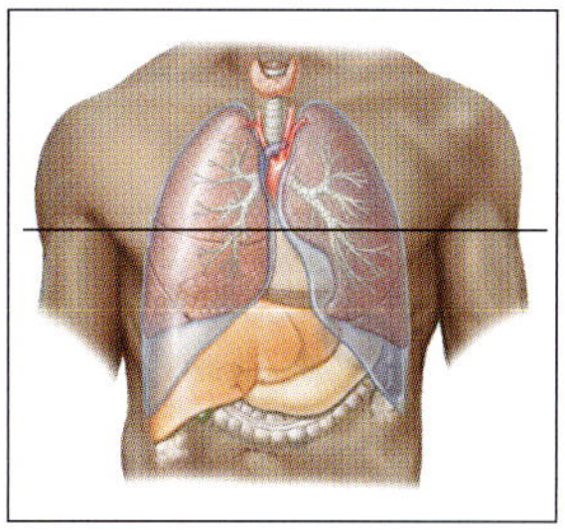

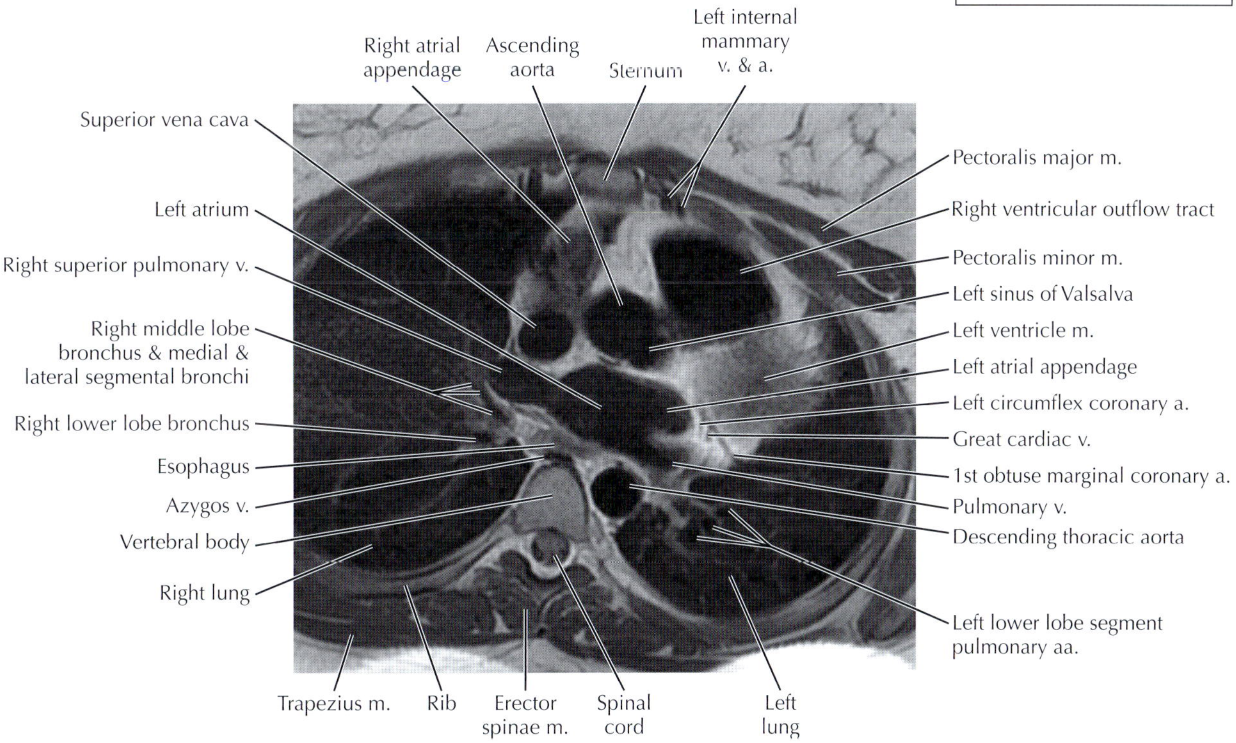
Right atrial appendage
Ascending aorta
Sternum
Left internal mammary v. & a.
Superior vena cava
Left atrium
Right superior pulmonary v.
Right middle lobe bronchus & medial & lateral segmental bronchi
Right lower lobe bronchus
Esophagus
Azygos v.
Vertebral body
Right lung
Pectoralis major m.
Right ventricular outflow tract
Pectoralis minor m.
Left sinus of Valsalva
Left ventricle m.
Left atrial appendage
Left circumflex coronary a.
Great cardiac v.
1st obtuse marginal coronary a.
Pulmonary v.
Descending thoracic aorta
Left lower lobe segment pulmonary aa.
Trapezius m.
Rib
Erector spinae m.
Spinal cord
Left lung

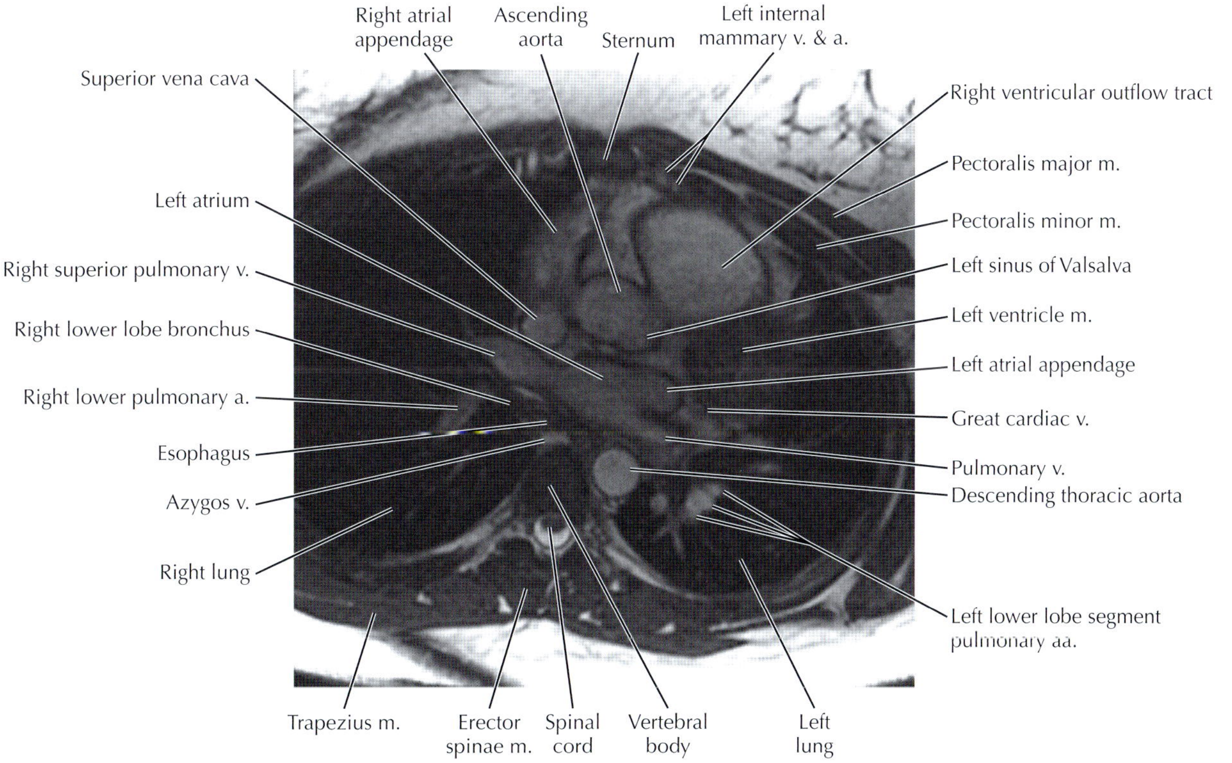
Right atrial appendage
Ascending aorta
Sternum
Left internal mammary v. & a.
Superior vena cava
Left atrium
Right superior pulmonary v.
Right lower lobe bronchus
Right lower pulmonary a.
Esophagus
Azygos v.
Right lung
Right ventricular outflow tract
Pectoralis major m.
Pectoralis minor m.
Left sinus of Valsalva
Left ventricle m.
Left atrial appendage
Great cardiac v.
Pulmonary v.
Descending thoracic aorta
Left lower lobe segment pulmonary aa.
Trapezius m.
Erector spinae m.
Spinal cord
Vertebral body
Left lung

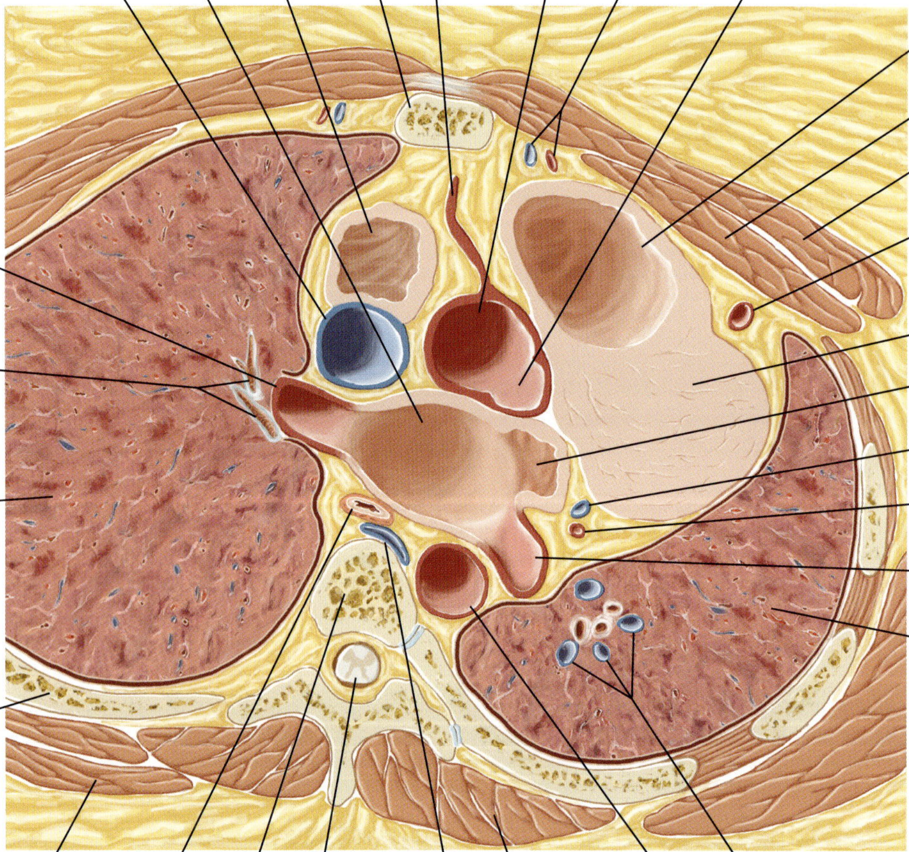

Right atrial appendage
Left atrium
Superior vena cava
Right coronary a.
Sternum
Ascending aorta
Left internal mammary v. & a.
Left sinus of Valsalva
Right ventricular outflow tract
Pectoralis minor m.
Pectoralis major m.
Left anterior descending coronary a.
Left ventricle m.
Left atrial appendage
Great cardiac v.
Left circumflex coronary a.
Left inferior pulmonary v.
Left lung
Right superior pulmonary v.
Right middle lobe medial & lateral segment bronchi
Right lung
Rib
Trapezius m.
Esophagus
Vertebral body
Spinal cord
Azygos v.
Erector spinae m.
Descending aorta
Left lower lobe segment pulmonary aa.

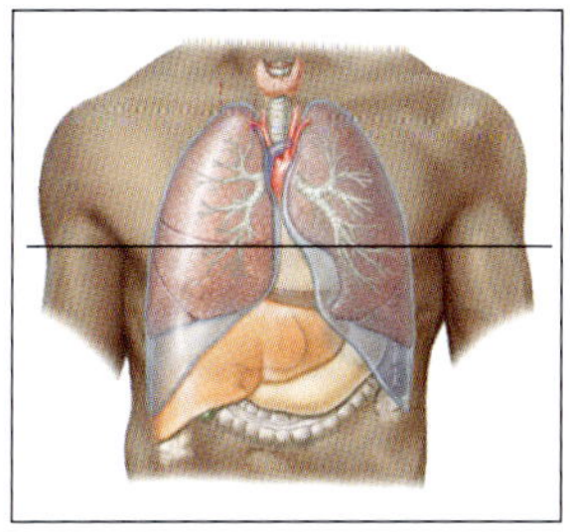

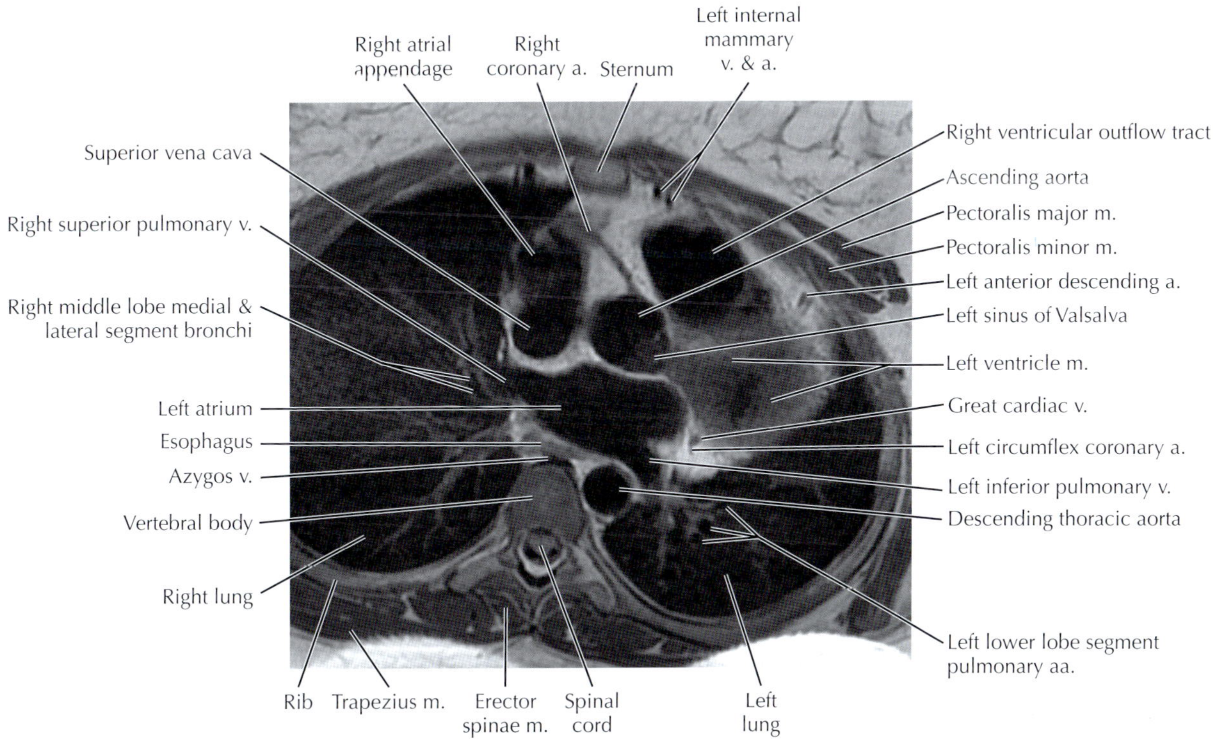
Right atrial appendage
Right coronary a.
Sternum
Left internal mammary v. & a.
Superior vena cava
Right superior pulmonary v.
Right middle lobe medial & lateral segment bronchi
Left atrium
Esophagus
Azygos v.
Vertebral body
Right lung
Right ventricular outflow tract
Ascending aorta
Pectoralis major m.
Pectoralis minor m.
Left anterior descending a.
Left sinus of Valsalva
Left ventricle m.
Great cardiac v.
Left circumflex coronary a.
Left inferior pulmonary v.
Descending thoracic aorta
Left lower lobe segment pulmonary aa.
Rib
Trapezius m.
Erector spinae m.
Spinal cord
Left lung

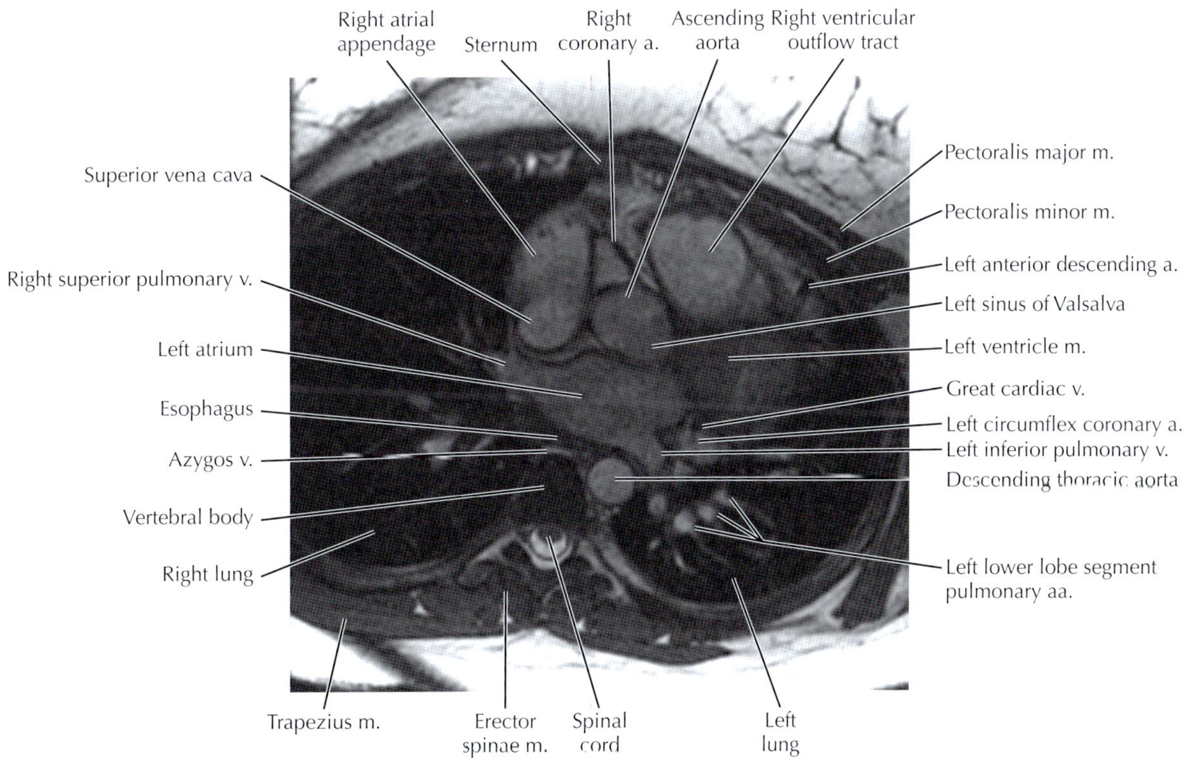
Right atrial appendage
Sternum
Right coronary a.
Ascending aorta
Right ventricular outflow tract
Superior vena cava
Right superior pulmonary v.
Left atrium
Esophagus
Azygos v.
Vertebral body
Right lung
Pectoralis major m.
Pectoralis minor m.
Left anterior descending a.
Left sinus of Valsalva
Left ventricle m.
Great cardiac v.
Left circumflex coronary a.
Left inferior pulmonary v.
Descending thoracic aorta
Left lower lobe segment pulmonary aa.
Trapezius m.
Erector spinae m.
Spinal cord
Left lung

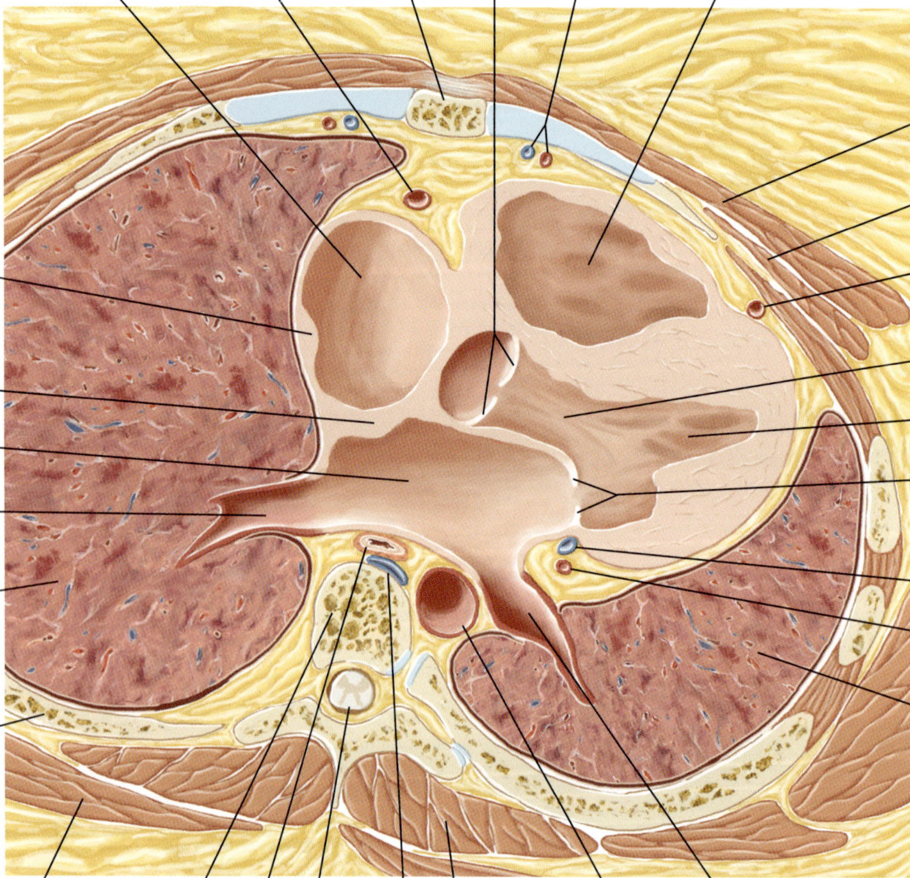
Aortic valve
Left internal mammary v. & a.
Right coronary a.
Sternum
Right ventricle
Right atrium
Pectoralis major m.
Pectoralis minor m.
Crista terminalis
Left anterior descending coronary a.
Interatrial septum
Left ventricular outflow tract
Left atrium
Left ventricle
Right inferior pulmonary v.
Mitral valve, anterior & posterior leaflets
Right lung
Great cardiac v.
Left circumflex coronary a.
Left lung
Rib
Trapezius m.
Vertebral body
Esophagus
Spinal cord
Azygos v.
Erector spinae m.
Descending aorta
Left inferior pulmonary v.

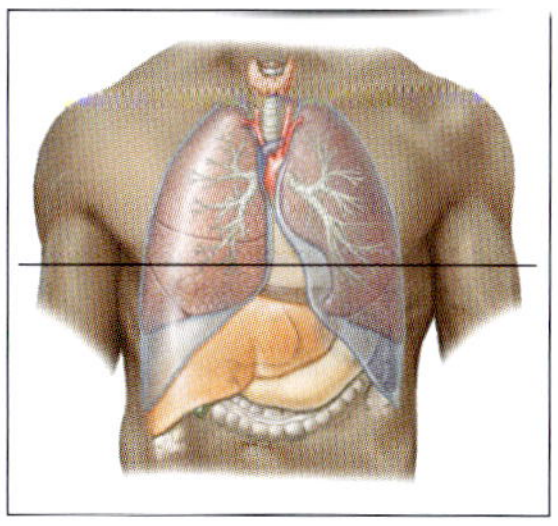

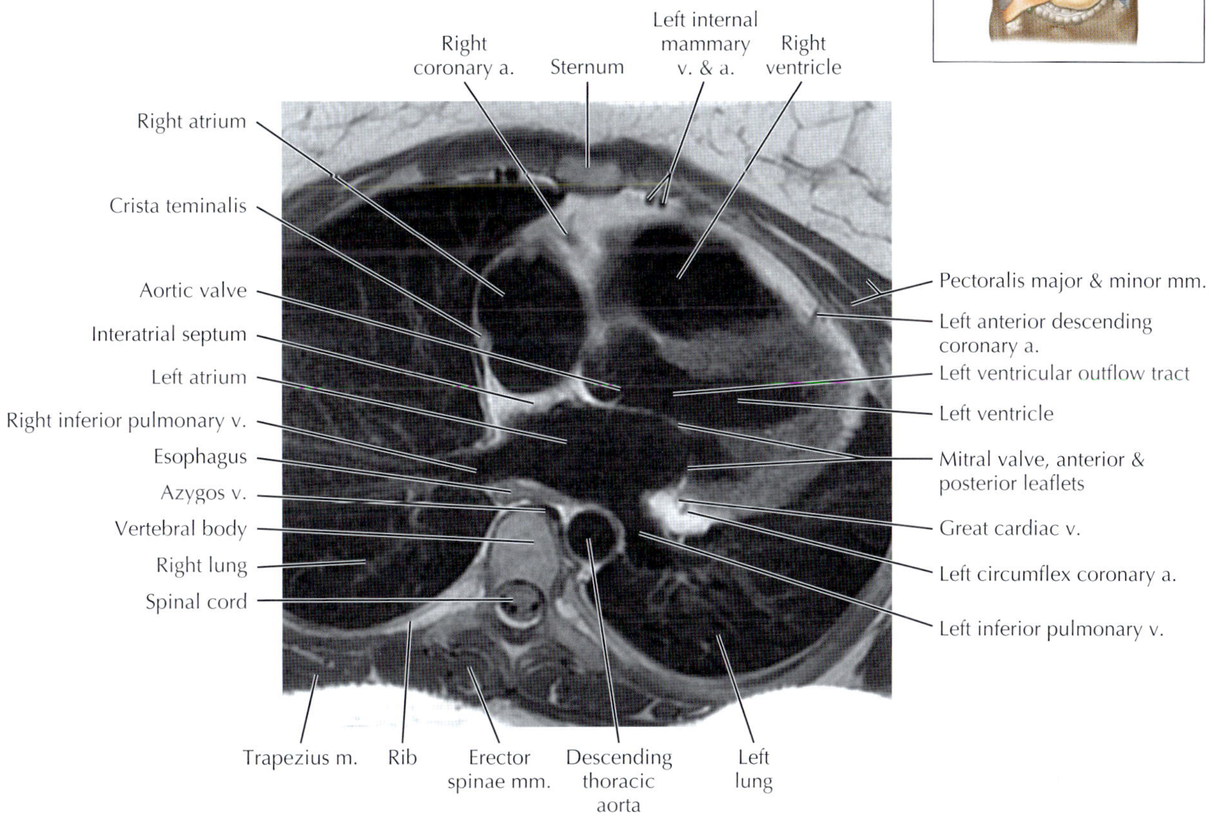
Right coronary a.
Sternum
Left internal mammary v. & a.
Right ventricle
Right atrium
Crista teminalis
Aortic valve
Interatrial septum
Left atrium
Right inferior pulmonary v.
Esophagus
Azygos v.
Vertebral body
Right lung
Spinal cord
Pectoralis major & minor mm.
Left anterior descending coronary a.
Left ventricular outflow tract
Left ventricle
Mitral valve, anterior & posterior leaflets
Great cardiac v.
Left circumflex coronary a.
Left inferior pulmonary v.
Trapezius m.
Rib
Erector spinae mm.
Descending thoracic aorta
Left lung

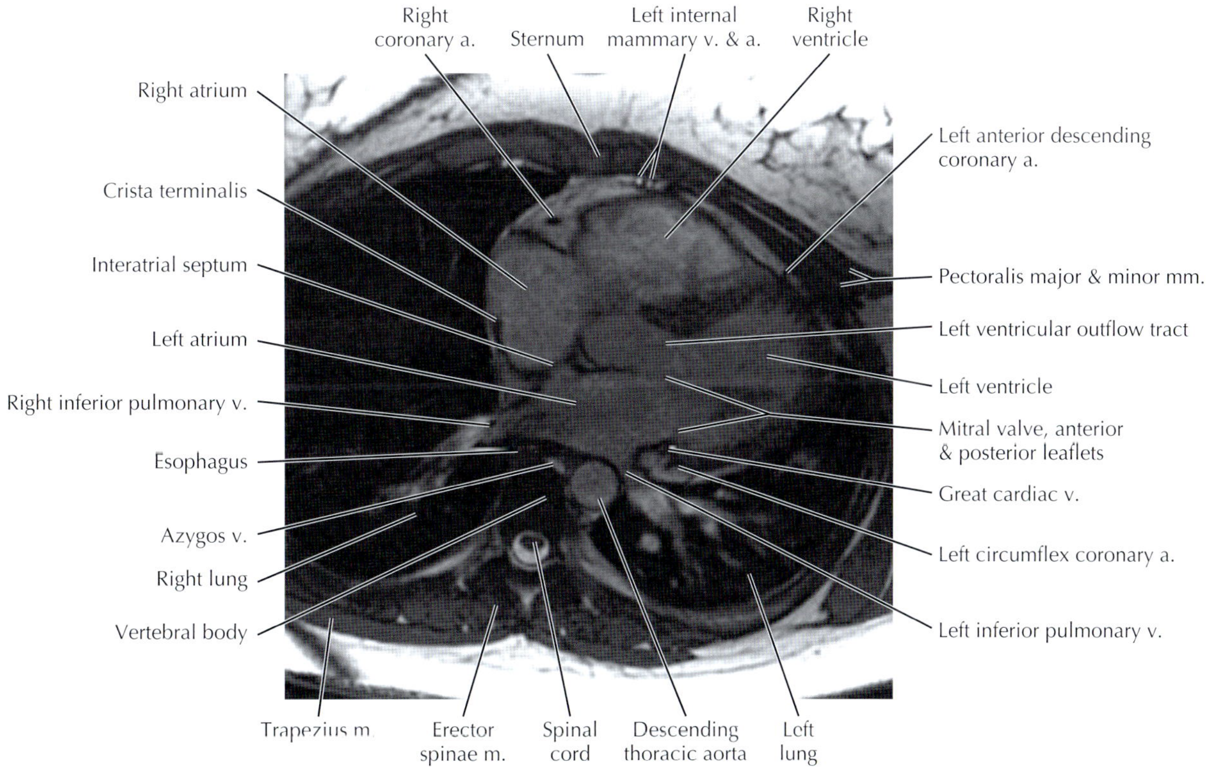
Right coronary a.
Sternum
Left internal mammary v. & a.
Right ventricle
Right atrium
Crista terminalis
Interatrial septum
Left atrium
Right inferior pulmonary v.
Esophagus
Azygos v.
Right lung
Vertebral body
Left anterior descending coronary a.
Pectoralis major & minor mm.
Left ventricular outflow tract
Left ventricle
Mitral valve, anterior & posterior leaflets
Great cardiac v.
Left circumflex coronary a.
Left inferior pulmonary v.
Trapezius m.
Erector spinae m.
Spinal cord
Descending thoracic aorta
Left lung

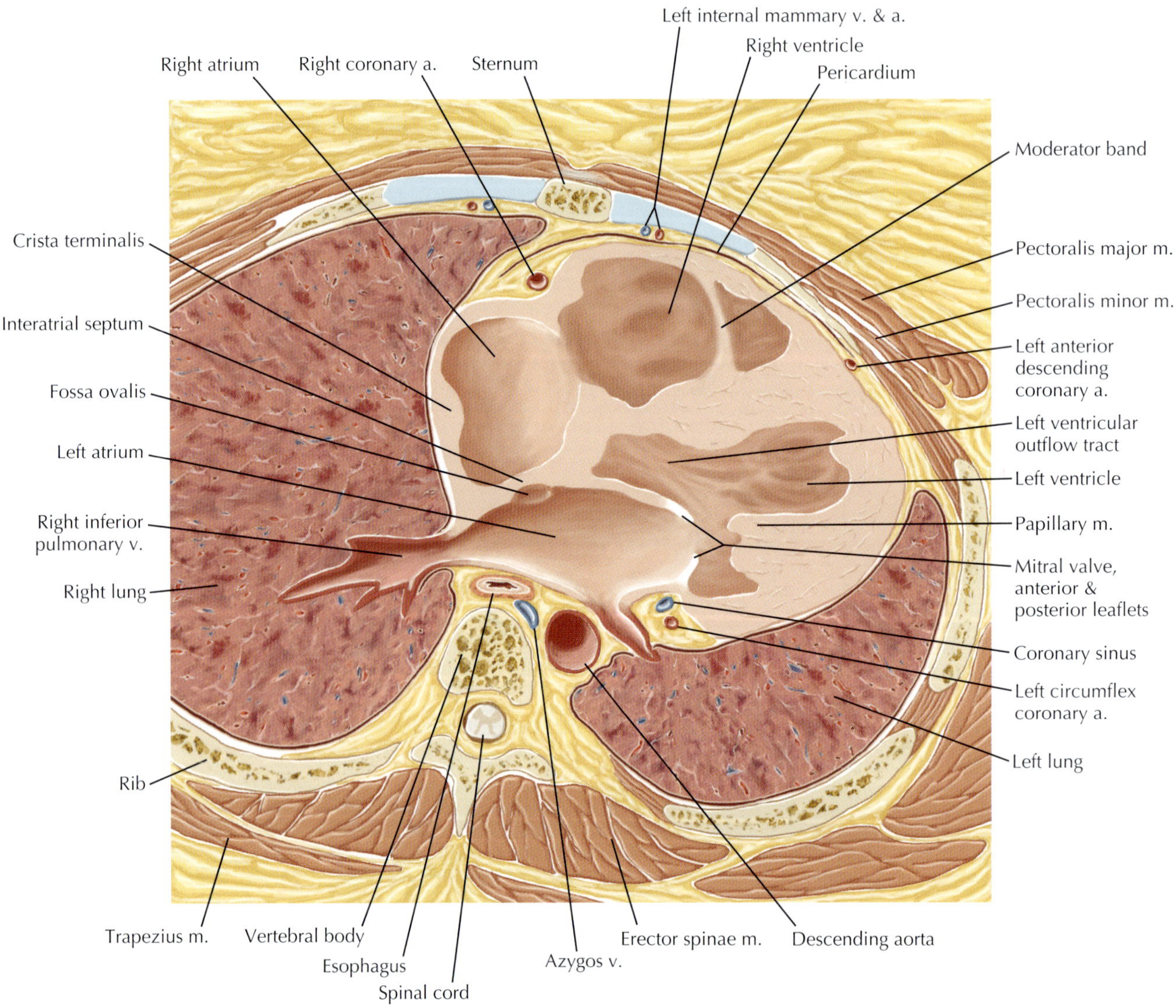
Left internal mammary v. & a.
Right ventricle
Pericardium
Right atrium
Right coronary a.
Sternum
Moderator band
Crista terminalis
Pectoralis major m.
Pectoralis minor m.
Interatrial septum
Left anterior descending coronary a.
Fossa ovalis
Left ventricular outflow tract
Left atrium
Left ventricle
Right inferior pulmonary v.
Papillary m.
Mitral valve, anterior & posterior leaflets
Right lung
Coronary sinus
Left circumflex coronary a.
Left lung
Rib
Trapezius m.
Vertebral body
Esophagus
Spinal cord
Azygos v.
Erector spinae m.
Descending aorta

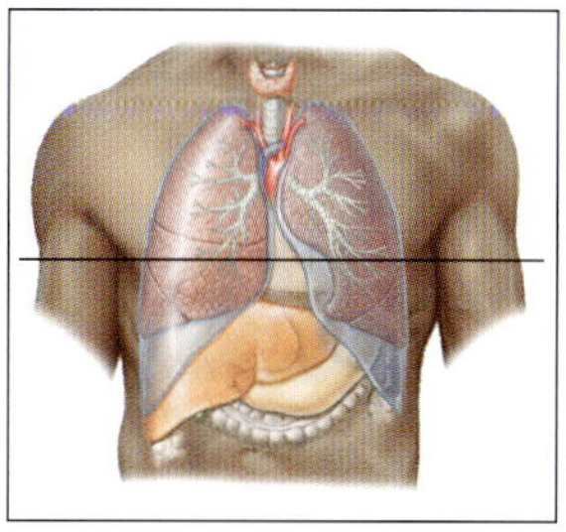

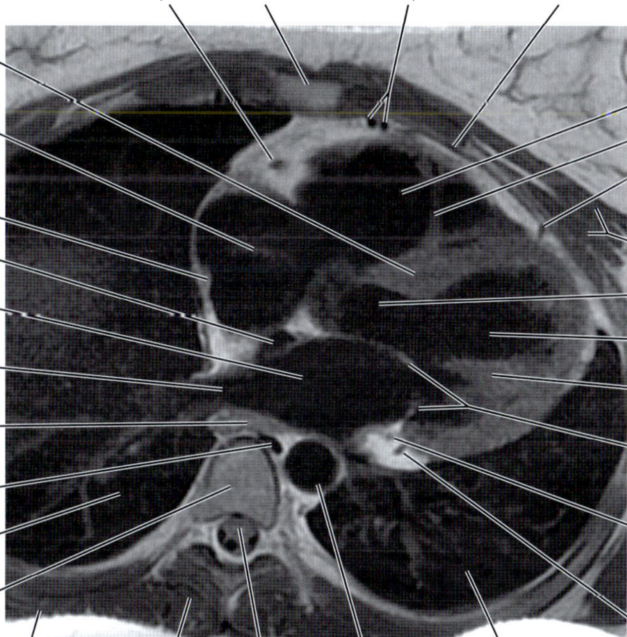
Right coronary a.
Sternum
Left internal mammary v. & a.
Pericardium
Interventricular septum
Right atrium
Crista teminalis
Fossa ovalis
Left atrium
Right inferior pulmonary v.
Esophagus
Azygos v.
Right lung
Vertebral body
Right ventricle
Moderator band
Left anterior descending coronary a.
Pectoralis major & minor mm.
Left ventricular outflow tract
Left ventricle
Papillary m.
Mitral valve, anterior & posterior leaflets
Coronary sinus
Left circumflex coronary a.
Trapezius m.
Erector spinae m.
Spinal cord
Descending thoracic aorta
Left lung

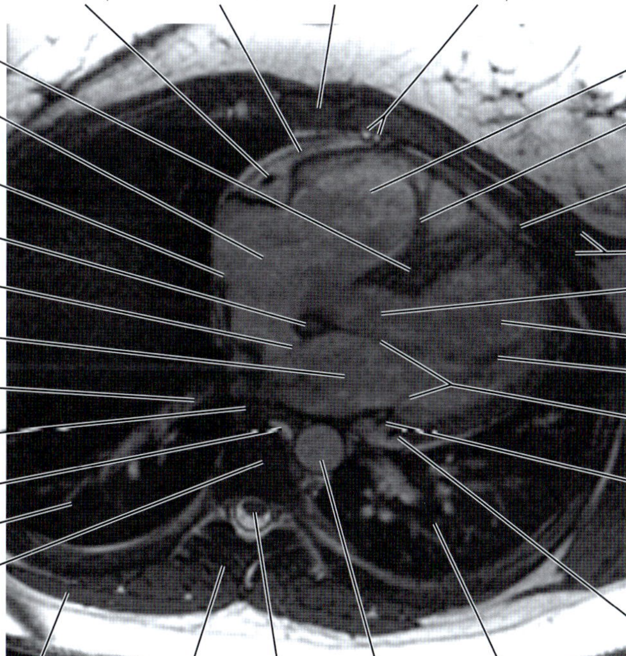
Right coronary a.
Pericardium
Sternum
Left internal mammary v. & a.
Interventricular septum
Right atrium
Crista terminalis
Interatrial septum
Fossa ovalis
Left atrium
Right inferior pulmonary v.
Esophagus
Azygos v.
Right lung
Vertebral body
Right ventricle
Moderator band
Left anterior descending coronary a.
Pectoralis major & minor mm.
Left ventricular outflow tract
Left ventricle
Papillary m.
Mitral valve, anterior & posterior leaflets
Coronary sinus
Left circumflex coronary a.
Trapezius m.
Erector spinae m.
Spinal cord
Descending thoracic aorta
Left lung

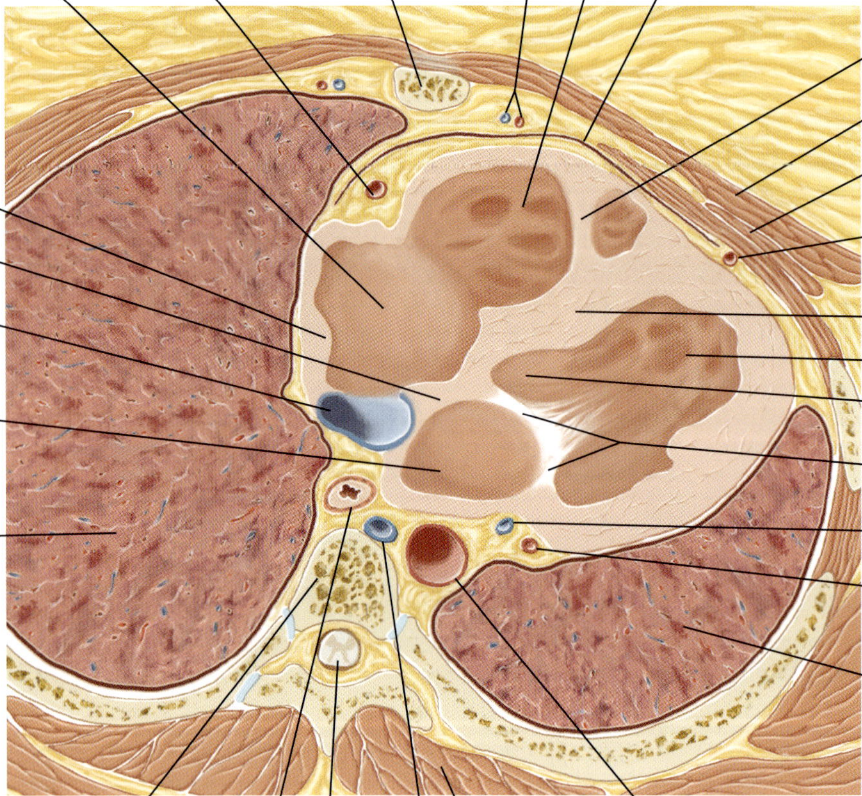

DIAGNOSTIC CONSIDERATION

Right ventricular anatomy with MR is shown. Cardiac CT requires the injection of iodinated contrast material to opacify the cardiac chambers and vessels to allow adequate visualization of these structures, but dense contrast within the right atrium and ventricle can often obscure adjacent anatomy, such as the right coronary artery, on CT. For this reason, cardiac CT examinations are often conducted with an injection of saline or saline-contrast mixtures following the injection of undiluted iodinated contrast to clear the dense contrast from the right cardiac chambers. Although this technique results in excellent imaging for left-sided cardiac structures and the right coronary artery, it may result in suboptimal visualization of right chamber anatomy (see Cardiac CTA plates). However, note the excellent demonstration of right chamber anatomy on MR—the trabeculae carneae, papillary muscles, and moderator band of the right ventricle and the tricuspid valve are readily visible, and intravenous contrast administration is not required for MR to demonstrate such detail.

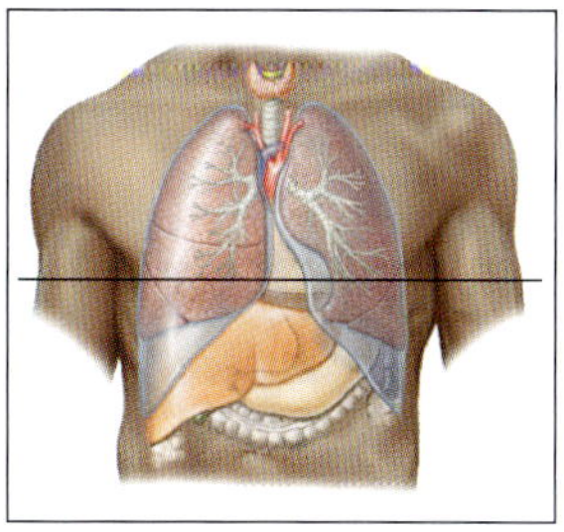

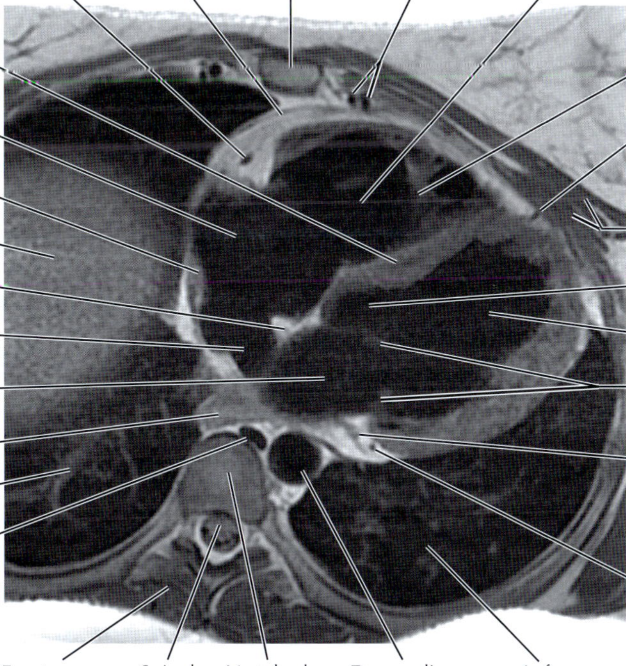
Right coronary a.
Pericardium
Sternum
Left internal mammary v. & a.
Right ventricle
Interventricular septum
Right atrium
Crista teminalis
Liver
Interatrial septum
Inferior vena cava
Left atrium
Esophagus
Right lung
Azygos v.
Moderator band
Left anterior descending coronary a.
Pectoralis major & minor mm.
Left ventricular outflow tract
Left ventricle
Mitral valve, anterior & posterior leaflets
Coronary sinus
Left circumflex coronary a.
Erector spinae m.
Spinal cord
Vertebral body
Descending thoracic aorta
Left lung

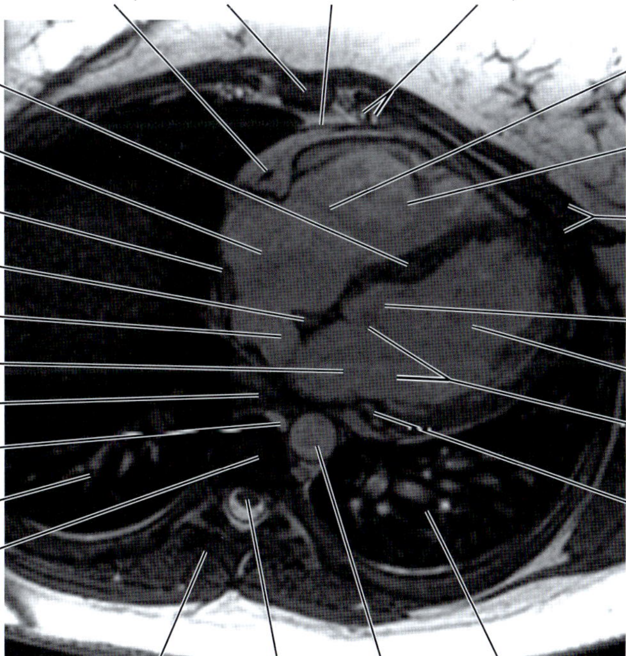
Right coronary a.
Sternum
Pericardium
Left internal mammary v. & a.
Interventricular septum
Right atrium
Crista terminalis
Interatrial septum
Inferior vena cava
Left atrium
Esophagus
Azygos v.
Right lung
Vertebral body
Tricuspid valve
Right ventricle
Pectoralis major & minor mm.
Left ventricular outflow tract
Left ventricle
Mitral valve, anterior & posterior leaflets
Coronary sinus
Erector spinae m.
Spinal cord
Descending thoracic aorta
Left lung

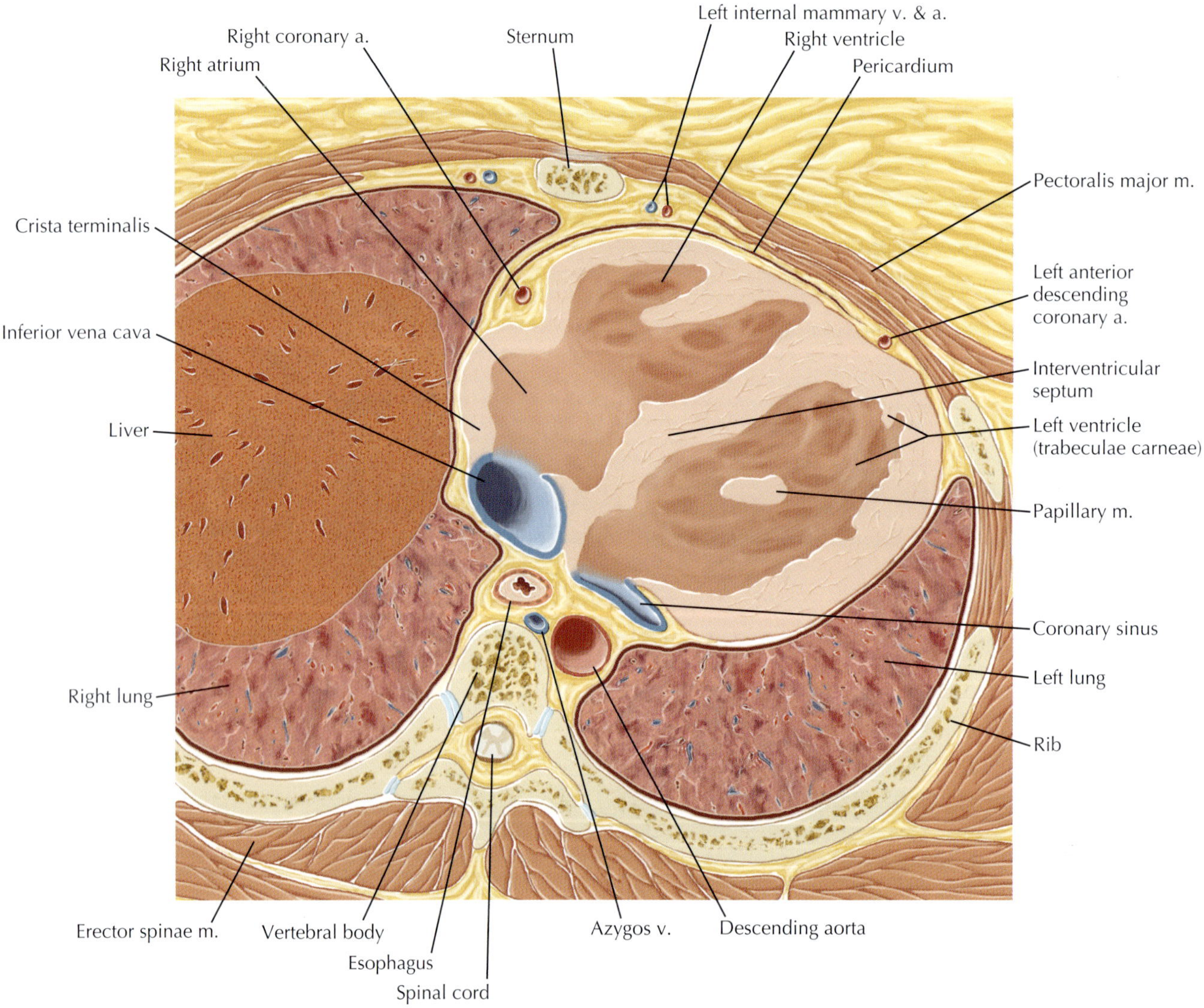
Left internal mammary v. & a.
Right coronary a.
Sternum
Right ventricle
Right atrium
Pericardium
Pectoralis major m.
Crista terminalis
Left anterior descending coronary a.
Inferior vena cava
Interventricular septum
Liver
Left ventricle (trabeculae carneae)
Papillary m.
Coronary sinus
Left lung
Right lung
Rib
Erector spinae m.
Vertebral body
Azygos v.
Descending aorta
Esophagus
Spinal cord

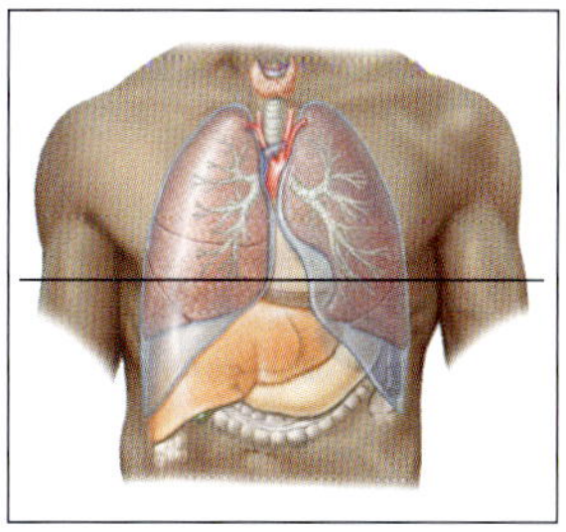

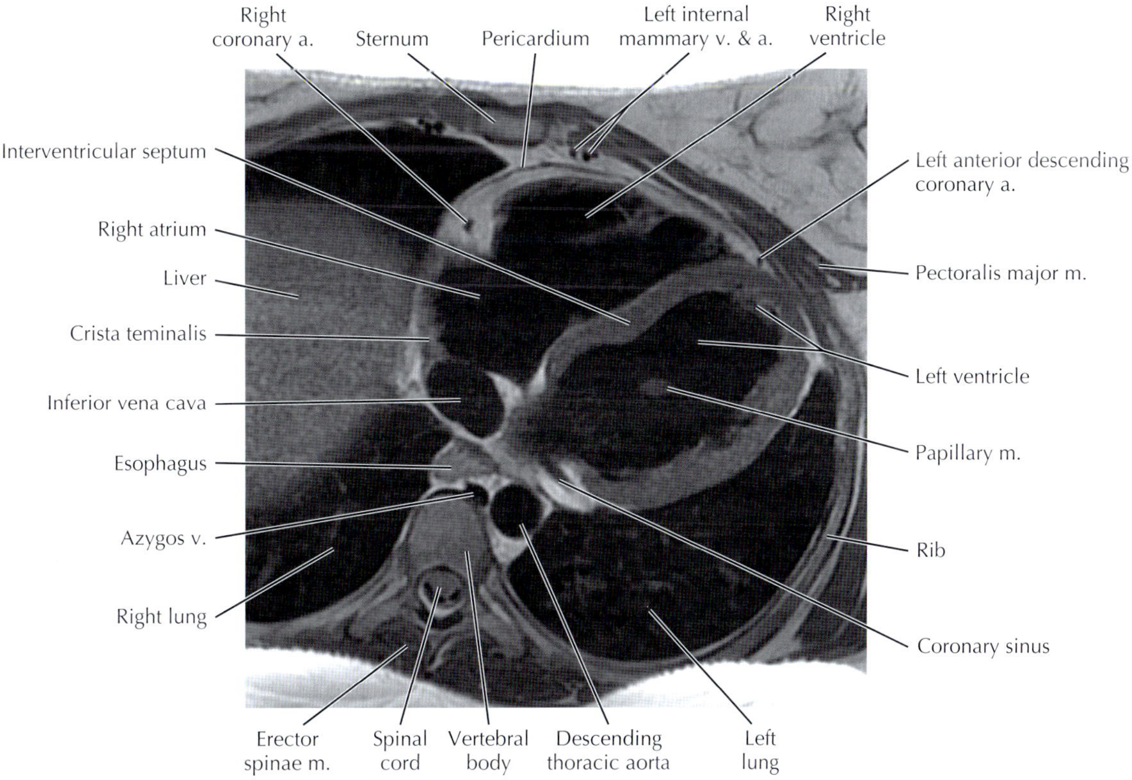
Right coronary a.
Sternum
Pericardium
Left internal mammary v. & a.
Right ventricle
Interventricular septum
Right atrium
Liver
Crista teminalis
Inferior vena cava
Esophagus
Azygos v.
Right lung
Left anterior descending coronary a.
Pectoralis major m.
Left ventricle
Papillary m.
Rib
Coronary sinus
Erector spinae m.
Spinal cord
Vertebral body
Descending thoracic aorta
Left lung

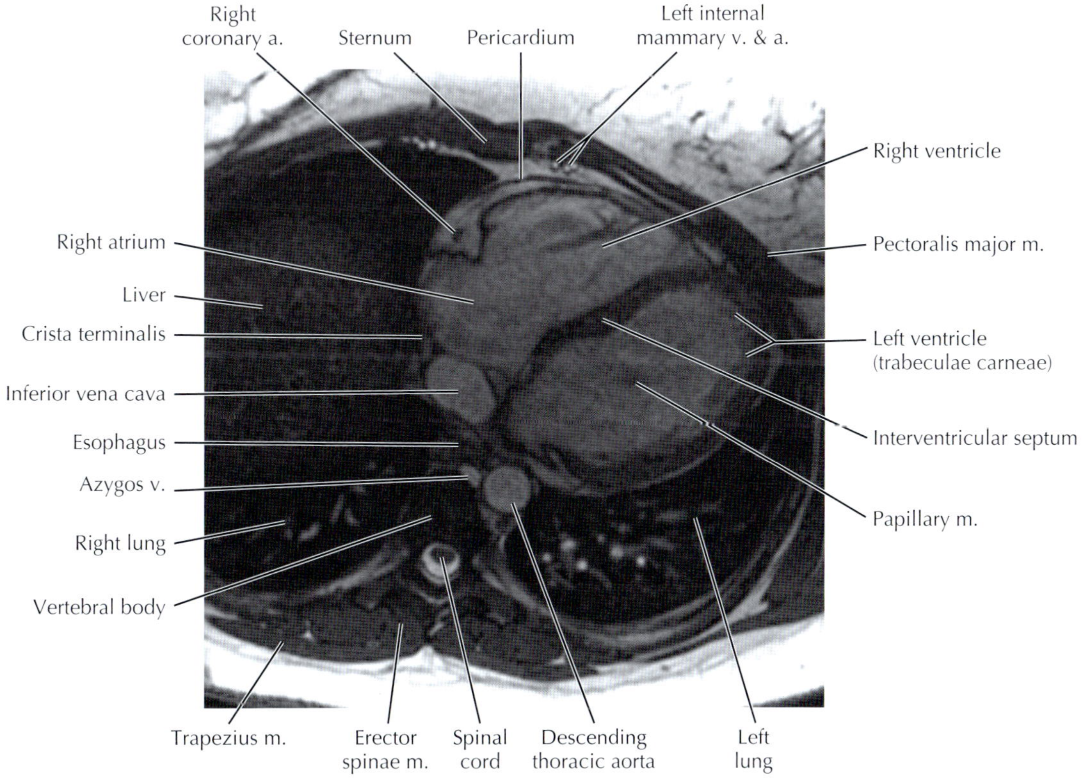
Right coronary a.
Sternum
Pericardium
Left internal mammary v. & a.
Right atrium
Liver
Crista terminalis
Inferior vena cava
Esophagus
Azygos v.
Right lung
Vertebral body
Right ventricle
Pectoralis major m.
Left ventricle (trabeculae carneae)
Interventricular septum
Papillary m.
Trapezius m.
Erector spinae m.
Spinal cord
Descending thoracic aorta
Left lung

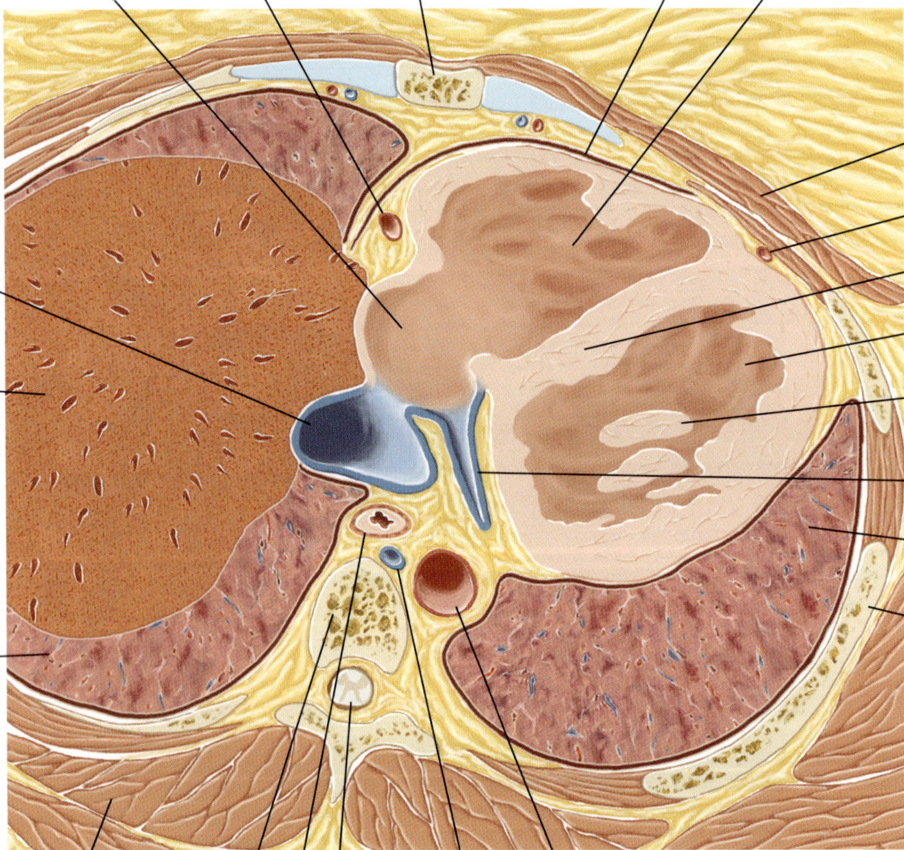
Right coronary a.
Sternum
Pericardium
Right atrium
Right ventricle
Pectoralis major m.
Left anterior descending coronary a.
Interventricular septum
Inferior vena cava
Left ventricle (trabeculae carneae)
Liver
Papillary m.
Coronary sinus
Left lung
Rib
Right lung
Erector spinae m.
Vertebral body
Esophagus
Spinal cord
Azygos v.
Descending thoracic aorta

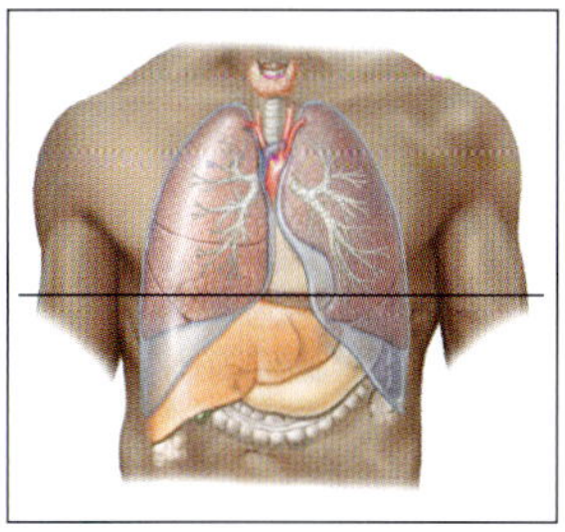

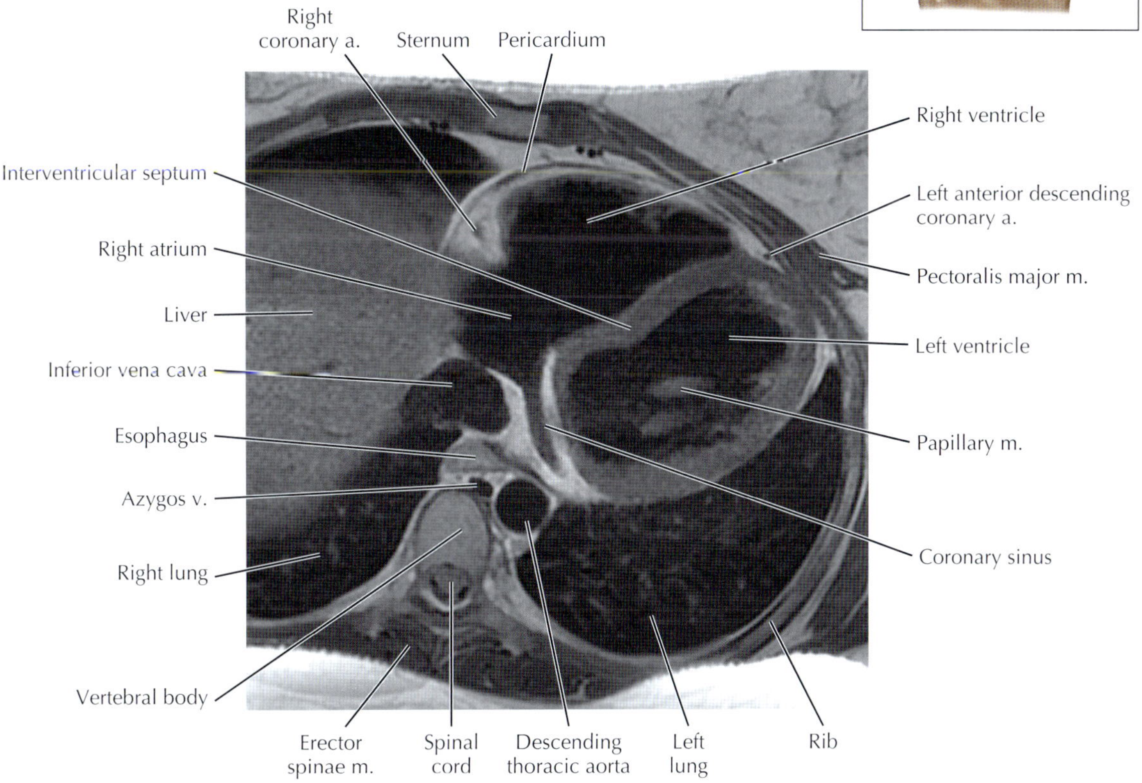
Right coronary a.
Sternum
Pericardium
Interventricular septum
Right atrium
Liver
Inferior vena cava
Esophagus
Azygos v.
Right lung
Vertebral body
Right ventricle
Left anterior descending coronary a.
Pectoralis major m.
Left ventricle
Papillary m.
Coronary sinus
Erector spinae m.
Spinal cord
Descending thoracic aorta
Left lung
Rib

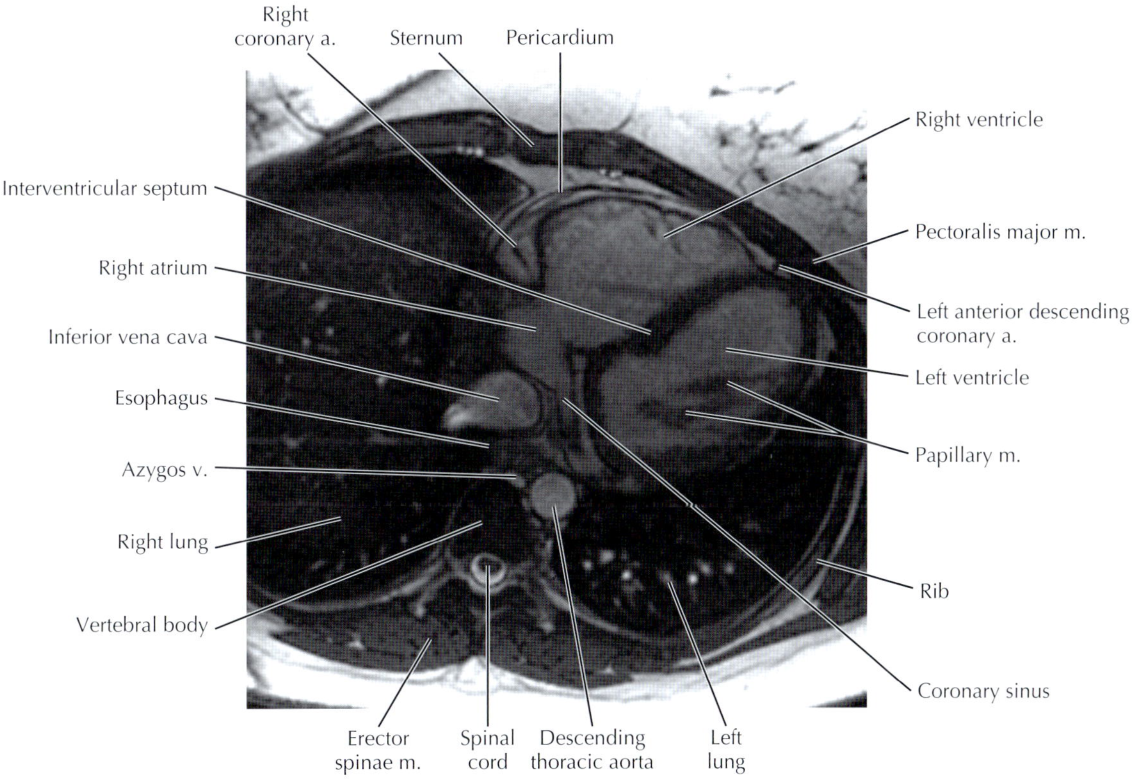
Right coronary a.
Sternum
Pericardium
Interventricular septum
Right atrium
Inferior vena cava
Esophagus
Azygos v.
Right lung
Vertebral body
Right ventricle
Pectoralis major m.
Left anterior descending coronary a.
Left ventricle
Papillary m.
Rib
Coronary sinus
Erector spinae m.
Spinal cord
Descending thoracic aorta
Left lung

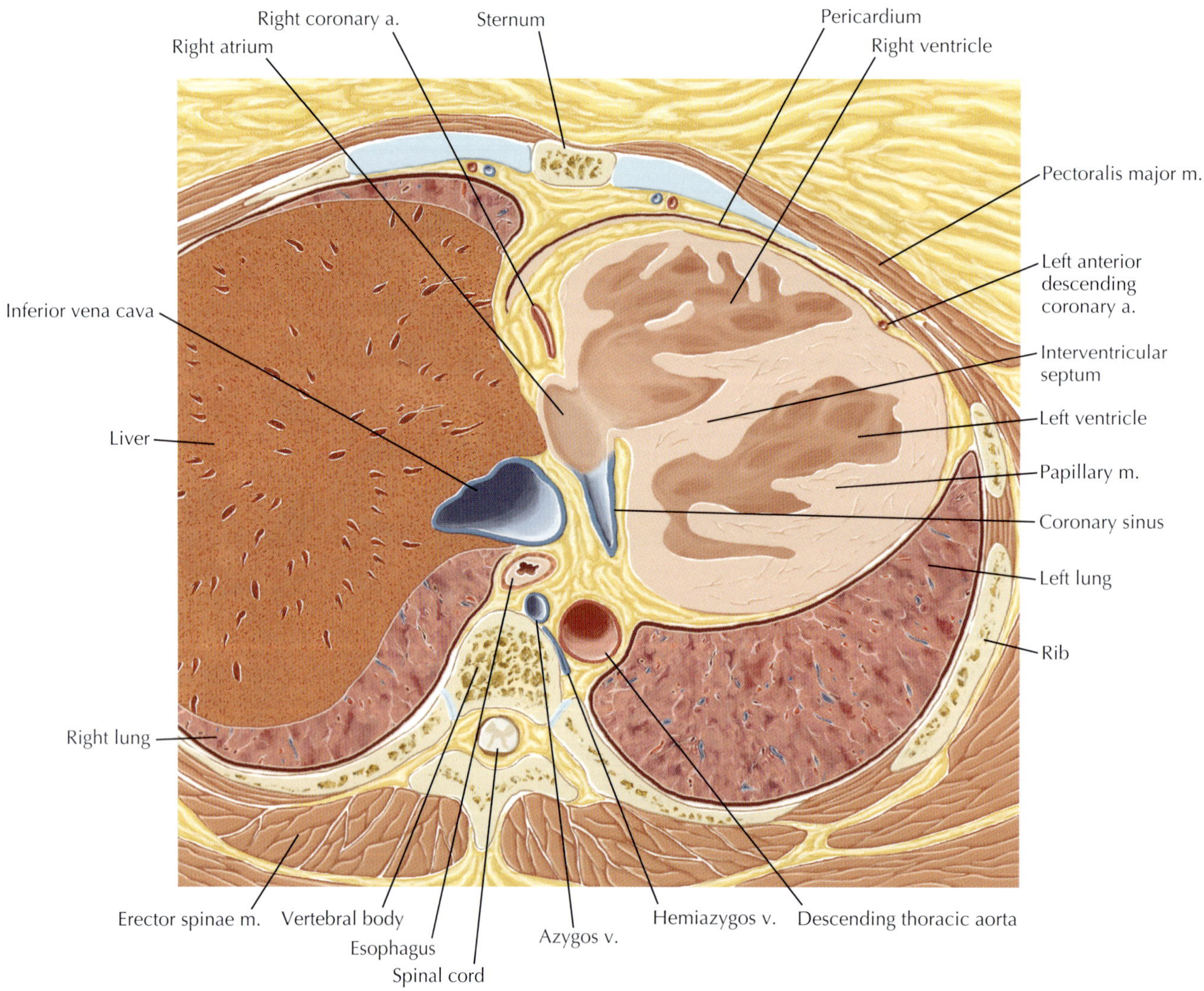
Right coronary a.
Sternum
Pericardium
Right atrium
Right ventricle
Pectoralis major m.
Left anterior descending coronary a.
Inferior vena cava
Interventricular septum
Left ventricle
Liver
Papillary m.
Coronary sinus
Left lung
Rib
Right lung
Erector spinae m.
Vertebral body
Esophagus
Spinal cord
Azygos v.
Hemiazygos v.
Descending thoracic aorta

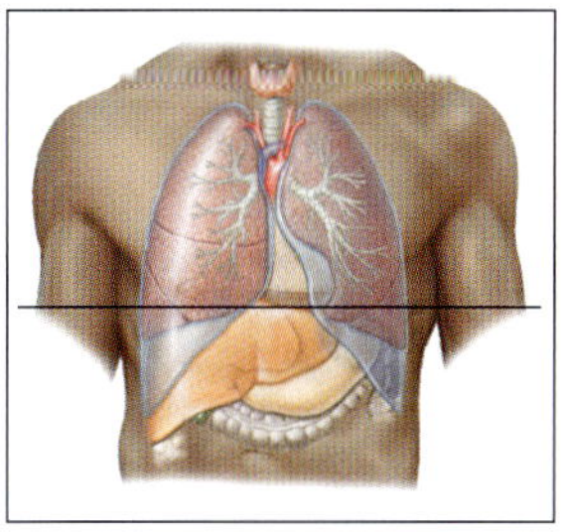

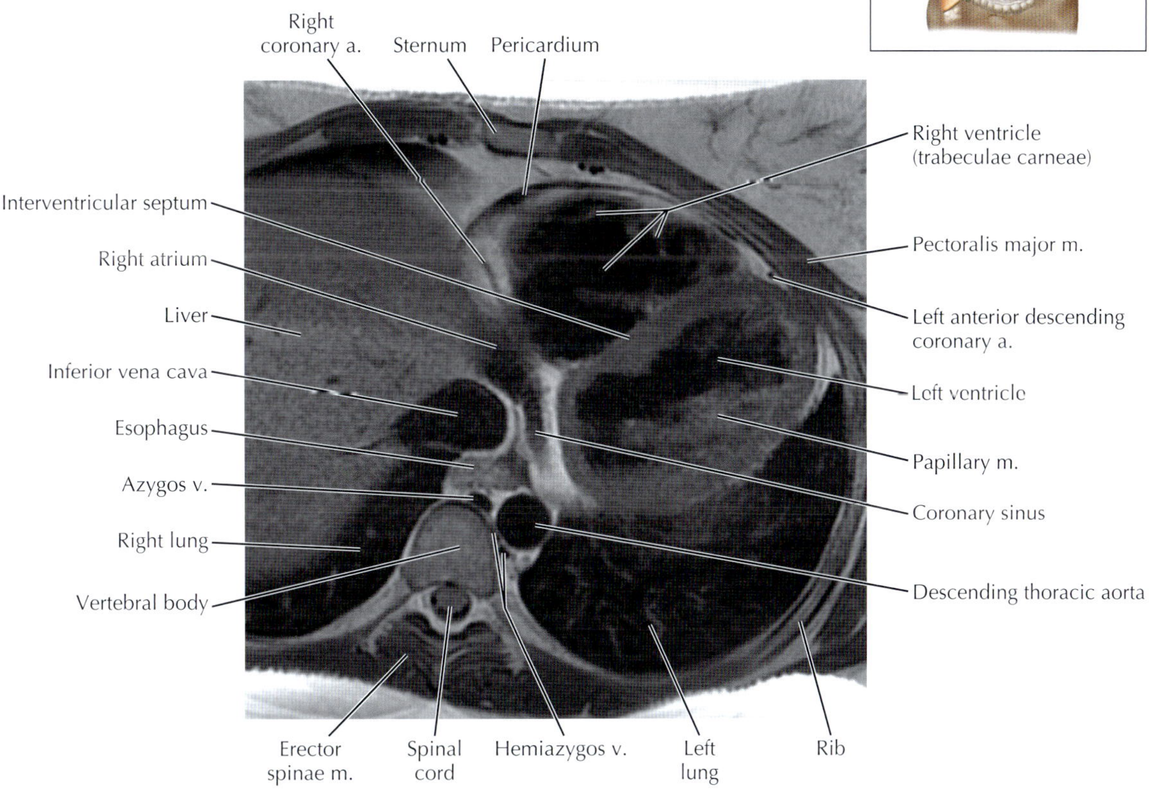
Right coronary a.
Sternum
Pericardium
Interventricular septum
Right atrium
Liver
Inferior vena cava
Esophagus
Azygos v.
Right lung
Vertebral body
Right ventricle (trabeculae carneae)
Pectoralis major m.
Left anterior descending coronary a.
Left ventricle
Papillary m.
Coronary sinus
Descending thoracic aorta
Erector spinae m.
Spinal cord
Hemiazygos v.
Left lung
Rib

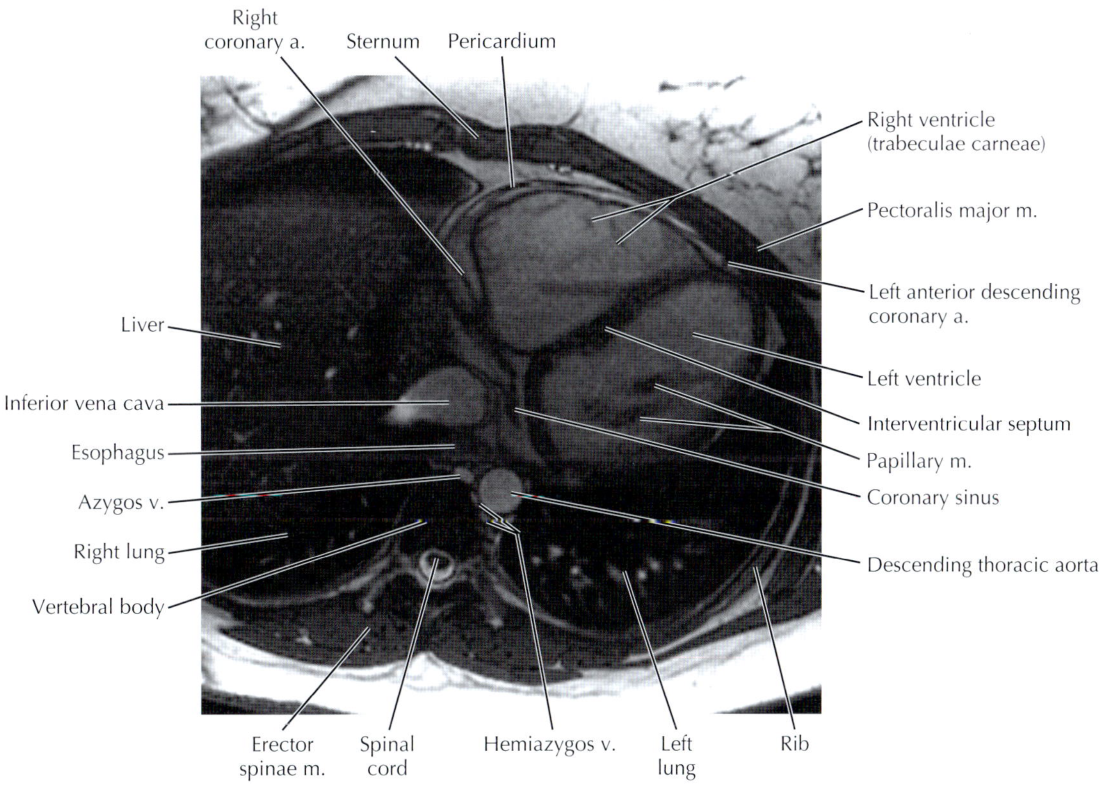
Right coronary a.
Sternum
Pericardium
Liver
Inferior vena cava
Esophagus
Azygos v.
Right lung
Vertebral body
Right ventricle (trabeculae carneae)
Pectoralis major m.
Left anterior descending coronary a.
Left ventricle
Interventricular septum
Papillary m.
Coronary sinus
Descending thoracic aorta
Erector spinae m.
Spinal cord
Hemiazygos v.
Left lung
Rib

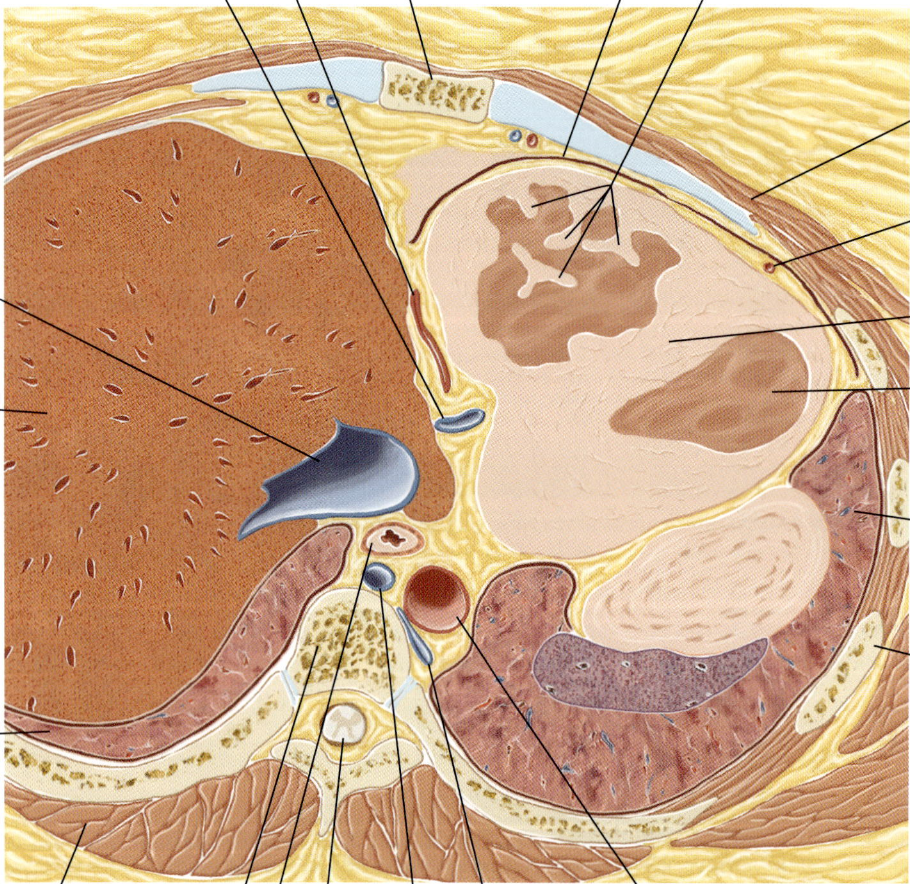
Right coronary a.
Sternum
Posterior interventricular v. (middle cardiac v.)
Pericardium
Right ventricle (trabeculae carneae)
Pectoralis major m.
Left anterior descending coronary a.
Inferior vena cava
Interventricular septum
Left ventricle
Liver
Left lung
Rib
Right lung
Erector spinae m.
Vertebral body
Esophagus
Spinal cord
Azygos v.
Hemiazygos v.
Descending thoracic aorta

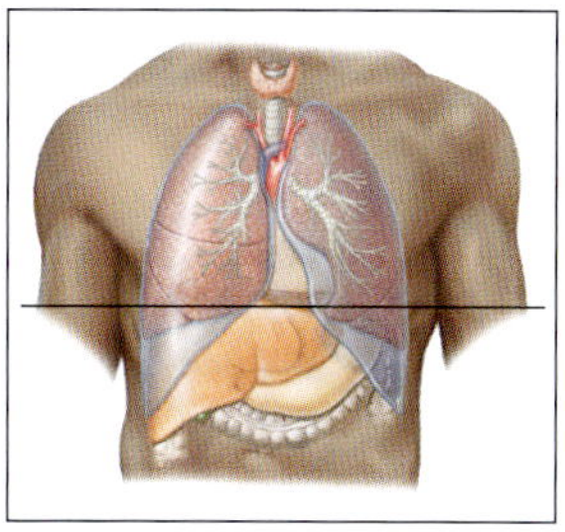

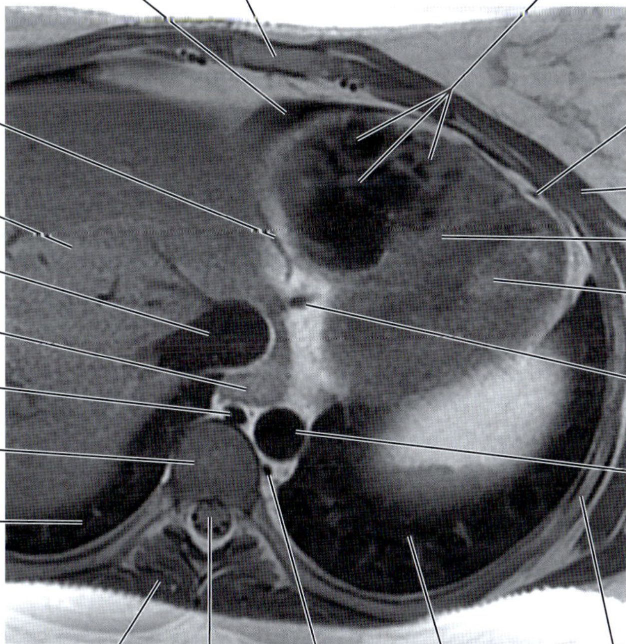
Pericardial fluid (normal)
Sternum
Right ventricle (trabeculae carneae)
Right coronary a.
Liver
Inferior vena cava
Esophagus
Azygos v.
Vertebral body
Right lung
Left anterior descending coronary a.
Pectoralis major m.
Interventricular septum
Left ventricle
Posterior interventricular v. (middle cardiac v.)
Descending thoracic aorta
Erector spinae m.
Spinal cord
Hemiazygos v.
Left lung
Rib

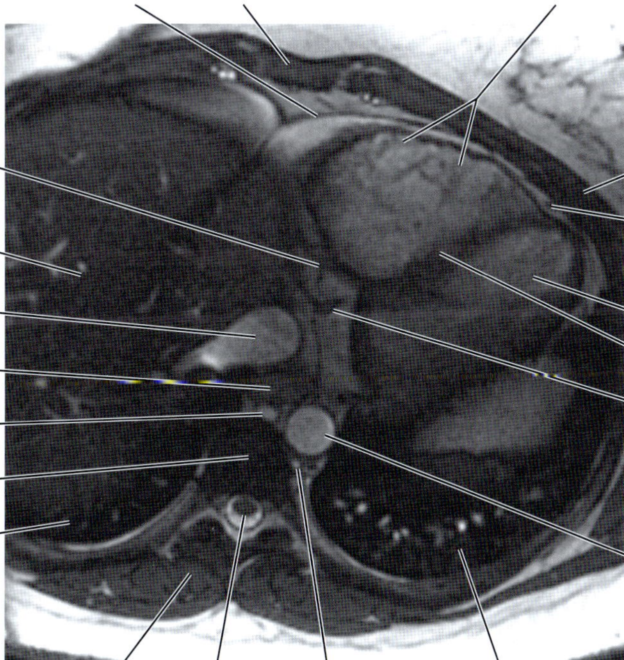
Pericardium
Sternum
Right ventricle (trabeculae carneae)
Right coronary a.
Liver
Inferior vena cava
Esophagus
Azygos v.
Vertebral body
Right lung
Pectoralis major m.
Left anterior descending coronary a.
Left ventricle
Interventricular septum
Posterior interventricular v. (middle cardiac v.)
Descending thoracic aorta
Erector spinae m.
Spinal cord
Hemiazygos v.
Left lung

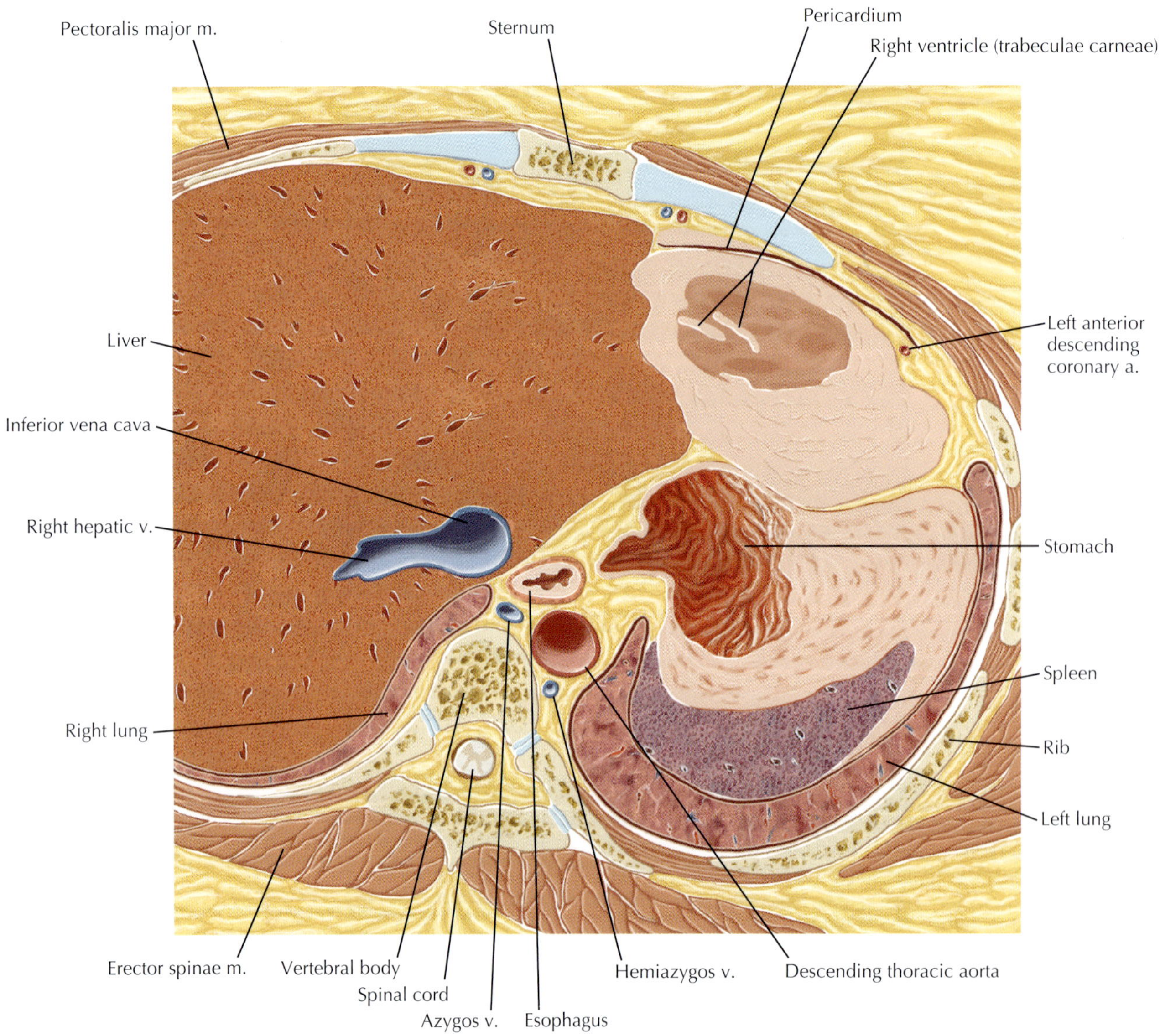
Pectoralis major m.
Sternum
Pericardium
Right ventricle (trabeculae carneae)
Liver
Left anterior descending coronary a.
Inferior vena cava
Right hepatic v.
Stomach
Spleen
Right lung
Rib
Left lung
Erector spinae m.
Vertebral body
Spinal cord
Azygos v.
Esophagus
Hemiazygos v.
Descending thoracic aorta

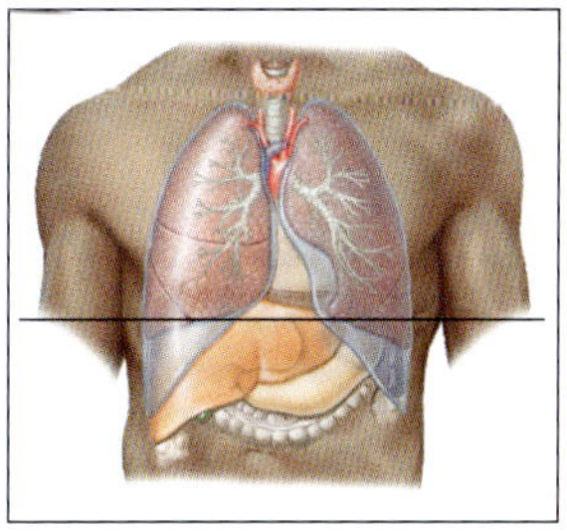

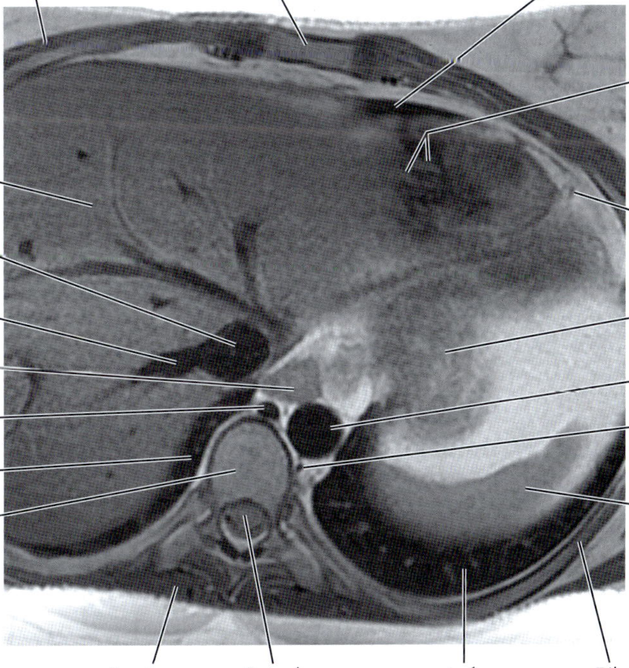
Pectoralis major m.
Sternum
Pericardial fluid (normal)
Right ventricle (trabeculae carneae)
Liver
Left anterior descending coronary a.
Inferior vena cava
Right hepatic v.
Stomach
Esophagus
Descending thoracic aorta
Azygos v.
Hemiazygos v.
Right lung
Vertebral body
Spleen
Erector spinae m.
Spinal cord
Left lung
Rib

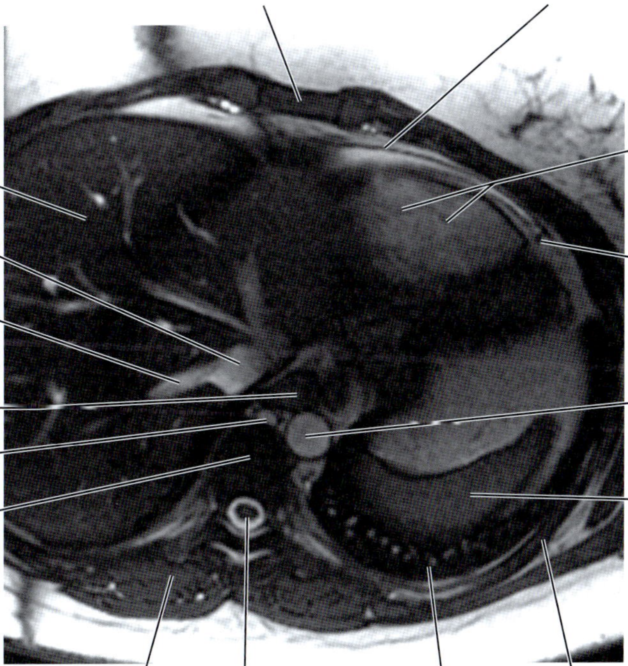
Sternum
Pericardium
Right ventricle (trabeculae carneae)
Liver
Left anterior descending coronary a.
Inferior vena cava
Right hepatic v.
Esophagus
Descending thoracic aorta
Azygos v.
Vertebral body
Spleen
Erector spinae m.
Spinal cord
Left lung
Rib

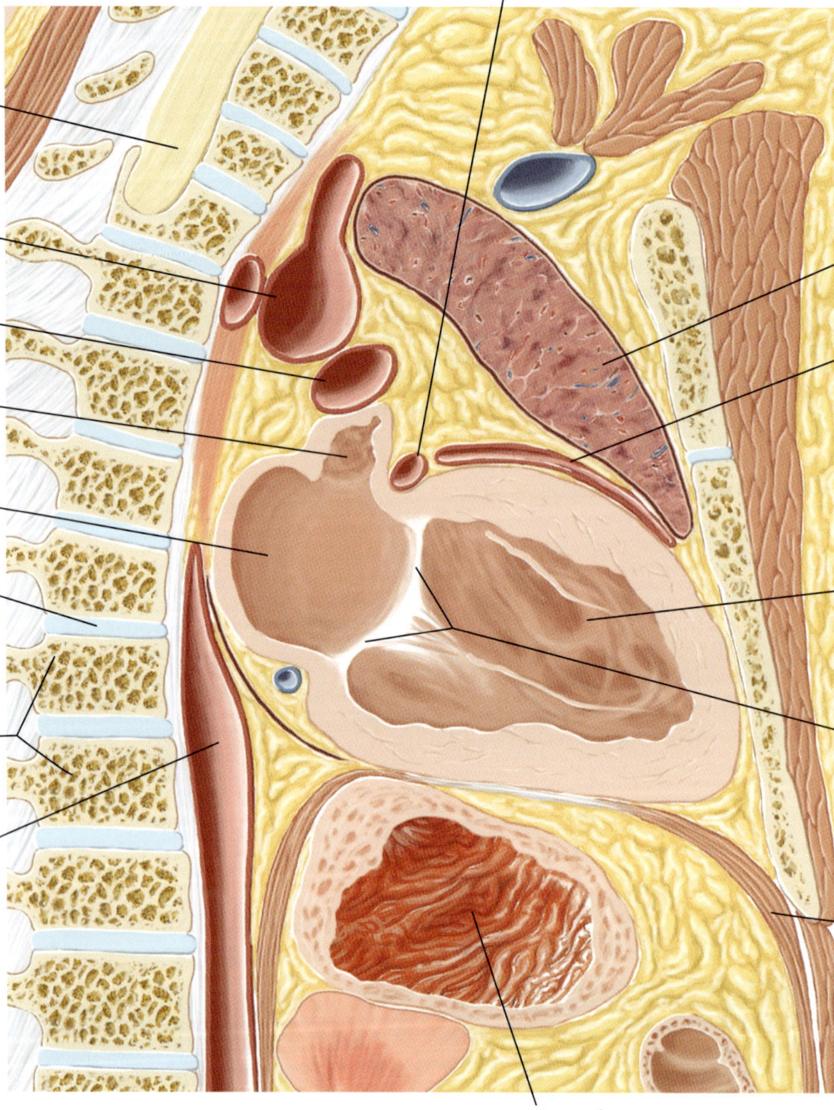

TECHNICAL CONSIDERATION

Cardiac imaging is often interpreted with images displayed in planes oriented with reference to the cardiac axis, as opposed to the axes of the body as is typical for most imaging applications (the axial, coronal, and sagittal planes). Cardiac imaging planes typically include "two-chamber," "three-chamber," "four-chamber," and "short axis" planes, and are commonly used for cardiac CT, MRI, nuclear medicine, and echocardiography. This "two-chamber" or "vertical long axis" view of the heart is useful for assessing the left ventricular cavity, left ventricular inferior and anterior wall motion, the mitral valve, and the left atrial appendage.

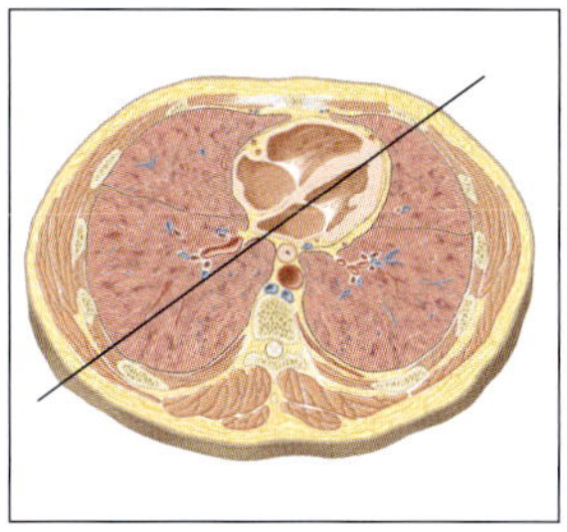

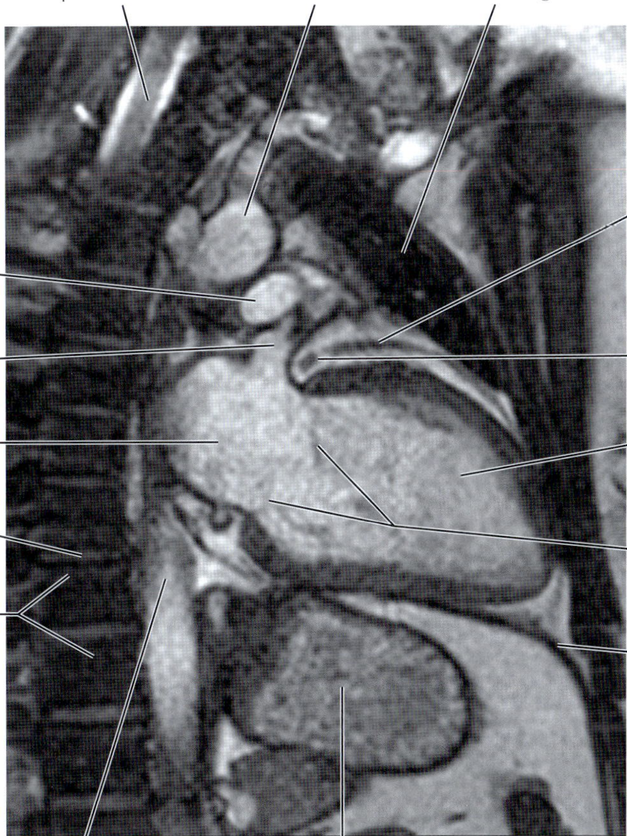
Spinal cord
Proximal descending thoracic aorta
Left lung
Left anterior descending coronary a.
Left superior pulmonary v.
Left atrial appendage
Left circumflex coronary a.
Left atrium
Left ventricle
Intervertebral disc space
Mitral valve, anterior & posterior leaflets
Thoracic spine vertebral bodies
Diaphragm
Descending thoracic aorta
Stomach

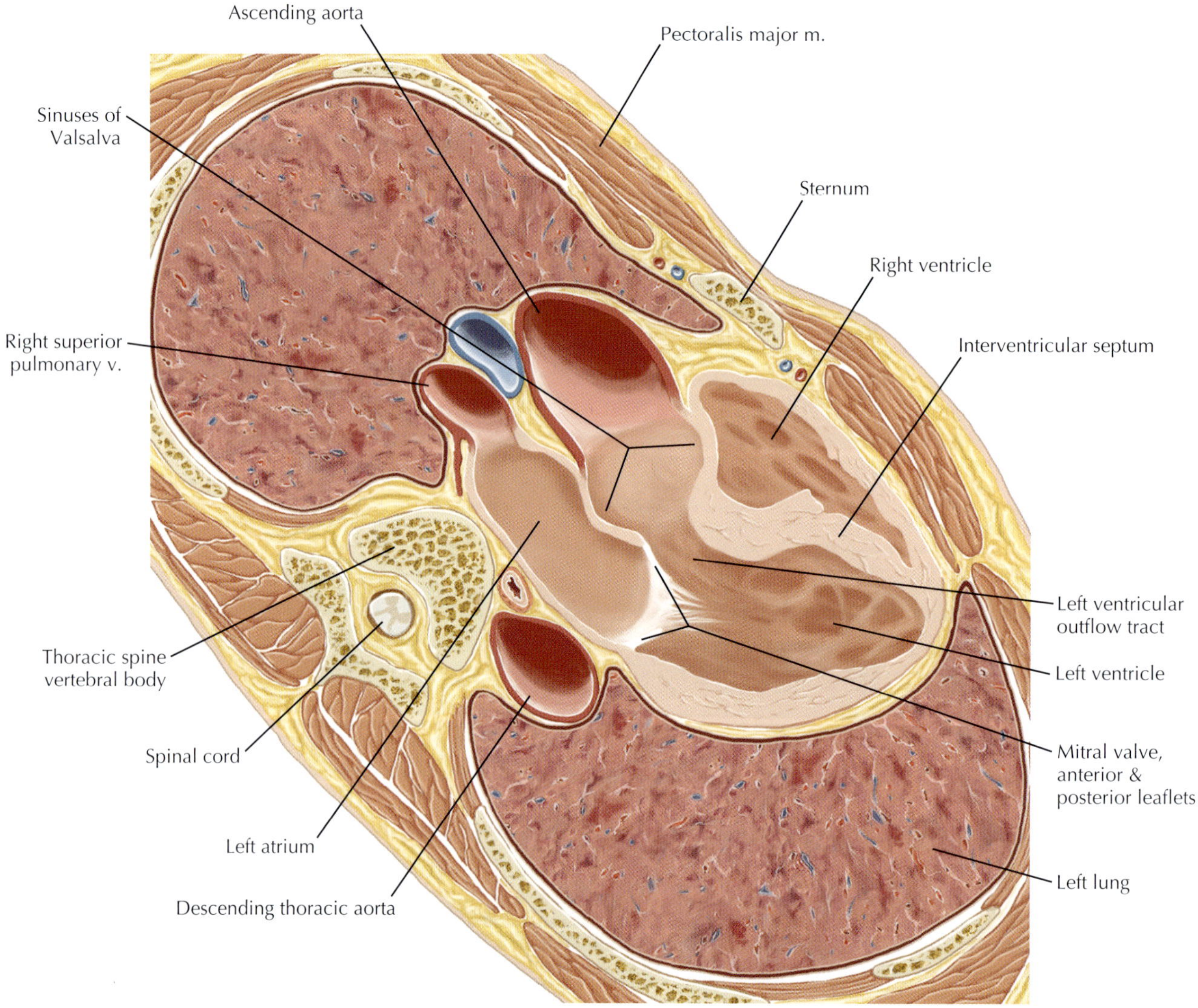

TECHNICAL CONSIDERATION

This is commonly referred to as a "three-chamber" view of the heart; it is useful for displaying the left ventricular outflow tract, left atrium, and mitral and aortic valves. The anteroseptal and inferolateral walls of the left ventricle are also well seen. Note how the continuity between the aortic root and anterior mitral valve are well shown in this view.

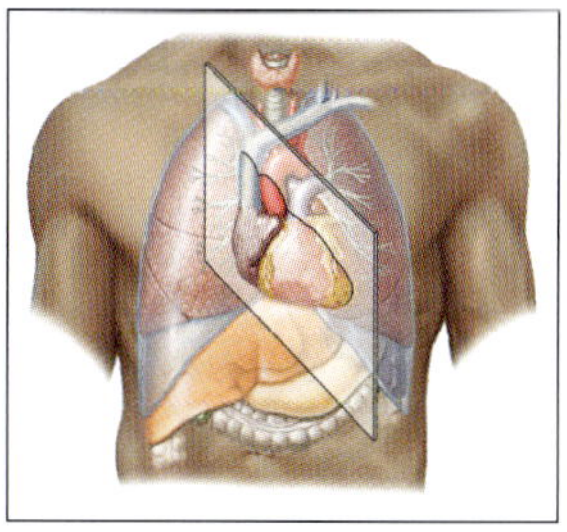

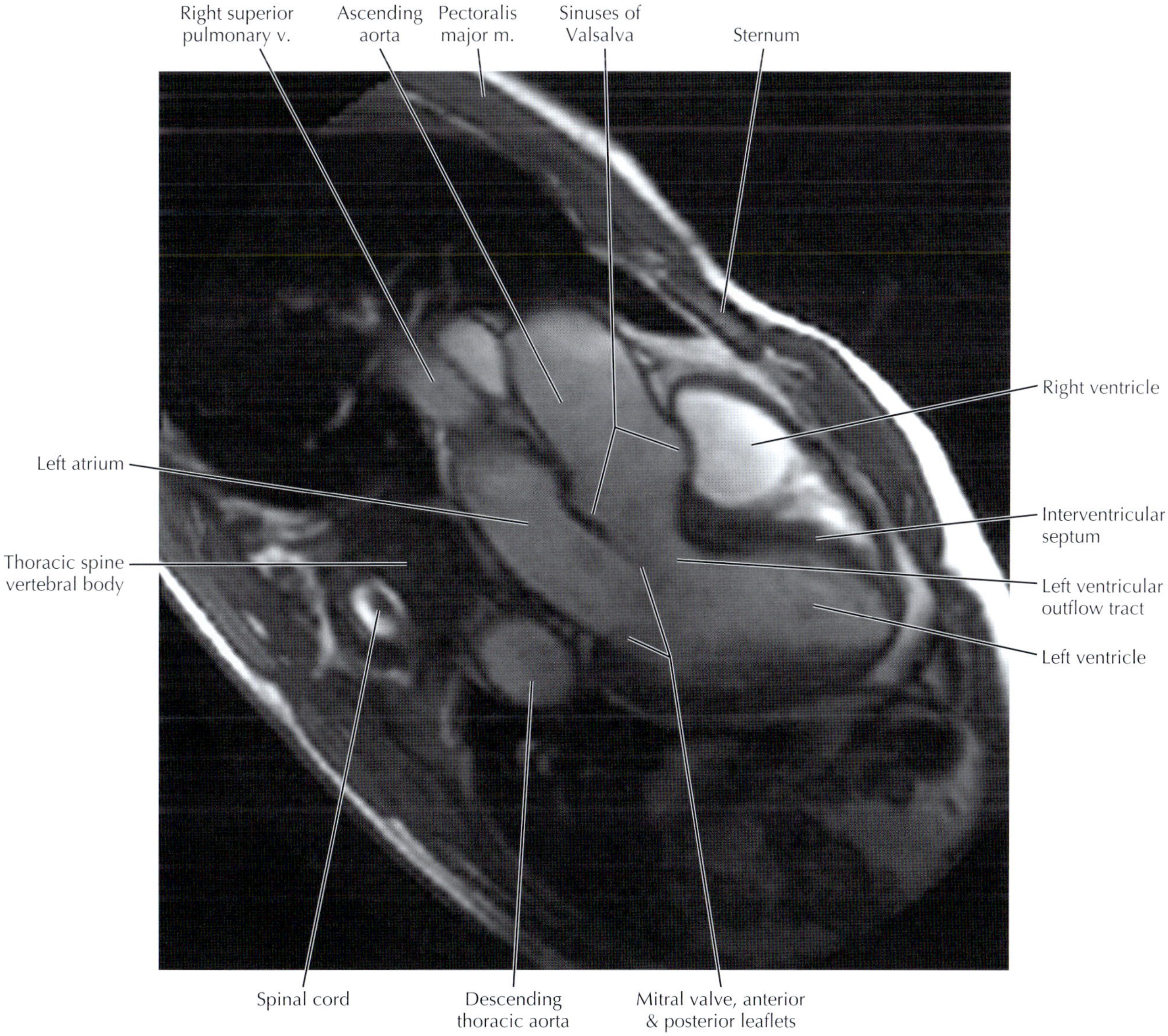
Right superior pulmonary v.
Ascending aorta
Pectoralis major m.
Sinuses of Valsalva
Sternum
Right ventricle
Left atrium
Interventricular septum
Thoracic spine vertebral body
Left ventricular outflow tract
Left ventricle
Spinal cord
Descending thoracic aorta
Mitral valve, anterior & posterior leaflets

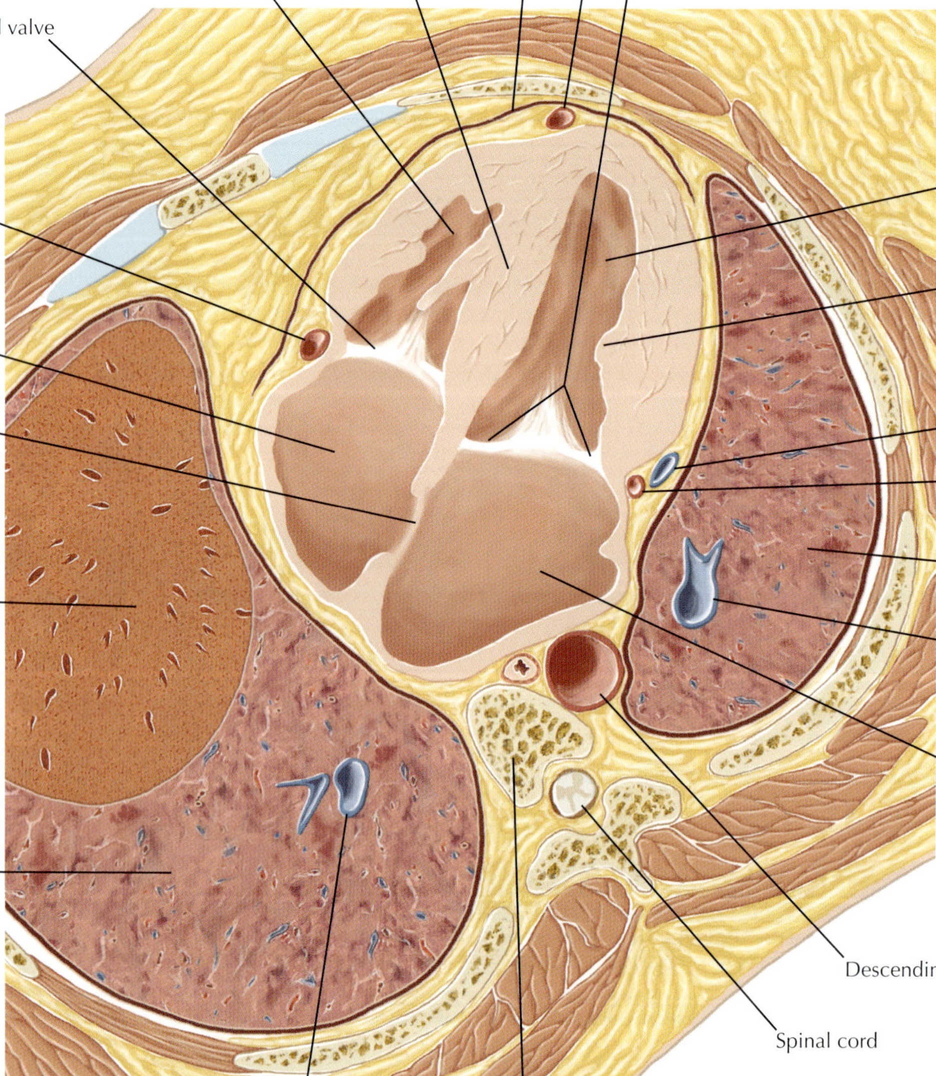

TECHNICAL CONSIDERATION

This view, often referred to as a "four-chamber" or "horizontal long axis" view, is oriented through the mid portions of the right and left ventricles, along a plane extending through the mitral valve to the apex of the heart. This projection provides a more precise analysis of ventricular size and morphology than standard axial, coronal, or sagittal imaging and is useful for assessing the function of the mitral and tricuspid valves. Left ventricular septal and lateral wall motion is also evaluable in this view.

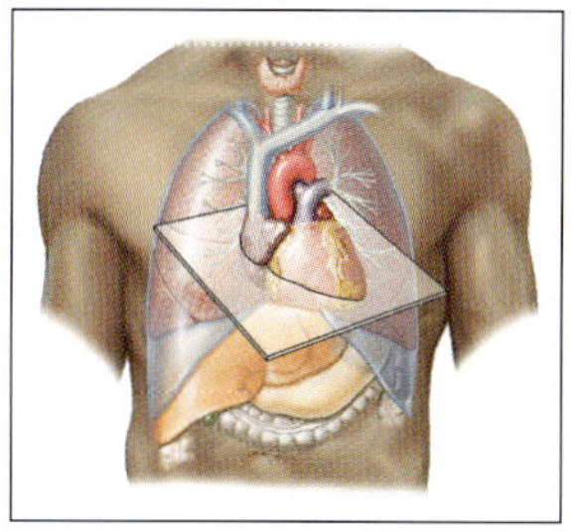

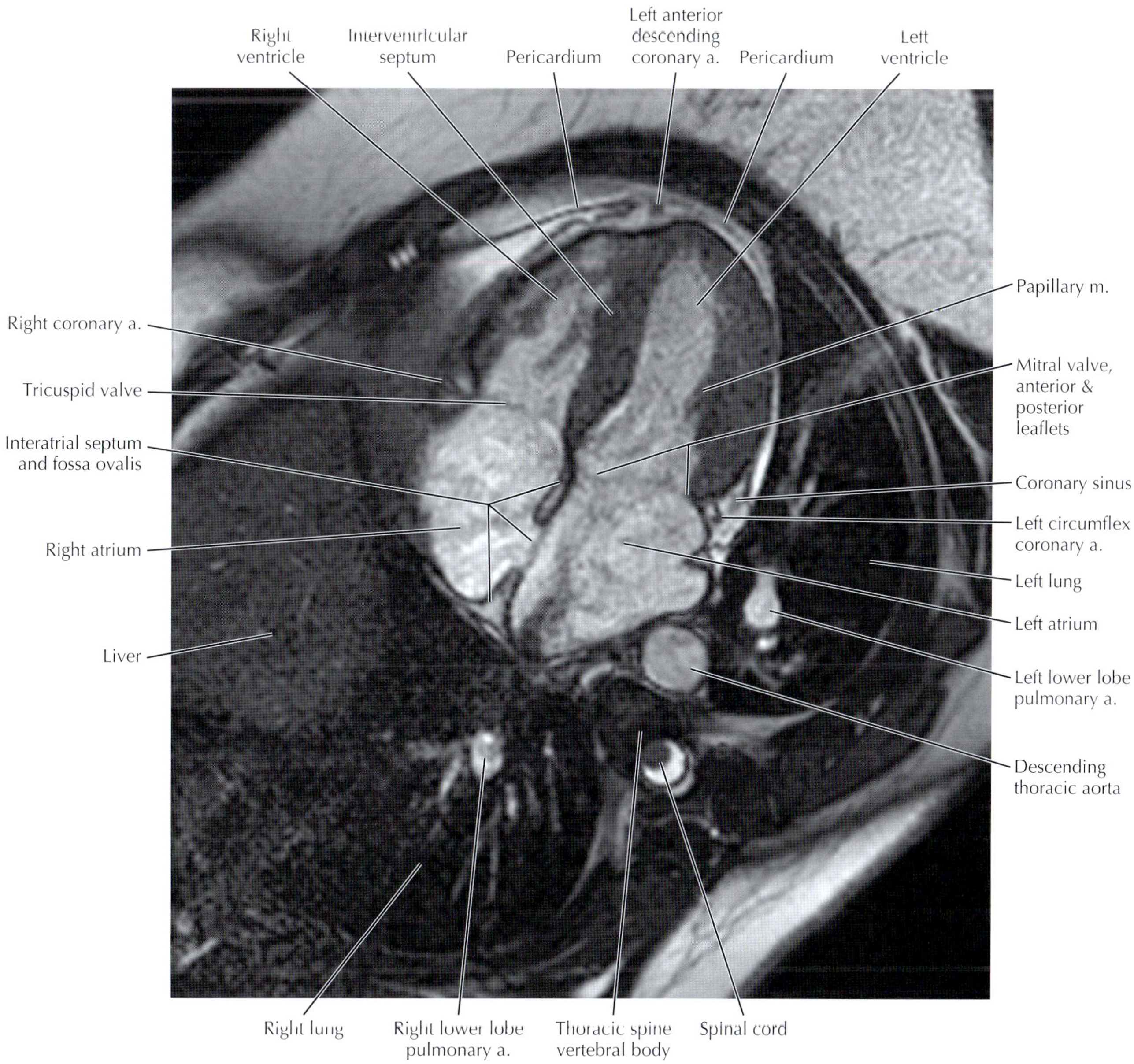
Right ventricle
Interventricular septum
Pericardium
Left anterior descending coronary a.
Pericardium
Left ventricle
Papillary m.
Right coronary a.
Tricuspid valve
Mitral valve, anterior & posterior leaflets
Interatrial septum and fossa ovalis
Coronary sinus
Left circumflex coronary a.
Right atrium
Left lung
Left atrium
Liver
Left lower lobe pulmonary a.
Descending thoracic aorta
Right lung
Right lower lobe pulmonary a.
Thoracic spine vertebral body
Spinal cord

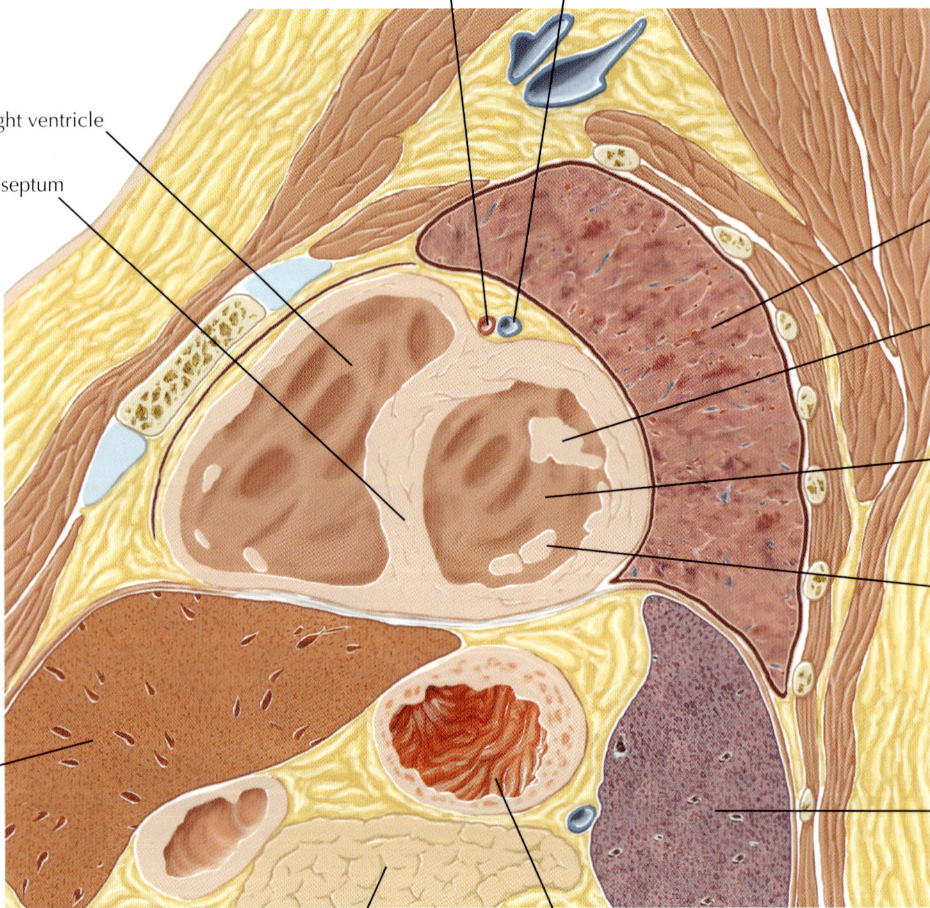

TECHNICAL CONSIDERATION

This view, often referred to as a "short axis" view, is oriented orthogonal to the four-chamber view, perpendicular to the long axis of the left ventricle from the mitral valve to the apex of the heart. This view is used for calculation of ventricular volumes and ejection fraction as well as assessment of left ventricular wall motion.

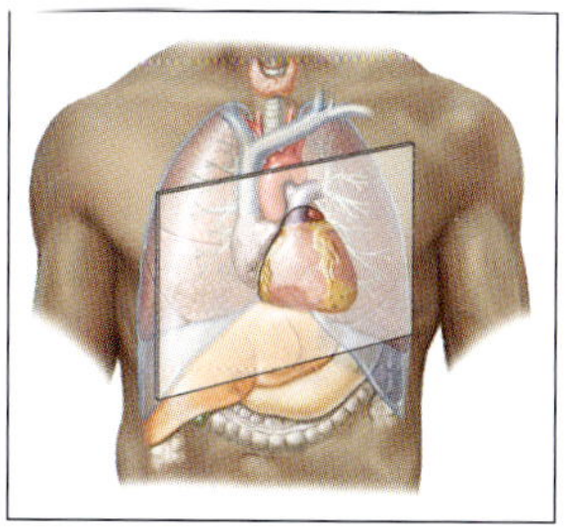

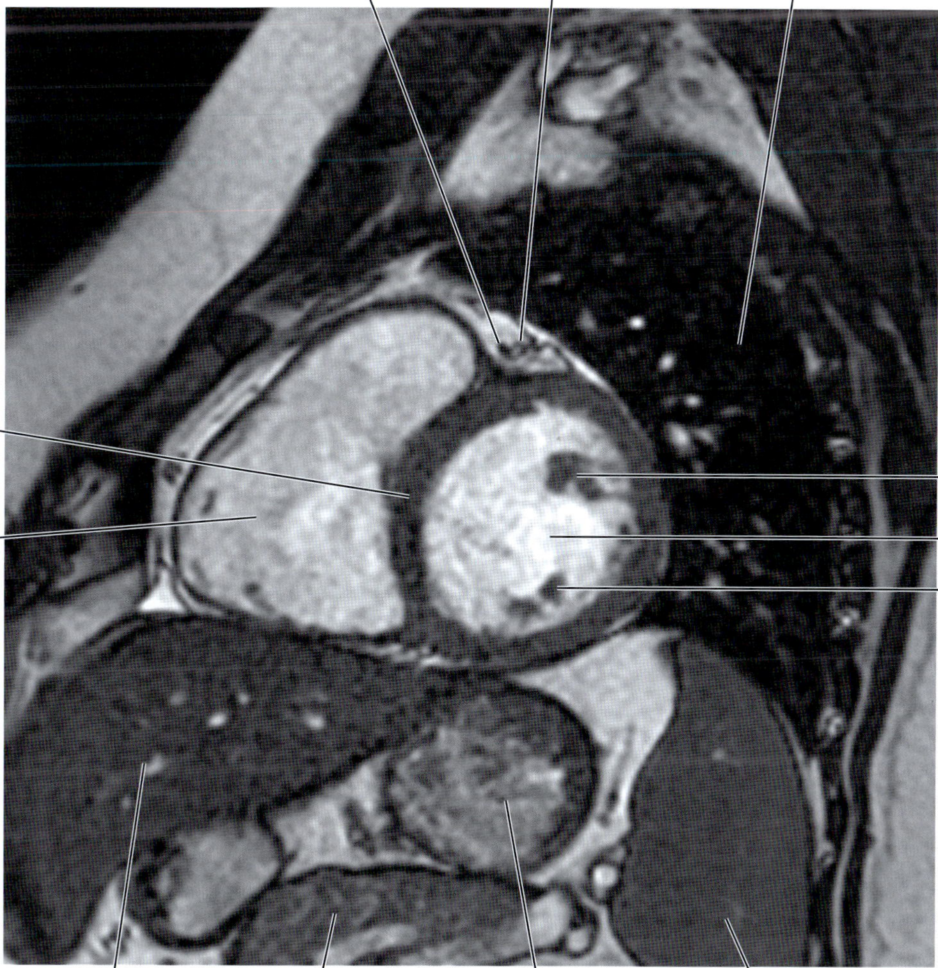
Left anterior descending coronary a.
Anterior interventricular v.
Left lung
Interventricular septum
Right ventricle
Papillary m.
Left ventricle
Papillary m.
Liver
Pancreas
Stomach
Spleen

Index

A

Page numbers followed by a f, figures; t, tables; b indicates boxes.

C

D

M

N

O

P

R

S

X

Z